Family Guide to Natural Medicine

Family Guide to Natural Medicine

HOW
TO STAY
HEALTHY
THE
NATURAL
WAY

Reader's Digest®

The Reader's Digest Association, Inc., Pleasantville, New York/Montreal

Family Guide to Natural Medicine

EDITOR: Alma E. Guinness

ART EDITOR: Robert M. Grant

SENIOR RESEARCH EDITOR: Christine Morgan

SENIOR ASSOCIATE EDITOR: Megan Newman

ART ASSOCIATE: Judith Carmel

RESEARCH ASSOCIATES: Christina Schlank, Sylvia Steinert

ASSOCIATE EDITORS: Donna Campbell, Elisabeth Jakab

LIBRARY RESEARCH: Nettie Seaberry

CONTRIBUTORS

WRITERS: John Banta, Peter Burchard, Jean Callahan, Jacqueline Damian, Thomas Dworetzky, Rosalie Brody Feder, Marjorie Flory, Beth Howard, Pam Lambert, Molly McKaughan, Donald Moffit, Wendy Murphy, Lew Petterson, Don Pfarrer, Joshua Rosenbaum, Cathy Sears, Joan Tedeschi, Joseph Wilkinson

CONTRIBUTING EDITOR: Susan Bronson

RESEARCHER: Emily Bradshaw

PICTURE RESEARCHERS: Linda Patterson Eger, Sybille Millard

EDITORIAL ASSISTANT: Troy Dreier

ART ASSISTANT: Lisa Drescher

PROOFREADER: May Dikeman

INDEXER: Sydney Wolfe Cohen

READER'S DIGEST GENERAL BOOKS

EDITOR IN CHIEF: John A. Pope, Jr.

MANAGING EDITOR: Jane Polley

EXECUTIVE EDITOR: Susan J. Wernert

ART DIRECTOR: David Trooper

GROUP EDITORS: Will Bradbury, Sally French, Norman B. Mack, Kaari Ward

GROUP ART EDITORS: Evelyn Bauer, Robert M. Grant, Joel Musler

CHIEF OF RESEARCH: Laurel A. Gilbride

COPY CHIEF: Edward W. Atkinson

PICTURE EDITOR: Richard Pasqual

RIGHTS AND PERMISSIONS: Pat Colomban

HEAD LIBRARIAN: Jo Manning

The information, recommendations, and visual material in this book are for reference and guidance only; they are not intended as a substitute for a physician's diagnosis and care. The editors urge anyone with continuing medical problems or symptoms to consult a qualified physician.

CHIEF CONSULTANTS

Andrew Weil, M.D.
College of Medicine, Division of Social Perspectives in Medicine, University of Arizona, Tucson, AZ

Norman R. Farnsworth, Ph.D.
Director, Program for Collaborative Research in the Pharmaceutical Sciences, University of Illinois at Chicago

Steven Freedman, M.D.
Chief of Family Practice and Health Education, Kaiser Permanente Medical Group, Fairfield, CA

Herbert Krauss, Ph.D.
Professor of Psychology, Hunter College, City University of New York

Marion Nestle, Ph.D.
Professor and Chair, Department of Nutrition, Food, and Hotel Management, New York University

CONTRIBUTORS/CONSULTANTS

ACUPUNCTURE
Leung Soon Jack, M.D.
New York, NY

ALEXANDER TECHNIQUE
Deborah Caplan, M.A., P.T.
American Center for the Alexander Technique, New York, NY

ANTHROPOLOGY
Helen Fisher, Ph.D.
Department of Anthropology, American Museum of Natural History New York, NY

AYURVEDISM
Rudolph Ballentine, M.D.
Director of Combined Therapy and President, Himalayan Institute Honesdale, PA

CHINESE MEDICINE
Qingcai Zhang, M.D., New York, NY

CHIROPRACTIC
Allan Weisberg, D.C., New York, NY
Peri L. Dwyer, D.C., Tallahassee, FL

EXERCISE
Elyse McNergney, M.A.
Fitness Consultant, Center for Holistic Medicine, New York, NY

HERBAL MEDICINE
Mark Blumenthal
Executive Director, American Botanical Council, Editor, *HerbalGram*, Austin, TX

HOMEOPATHY
Dana Ullman, M.P.H.
President, Homeopathic Educational Services, Berkeley, CA

MASSAGE
Lucy Liben, L.M.Th.
Director of Education, Swedish Institute of Massage, New York, NY

NATUROPATHY
Kaiya Montaocean
Co-director, Center for Natural and Traditional Medicines, Washington, DC

Michael Murray, N.D.
Faculty Member, Bastyr College of Natural Health Sciences, Seattle, WA

OPHTHALMOLOGY
George Dever, O.D., Seattle, WA

OSTEOPATHY
Steven J. Weiss, D.O., New York, NY

POLARITY
Ellen Krueger, M.Th., R.P.P.
American Polarity Therapy Association Astoria, NY

REFLEXOLOGY
Laura Norman, M.S.
Certified Reflexologist, New York, NY

SHIATSU/ACUPRESSURE
Gina Martin, L.M.Th.
Senior Faculty Member, Swedish Institute of Massage, New York, NY

THERAPEUTIC TOUCH
Dolores Krieger, Ph.D., R.N.
Professor Emerita, New York University

T'AI CHI
Bryant Fong
Instructor, University of California at Berkeley Martial Arts Program

VITAMIN THERAPY
Alan R. Gaby, M.D., Baltimore, MD

YOGA
Beryl Bender Birch
Yoga Therapist, Wellness Director, New York Road Runners Club, New York, NY

Library of Congress Cataloging in Publication Data

Family guide to natural medicine : how to stay healthy the natural way / Reader's Digest.
        p.   cm.
    Includes bibliographical references and index.
    ISBN 0-89577-433-X
    1. Alternative medicine. I. Reader's Digest Association
R733.F36 1993
615.5—dc20   92-6163

TABLE OF CONTENTS

INTRODUCTION

Why a Book on Natural Medicine? 8

CHAPTER ONE

The Realm of Natural Medicine 16

Staying Healthy the Natural Way 18
Excerpt: Our Incredible Balancing Act 23
Case History: Taking a Hand In Your Own Care 24
Excerpt: You Are Healthier Than You Think 29
The Ancient Roots of Medicine 30
Case History: A Workshop in Shamanism 35
Native American Medicine 36
Excerpt: The Healing Power of Rituals 39
Picture Essay: A Sioux Ceremony of Healing 40
Balancing Yin and Yang 42
Case History: Acupuncture as Anesthesia 48
Ayurveda's Healthful Balance 52
Picture Essay: Creating Mandalas from Colored Sand 58
Homeopathy: Where Less Is More 60
Excerpt: Like Cures Like 63
Whole-Body Healing 66
Case History: A Wider View of Osteopathy 70
Making a Healthy Adjustment 72
When Nature Is the Healer 76
Case History: A Different Way of Healing 79
Vision Therapies and Iridology 82
Case History: Learning to See 84

CHAPTER TWO

The Mind and Health 86

The Mind-Body Connection 88
Case History: One Body with Many Minds 90
Excerpt: The Riddle of Vanishing Warts 92
The Healing Touch 94
Excerpt: Out of Touch 98
Meditation East and West 100
The Art and Science of Relaxation 106
Time Out for Relaxation 112

Biofeedback and Visualization **114**
Case History: Combining Therapies to Ease Pain **116**
Case History: Picturing Perfection **119**
The Intriguing State of Hypnosis **120**
Case History: Using Hypnosis for Surgery **124**
The Stuff of Dreams **126**
Picture Essay: Dreamtime in Aboriginal Australia **130**
Looking Inward: Psychotherapies **132**
Sharing Professional Help: Group Therapy **136**
The Magic of Creative Therapies **138**
Out-of-Control Habits: Addiction **142**
Excerpt: The Search for Gratification **145**
"We're All in the Same Boat": Self-Help Groups **146**
Case History: Overeaters Anonymous **149**
Primal Therapy and Rebirthing **150**

CHAPTER THREE
Bodywork 152

The Art of Bodywork **154**
The Many Benefits of Massage **156**
Pressure-Point Massage **164**
Case History: Freeing Energy Blockages **167**
Discovering Reflexology **168**
Energy in Motion: Polarity **176**
Excerpt: Attaining a Healthy Self-Awareness **179**
The Alexander Technique **180**
Excerpt: A Life Transformed **183**
New Directions in Bodywork **184**
Case History: Relearning Body-Awareness **186**
More Than Skin-Deep **188**

CHAPTER FOUR
Movement 190

Why You Should Exercise **192**
Case History: Setting the Clock Back **196**
A Basic Exercise Routine **200**
Water, Water Everywhere **206**
Case History: A Sudden Cure **211**
Picture Essay: Cleansing with Mud, Sand, and Sweat **212**
The Ancient Practice of Yoga **214**

Case History: The Insight of a Yoga Therapist **221**
The Martial Arts **222**
Excerpt: Portal to the Spirit **229**
T'ai Chi: The Supreme Ultimate **230**

CHAPTER FIVE

Eating Well 238

The New Nutrition **240**
Case History: The Perils of a Modern Diet **244**
Excerpt: The Truth About Cholesterol **246**
Protecting Your Health Naturally **248**
Excerpt: New Studies, Old Wisdom **253**
What Else is in Food? **254**
Understanding Food Sensitivities **258**
Case History: Searching Out Food Sensitivities **259**
Shopping, Storing, Cooking **260**
Putting Diets in Perspective **264**
Case History: Running on Empty **266**
The New Vegetarian **268**
Macrobiotics: A Matter of Balance **270**
Picture Essay: Healthy Eating Around the World **272**
The Role of Vitamins and Minerals **274**
Vitamins and Minerals as Therapy **282**

CHAPTER SIX

Herbal Medicine 288

Healing with Herbs **290**
Excerpt: The Value of Using Whole Plants **295**
Aromatherapy: Soothing Scents **328**
Bach Flower Remedies **330**

CHAPTER SEVEN

Ailments and Remedy Options 332

Complementary Therapies **334**
Case History: The Dangers of Self-Diagnosis **336**

Index **392**   Sources **413**   Credits and Acknowledgments **414**

Why a Book on Natural Medicine?

Dr. Andrew Weil, chief consultant for Family Guide to
Natural Medicine, *explains why alternative therapies are attracting so
much attention, and how they mesh with orthodox medicine.*

HEALING IS A NATURAL PROCESS, common to all life. Wounds heal
by themselves in people just as in animals and plants. If we
want to foster healing and promote health, we should pay attention to the ways of nature and learn to encourage the body's own,
innate mechanisms of self-repair. This is the basic principle of natural
medicine. Regrettably, orthodox medicine has moved away from nature.

The meteoric rise of scientific medicine in the 20th century—discovery of effective drugs for bacterial infections and development of
immunizations and modern surgical techniques—helped foster belief
in a technological utopia, a Golden Age in which science and technology would conquer poverty, illiteracy, hunger, and disease.

Sometime after 1960 the idea of a technological utopia faded, as
people in developed countries began to see that science and technology created as many problems as they solved. We were also forced to
confront the limitations of our power to change many human ills. For
example, as medicine succeeded in reducing the amount of sickness
and premature death caused by infectious illness, it had to deal with
more difficult kinds of illness prevalent in an aging population, such as
chronic degenerative diseases and cancer. Orthodox medicine has no
magic bullets for these conditions. Nor does it have effective treatments
for viral infections, allergies and autoimmune diseases, mental illnesses, metabolic diseases, and functional and psychosomatic diseases.

As public realization of the limitations of orthodox medicine has
grown, so too has interest in alternatives to it. Many systems of treatment that went into eclipse in the first half of this century are now re-

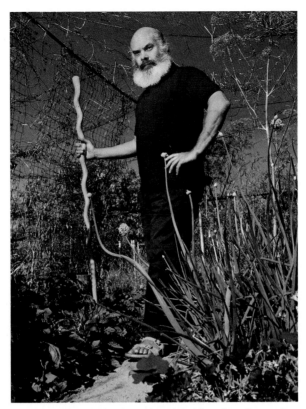

Dr. Andrew Weil is the author of Health and Healing *and*
Natural Health, Natural Medicine.

surgent, attracting large numbers of patients, including the educated
and affluent. Alternative medicine is a hot topic in the media, a source
of irritation to conservative doctors, and an interesting challenge to orthodox philosophy.

Alternative, Complementary, Holistic. Alternative medicine is a
vast collection of theories and practices, some very ancient,
some very recent, some sensible and worthy of study, others
not so sensible. You will find many of them described in detail in this
book along with suggestions for how and when to use them. Some
doctors refer to orthodox medicine as "traditional" medicine, imply-
ing that all the alternative forms of treatment are nontraditional. But
this label is a misnomer. For example, the origins of acupuncture are
lost in prehistory; it would be hard to imagine a more traditional healing practice. Herbalism is also an ancient folk tradition, handed down
from mother to daughter, father to son in most cultures around the
world. Such folk practices are the really traditional forms of healing.
What most M.D.s do is better called "orthodox" medicine.

At the same time, it is also fair to describe many of the practices
covered in this book as true alternatives to orthodox medicine. Osteopathic manipulation, yoga, and acupuncture may be better than anal-

gesic, anti-inflammatory, and muscle-relaxant drugs in the treatment of acute back pain. A dairy-free diet, daily nasal irrigation with saline, and hot compresses over the face may relieve chronic sinusitis better than regimens of antibiotics and decongestants.

Some people suggest using the term "complementary" medicine for the practices described in this book. The idea is that these treatments are best used as adjuncts or complements to orthodox methods. In some cases combining therapies makes good sense. A woman with early breast cancer might have surgery and radiation to deal with the actual tumor. She should then follow an anticancer diet, use vitamins and herbs that reduce the chance of a recurrence, start an exercise program, and practice some kind of mental technique, such as visualization, to speed her recovery and strengthen her immunity.

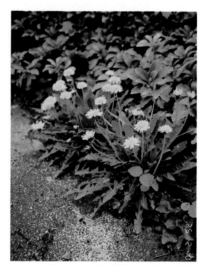

Even the common dandelion can be used in natural healing (see page 303).

The holistic medical movement of recent years emphasizes self-care and personal responsibility for wellness. Holistic medicine started as a reaction to the narrow, body-focused approach of the orthodox system. It looks at *whole* people as bodies, minds, and spirits and is open to using all forms of treatment, whether alternative or not. Holistic doctors like to enter into partnerships with patients, encouraging them to learn about how to reduce the risks of illness and how to choose the best therapies.

*T*he Realm of Orthodox Medicine. Interest in natural medicine in no way denies the solid achievements of orthodox medicine. Doctors can now treat victims of trauma more effectively than ever. They can cure many acute bacterial infections, like pneumococcal pneumonia, that frequently killed people in the recent past. They can often prevent untimely death in cases of medical and surgical emergencies, like heart attacks and appendicitis. They can rescue babies from obstetrical complications that used to be fatal, and they can perform miracles of reconstructive surgery, such as giving new hips and knees to those with joints destroyed by injury or illness. Through immunization, they can also prevent some infectious diseases like polio, diphtheria, and tetanus that once were major killers.

It would be foolish to seek alternative therapy for conditions that orthodox medicine treats very well. If I were in a serious automobile accident or had a bleeding duodenal ulcer, I would want to be taken straight to a hospital emergency room, not to a shaman, homeopath, or shiatsu practitioner. The first requirement for taking more responsibility for your own health is to know when a problem demands immediate intervention by orthodox medical methods.

High-Tech, High-Cost. I majored in botany as an undergraduate at Harvard in the 1960s, then went on to Harvard Medical School and a career that has included the study and use of medicinal plants. No one else in my medical school class had studied botany, and I know only two physicians who majored in botany as undergraduates.

Not that long ago, medicine and botany were closely allied fields, because most remedies came from plants. Some pharmaceutical drugs in common use today are still of plant origin, but they are available only as highly refined chemical derivatives. The idea of using actual preparations of plants to treat sick people now seems hopelessly old-fashioned and unscientific to most physicians, and there is virtually no communication between the worlds of botany and medicine.

Not only did my medical education slight nature, it gave me very little information about health and healing. Even today the medical school curriculum focuses entirely on disease. Students learn how to diagnose and treat disease once it is established in the body. They do not learn much about how to prevent disease, and they learn even less about how to maintain health and encourage the body's natural healing mechanisms.

Rejection of simple, natural methods in favor of reliance on technology is expensive. Orthodox medicine has now become so expensive that many people cannot afford it. More than any other factor, the cost crisis in health care is forcing doctors and patients to question the philosophy and practices of the dominant system.

Not only is high-tech medicine expensive, it can also be dangerous. Its methods are potent and invasive, and it is frequently harmful. This tendency is nowhere more evident than in the amount of drug toxicity caused by modern prescribing practices. Adverse drug reactions are now so common that most patients will experience one sooner or later. These reactions can be as minor as hives and as major as permanent disability or death. In my own private practice of natural and preventive medicine, I frequently use medicinal plants. For every prescription I write for a pharmaceutical drug, I give out 40 or 50 for botanical remedies. In almost 10 years of prescribing in that way, I have not yet seen a serious adverse reaction in any patient taking a medicinal plant. No physician who uses pharmaceutical drugs exclusively can match that record of safety.

The problem is that most pharmaceutical drugs are too strong. Doctors have come to like drugs that produce very intense effects very rapidly. Certainly, there is a place for such products, particularly for the treatment of emergency conditions, where time is of the essence, but for the routine management of common illnesses, exclusive use of these strong drugs is technological overkill and a clear violation of the famous precept of Hippocrates to physicians: *Primum non nocere*— First, do no harm.

One of the complaints I hear from patients today is that doctors are too ready to hand out drugs. In the last years of the 20th century, as people become disillusioned with technology, they are also becoming uneasy about synthetic chemicals and much more interested in natural products. A huge market for vitamins, herbs, and natural foods has developed, along with a strong consumers' movement opposed to the excesses of science and technology. Very slowly and sometimes very reluctantly, the medical profession is beginning to respond to demands from consumers for changes in the way medicine is practiced.

T**he Role of Nutrition.** Virtual omission of any instruction in nutrition in the medical curriculum is a glaring defect in the training of doctors. In my four years at Harvard Medical School and one year of internship, I received a total of 30 minutes of nutritional instruction, grudgingly allocated to a dietitian to tell us about the special diets we could order for hospitalized patients. There has been little improvement since I graduated.

When I was in school, medical doctors were quick to brand as a quack anyone who argued that diet could be a risk factor for cancer. It is now generally accepted that high-fat, low-fiber diets, especially those high in meat and low in vegetables, predispose people to cancer of the colon, breast, uterus, and prostate. Those who argued that vitamins had any benefits other than preventing deficiency diseases in "recommended daily allowances" also risked the charge of quackery, but we now find that beta-carotene, a precursor of vitamin A, has strong cancer-inhibiting effects, especially against lung and cervical cancer. High doses of niacin (vitamin B$_3$) lower cholesterol. High doses of vitamin E can help treat fibrocystic breast disease. Researchers are beginning to document the therapeutic effects of these and other vitamins and minerals.

Many of the methods described in these pages remain unproved, controversial, even suspect in the eyes of conventional doctors. But the world and medicine are changing. Researchers are documenting the effectiveness of folk treatments once disavowed by professionals. Garlic, one of the most prominent healing herbs in the folk traditions of many cultures, really does have powerful antibiotic properties; it also lowers blood pressure. Some physicians are learning how to use diet and nutritional supplements to treat disease. I predict that we will see ever-widening interest in natural and preventive medicine.

Turnabout on Birth and Nursing. In the mid-20th century, many doctors convinced women that breast feeding was old-fashioned and unscientific. Formula feeding was supposed to be modern and better. Doctors also discredited natural childbirth and many forms of natural treatment, from vitamin therapy to massage, branding them worthless, harmful, and, always, unscientific.

In 1967, when I did my obstetrical training in Boston, natural childbirth was rare in university hospitals, and doctors tried to convince women who wanted it that they were being irrational. All but one of the births I attended at the Boston Lying-In Hospital in that year were done with full technological intervention: anesthesia (often rendering the mothers unconscious), scopolamine (a dangerous, delirium-inducing drug given to make women amnesic for the experience), episiotomies (surgery to prevent tearing of the birth canal), strong drugs to induce uterine contractions, frequent use of forceps, and, of course, hormone injections to prevent normal milk development so that new mothers could choose formula instead.

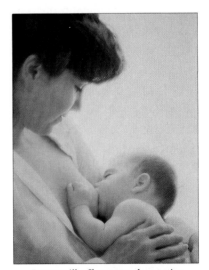

Breast milk offers natural protection from a host of infectious diseases.

Of course, we know now that colostrum, the first fluid secreted by the breasts after birth, is an important source of maternal antibodies that gives newborns passive immunity against many infections until their own immune systems begin to function. Breast feeding is one way of establishing an intimate bond between mother and baby that provides a good foundation for emotional well-being in later life. Some studies suggest that, on average, breast-fed infants show higher intelligence and may be less prone to develop allergies than their formula-fed counterparts. Nature does appear to know best.

The world has changed greatly since the 1960s. Breast feeding is back in fashion, and natural childbirth is common. Some of the obstetrical practices that were the rule in 1967 are now considered barbaric.

Enlisting Mind Power. Health care consumers want doctors to pay attention to the mental, emotional, and spiritual aspects of health, not just the physical body. Orthodox medicine gives lip service to the mind but, in practice, acts as if the mind is not as real or as important as the liver. For this reason it undervalues or ignores therapies like hypnosis and visualization that claim to be able to change physical conditions through purely mental interventions. Such therapies are often safer than invasive procedures, and when they work, are also much less costly.

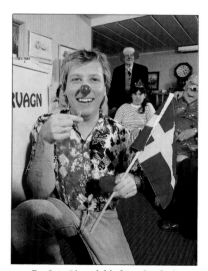

Dr. Lars Ljungdahl of Sweden finds that humor is an effective therapy.

The public's impatience with the purely physical preoccupations of most doctors is evident in the popularity of books and television productions about the power of the mind. One example is Norman Cousins' 1979 book, *Anatomy of an Illness*, describing his dramatic recovery from a mysterious and severe connective-tissue disease. Cousins came down with fever, malaise, and joint pains on returning to the United States from a trip to Moscow. His condition soon worsened—he could not move his limbs; nodules appeared on his body; and his jaws almost locked. Hospitalization in New York City failed to provide relief. Doctors could only offer him suppressive treatment in the form of painkilling and anti-inflammatory drugs.

Acting on an intuitive sense of the importance of emotional well-being to physical health, Cousins checked himself out of the hospital and into a comfortable hotel suite, where he could get food that he liked. The hospital food had seemed unhealthy as well as unappetizing to him. He took large doses of vitamin C. Most significantly Cousins worked at getting himself into good moods by renting funny movies and watching them for hours. The result was a seemingly miraculous restoration of good health: Cousins laughed his way to a cure. He first wrote about his experience in an article in the *New England Journal of Medicine*; later he expanded the account into a best-selling book. For the rest of his life he tried to remind doctors and patients that the body has a head, and the head should come first. One effect of his efforts has been the appearance of laughter therapists who work with sick people both in and out of hospitals.

Your Role in Your Own Care. If you are reading this book, you probably want to be more independent of doctors, pharmacies, and hospitals, and you are probably motivated to keep yourself healthy. It is very much in your interest to explore the material presented here, to think in terms of staying well rather than looking for cures, and to assume full responsibility for your health. Not only will that attitude save you money, it will cut your risks of medical toxicity, and help you avoid future health problems.

Just as it would be foolish to consult alternative practitioners for problems that today's orthodox treatments can best address, so it is foolish to expect help from orthodox medicine with problems that it cannot treat well.

I recommend that you keep a record of your health history, including tests you have had and treatments you have received. It is up to you to learn when and when not to use orthodox physicians. It is up to you to become informed about simple, natural treatment alternatives.

If many doctors do not understand how to use natural healing methods, how are laypeople to know when to use them and how (or how not) to combine them with standard treatments? I am afraid I have no simple answer to that question, except to remind you that the responsibility for health is yours. You must learn to be an active participant in your well-being, not a passive recipient of medical care.

Remember that your body has remarkable powers of healing and self-repair. Natural medicine begins and ends with that simple truth. It is your job to make intelligent choices of methods to activate and enhance those powers. ❏

CHAPTER ONE

The Realm of Natural Medicine

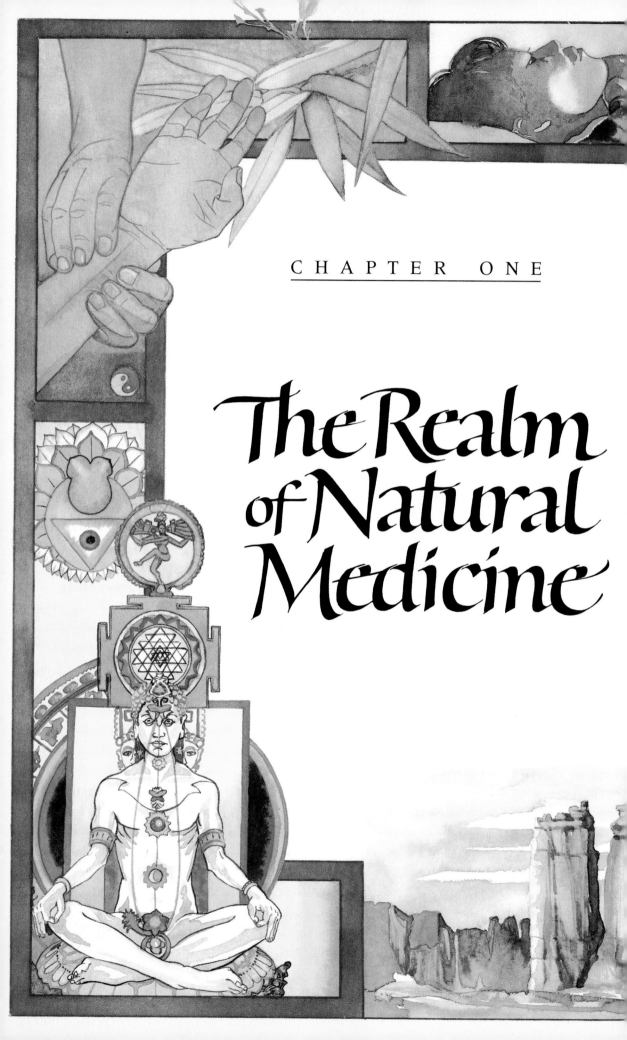

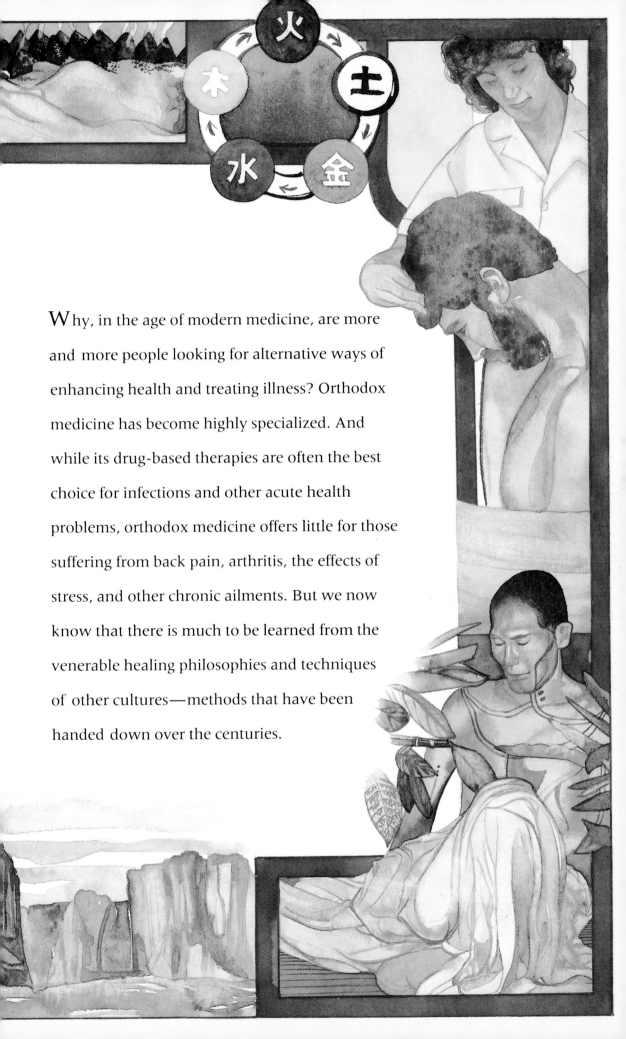

Why, in the age of modern medicine, are more and more people looking for alternative ways of enhancing health and treating illness? Orthodox medicine has become highly specialized. And while its drug-based therapies are often the best choice for infections and other acute health problems, orthodox medicine offers little for those suffering from back pain, arthritis, the effects of stress, and other chronic ailments. But we now know that there is much to be learned from the venerable healing philosophies and techniques of other cultures—methods that have been handed down over the centuries.

Staying Healthy the Natural Way

Eager to take charge of their own health, more and more people are exploring the wide array of healing options that natural medicine has to offer. For many, it marks the beginning of a new perspective on health.

AS INVIGORATING AS the first breeze of spring, a feeling is sweeping the land that good health may be within nearly everyone's reach. People who have spent most of their lives believing that wellness is a matter of luck and illnesses almost inevitable, and that physicians alone hold the key to health, are now rejecting these assumptions.

We have become accustomed to not understanding the medical treatment we receive—and have learned not to ask a busy doctor too many probing questions. In fact, we have more or less been trained to turn the care of our bodies over to physicians, with the understanding that they know best. This inequality contributes to a feeling of helplessness on the part of many patients, which, in turn, has fueled an interest in alternative healing methods.

The Healing Powers Within. The treatments discussed in this book range from complete systems of medicine, such as traditional Chinese medicine, to more specific bodywork therapies, like the Alexander technique. But what actually sets natural medicine apart from orthodox medicine? Part of the answer lies in the belief that our bodies are remarkably resilient machines, capable, with some occasional prodding or intervention, of healing themselves. Health, therefore, is a matter of balance.

For most of us, body temperature is a familiar example of the idea of balance. Human beings have a strong tendency to maintain balance in a changing environment. When it is cold we shiver, when it is too warm we sweat—and both strategies help to keep our body temperature at about 98.6 degrees F (37 degrees celsius). This average temperature is genetically programmed and differs little from person to person, and neither diet, exercise, nor mood has any significant effect on it. However, a moderate fever is one way our bodies deal with invading organisms because at 101 degrees F (38.3 degrees celsius), our systems still function, but bacteria and viruses may be destroyed, thus restoring our balance and our health.

For practitioners of Eastern therapies, such as acupuncture or shiatsu, balance means that our vital energy (qi) is flowing unimpeded along a series of pathways that connect all of our organs and bodily systems. Stress and other factors can interrupt the flow, creating an imbalance in the system. A traditional Chinese doctor, for instance, won't just treat the symptoms of an illness, but will treat the imbalance that is producing the symptoms.

According to practitioners of natural medicine, this perspective of dynamic balance is more useful and comprehensive than a symptom-oriented view. Consider chronic indigestion, for example. An antacid may ease the symptoms, but a better long-term solution would be to rebalance

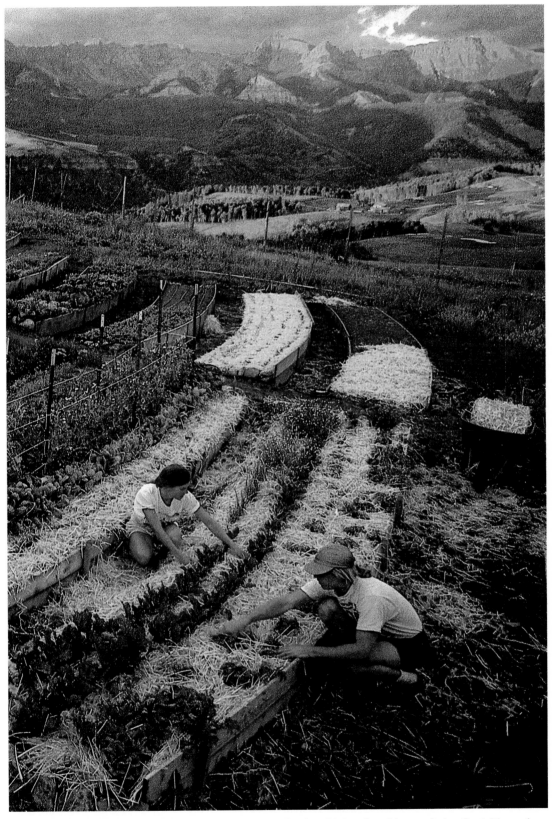

More and more *people are actively pursuing a healthy lifestyle. This is reflected in our choice of activities and foods, and in our concern about the overuse of chemical fertilizers and pesticides. This verdant organic garden high in the mountains near Telluride, Colorado, testifies to the success of natural methods of cultivation.*

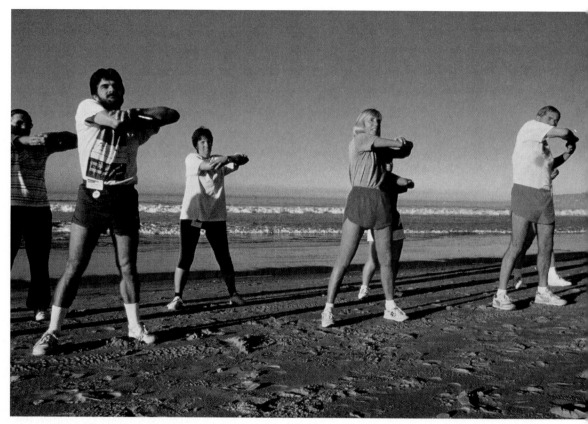

A regular program of exercise is the cornerstone of preventive medicine. A program should be varied, to include more than one kind of activity. The aim is to stretch and strengthen muscles and to increase cardiovascular efficiency. A further health dividend may be loss of excess weight.

the system with a change in diet and some stress-reduction techniques—and so eliminate a chronic problem.

The Balance of Mind and Body. The immune system is an around-the-clock defense network that protects the body from infection. However, it, too, can get worn down from overuse or chronic abuse. Aside from getting adequate amounts of rest and eating properly, are there active steps we can take to keep our immune systems functioning at peak efficiency? One premise of natural medicine is that we can bolster our immune systems and generally enhance our health by making a few simple changes. For instance, regular exercise strengthens immune function, while also lowering the risk of coronary heart disease, diabetes, hypertension, osteoporosis, and obesity. In addition, there is a growing body of evidence indicating that certain foods may help our bodies fend off diseases.

People are finally recognizing that stress can take a tremendous toll on the body, leaving us prey to a range of health problems. According to practitioners of natural medicine, the effects of stress—which can include everything from migraines to heart disease—illustrate the role of the mind in health. So, too, the mind can play a role in healing. Meditation, breathing exercises, and other relaxation techniques offer natural ways of coping with stress, inexpensively and without side effects. In fact, orthodox medicine is beginning to embrace some of these techniques. And well it should, for it has been estimated that up to two-thirds of all office visits are for stress- or anxiety-related ailments.

Listening to Our Bodies. Staying well the natural way means becoming more informed and more self-aware about our bodies. As a first step, we should take a more active role in our health—by eating sensibly, exercising, and breaking habits or abandoning activities that are harmful to body and mind. But if something does go wrong and we need medical care, it helps to be an informed consumer.

Unlike most orthodox physicians, many alternative practitioners view healing as a partnership. For the consumer, this approach has tradeoffs as well as benefits. For starters, by participating in your own care you are also accepting some responsibility for your own wellness. Consider coronary heart disease, our nation's leading cause of death. While it used to be that physicians scoffed at the idea of disease prevention, today orthodox and natural practitioners agree that a sensible diet and regular exercise play a large role in lowering the risk of heart disease. But it falls to the patient to make the necessary adjustments to prevent or reverse the course of disease.

Benefits of this healing partnership include a more positive, take-charge attitude, which can renew both body and mind—a notion that has not been completely lost on the medical establishment. In fact, a number of reputable studies have explored the link between a patient's emotional outlook and rate of recovery—a territory that would have been dismissed as woefully unscientific just a few years ago.

Complementary Care. Many people go to their doctors with vague complaints hoping for emotional support or reassurance, and often leave the office a little disappointed. Others go seeking relief from chronic conditions, such as back pain or arthritis, for which mainstream medicine has few long-term solutions.

For the most part, orthodox physicians are trained to deal with specific symptoms or illnesses, and are less comfortable when a pill or procedure is not available to fix the problem. On the other hand, natural practitioners, who take a more "holistic" view of health, tend to spend more time listening to a patient's concerns and many use a battery of hands-on techniques that are, by their very nature, therapeutic.

Choosing an alternative or natural treatment does not imply rejection of orthodox care—in any health emergency (bone fracture, chest pains, a high fever), orthodox

A Medical Glossary

With the growing popularity of alternative forms of health care, discussions of medicine sometimes include new and unfamiliar vocabulary. Here are some commonly used terms.

- *Alternative:* Virtually any form of medicine that remains outside the realm of conventional modern medicine may be labeled alternative. Examples are naturopathy, chiropractic, and homeopathy.

- *Folk:* Varying from culture to culture, folk medicine involves a belief in the effectiveness of a chosen cure. Remedies based on plants, charms, and rituals are common elements.

- *Holistic:* Holistic therapies treat the whole person — body and mind — as opposed to focusing only on the part of the body where symptoms occur. The importance of self-care and preventing illness are stressed.

- *Natural:* Any therapy that relies on the body's own healing powers may be considered natural medicine. These include herbal remedies, diet, and water therapies.

- *Orthodox:* This refers to conventional modern, or Western, medicine, which is the dominant type of health care in most developed countries.

- *Traditional:* Any medical system with ancient origins, strong cultural ties, trained healers, and an underlying theory of health care can be considered traditional medicine. This includes shamanism and Chinese medicine.

medical care should be sought immediately. But many of the therapies in this book are suitable complements to standard medical treatment. For instance, a migraine sufferer may consult a neurologist for a diagnosis of the problem, while also using meditation or biofeedback for more immediate pain relief.

The Overuse of Drugs and Technology. When it comes to wiping out bacterial infections or dulling sharp pain, prescription drugs can be invaluable. But alternative practitioners, and a growing number of orthodox physicians, say that drugs are overused. In addition, there are serious questions about the ways drugs are tested. For example, while the elderly take more prescription medications than other age groups, most drugs are tested on younger people whose physiology is quite different. Some drugs affect the absorp-

Hypnotherapy, which is based in part on the power of suggestion, has been used to relieve pain. It can also be valuable for stress reduction. Hypnosis was once regarded as quackery, but the American Medical Association has recognized it as a form of treatment for over thirty years.

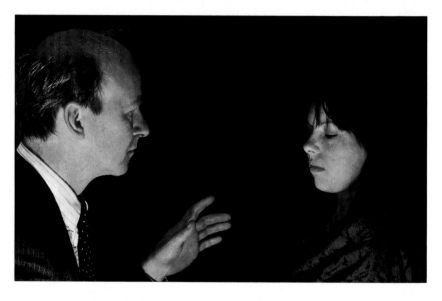

tion of vitamins and minerals, which can lead to further problems, particularly among the elderly, whose diets tend to be deficient in nutrients. Finally, the side effects of some prescription drugs are almost as unpleasant as the symptoms they are meant to treat, which has led many people to seek alternatives.

The Ailments and Remedy Options section of this book (pages 332-391) describes some natural remedies that are suitable for treating a number of common ailments. For example, an occasional insomniac may be better off with a warm bath than a sleeping pill, which can produce dizziness, daytime drowsiness, and, over time, dependency. Of course, there are those who feel let down if they don't emerge from an office visit with a prescription for pills—and there is no shortage of physicians willing to comply.

In addition to an overreliance on drugs to "fix" health problems, many orthodox physicians are using costly tests more often than is necessary. Part of this trend is the result of specialization. When health problems arise, even relatively minor ones, patients are often referred to specialists.

Our Incredible Balancing Act

We are constantly besieged, writes Dr. Andrew Weil, by stress and changes within us and around us, so it is essential for our health to achieve a harmonious inner balance.

Balance is truly a mystery. Learn to stand on your head or to walk a tightrope, and you will experience the mystery. The balance point is non-dimensional but quite real. At first you overshoot it grossly, then over-correct and miss it again. Your movements are exaggerated and jerky, anything but harmonious. Eventually, you become conscious of the special point, if only momentarily while falling through it. Soon you can stay in it for several moments, becoming familiar with the distinctive feeling of effortlessness it provides. Lose it even slightly, and you must put out tremendous effort to regain it, but when you are on target, there is no work to be done. You can just enjoy the grace of a magical zone where all external forces cancel out by virtue of precise arrangement, one against another. In balance there is stillness and beauty in the very midst of chaos.

This stillness and beauty at the heart of change is the magic of the hurricane's eye, of the moment of totality of a solar eclipse, and indeed, of the very stability of the earth itself. The equinoxes of the seasonal cycle are magical points, as are the moments of sunrise and sunset, the *equilibrated* times of day, when reflection and meditation are possible with least effort.

The balance of health is also dynamic. The elements and forces making up a human being and the changing environmental stresses impinging on them constitute a system so elaborate as to be unimaginable in its complexity. We are islands of change in a sea of change, subject to cycles of rest and activity, of secretion of hormones, and of the rise and fall of powerful drives, subject to noise, irritants, agents of disease, electrical and magnetic fields, the deteriorations of age, emotional tides. The variables are infinite, and all is in flux and motion. That equilibrium occurs even

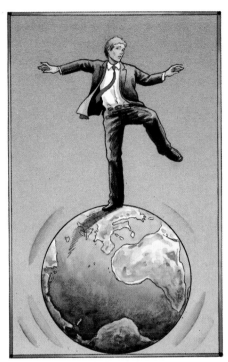

Stability can be hard to maintain

for an instant in such a system is miraculous, yet most of us are mostly healthy most of the time, our mind-bodies always trying to keep up the incredible balancing act demanded by all the stresses from inside and out. Moreover, they do it dynamically, since equilibrium is constantly destroyed and re-created.

The achievement of balance adds an extra quality to a whole. It makes the perfect whole greater than the sum of its parts. Health is wholeness—wholeness in its most profound sense, with nothing left out, and everything in just the right order to manifest the mystery of balance. Far from being simply the absence of disease, health is a dynamic and harmonious equilibrium of all the elements and forces making up and surrounding a human being.

Excerpted from Health and Healing *by Andrew Weil, M.D.*

Their expertise can often prevent severe, life-threatening health crises, but it does not come cheap. A recent study found that cardiologists and endocrinologists ordered more drugs and tests, and hospitalized patients more often than family doctors and internists who were treating patients for nearly identical ailments. The net result of these trends is that for many patients, orthodox medicine is simply too costly for everyday complaints. Such people have an urgent need for sensible alternatives.

CASE HISTORY

TAKING A HAND IN YOUR OWN CARE

A new approach to health care sees the individual, not the physician, as the key player in health care. In an article from Medical Self-Care, *Tom Ferguson, M.D., gives this case history.*

"Let me tell you about a 62-year-old friend I'll call Dorothy. Three years ago, Dorothy developed pains in her legs and shoulders. Dorothy visited her doctor and accepted his advice without question. The prescription she received produced unpleasant side effects. Her doctor substituted another, which produced a different set of side effects. A third drug produced some relief, accompanied by annoying side effects. After three months of medical treatment, Dorothy's pain was markedly reduced. Her medical expenses for that period looked like this: Doctor's visit — $215. Medical tests — $92. Drugs — $86. Total — $393.

"Earlier this year, Dorothy experienced similar pain. But by this time she had become a self-care enthusiast. She resolved not to leave things totally up to the doctor.

"She began, again, by visiting her physician. 'We're still not sure exactly what it is,' he told her. But when he reached for his prescription pad, Dorothy held up her hand to stop him.

"'Please write down what my choices are,' she told him. 'I want to read up on them.'

"Her doctor wrote down the names of three drugs, the same ones she had taken three years before. Dorothy went to the library to research them. She was surprised to find that aspirin often produced equal or superior results, so she began to take it.

"A friend suggested acupuncture. She visited an acupuncturist and had a short course of treatments, with good results. An in-law from out of town loaned her a relaxation/healing tape. She subscribed to two health magazines and began taking a multiple vitamin/ mineral insurance formula. She listened to the healing tape every night at bedtime. It eased the pain and helped her get to sleep.

"At a friend's suggestion, Dorothy began an early-morning exercise class at the local pool. It seemed to help. She ordered a book on rheumatism and an information packet on rheumatic conditions from a consumer health information center. This time her medical expenses looked like this: Doctor's visit — $45. Acupuncturist — $60. Aspirin — $4. Self-care information (three books, two magazine subscriptions, one information packet, one cassette tape) — $51. Self-care tools (heating pad) — $36. Total — $196.

"At the end of three months her symptoms had improved remarkably."

Excerpted from *Medical Self-Care,* March — April 1987, by Tom Ferguson, M.D.

How Thorough Is Too Thorough? Even those who are fully equipped to deal with high-tech medicine—physicians—can get pulled into the maelstrom of overtesting. The following, a dramatic example of how the tools of modern medicine can actually get in the way of an accurate (and speedy) diagnosis, was reported by Lawrence K. Altman, M.D. in *The New York Times* (May 12, 1992).

After playing a round of golf, Dr. Franklin K. Yee, a surgeon from Sacramento, California gradually developed a fever, nausea, and pain in his abdomen. Thinking he was coming down with the flu, he went home to bed. But in the morning when the pain was worse, he called a gastroenterologist he had worked with for many years.

Yee suspected that he had an ulcer; but after examining him, the specialist concluded that Yee had a viral infection—however, the doctor ordered an electrocardiogram just in case. Though the test looked normal, the cardiologist who had been brought in thought he detected something slightly unusual on the EKG, and as a precaution Dr. Yee was hospitalized.

While he agreed to being hospitalized, Dr. Yee did not believe there was anything wrong with his heart. However, he was cautious about second-guessing his physicians, and was mindful of the traditional warning that "a doctor who treats himself has a fool for a patient."

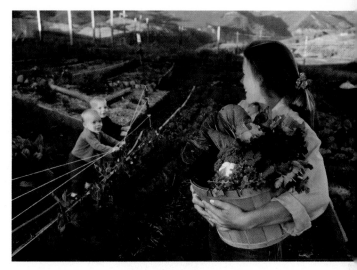

Fresh-picked vegetables provide not only a bounty of vitamins and minerals, but also a good source of dietary fiber, which is generally insufficient in the diet of many Americans. People who worry about the toxic effect of pesticides used on commercial crops may try growing their own produce using little or no pest-killing chemicals.

As he lay in the coronary care unit, the pain in his upper abdomen moved down to the lower right, and Dr. Yee began to feel bloated. Examining himself as he would a patient, Yee pressed his abdomen with his fingers and quickly let go. The pain he experienced was consistent with appendicitis. His son, also a doctor, examined him and confirmed his diagnosis. Yee called his gastroenterologist.

The specialist found the tenderness, but because Yee's white blood count was normal, he disputed the diagnosis. Yee stayed in the hospital over the weekend, his vital signs and blood pressure being monitored regularly. And while the pain got worse, the cardiologist on the case concluded that his heart was fine. Dr. Yee was sent home.

That evening the pain was more severe than ever, and Yee still had a fever. More convinced than ever that he had an appendicitis, he called a surgeon and told him to meet him in the emergency room. Still doubting Yee's diagnosis, the surgeon and gastroenterologist ordered kidney X rays to see if he was perhaps passing a kidney stone. The results were negative.

They next ordered a CAT scan of his abdomen, for which Yee had to drink a pint of barium solution—an unpleasant requirement for the test. The CAT scan seemed to indicate that Yee was suffering a very serious problem in

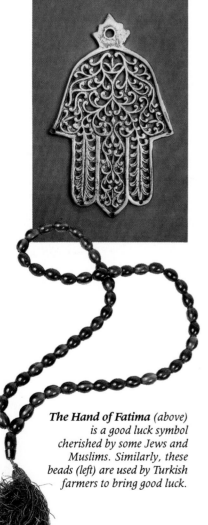

These golden walnuts are rolled in the palms to increase the circulation and relieve stress. A similar Chinese practice using metal balls dates back to antiquity.

The Hand of Fatima (above) is a good luck symbol cherished by some Jews and Muslims. Similarly, these beads (left) are used by Turkish farmers to bring good luck.

the blood vessels leading to his bowel. To confirm the diagnosis, they called in a vascular surgeon to perform an angiogram (in which dye is injected into the arteries so that they are highlighted on the X ray).

Yee still believed he had an appendicitis, and finally insisted that the doctors operate to confirm the diagnosis. The specialists agreed, all the while thinking that they would end up removing portions of his bowel. When Yee awoke, the doctors informed him that they'd removed his appendix—confirming his diagnosis. However, the delay in surgery (due to all the tests) gave his appendix time to rupture, sending bacteria spilling into his abdomen. As a result, Yee was put on three kinds of antibiotics, and was so ill he could barely turn his head to take a sip of water.

Eight days, and $30,000 later, Dr. Yee was discharged from the hospital. Had Yee had surgery when he first suspected the problem, he probably would have been hospitalized three or four days, and the bill would have been closer to $10,000.

Choosing a Therapy. The alternative therapies discussed in this book cover a wide spectrum of healing techniques. The aim of *Family Guide to Natural Medicine* is to examine these therapies under the lens of objective inquiry. But how is the average person to evaluate health care of any kind? Obviously, there is a limit to how much research most people are able to do. But you can keep abreast of developments by reading health columns in the newspapers and by subscribing to magazines and newsletters that regularly cover health topics.

When choosing a practitioner of natural medicine, ask other health professionals and your friends for recommendations—just as you would if seeking a referral for an orthodox physician. Don't forget to ask about their particular experiences with the practitioner they are recommending.

When you call for an appointment, ask the practitioner if he or she is certified or licensed by a state board or professional agency. Some of the natural medicine organizations willing to supply information are listed in the Sources section, on pages 413-414 of this book. Generally, the longer a therapy has been established, the easier it is to find reliable information.

Also, be sure to ask about the fee and time commitment when you call. Some therapies, such as the Alexander Technique or Rolfing, require quite a few sessions.

According to a recent poll, more than three out of five people surveyed who have never tried alternative medicine would give it a try if conventional therapy didn't help. Of those who have tried alternative medicine, the poll indicated, more than four out of five people would return to their practitioner. However, you must be the ultimate judge of any therapy. No discipline is free of incompetents or outright frauds, so, if you feel uncomfortable with any therapy or practitioner, do not continue.

The medical establishment has been quick to dismiss

many natural therapies, charging that the proof of their effectiveness rests solely on anecdotal evidence. Natural medicine practitioners respond that their approaches have withstood the test of time, even if they don't qualify for acceptance by orthodox medicine. However, in many cases, particularly in the area of herbal medicine, there is a growing body of scientific data to support therapeutic claims. It is well to remember that standards for acceptance sometimes shift. For example, osteopaths were denounced as frauds by the American Medical Association just a few decades ago. Today they are licensed to practice in all 50 states, and some orthodox physicians refer patients with chronic pain to osteopaths. In addition, acupuncture, hypnosis, and other therapies discussed in this book have been branded as quackery or dubious practices at one time or another, but are now gaining acceptance.

Innovation Versus Quack Cures. The distinction between outright scams and unproven but useful therapies is not always clear-cut. To skeptics, some types of natural healing seem to be merely exotic curiosities, while devotees swear that they work. An example includes Reiki, a hands-on healing technique whose advocates claim it can be used to cure a wide variety of ailments. The only explanation they offer is that there is a transfer of energy between practitioner and client.

Sales of over-the-counter medications have long been a profitable arena for those engaged in medical scams. Congressional passage of the Pure Food and Drugs Act in 1906 allowed the U.S. government to regulate the labeling of medical products. This act was the first federal statute intended to restrict sales of such products as Aromatic Lozenges of Steel, touted as a cure for "sexual weakness," patent medicines with high alcohol content, and medications that contained the radioactive element radium, which was said to cure cancer. This landmark legislation made a dent in the business but by no means brought it to a halt.

The subsequent passage of federal and state laws to curtail health fraud and ban outrageous advertising claims has been partly effective, at best. By several estimates, sales for cures that range from dubious to downright fraudulent exceed $10 billion annually in the United States. Authors of diet books sometimes promise weight loss with very-low-calorie diets that are nutritionally deficient and potentially harmful. Worse still, quacks often prey on arthritis sufferers, cancer patients, and others with serious ailments.

From the slightly offbeat to the truly bizarre, claims about new cures filter through the media daily. What is the

---

How to Avoid Quacks and Frauds

Suffering with a health problem that doesn't respond to conventional therapy can make one overly anxious to find a cure. Even the most cautious patient may find it hard to distinguish scams from legitimate treatments, and quacks from competent practitioners. Here are a few suggestions:

- Steer clear of health care practitioners who claim to possess secret knowledge. Safe and reliable treatments are never closely held secrets.

- Don't be awed by a lot of abbreviations after a practitioner's name. Find out if the abbreviations stand for degrees that were earned in accredited schools or training institutes.

- Regard skeptically medicines that promise to cure a wide range of serious ailments. This is especially true of treatments said to work for all types of arthritis or all forms of cancer.

- Don't assume that because an advertisement appears in a reputable magazine or newspaper, or on radio or TV, that the product or service must be good. Many advertisements are not subjected to close scrutiny.

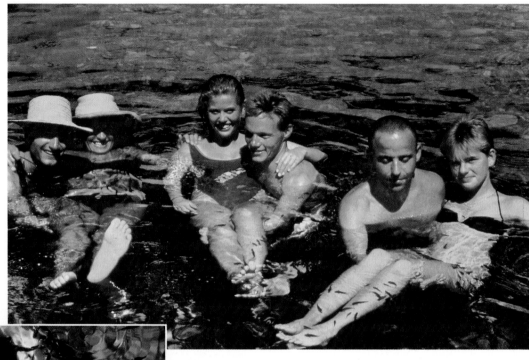

Bathers relaxing in this one-of-a-kind spa in a remote area of central Turkey suffer from psoriasis, a condition characterized by patches of thick, reddened skin covered with silvery scales. Fish that live in the sulfur-rich thermal pool nibble off scales and remove thickened skin. Patients who undergo the 21-day treatment report that it provides relief.

proper attitude to take about such reports? A healthy dose of skepticism is generally prescribed. One rule of thumb is that if a remedy or treatment sounds too good to be true, it probably is—this goes for orthodox as well as alternative care.

Still, a number of questionable-sounding treatments have proved to be legitimate. For example, thousands of years ago, Egyptians packed serious wounds with honey and other sweet substances. These treatments fell into disuse, particularly after the discovery of antibiotics. However, in Germany and elsewhere a few physicians are using sugar to treat bedsores and other stubborn wounds. Experts believe that the sugar works by drying the wound, dehydrating any infectious bacteria, and promoting the growth of healthy tissue. The advantage? The treatment is painless and inexpensive, and doctors who have used it say that sugar seems to heal wounds more quickly.

Things to Come. Proponents of natural medicine look to the day when alternative therapies are regularly used to complement standard medical treatment. Heart disease, obesity, and certain cancers are epidemic in our society. Yet if we look to other cultures, there is evidence that these conditions are not inevitable—instead they seem to be a result of poor eating habits, lack of exercise, stress, and other factors related to our fast-paced culture. Preventive care is at the heart of natural medicine—a strategy that entails adopting a healthy lifestyle and developing a positive outlook.

Readers of *Family Guide to Natural Medicine* will find some of the alternative health care approaches innovative, easy, and familiar. Others may seem too time-consuming or strange. Let intuition and information be your guide. When it comes to our own health, we are not powerless. ❏

You Are Healthier Than You Think

Writer and editor Norman Cousins believed that many of us rely too much on painkillers and other pills. We overestimate the threat of illness and underestimate the body's healing powers.

One of the unfortunate aspects of health education is that it tends to make us more aware of our weaknesses than of our strengths. By focusing our attention and concerns on things that can go wrong, we tend to develop a one-sided view of the human body, regarding it as a ready receiver for all sorts of illnesses. The most important health lesson of all to be learned is that the human body is a beautifully robust mechanism, capable of attending to most of its needs. But we know very little about the body's own processes for dealing with such needs. We have allowed pain to intimidate us unduly. We make the mistake of equating pain with disease; very little is said about the fact that most pain belongs to a warning system to tell us that we are doing something wrong.

Instead of understanding the message that pain is trying to give us, and attending to the cause, we reach almost automatically for this or that painkiller. . . . We have become a pill-popping and self-medicating society; in fact we are becoming a nation of weaklings and hypochondriacs, intimidated by the slightest pain and prepared to believe the worst. The trouble about believing the worst, of course, is that it has a tendency to invite the worst.

Proper health education should begin with an awareness of the magnificent resources built into the human system. We need to know that we possess mechanisms for warding off disease and for combating it. We need to become aware of the marvelous array of cells that circulate throughout the body, detecting the presence of invaders, reporting their presence and location to a command post in the brain that has the ability to activate the response forces—cells that go directly to the site of invasion, employing the body's own chemical system for combating infectious agents or correcting abnormal growths. This beautiful system can be impaired by all the self-medication we take in the mistaken notion that this is the only way we are going to subdue our pains.

Few things are more essential for the national future than the need for Americans to be reeducated about health: education about internal and external mechanisms for warding off disease or coping with it, should it occur; education that can teach us that panic and defeat are the great multipliers of illness; education about the importance of confidence in repair, restoration, recovery, regeneration; education in the need for partnership between patient and physician; education in what is meant by the human healing system and how it works best, . . . and, finally, education that can instruct us that what goes on in the mind can promote or retard health.

Excerpted from Head First, the Biology of Hope *by Norman Cousins*

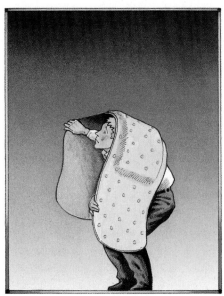

Worry about health is itself a problem

The Ancient Roots of Healing

The dramatic rituals of shamans and the healing plants of herbalists are widely used throughout the world. Though Western medicine is supremely effective in many respects, these alternate systems merit our attention.

FROM THE RAIN FORESTS of South America to the treeless tundra of Siberia, most of the world's people still rely on traditional healers to deliver their babies, treat their wounds, and quell vexatious spirits. Even in the United States, where the latest medical technology is readily available, traditional and folk medicine endures—particularly among Native Americans and in rural pockets of Appalachia. As more and more scientists are discovering, these healing traditions and remedies have survived not for reasons of ignorance or nostalgia, but because, more times than not, they work.

In many societies, disease is generally considered to be the physical manifestation of a spiritual miasma. As a result, healers assume varied roles in the community—from soothsayers and psychologists to priests and pharmacists. The terms shaman and medicine man are frequently used interchangeably, but shaman is the preferred usage. The shaman deals with the spiritual component of illness, while herbalists are expert in the use of healing plants.

From the Forest to the Laboratory. In recent years, a number of botanists, biologists, and chemists have turned their sights to tropical rain forests (where two-thirds of the world's plant species are found) to investigate the healing plants used by local healers, both shamans and herbalists. In South America, the search has a particular urgency since the rain forests there are rapidly being lost to deforestation and farming, and the tribal healers are beginning to die out as well.

To find out about an area's healing plants, researchers rely on the unrecorded wisdom of the local healers, whose own knowledge was acquired through years of study. For example, in Belize, a small country in Central America, the National Cancer Institute has funded an effort to collect plants for cancer and AIDS research. The scientists report that the lore of the shamans and herbalists has been invaluable in helping them to isolate suitable botanical species.

Communing with the Spirits. The world's oldest system of mind-body healing, shamanism continues to flourish in cultures the world over. From the remote regions of Alaska to the jungles of New Guinea, the beliefs, rituals, and methods of the shaman are strikingly similar from culture to culture. Traditionally, shamans have been highly trained individuals capable of healing the sick. What sets them apart from others in the community is their perceived ability to mediate between the ordinary world and the world of the spirits.

Shamanic societies attribute ill-defined illnesses to

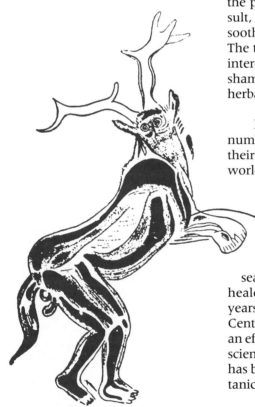

Prehistoric renderings of deerlike figures, found on cave walls in Europe, are offered as evidence that shamanism existed as much as 20,000 years ago. Even today, deer play a significant role in shamanic practices worldwide.

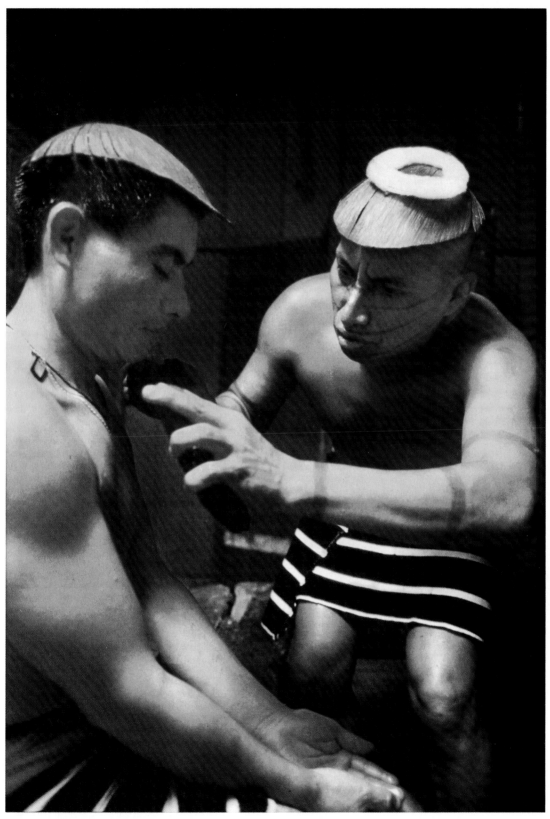

During a shamanic initiation rite, *a young member of the Colorado tribe of Ecuador receives special training from his teacher. Colorado shamans are known not just as skilled practitioners of the healing arts, but as intermediaries with the spirit world. They are responsible for preserving the religious traditions of the tribe.*

spirits, who must be placated to permit a cure. Perhaps the patient has offended them by breaking a taboo. Maybe a sorcerer has secretly bewitched the patient with "spirit darts." Or perhaps the soul has left the patient's body and fallen into the hands of ghosts, demons, or other evil spirits. The shaman's primary task is to discover the divine reason for the patient's illness.

In addition to performing healings, shamans (a word meaning wise ones) play a variety of important roles. They officiate at rites of passage, forecast the weather and the hunt, divine the location of missing persons and animals, identify criminals, and mediate disputes. In short, they are among those responsible for the integrity of the community.

Today's technological world is a far cry from the naturalistic world that gave rise to shamanism. Nowadays, diseases that might have wiped out entire villages can be prevented with inoculations. High-tech devices such as CAT scans and ultrasound enable doctors to see inside the body. So, what can we possibly learn from healers who blend mysticism with hands-on techniques to invoke healing? For one thing, shamans have long understood the importance of emotional factors and patient involvement in healing—and Western medicine is finally catching up.

An African healer and her trainees tend to a patient using a variety of traditional methods to diagnose and treat her illness. At the moment, the healer and her assistant (at right) pore over a collection of objects that they'll use for prescribing treatment, while the trainee at left waves a horse-mane whip to repel evil spirits.

Receiving the Call. Certain mental and physical characteristics are often thought to be indicative of shamanic gifts. In many areas, including Siberia, nervous disorders such as epilepsy are regarded as positive signs. Other cultures find minor deformities like six fingers significant. Most telling, however, is an active imagination and a propensity for visions, especially of spirits.

Traditionally, the role of shaman can be very dangerous for the practitioner. For instance, the initiation usually includes a period of

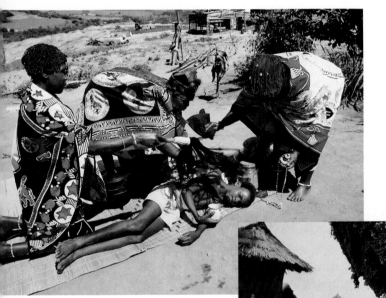

In the Ivory Coast nation of Africa, the village healer covers his earthen hut with the skulls of sacrificed animals, chicken feathers, and other symbolic figures. These objects offer protection against harmful spirits and other intruders.

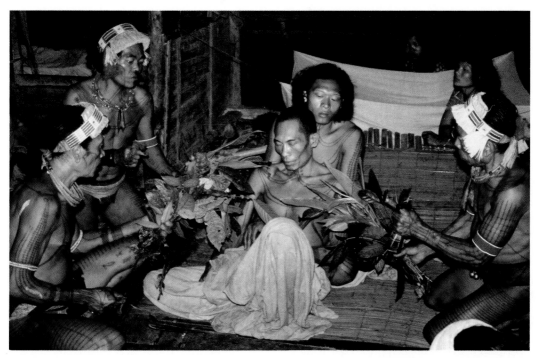

physical and mental testing that verges on torture. In addition, the shaman faces the peril of being punished if he fails to cure a patient. But despite the danger and discomfort inherent to the job, there is also considerable honor and financial reward that comes with the office—a shaman's services do not come cheap. In fact, they can be quite costly, which adds to the healer's prestige and power.

A circle of spirit helpers are believed to protect, guide, and assist the shaman in his healing duties. Often these guardian figures take the form of "power animals." Among Native Americans, bears and eagles are examples of typical power animals; Eskimo may call upon wolves, Malay shamans upon tigers.

The Trance. During a ceremonial healing, the shaman enters a trance for his journey to the spirit realm. Techniques for inducing the trance differ from culture to culture: some shamans rely on physical deprivation, such as fasting or working in darkness; others use hallucinogenic plants, such as the mescaline-containing San Pedro cactus. But the most notable trance-inducing tools are the monotonous elements of the rituals themselves—dancing, chanting, and especially drumming.

Over the ages shamans have regarded the drum as the "horse" that carries them to the Other World. So potent is the pulse of the drum that it appears capable of transporting even modern students of shamanism. Some research suggests the monotonous rhythm produces "theta" patterns in the brain, the kind of activity associated with dreams, hypnotic imagery, and creative thought. Shamans claim that while in the trance they can fly, turn into animals, and surmount any type of obstacle.

During a healing ceremony in Indonesia, village healers use sacred plants and cast spells in an effort to reunite a sick man with his soul. If this fails, the healers may ornament him with garlands and perform a wedding-like ceremony, complete with songs and dances, in order to convince his soul that it would be worthwhile to return to the world of the living.

The Healing. Healing ceremonies are usually conducted at night, with the patient, relatives, and other community members all in attendance. As the drumming and dancing starts, the shaman, who wears symbolic dress and carries a variety of tools and instruments, summons his spiritual guardians for the journey into the realm of the spirits. While there, he tries to discover the nature of breached taboos and intercede with the offended spirits. For instance, if the shaman determines that a harmful spirit has entered the patient, he may dramatically "suck" it from the patient's body.

Lasting from several hours to several days, these healing rituals are intense, draining, community affairs that show the patient that he or she is not alone in the struggle. Psychologists who have studied these ceremonies contend that such demonstrations of support boost the patient's spirits and restore health.

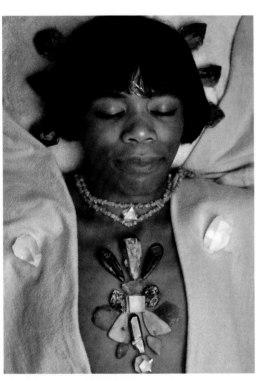

There is little evidence *that traditional shamans relied on crystals in their healing ceremonies. However, in recent years, neo-shamans of the New Age movement have blended the Ayurvedic idea of energy centers with the shamanic practice of using symbolic objects for healing. Here, crystals believed to have healing powers have been placed over energy points on this woman's body.*

A Potent Placebo. In shamanistic societies, faith takes on an important role in traditional healing. Some who have studied such phenomena, like Dr. Jerome Frank, author of *Persuasion and Healing*, believe that the effectiveness of shamanic healing is dependent upon the "heightened expectancy" of the person who is ill. Because the shaman's practice is so strongly connected to the belief system of the community as a whole, he is able to make use of the patient's faith in his perceived healing powers. The shaman does this in part by using a wide array of "symbolic" techniques and visual aids to create an atmosphere, which he feels will evoke the deepest feelings of trust and competence on the part of the patient. Examples of these techniques include the use of elaborate costumes, drums, rattles, and animal sounds.

During the healing ceremony, the shaman may choose to perform an extraction. Often, the shaman will secrete a twig or some other object in his mouth and pretend he has sucked it from the patient's body. For the healer, the object is merely symbolic, but to the patient such visual aids may be an essential part of the healing process.

Modern medicine views a cure elicited in this way strictly as a "placebo response," that is, a reaction that is the direct result of the expectations of the patient. However, as we learn more and more about the important interaction between the mind and body, the efficacy of shamanic healing practices becomes clearer.

Shamanism in a Modern Setting. While far from common, shamanic techniques, such as chanting, visualization, and drumming, have been used in a few clinics in the U.S. According to G. Frank Lawlis, a psychologist and researcher working with cancer patients at Stanford University in California, shamanistic methods can be useful for treating pain, anxiety, and stress. Lawlis has used rhythmic drumming, for example, to help patients break destructive thought patterns that were hindering their recovery.

Other proponents of shamanism, such as anthropologist Michael Harner, suggest that the ancient rituals and techniques are a way for us to reconnect with ourselves, our communities, and our planet. Considered from this perspective, modern shamanism is a way of achieving a kind of spiritual or emotional healing. ❏

CASE HISTORY

A WORKSHOP IN SHAMANISM

To understand the mystic experiences which lie at the core of shamanism, Nevill Drury participated in a shaman workshop. Here is his account of what happened.

"I vividly recall my first brush with shamanic consciousness. In 1980 I was involved as a lecturer at the International Transpersonal Conference, outside Melbourne, and it was the first time that many of the leading figures of the American human potential movement had visited Australia. Professor Michael Harner was a member of this group. He arrived at Tullamarine Airport carrying a shaman's drum, gourd rattles and a set of feathers and bones used by the Salish Indians for a mind-control game.

"Here was an opportunity to explore shamanic visualisation more thoroughly. I had already made use of magical techniques of visualisation and found it comparatively easy to hold images in my mind's eye. I was hopeful, therefore, that I could also gain some sort of experiential breakthrough into the 'shamanic reality.'

"As I recall, we went all day without eating much food and for the most part it was simply a matter of journeying inwardly on the drumbeat. For me the initial contact, in a mythic sense, had come through the form of a hawk. It had powerful deep black and yellow eyes and a mix of black and brown feathers.

"The climax came in the evening.

Harner asked us to imagine entering a smoke tunnel either by wafting upwards on smoke from a campfire or by entering a fireplace and soaring towards the sky up a chimney. As we entered the smoke tunnel, he explained, we would see it unfolding before us, taking us higher and higher.

"The room was quite dark as Harner began to beat on his drum. Here is a transcript of my notes from this particular journey.

" 'In the distance I see a golden mountain rising in the mist. As we draw closer I see that, built on the top of the mountain, is a magnificent palace made of golden crystal, radiating lime-yellow light. I am told that this is the palace of the phoenix, and I then see that golden bird surmounting the edifice.

" 'I feel awed and amazed by the beauty of this place, but the regal bird bids me welcome.

" 'The drum is still sounding but soon Michael asks us to return.'

"The journey was a very awesome one for me. I felt I had been in a very sacred space. My interest in shamanism has never waned since this particularly eventful day in my life."

Excerpted from *The Elements of Shamanism* by Nevill Drury.

Native American Medicine

Herbal remedies, medicine bundles, and sweat baths are among the therapies commonly used by Native Americans. And local healers are still very much involved in the health of their communities.

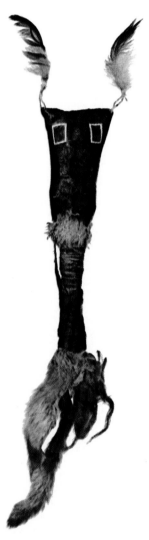

This Navajo rattle, *covered in deerskin and decorated with mountain lion fur and eagle feathers, was used by healers to keep the tempo during tribal chants.*

THE NATIVE TRIBES OF NORTH AMERICA, from the Eskimo of the Arctic, to the Sioux and Kansa of the Great Plains, to the Pima and Navajo of the Southwest, all have complex healing systems. And while these groups differ in many ways, they share a central philosophy that people are not separate from, or above, nature, but a part of it. Native Americans believe that everything in nature has a spirit—not just animals and humans, but rocks, and trees, and wind, for example—and these spirits are generally beneficial to people. But there are other realms of spirits that can cause harm. Illness occurs when these spirits feel angered or insulted. Fighting illness is more than treating physical symptoms; addressing the spiritual cause is just as important.

Many Native Americans first establish a relationship with the spirit world in their early adolescence. Among the Plains tribes, a boy will go alone on a vigil called a vision quest. During the quest he will fast and pray for several days in the hope that spirits will take pity on him. If successful, the spirit of an animal may appear, and that animal will have a special significance for the boy. Visions are important to these Native Americans; a vision of a powerful animal may foretell a life of leadership to the community.

This spirit stays with the boy all his life, first giving instructions on how to make an important healing object, the medicine bundle. The bundle is a collection of items that are believed to be the physical homes of these spirits. A bundle may contain animal skins, powders, or stones. It is to this personal medicine bundle that he may first turn when sick, asking the spirits for help in fighting illness.

Herbalists and Shamans. When illness strikes, a person will first try self-medication with herbs, or perhaps an herbalist will be consulted. Of the many kinds of Native American healers, herbalists are the ones who treat common minor ailments, such as sore throats, wounds, toothaches, and broken bones. Many herbalists are women, and they frequently specialize in certain types of illness. For more poorly defined illnesses, which are considered due to supernatural forces, a shaman is hired. A variety of healing devices are associated with specific shamanic cures, such as songs, rituals, and tokens of power. These can be bought, exchanged, or handed down, and many individuals in a community may have limited shamanic powers.

When treating an illness, these healers seldom don elaborate dress, as the group's most powerful shaman does. They may bring their own medicine bundle and rattles. The air is purified by burning special plants, and an herbal treatment is sometimes administered. The events of the session are important, and can involve singing and placing the patient in a sweat bath.

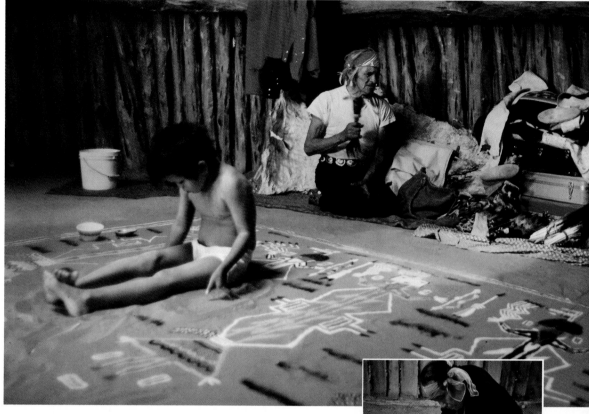

During a healing ceremony this Navajo boy sits on a sand painting so that the healing power of the painting can flow through him.

Sweat baths are often used, by themselves or as a part of healing or religious ceremonies. The bath takes place in a dome-shaped building made from bent willow sticks covered with animal skins. Hot rocks are placed inside, and water poured over them. The lodge heats quickly, and the occupants sweat profusely. Once finished, they may rub themselves with dry sage leaves, or perhaps they jump into a cooling river or snowbank.

The Uses of Plants. As with other traditional healing systems, plants are an important part of Native American medicine. Native Americans have developed an effective pharmacopoeia, using plants either internally or externally to speed healing and fight disease. For example, many groups have used species of willow, such as pussy willow, for healing. The Eskimo used a tea made from the boiled bark of one willow as a gargle for sore throats, and the leaves of another species on wounds. The Creek bathed in, or drank, a willow tea to ease aching joints. We now know that willow contains salicin, which is the natural precursor of acetylsalicylic acid, the active ingredient in aspirin. Thus a form of the popular painkiller was in use long before aspirin was developed by modern science.

The uses of medicinal plants were never standardized across the continent, varying widely from one group to an-

Sand-painting rituals are a common feature of Navajo medicine, remedying the spiritual causes of illness. The various colored powders are made from ground minerals or vegetable matter.

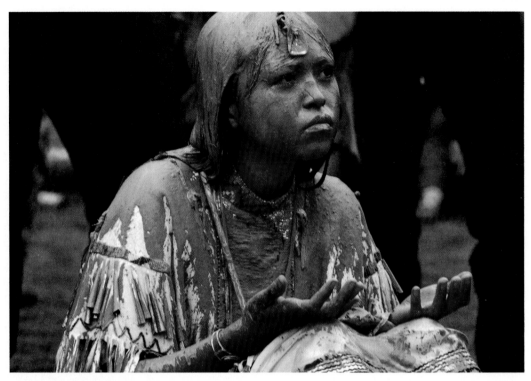

This young Apache woman has just been sprinkled with yellow cattail pollen, a symbol of fertility. The community has gathered for a four-day ceremony that marks her becoming an adult. The event serves to commemorate her new status and responsibilities.

other. For example, after dandelion was introduced by Europeans to the New World, Native Americans found many uses for it. The Fox used it for chest pain, and the Tewa used the ground leaves to speed the healing of broken bones. The Mohegans used it in a tonic.

Herbal remedies are often passed down within a family, and herbalists, of course, know of many healing plants. Traditionally, shamans are believed to be channels through which a still greater healing power could flow. In the past, they often claimed that their herbal remedies came to them in dreams, by means of spirit informers. Sometimes ailing animals were followed to see what plants they ate to get well. The favorite animal to follow was the bear, revered for its intelligence, and considered a reliable source of herbal remedies.

Curing with Grains of Sand. Unique to the Navajo is a healing ceremony centered around symbolic drawings made of colored sand. The Navajo exorcise the influences of evil spirits through this ritual. The symbolic design can be quite elaborate, perhaps taking many helpers a full day to complete, and will vary depending on what is seen as the cause of the illness. The sick person then sits at the center of the painting, absorbing the healing power it contains, while the Navajo healer shakes a rattle, prays, and chants. The painting is destroyed immediately after the ceremony. Each person who is present is allowed to take a pinch of the healing sand with them. They might touch it to an ailing part of their body, or save it for use in the future. In this, as in much of Native American medicine, belief is crucial for the benefits of healing. ❏

The Healing Power of Rituals

*We heal more quickly when we believe in the effectiveness
of the treatment used. For the Navajo, that means having Singers
perform their time-honored healing ceremonies.*

It is difficult for many white people to understand why, when the resources of white medicine are available to Navajos in government hospitals and dispensaries, the Navajos continue to patronize "ignorant medicine men." The answer is that native practice brings good results—in many cases as good as those of a white physician or hospital.

In the hospital a Navajo is lonely and homesick, living by a strange routine and eating unfamiliar foods. During the chant [a Navajo healing ritual] the patient feels himself personally being succored and loved, for his relatives are spending their substance to get him cured, and they are rallying to aid in the ceremonial.

Some of the help which [the healing ceremonies] give has a straightforward physical explanation. But there can be no doubt that the main effects are psychological. There is nothing too mysterious about this. Physicians have long known that the will to get well, the belief that one is going to recover, can be more than half the battle.

Then there is the prestige and authority of the Singer assuring the patient that he will recover. In his capacity as Singer, gifted with the learning of the Holy People, he is more than mortal and at times becomes identified with the supernaturals, speaking in their voices and telling hearers that all is well. The prestige, mysticism, and power of the ceremonial itself are active, coming directly from the supernatural powers that build up the growing earth in spring, drench it with rain, or tear it apart with lightning.

In the height of the chant the patient himself becomes one of the Holy People, puts his feet in their moccasins, and breathes in the strength of the sun. He comes into complete harmony with the universe and must of course be free of all ills and evils. There will be an upswing of reawakened memories, like

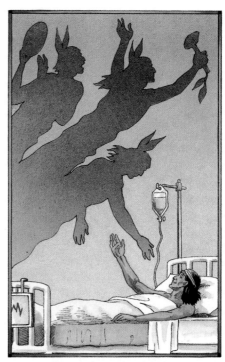

Calling on the powers of tradition.

old melodies bearing him on emotional waves to feelings of security.

As well as this reassurance, occupation and diversion are supplied to the patient. He has the sense of doing something about a misfortune which otherwise might leave him in the misery of feeling completely helpless. During the ceremonial the patient's thoughts are busy following the Singer's instructions, pondering over the implications in the songs and prayers, the speeches and side remarks of the Singer. The period of being quiet and aloof after the ceremonial is a splendid opportunity for rumination and for development of the conviction that the purposes of the chant have been achieved.

Excerpted from The Navaho *by Clyde Kluckhohn
and Dorothea Leighton*

A Sioux Ceremony to Heal Veterans

On Memorial Day, 1990, a group of Vietnam veterans began a 700-mile march that would bring them from Angel Fire, New Mexico, to the Pine Ridge Indian Reservation in South Dakota. Still haunted by the war in Vietnam, these veterans hoped to find relief in the traditional ceremonies of the Sioux.

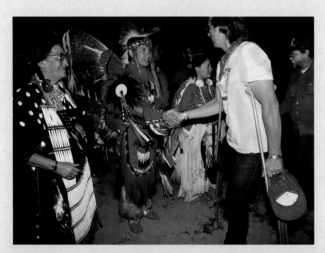

Hundreds of people greeted the marchers when they arrived for the five-day ceremony. The Sioux have long celebrated the return of their warriors from battle. These traditional rituals have been effective for some Vietnam veterans, allowing them finally to confront the intense emotions they have experienced.

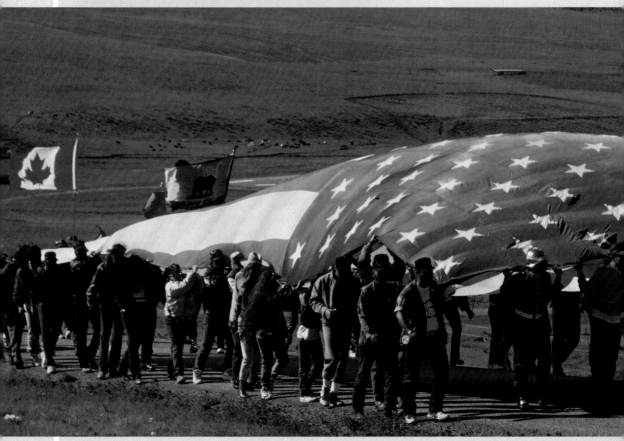

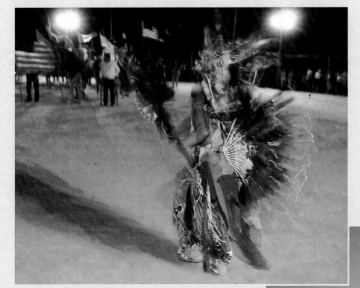

On the first night the veterans were greeted with a traditional dance. They would later take part in rituals such as sweat lodge ceremonies and vision quests, which offered them a time for introspection.

Here a Native American veteran leads the morning prayer, holding his own pipe and a sacred eagle feather. In front of him is a sacred pipe that was carved for one of the vets and carried on the march from New Mexico.

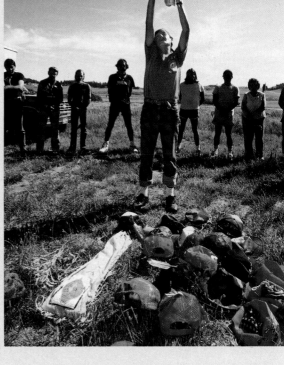

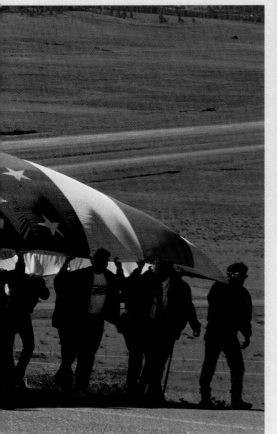

A large group of veterans carried this giant flag to the Disabled American Veterans Memorial in Angel Fire, New Mexico. Most of the month-long march that followed was made by a core group of about eight. The march was conceived of by a vet who had visited the Pine Ridge reservation and learned of their ceremonies.

Balancing Yin and Yang

Practitioners of traditional Chinese medicine use herbal concoctions, acupuncture, and other methods to promote the smooth flow of energy, or qi, along the body's internal pathways, or meridians.

AN ANCIENT, BUT STILL VITAL SYSTEM of health and healing, traditional Chinese medicine is based on the notion of harmony or balance. Accordingly, a healthy person is someone in complete harmony, both internally and with nature.

A central tenet of traditional Chinese medicine is prevention. Two thousand years ago, physicians were already emphasizing the importance of moderation—in lifestyle, diet, and exercise—in maintaining health and preventing illness. In fact, classical Chinese physicians taught patients how to live a moderate and balanced life, and were paid only as long as their patients remained healthy.

China's first physicians were also philosophers, and their theories on health were firmly rooted in the Taoist tradition, which stresses the oneness of all things in nature. The human body is seen as a microcosm of the universe, and as such, operates according to the same principles. *The Yellow Emperor's Classic of Internal Medicine*, written over 2000 years ago, was the first book to lay forth the ideas of traditional Chinese medicine.

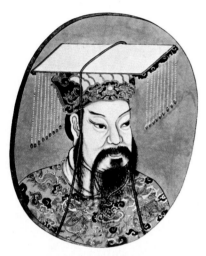

China's Legendary Yellow Emperor

Huang-di, the Yellow Emperor, is credited with writing the classic text on traditional Chinese medicine over 2000 years ago. However, it is more than likely that *The Yellow Emperor's Classic of Internal Medicine* is a composite, compiled and amended by unknown authors over hundreds of years. Regardless of its authorship, the book represents the first attempt to codify Chinese medicine. And while no longer consulted as a primary text, the wisdom set forth in the book still serves as the basis for this Eastern system of medicine.

Yin and Yang. Within traditional Chinese medicine, health is defined as a balance of the body's yin and yang aspects. These terms refer to the complementary but opposing qualities that make up everything in the natural world. All things have a yin aspect as well as a yang—and these interdependent qualities comprise the parts of any whole. For example, time consists of day (yang) and night (yin), the body has yin organs as well as yang, and so forth.

Harmony, and therefore health, depends on balancing yin and yang. This concept promotes a clinical perspective. Since our bodies are in dynamic balance internally as well as externally (with nature), we are constantly making minor adjustments to maintain equilibrium. In other words, perfect health is not some static state we can hope to achieve; instead, our bodies stay well by making changes in response to various influences. When we are unable to adapt—whether to a change in weather or the invasion of a virus—we fall ill.

The Human Anatomy. The Chinese view of anatomy emerged from the idea that the body is an integrated whole, composed of both yin and yang aspects. Accordingly, the organs operate in pairs with each of the five *zang* organs (heart, kidney, liver, lungs, and spleen) paired with an opposing *fu* organ. These pairs work together as a unit, regulating each other's activities. The *fu* organs, which include the gallbladder, small intestine, stomach, large intestine, and bladder, serve primarily to transform food into energy and eliminate wastes, and are considered yang. The five *zang* organs are said to control the storage of vital sub-

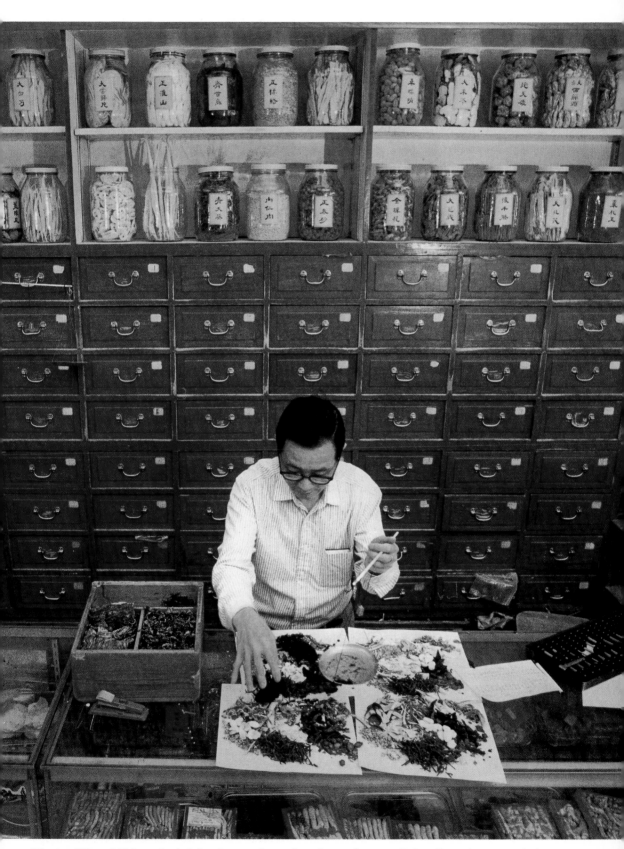

The traditional Chinese herbal shop has not changed much over the years. Before dispensing a prescription, herbalists prepare and measure ingredients by hand, mixing the remedies according to precise instructions.

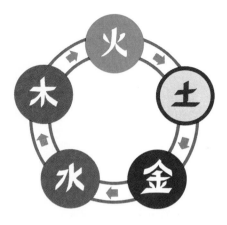

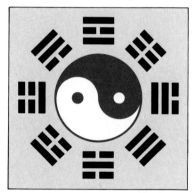

These Chinese symbols, the Five Elements (top) and the yin and yang (bottom), represent the rhythms of life—the constant movement and transformation that are central to the cycles of nature. According to the tenets of Chinese medicine, good health is a function of maintaining a balance between the body's vital energy and the forces of nature.

stances, and are considered yin. In addition, Chinese medicine recognizes a number of miscellaneous organs, including the brain and blood vessels, which both store and transport materials.

It is important to note that in Chinese medicine, the term "organ" refers to a whole network—not just the organ itself. For example, when a Chinese physician speaks of the "liver," he's referring not just to the organ, but to a whole system of structures—tissues, skin, tendons, bones—that form an energy network in the body. Emphasis is less on form (shape, size, location), and more on function—how the organ interacts with and affects the rest of the body. While each internal organ has a specific function, it is also linked to the rest of the body by an intricate network of energy channels, known as meridians.

Tapping Vital Energy. The energy network that links the organs also serves as the pathway for qi, the body's vital energy. Invisible, formless, and indispensable, according to Chinese theory, qi is said to spring from several sources, and to perform a range of functions. Qi circulates through the body, warming us, offering protection against illness, giving us vitality. Some of the energy comes from our parents at conception, and some is derived from food and air (which is one reason diet and breathing exercises are so important to Chinese medicine).

Like qi itself, the energy meridians that transport it are invisible. However, according to theory, they serve three primary purposes. The meridians transport qi; they are the communication link for all the parts of the body; and they regulate the *zang-fu* organ systems. The meridians also connect the exterior and interior of the body, which is why acupuncture is able to have effects deep within the body. When viewed from this perspective, meridian theory explains why a problem with the liver, for example, can reverberate throughout the body—by disrupting the normal flow of qi and causing imbalances elsewhere in the body.

Making an Assessment. Chinese practitioners have mapped an elaborate system of meridians, each of which can be used to both diagnose and treat disease. According to theory, a number of precipitating factors may contribute to the onset of symptoms. They include external or "pernicious influences" such as wind and dampness, internal disturbances, and unhealthy lifestyles. Chinese medicine also recognizes other factors in illness, including insect bites, parasites, and trauma.

However, these precipitating influences are not seen as causing illness. Rather, each factor is part of a general pattern of disharmony that is disrupting the system. As one classic text puts it, "wind, rain, cold, and heat alone can hurt no man without weak points." So the focus of treatment is not on eliminating symptoms, but on using them to discover and treat underlying imbalances.

Because internal imbalances are reflected externally, traditional Chinese doctors assess patients using four techniques: looking, listening and smelling (these are the same word in Chinese), asking, and touching. First, the physician looks at the patient, noting general appearance, complexion, manner, and "spirit," as indicated by these signs, including posture and facial expression.

Next, and of great importance, the physician examines the patient's tongue. According to traditional theory, the tongue is a barometer of health because of its close connection to the internal organs through the meridian system. Changes in the tongue—color, texture, coating, size, and motion—are said to be clues to the nature of an imbalance. By studying hundreds of tongues (and replicas used as educational tools), the traditional doctor learns to recognize the diagnostic significance of these changes.

During the "listening" phase, the practitioner assesses the sound of the patient's breathing (including coughing) and voice. The "smelling" assessment takes into account two types of bodily odors—one foul, the other pungent. The presence of either is an important indicator of illness. In the "asking" examination, the physician poses questions about the patient's medical history, symptoms, lifestyle, and other areas deemed significant. For example, the doctor will ask specific questions about the patient's perspiration, thirst and appetite, and sensitivity to heat and cold.

The last part of the assessment is "touching." This includes palpating different areas of the body, including acupuncture points, to detect swelling and any sensitivity. The key to touching, and indeed to Chinese diagnostics, is the taking of the pulse. In fact pulse diagnosis is so significant that many Chinese call visiting the doctor "going to have my pulse felt."

Chinese pulse-taking is much more complex than the Western method. While Chinese doctors also use the radial artery near the wrist, they feel for the pulse at three positions on each wrist, rather than just one. Each pulse is said to reflect the condition of different areas of the body. In addition, traditional theory recognizes some 28 different pulse qualities, each of which reflects a distinct type of imbalance.

Based on the four-point examination of the patient, the traditional practitioner tries to discern the patterns of disharmony—a very complex task. For instance, the Western diagnosis of diabetes may, according to Chinese medicine, result from lung "fire," stomach "fire," or kidney "fire," depending upon the configuration of the other bodily signs, including the precise degree of thirst, the strength and quali-

This modern chart of acupuncture points illustrates the complexity of meridian theory. While charts are useful as teaching tools or general reference, acupuncturists always feel for the points since their precise location differs from person to person.

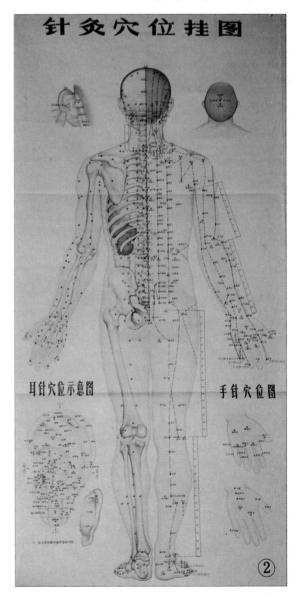

ty of the pulse, and the general appearance of the tongue.

Finally, after the physician has meshed each part of the assessment and determined the source of the disharmony, he formulates a treatment plan. Treatment may include herbal remedies, acupuncture, massage, exercise, diet, or, frequently, a combination of these and other traditional methods.

The tongue exam is considered to be one of the most useful and reliable diagnostic tools. The physician looks at the shape and color of the tongue, as well as at its coating.

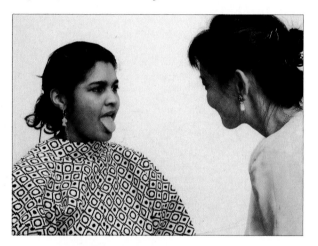

Acupuncture. An ancient Chinese healing art, acupuncture aims to restore the smooth flow of qi. Though this energy circulates within the body, it can be accessed at many superficial points located along the major meridians. Each of these meridians is associated with specific organs, and every acupuncture point is considered to have a particular therapeutic effect.

Classical texts describe 365 acupuncture points. But today, some practitioners claim that the total is more than 2000. Acupuncturists are trained to select points and insert needles, but many also use other therapeutic techniques—not all of which require the insertion of needles.

The most common acupuncture method involves insertion of one slender needle at each selected point. Traditionally, needles are twirled for greater stimulation. However, a number of practitioners also use a weak electric current, sent through conventional needles, to produce the same effect. This method is especially useful when continued stimulation (15 to 20 minutes) of a point is indicated.

Acupuncture points can also be stimulated by heat or pressure. During moxibustion, for instance, the practitioner places small cones of the herb mugwort ("moxa") on the needle or acupuncture point. The cones are then burned to produce a penetrating heat (and removed before causing pain). Or for gentler warming, a large cigar-shaped moxa stick may be lit and slowly rotated above the spot. Deep finger pressure, known as acupressure, is another therapeutic technique used by some acupuncturists. Similar to the Japanese massage technique shiatsu, it can be used to relieve headaches and menstrual discomfort.

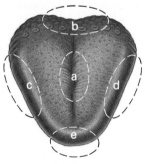

Certain areas of the tongue are thought to correspond to specific organ systems in the body. For instance, area a of this diagram relates to the stomach, b to the kidneys, c and d to the liver and gallbladder, and e to the heart/lung system.

Traditional and Newer Usages. Many Westerners associate acupuncture with pain relief. However, in Chinese medicine it plays a much broader role. Because acupuncture is thought to regulate the flow of qi, it may be used preventively, as well as therapeutically. For instance, some traditional Chinese practitioners give seasonal "balancing treatments" to avert colds and flu associated with climatic changes. To treat an imbalance in a particular organ system, the acupuncturist would stimulate points along the appropriate meridians.

Acupuncture has generated a lot of interest, even

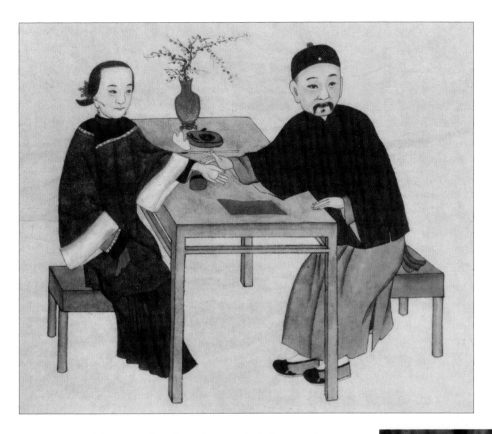

among practitioners who do not accept qi theory. Among the most widely publicized of newer uses is acupuncture analgesia, which is used to reduce pain during surgery. Though the technique originated in China during the fifties, it has little to do with traditional Chinese medicine (where surgery was virtually unknown). The treatment is sometimes used along with chemical anesthesia, which allows for lower doses—resulting in fewer side effects.

Among Western practitioners, by far the most common use for acupuncture is in the treatment of chronic pain. Many people report finding relief from such intractable conditions as arthritis, chronic headaches, and back pain. Acupuncture has also been used to treat drug addiction, alcoholism, and smoking. While early reports have been promising, it is too early to tell if acupuncture is truly useful for treating addictions.

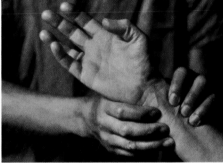

*A **highly developed** and refined diagnostic method, pulse-taking has been a primary tool of Chinese medicine for at least 2000 years. The pulse is taken at three different points on each wrist, and based on the quality of the beats, the physician is able to assess the condition of the body's organ systems and vital energy.*

How Does It Work? Chinese and Western investigators are searching for scientific explanations of acupuncture. Dr. Bruce Pomeranz, a physiologist at the University of Toronto, suggests that acupuncture works by stimulating the body's production of various pain-blocking neurochemicals. The effectiveness of the treatment seems to depend on which points are stimulated.

For instance, Dr. Pomeranz reports that needling at the site of pain prompts the spinal cord to generate chemicals that work locally. In contrast, points stimulated at a distance from the pain appear to stimulate pain blockers in the brain. Many people are still unconvinced by such research and consider any benefits from acupuncture to be the result of the placebo effect. But the many patients who have found relief from chronic pain and other afflictions would undoubtedly disagree.

Finding a Practitioner. During the past decade it has become increasingly easy to find an acupuncturist—though not necessarily a qualified one. In the U.S., many states now license practitioners (a requirement of three

---

CASE HISTORY

ACUPUNCTURE AS ANALGESIA

When David Eisenberg went to China to study traditional medicine, he was allowed to observe an operation for a brain tumor. Throughout, the patient was conscious and free of pain.

"A fifty-eight-year-old professor of history named Lu had a brain tumor. He was referred to the Beijing Neurological Institute, where an X ray of his skull revealed a chestnut-size growth located in the center of his brain.

"Lu's surgeon, Dr. Wang Zhong-cheng, suggested he have the procedure done under acupuncture analgesia. At first, Lu was not too enthusiastic about the idea. He was understandably unnerved by the prospect of being totally awake and responsive during brain surgery. However, after Dr. Wang told him that more than 90 percent of all head and neck surgeries at the Neurological Institute were performed successfully under acupuncture, Professor Lu agreed to give it a try.

"Lu had an intravenous line in place and through it received mild preoperative sedatives. These medications would relax and sedate the patient, but they would not provide adequate anesthesia.

"The next step was the insertion of needles and the beginning of acupuncture stimulation. The needle was twisted by hand for initial stimulation until Comrade Lu 'obtained the Qi' — that is, experienced a sensation of fullness, distention, and mild electric shock.

"The anesthesiologist then attached

a low-voltage electric stimulator to the protruding end of the needle in order to send electric current through it at fixed intervals.

"The doctors gave me a seat next to the operating table so that I could monitor his pulse and blood pressure during the procedure.

"The surgeons took up their scalpels. At the moment of incision, Lu failed to wince, grimace, or give any hint of pain. His pulse and blood pressure remained at their preoperative levels.

"The manipulation of bony surfaces is usually extremely painful. Lu said he felt no pain. His pulse and blood pressure remained unchanged. He was calm, responsive, and talkative.

"Throughout the entire procedure, which continued for more than four hours, Lu remained conscious, and his vital signs remained stable.

"After the completion of the surgery, Lu shook the hand of his surgeon, thanked him profusely, then walked out of the operating room unassisted. The large tumor had been successfully removed, and it subsequently proved to be benign."

Excerpted from *Encounters with Qi* by David Eisenberg, M.D.

years of full-time study is typical), but in others anyone can call himself or herself an acupuncturist. And almost all states allow physicians to perform the procedure even if the only training they've had is a brief extension course.

Though there are exceptions, Western-trained physicians tend to use acupuncture to relieve local symptoms, particularly pain. In contrast, traditional acupuncturists first make a diagnosis of underlying imbalances, then they rely on meridian theory to select appropriate points.

Treatment details—including number, length, and thickness of needles; angle and depth of insertion; use of electrical or heat stimulation—depend on the practitioner and the particular points selected. Many acupuncturists will insert one to 15 needles during a treatment. Insertion of the fine, sterile steel doesn't usually hurt, though some ailments may increase sensitivity.

The needles are generally left in place for 15 to 20 minutes. Patients report a variety of sensations, including soreness, pins and needles, and numbness. Afterward some people feel exhilarated; others want to sleep. Some patients report that their symptoms temporarily flare up following a session. Acupuncturists say that this reaction is a sign that the body is becoming energized to overcome the problem or illness.

Herbal Medicine. While acupuncture has mesmerized the media, herbal medicine is actually the mainstay of Chinese medicine. So complex and highly regarded is herbalism that students of traditional Chinese medicine must spend at least six years studying it.

Like other Chinese therapies, herbal medicines are used to restore balance to the system. Many herbal remedies seem particularly suited to such a regulatory role because of their potential for dual action. For instance, dang gui is said to relax the uterus when it's tight and contract it when slack. In addition to restoring the balance of yin and

Moxa cones burn very slowly, and many patients find the penetrating heat relaxing. Although the cones may be placed directly on the patient's skin, they are sometimes set on a thin bed of ginger so they can be kept burning longer without causing discomfort.

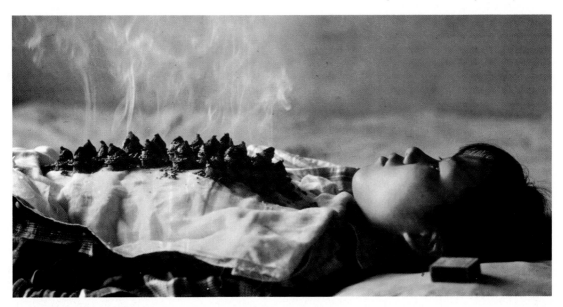

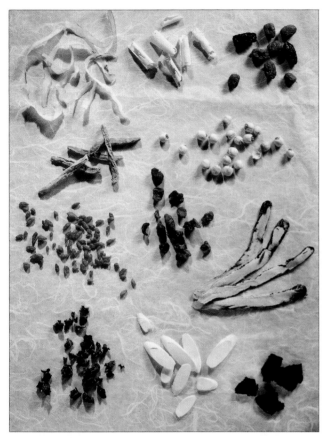

Many Chinese healing herbs and foods are used to fortify the immune system, increase stamina, and ease stress. The items pictured above include lotus seeds, astragalus, and red and black dates. While somewhat difficult to find, they are generally available in Chinese shops in larger American cities.

yang, herbs may also be used to increase the body's resistance to illness.

Food Cures. Before prescribing any herbs, a traditional practitioner may well try an allied form of treatment—food therapy. This approach dates back to the earliest Chinese medical texts, which urged doctors to "use medicine as a last resort only when food fails."

Food therapy is not about cutting down on fat and calories. Instead, traditional Chinese physicians use specific foods as another way of balancing an individual's yin and yang aspects. Like herbs, foods are categorized and prescribed according to qualities including their "hotness" or "coolness," general effect on the body, and flavor—hot, sour, bitter, sweet, or salty. Different flavors are considered to have affinities for specific organ systems—for example, salty with the kidneys, sour with the liver.

Food plays a fundamental role in Chinese medicine in preventing as well as treating disease. If dietary guidelines are followed, disease is less likely to develop. Ideally, meals should strike a balance of tastes, textures, smells, colors, and other qualities that will promote internal harmony among the organ systems.

Finding the Right Formula. Restoring balance may sound straightforward in theory, but it can prove tricky in practice. For instance, the same general symptoms may stem from very different underlying disorders—requiring quite different herbal remedies. For instance, a low back pain due to damp cold (after one has been caught in the rain or sat on cold, wet ground) would be treated with herbs to dispel the dampness and unblock the meridians. On the other hand, a low back pain caused by strain or trauma would be treated with herbs that restore the smooth flow of qi.

Generally speaking, Chinese herbs are far less toxic than chemical drugs (and truly toxic herbs are few), but self-diagnosis and prescription is not recommended. However the trained herbalist has centuries of clinical experience at his fingertips, in a library of time-tested remedies. Herbalists have literally tens of thousands of formulas to choose from, but in practice 500 classical remedies are routinely used.

Chinese practitioners recognize close to 6000 medicinal substances—not only botanicals but also minerals and animal products—and the average prescription formula contains between five and 15 of them. In addition to the principal agent selected to treat the illness, herbal remedies generally incorporate several other types of ingredients. These may include "conductants" to channel the medication and "correctants" to counter side effects. In addition, the practitioner can fine-tune the remedy by choosing how it will be prepared and administered. The eight most common types of preparations—among them concentrated extracts, broths (also known as decoctions), pills, pastes and medicine-wines—vary in strength and rate of absorption. In addition, physicians in China have developed injectable forms of some herbal preparations.

Validating Claims. While China has encouraged Western-trained doctors and scientists to study their medicinal herbs, there have been relatively few independent clinical studies to date. However, some of the most commonly used herbs have been researched in China and the West, and their pharmacologic bases are known. Ma huang (ephedrine), for example, a popular antiasthmatic herb in China, is also a common ingredient in Western drugs used for the same purpose.

Other Chinese herbs have yielded new drugs or show promise of doing so. For instance, the popular Chinese herbal qinghao has generated a new antimalarial agent. And the sour date kernel, used as a sedative/hypnotic by the Chinese for 3000 years, is showing the same effects in lab experiments. Common foxglove, which yields the cardiac drug digitalis, is also used in a Chinese heart medication—not just for the digitalis, but for another active ingredient, verodoxin. This substance reinforces the effects of digitalis, allowing smaller doses to be used. Verodoxin is refined out of the Western derivative.

Many herbal formulas contain dozens of ingredients, so it is difficult to design experiments that can evaluate which herbs are producing medicinal effects. Differences between Chinese and Western diagnostic techniques create roadblocks to research as well. Even so, Chinese medicinal herbs are continuing to attract interest and gain scientific support around the world.

Movement. Over the centuries, exercise has remained a key part of Chinese preventive medicine. Every morning, millions of Chinese start the day with the flowing movements of t'ai chi and the breathing techniques of qi dong. Both are used to promote the smooth flow of qi through the body, as well as to relieve stress. (For more on t'ai chi see pages 230-237.)

Through exercise, diet, and general moderation in all things, traditional Chinese medicine aims to make the body sufficiently strong and well-balanced to resist disease and infection. The emphasis on lifestyle and self-care also makes the individual an active partner in his or her health care—and in this way this ancient system of healing is at the fore of modern medicine. ❑

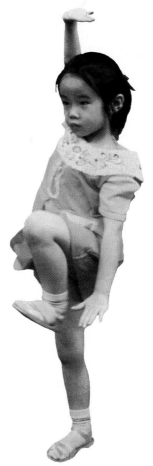

In China, regular exercise starts early. This child is learning t'ai chi. Because the exercises are performed slowly and rhythmically, t'ai chi is suitable for people of all ages.

Ayurveda's Healthful Balance

Emphasizing the need for using all the physical and mental powers at our command, this system, derived from Indian philosophy and practice, bids us keep ourselves in harmony with our bodies and our environment.

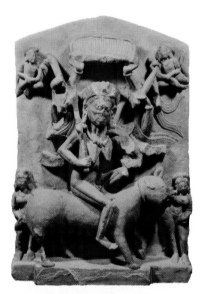

The Hindu goddess *Sitala was worshipped for centuries to protect the community against smallpox. Herbs were burned before statues of Sitala, in the hope of warding off this devastating disease. This sculpture from northern India is believed to date from the 10th century.*

THE BODY'S INNATE ABILITY TO HEAL ITSELF provides the unifying force behind Ayurvedic medicine, which arose in India at least 2500 years ago. Ayurveda is considered the first organized approach to health based on natural phenomena, rather than on magic, superstition, or spiritual forces. Illness develops as a result of internal disharmony, according to Ayurveda, which can be translated as the science of life or longevity. Its emphasis is on teaching preventive health care so that we can enjoy longer, healthier lives.

According to Ayurvedic thinking, too often we fail to take advantage of our own healing powers: in effect, we allow ourselves to become sick. Stressful lifestyles, unsuitable diets, and engaging in activities out of tune with the seasons can upset the delicate balance required for healthful living. Of course, other things such as infectious diseases can also be disruptive. But when we are in balance with ourselves and our environments, we are far less likely to succumb to ailments of any kind.

The Triumvirate of Health. The crucial balance, according to Ayurveda, depends on three basic life forces, or doshas. Sometimes compared to the Greek notion of humors or the Chinese precepts of yin and yang, the doshas are thought of as the fundamental elements underlying human functioning.

Vata, symbolized by air, is viewed as the dosha that produces movement. At the other end of the life-force spectrum is kapha, allied with earth, which is seen as a stabilizing force that is responsible for bodily structure. Pitta, the fire dosha, is associated with heat, dehydration, and digestion, and perhaps more importantly, serves as a transformative interface between kapha and vata: it is fire that converts the kaphic or material substance into the vatic or gaseous force that activates and animates.

Each of us is born with a unique ratio of the three doshas, though often one predominates. Ayurveda holds that this basic constitution is reflected in body type, temperament, even the kind of chronic disorders to which one is most susceptible. For example, predominantly pitta types tend to be passionate, argumentative, and quick to anger, as well as likely to have "fiery" ailments such as rashes, heartburn, and peptic ulcers. However, in someone with another constitutional profile, these disorders could also reflect a temporarily unbalanced pitta.

According to Ayurveda, the doshas also characterize the world around us—foods, seasons, time of day. These correspondences suggest a diet, daily routine, and activities that will help each individual maintain balance. For instance in spring, a kapha season, predominantly kapha types will probably be advised to go light on kapha-aggra-

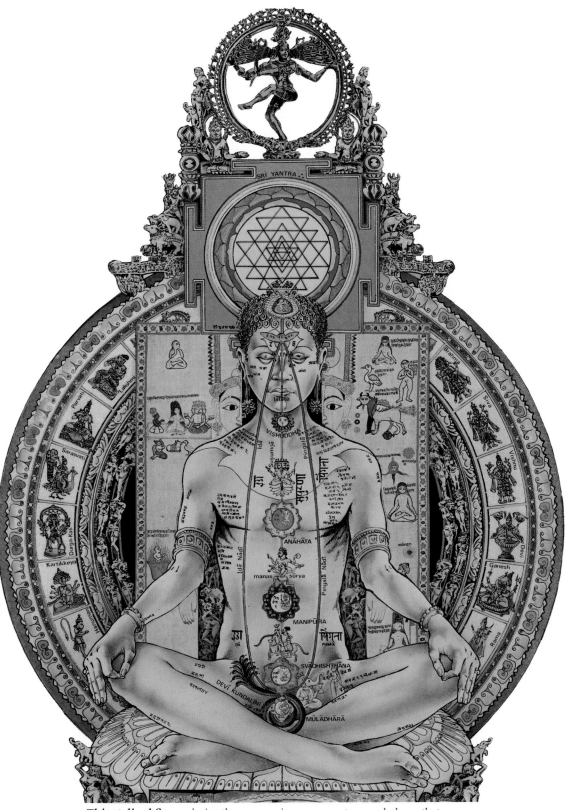

This stylized figure depicts the seven major energy centers, or chakras, that span the body from the base of the spine to the head. Each is linked, conceptually, to a specific organ, natural element, color, shape, and deity. The ultimate aim of yoga is to draw energy up to the topmost chakra and achieve self-illumination.

vating foods such as heavy dairy products. Otherwise the body will be forced to divest itself of the excess kapha as mucus: a "spring cold." Foods and herbs can be easily tested by taste to see which ones will increase or subdue each dosha. Pungent chilies increase pitta, of course, while sweet or starchy foods cause a welling up of kapha.

When illness strikes, despite a person's effort to take all necessary precautions to guard against it, Ayurveda offers an arsenal of cures, including thousands of herbal potions and even surgery. Texts dating back several centuries before the Christian era attest to the skill of Ayurvedic practitioners in a variety of major and minor surgical procedures, from cosmetic surgery to skin grafting and the removal of gallbladders and tumors.

Western Medicine's Eastern Roots. References to Ayurveda are contained in some of India's most ancient scriptures, written several thousand years ago. These teachings spread beyond the Himalayas, most notably to China; those familiar with traditional Chinese medicine can trace the lineage of such similarities as pulse diagnosis and the importance of keeping energy forces in balance. Through its impact on Persian and eventually Greek medicine, Ayurveda served as a wellspring from which Western medicine developed as well.

But whereas Western medicine veered off toward a focus on physical causes and cures and a total, passive reliance of the patient on the physician, Ayurveda retained its dual emphasis on treatment and prevention.

There are really two Ayurvedas. One is practiced by Ayurvedic physicians and is applied to those who are sick. The other is practiced by each and every person as a way of staying healthy. In this case the observation of the three doshas is a matter of individual introspection, and as soon as one notices any disturbance in them, appropriate adjustments are made in diet, or exercise, or even patterns of thought and emotion. This brings the doshas back into balance, and illness is elegantly sidestepped.

A major upheaval in Ayurvedic medicine began in the 1800s when the influence of Western medicine began to be felt with increasing force. Recognizing the need to preserve the best aspects of its own traditions, in 1947 the newly independent Indian government established national councils to oversee Ayurvedic training, practice, and research.

Today in India the old medicine, which has been formally recognized by the World Health Organization, and the new exist side by side. Ayurveda remains firmly rooted in the villages and everyday life of most Indians, whereas modern Western medicine has taken its place alongside Ayurvedic clinics and hospitals to provide, quite appropriately it would seem, high-tech care for acute or advanced illness or trauma.

Holistic Traditions. Unlike its Western counterpart, Ayurvedic medicine deals in an integrated way with body and mind. Whereas orthodox medicine acknowledges that

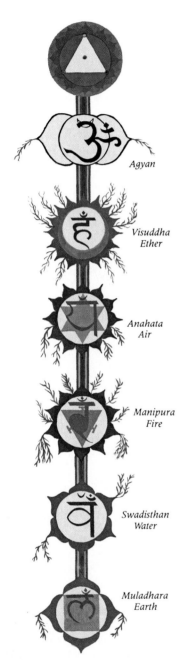

Agyan

Visuddha
Ether

Anahata
Air

Manipura
Fire

Swadisthan
Water

Muladhara
Earth

This drawing *of a chakra column relates the energy sources to specific areas of the body, such as the navel, heart, and head. The lowest chakra is represented by a four-petal lotus, while an inverted lotus with 1000 petals tops the head.*

the physical can affect the mental or that sometimes, at least, the mental may affect the physical, Ayurvedic thinking is more complex. Any disturbance of one of the three doshas (vata, pitta, or kapha) will be reflected on both mental and physical levels.

For example, a disturbance of vata can produce both numbness and pain (physically) and anxiety (mentally). Moreover, either a mental event, such as worry, or a physical one, such as fasting, can aggravate the corresponding dosha—in this case, vata. This vatic disturbance in turn causes further symptoms, both physical and mental. This spiraling feedforward/feedback interaction between different levels of functioning in Ayurveda contrasts sharply with the simple (and perhaps simplistic) cause-and-effect thinking of modern orthodox medicine.

Because of the comparatively sophisticated conceptual framework Ayurveda offers, its major usefulness may turn out to be as an integrating perspective for bringing together different holistic therapies. As perhaps the oldest system in use today, it has seen many ideas come and go, and has assimilated the best of many. Ayurvedic thinking easily accommodates therapies as diverse as antibiotics, surgery, nutrition, massage, meditation, and even acupuncture. (In fact, one of the oldest acupuncture charts is of an elephant—with the points labeled in Sanskrit.)

Modern-day Practitioners. While Ayurveda and yoga come from the same ancient roots, they have for some time been considered distinct. Nowadays, however, there is a trend toward bringing the two back together. A modern

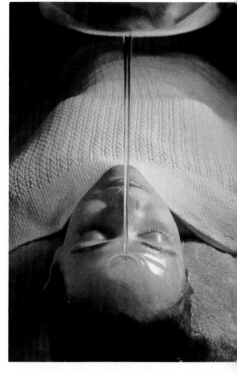

At an American health center *devoted chiefly to Ayurvedic medicine, new practices are added to old healing traditions. Here, warmed sesame oil is poured on a patient's forehead to reduce stress.*

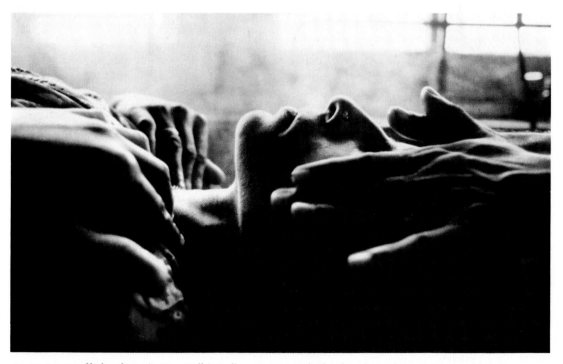

At an Ayurvedic institute *in New Delhi, India, massage and other hands-on therapies are used to help patients regain the internal equilibrium needed to heal. Such therapies are also used to prevent illness.*

practitioner of Ayurveda may well prescribe meditation and yoga exercises as well as the customary diet and herbal remedies. The new emphasis on yoga is probably a desirable development in Ayurveda since it helps bridge the gap between Ayurveda as a treatment and Ayurveda as a system of prevention. Patients who learn techniques of meditation, relaxation, breathing, and yoga postures are prepared to maintain—and even increase—their health once it is regained. The Ayurvedic practitioner who tailors exercise prescriptions or dietary recommendations to the patient's specific makeup, rather than simply providing exotic herbal remedies or elaborate massage and oil baths, will prepare the patient to manage himself well. For example, while on-the-go vata types might be advised to add butter and sweet foods to their diet, such a recommendation would not suit the needs of a sedentary kapha type.

Assessing a Patient's Constitution. In order to understand your doshic profile, the Ayurvedic practitioner will ask you about your habits, preferences, and even dreams. The physical exam that follows involves an assessment of

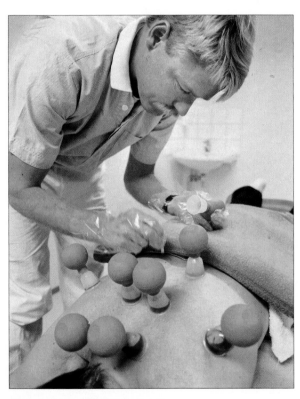

the body's *dhatus* or tissues and *srotases* or passageways through which cleansing and elimination take place. The entire body and even waste products like urine and stool are considered, but a key signpost is the pulse. Ayurvedic practitioners feel it at both wrists, using the first three fingers. Pace, strength, and patterns of movement are said to vary greatly from one body type to another; for instance a pulse that bounds like a frog points to a pitta person, while one with a swanlike glide signals a kapha. Experienced diagnosticians claim to be able to assess the condition of an organ by exerting light or deep pressure at each pulse point, detecting imbalances before they develop into diseases. Signs of a kapha imbalance may include mental inertia and depression, such behavioral patterns as procrastination and a resistance to change, and physical complaints such as sinus or chest congestion, aching joints, and skin pallor. Such an imbalance can lead to allergies, coughs, sore throats, and even diabetes. Based on the diagnostic assessment, a practitioner may recommend a variety of therapies for treating both body and mind.

Cupping is an ancient Ayurvedic and Chinese healing technique. A therapist performs wet cupping by making punctures in the skin and placing heated cups over them. The aim is to lower blood pressure, relieve muscle pain, and boost circulation.

Prescribing Treatment. While adjusting your diet to suit your constitutional type and the season of the year is commonly suggested, herbal remedies may also be advised, either to correct specific imbalances or as general rejuvenating supplements. Although some herbal preparations

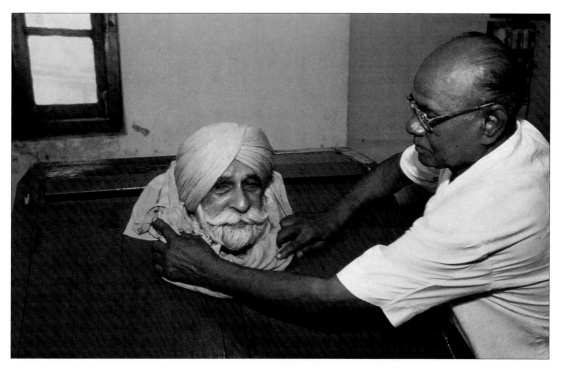

are rather elaborate, others employ spices available at many local markets, such as turmeric to dry up phlegm.

To cleanse the body of accumulated wastes, Ayurveda has developed several procedures collectively known as *panchakarma*. These include herbalized steam treatments, oil massage, nasal purging, and the use of laxatives and medicated enemas. Some procedures should be performed only by trained practitioners or under their supervision; they can be dangerous for people with certain conditions. For example, one should not try to remove an excessive dosha until it is returned to its *kosht* or customary location. Ayurveda offers elaborate guidelines for using these techniques, based on more than a thousand years' experience.

If *panchakarma* is recommended by your practitioner, you may decide to visit an Ayurvedic institute. Such facilities offer expanded versions of therapies you may be performing at home. For example, instead of the light do-it-yourself massage suggested as part of the morning routine, at an institute you can experience a "detoxifying" with two full-body therapists kneading in tandem.

Finding a Practitioner. Since Ayurvedic medicine is not licensed in the United States, those who practice this specialty must be accredited in medicine, chiropractic, nutrition, or another health-care field. Consulting a practitioner who has a license in another field makes it all the more likely that patients will be referred for any specialized care that is needed. Several hundred physicians have trained in the United States at Ayurvedic institutes. Such training generally lasts a few months; however, physicians in India educated in Ayurvedic medicine complete a five-and-a-half-year program of study and hospital residency. ❏

Sitting in a steam-filled sweatbox looks daunting, but it's highly regarded as a way of cleansing the body, which Ayurvedic medicine considers an important step in the healing process. Sweating your way back to health is not exclusively an Eastern practice. Some Native Americans, for example, believe that a session in a sweat lodge will produce similar results.

Creating Mandalas from Colored Sand

Through meditation the mind may tap into its healing powers, while creating a deep sense of peace. In Buddhist rituals, followers concentrate on symbolic designs, known as mandalas, contemplating the wisdom of a particular deity. While they may be painted or built from wood, sand is the preferred medium for these ornate patterns. The work is meticulous, often progressing grain by grain.

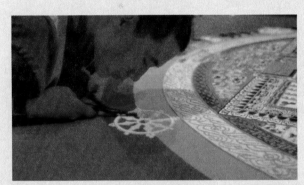

The pattern *of a mandala is dictated by ancient teachings, and its creation may take two or three weeks. The honor of viewing the completed work is usually reserved for those who have been initiated into Buddhist teachings.*

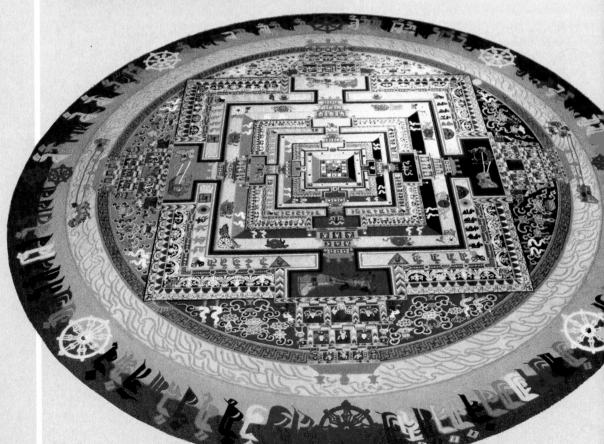

The Kalachakra mandala is rare in that it may be viewed by the uninitiated.

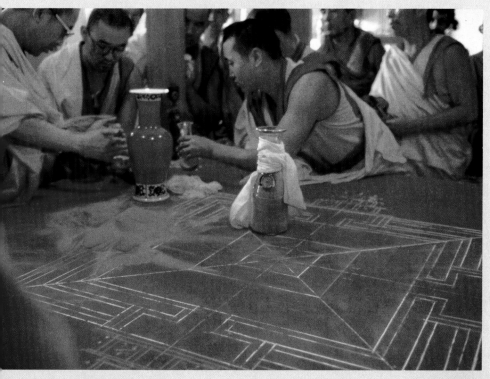

Ideally, a particle mandala would be made from ground jewels, but is more commonly made from dyed sand. This mandala symbolizes the ultimate wisdom of the Kalachakra deity. But the observer does not have to understand the symbolism in order to perceive the beauty of the form, and perhaps gain from it a feeling of peace. Here Buddhist monks sweep up the finished mandala.

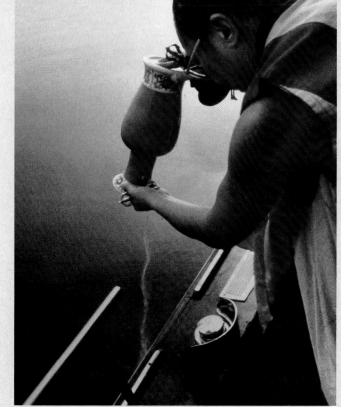

The ritual destroying of the finished mandala is a symbol of the impermanence of worldly things. The swept particles are collected and emptied into a nearby river or pond, so that the great blessings in the sand may then flow into nature.

Homeopathy: Where Less Is More

*In this two-hundred-year-old system of medicine,
symptoms are treated with minute quantities of drugs that would
normally bring on those very same symptoms.*

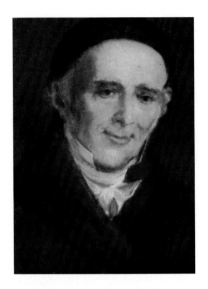

The Founding Father of Homeopathy

Samuel Hahnemann (1753-1843), a German physician and chemist, developed homeopathy in the early 19th century. Deploring most popular medical procedures, Hahnemann studied the potential healing properties of a variety of substances, ranging from herbs to snake venom. Today, homeopaths look at each patient's unique pattern of symptoms, and treat ailments with a host of dilute preparations.

HOMEOPATHY BEGAN IN THE EARLY 19TH CENTURY as a reaction against the "heroic measures" commonly used to treat disease, including bloodletting, induced vomiting, purging of the intestines, and application of massive doses of poorly understood drugs. Dr. Samuel Hahnemann, a German physician who had received a conventional medical education, later became disillusioned with what he perceived as the excesses of orthodox medicine.

Hahnemann put his trust in the healing powers of exercise, fresh air, and a nourishing diet—a then-radical approach to patient care. However, not satisfied with the results of these measures, he began to explore other means of treatment. Besides being a physician, Hahnemann was also a chemist and the author of a text widely used by German pharmacists. Thus he was thoroughly familiar with a wide variety of medicinal substances and with up-to-date methods of preparation.

As an avid experimenter, Hahnemann began to test some common remedies on himself. One of the first medicines he investigated was cinchona, also called Peruvian bark, and the natural source of quinine, which was used to treat malaria. Taking cinchona when he was healthy produced fever, chills, thirst, and a throbbing headache—the symptoms of malaria. Hahnemann decided that the effectiveness of the drug in the treatment of malaria came from its ability to cause symptoms similar to those of the disease.

"Like Cures Like." This experiment—along with others like it using different substances—led Hahnemann to formulate his first theory, "The Law of Similars," or "like cures like." According to this idea, a substance that produces certain symptoms in a healthy person can cure a sick person who shows the same symptoms. Hahnemann coined the term homeopathy from the Greek words *homoios* and *pathos,* meaning "similar sickness" to describe treatment based on this belief.

Hahnemann used minute doses because he found that large amounts of substances caused a host of side effects. He found he could preserve the healing properties of a medication and eliminate potential side effects through a pharmacological process he called "potentization." This is a process of serial dilution, in which a substance is mixed with distilled water, then vigorously shaken, then diluted and shaken a number of times more. Much to Hahnemann's surprise, he found that this process increased the strength of the medication and the duration of its effect. Hahnemann called this effect the "Law of Infinitesimals." Despite the controversy that has gone on since its first application, extremely small doses are still used daily all over the world by millions of people.

Rapid Spread in the 19th Century. Success in treating infectious disease, especially epidemic diseases such as cholera, typhoid, yellow fever, and scarlet fever, led to wide acceptance of homeopathy by the public. The first homeopathic college opened in Philadelphia in 1836, and others soon followed. In 1844, the American Institute of Homeopathy was formed, the first national medical organization in the country. By the end of the century, there were 15,000 practitioners and 22 homeopathic schools in the U.S.

Homeopathic treatment enjoyed the support of many prominent Americans of the day, including philosopher William James, poet Henry Wadsworth Longfellow, writer Nathaniel Hawthorne, journalist Horace Greeley, and industrialist John D. Rockefeller. Homeopathy also flourished in Europe, particularly in Britain, where it counted among its supporters writer Charles Dickens, prime minister Benjamin Disraeli, and members of the British royal family.

The American Medical Association was strongly opposed to homeopathy for scientific and economic reasons. From the 1860s until after the turn of the century, medical groups attempted to expel any physician who practiced homeopathy or who even consulted with a homeopath about the care of a patient. In the 20th century, because of AMA opposition, and also because of advances in modern medicine such as antibiotics, homeopathy virtually died out. By the 1920s, only two homeopathic medical schools in the U.S. were still functioning, and there were just a few homeopaths in practice nationwide. Only in the last 20 years, with the general resurgence of interest in alternative health care, has there been a revival of interest in homeopathy.

A Different Approach to Symptoms. Advocates and practitioners of homeopathy see major differences in philosophy and practice between their treatment and conventional, or orthodox, medicine. Homeopaths consider their method to be holistic since they believe illness is not localized in one organ, but instead involves the entire person—both body and mind. Their concern, they say, is to treat the whole patient instead of the disease. Homeopaths also say they differ from conventional physicians in their attitude toward symptoms of illness. Orthodox doctors, they claim, will try to suppress symptoms by prescribing drugs. Homeopaths see symptoms as positive signs that the body is trying to defend itself against an underlying disease. In fact, they say, homeopathic drugs may sometimes temporarily aggravate symptoms as they stimulate the body's self-healing mechanism.

For recurrent or potentially dangerous symptoms, advocates of homeopathy strongly recommend a consulta-

Hahnemann's own pocket-size medical kit, with its four tiers containing some 200 vials of homeopathic remedies, has been carefully preserved at the National Museum of American History in Washington, D.C.

tion with a trained homeopath. The direct purchase of homeopathic remedies from pharmacies or health food stores should be only for relatively minor ailments.

Visiting a Homeopathic Practitioner. A homeopath generally begins by asking the patient a long list of detailed questions, not only about his or her medical history, but also about such things as overall energy, sensitivity to temperature and weather, sleep habits, food preferences, and various kinds of subtle but vital information that describes the sick person's unique response to illness. These and other factors, as well as various emotional symptoms, they say, must be taken into account when deciding which remedy to prescribe.

There are more than 2000 homeopathic remedies in use, all derived from various plant, mineral, animal, or chemical sources. These substances are then highly diluted and taken in the form of tablets, granules, liquids, or ointments. Some examples of homeopathic medicines are marigold flowers; onions; calcium carbonate derived from oyster shells; graphite, a gray mineral that is commonly used in lead pencils; sepia, the inky fluid from cuttlefish; snake venom; and honeybee extract. Though some of these substances might seem to be dangerous, the doses that homeopaths use are so diluted that they are widely recognized as safe.

Dr. Edward Jenner (1749-1823), a British physician, found that injecting small amounts of material from a cowpox lesion could immunize a person against smallpox. It was in 1796 that Jenner performed his first vaccination. That same year, Hahnemann experimented with the malaria cure, cinchona, which led to the formulation of his theory of homeopathy. Though in both cases small amounts of a substance were used to stimulate the body's defenses, the similarity of the work was not appreciated. Jenner's work was acclaimed by orthodox physicians; Hahnemann's was rejected.

Homeopaths learned which remedies to prescribe through a process of drug trials, called "provings," in which doses were given to healthy individuals and their reactions were studied. This information is compiled in "materia medica," encyclopedias of homeopathic drug effects, and "repertories," books that list symptoms and the drugs that have been shown to cause and cure them. While homeopaths rely on these reference books as guidelines, they emphasize that each individual is unique; remedies must always be tailored to individual needs. After administering the remedy, a homeopath will generally wait four to six weeks before the next appointment to allow the healing process to take place.

When Homeopathy Works Best. Practitioners especially recommend the treatment for chronic problems like allergies, headaches, arthritis, colitis, peptic ulcer, high blood pressure, and obesity; deficiencies like anemia or hormone imbalance; and some infections. They also recommend homeopathy as a safer alternative to conventional drugs for pregnant women, and for infants and children. Homeopaths acknowledge that severe infections and highly infectious diseases should be treated by antibiotics, though homeopathic medicines can be used concurrently to augment the person's natural defenses, thereby reducing the chance of complications or repeated infections. Similarly, it is widely recognized that conventional medicine should be used in the treatment of injuries or emergency conditions,

Like Cures Like

*Revolted by the brutality of 18th century medicine—
which indeed was often violent—Samuel Hahnemann originated a
new and gentle form of therapy. He called it homeopathy.*

To explain his medical treatment, the German doctor, Samuel Hahnemann, wrote *Organon of Medicine.* As well as giving specific methods of homeopathic treatments, he also forcibly expressed his opinion of the accepted treatments of his day, which he believed often harmed rather than healed the patient.

"In recent times the old school practitioners have quite surpassed themselves in their cruelty towards their sick fellow creatures, and in the unsuitableness of their operations, as every unprejudiced observer must admit, and as even physicians have been forced, by the pricks of their conscience, to confess before the world.

"It was high time for the wise and benevolent Creator and Preserver of mankind to put a stop to these abominations, to command a cessation of these tortures, and to reveal a healing art at the very opposite of all this, which would not waste the vital juices and powers by emetics, perennial scourings out of the bowels, warm baths, diaphoretics or salivation; nor shed the life's blood, nor torment and weaken with painful appliances; nor, in place of curing the patients, suffering from diseases, render them incurable by the addition of new, chronic medicinal maladies by means of the prolonged use of wrong, powerful medicines of unknown properties; nor yoke the horse behind the cart, by giving strong palliatives, nor, in short, in place of lending the patient aid, to guide in the way to death as is done by the merciless routine practitioner;—but which, on the contrary, should spare the patient's strength as much as possible, and should, rapidly and mildly, effect an unalloyed and permanent cure, and restore to health by means of smallest doses of few simple medicines carefully selected according to their proven effects, by the only therapeutic law conformable to nature: *similia similibus*

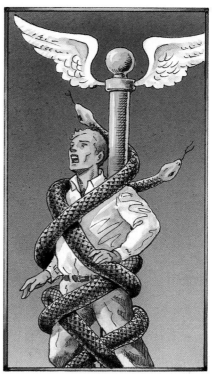

Breaking away from traditional medicine

curentur (in English, like cures like.)

"By observation, reflection and experience, I discovered that, contrary to the old method, the true, the proper, the best mode of treatment is contained in the maxim; *To cure mildly, rapidly, certainly, and permanently, to choose, in every case of disease, a medicine which can itself produce an ailment similar to that sought to be cured.*

"How close the great truth was at times to being understood! But it was dismissed with a mere passing thought, and thus the indispensable change of the antiquated medical treatment of disease, of the improper therapeutic system hitherto in vogue, into a real, true, and certain healing art, remained to be accomplished in our own times."

Excerpted from Organon of Medicine *(6th edition) by Dr. Samuel Hahnemann.*

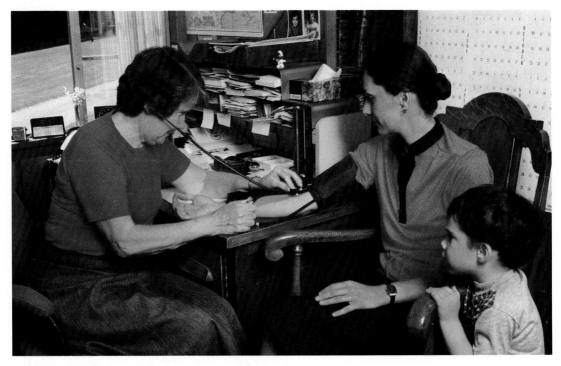

Practitioners of homeopathy in the United States may also be chiropractors or naturopaths, but most, like Dr. Maesimund Panos of Ohio, are medical doctors. Although both homeopaths and orthodox physicians take blood-pressure readings and use many of the same diagnostic procedures, they differ in their views of symptoms and treatment.

such as broken bones, a burst appendix, or a hernia. Again, homeopathic medicines may be used to complement conventional medical treatment.

The Controversy Continues. Although there are medical doctors who practice homeopathy, M.D.s in general are adamantly opposed to the treatment. They say that there is no scientific basis for homeopathy's claims and that, if treatments work at all, it is probably because the remedies act as placebos—in effect, "sugar pills" of no medicinal value. Many conventional physicians can accept, in theory at least, the idea behind the Law of Similars. There are analogies to the idea that "like cures like" in conventional medicine, such as vaccination or allergy desensitization. However, the second homeopathic principle, the Law of Infinitesimals, is more difficult for medicine to accept because it appears to contradict scientific understanding. Homeopathic remedies are often so diluted that not one molecule of the initial substance remains. How then, orthodox doctors and scientists ask, can the remedies possibly work?

Homeopaths have yet to come up with a convincing explanation of why small doses work, but some theorize that as the formula is diluted, the initial substance leaves some kind of imprint in the solution by changing the molecular structure. Perhaps, even though the physical substance doesn't remain, its energy or pattern might still be there. They liken it to the musical phenomenon of playing one note on a piano and hearing it reverberate elsewhere. In the same way, homeopaths say, an infinitesimal dose of some substance will "resonate" with symptoms biologically throughout a person's body. And homeopaths believe that there is a "life force" or "vital force," similar to the Chi-

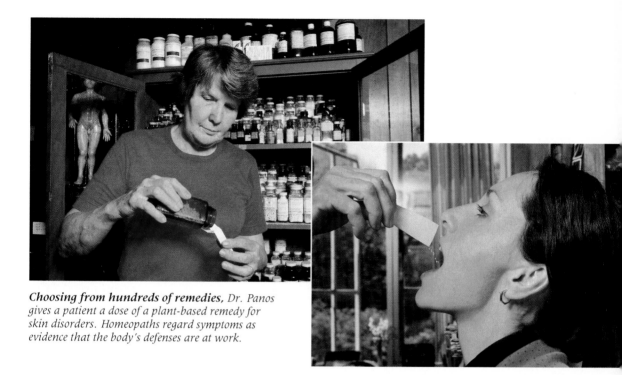

Choosing from hundreds of remedies, *Dr. Panos gives a patient a dose of a plant-based remedy for skin disorders. Homeopaths regard symptoms as evidence that the body's defenses are at work.*

nese concept of qi that flows through the body and is the self-healing process. This life force, they say, may somehow be sensitive to submolecular homeopathic medicines.

Advocates of homeopathy cite the effectiveness of homeopathy in treating infants and animals, who don't realize they're taking medicine and thus wouldn't have a psychological reason for responding to a placebo. They also note that homeopathic remedies do create symptoms, which they say indicates that biological action is taking place. In any case, advocates of homeopathy argue that theories are not as significant as clinical results. What matters, they say, is that homeopathy works.

Long-Standing Acceptance. In the U.S., homeopathic remedies have had legal status since 1938. Because of this, in most states anyone who is a licensed health care professional can practice homeopathy. According to the National Center of Homeopathy in Alexandria, Va., there are only about 3000 recognized practitioners nationwide, about half of whom are physicians, with the rest mostly dentists, naturopaths, chiropractors, and veterinarians. Nurses and physician assistants have also begun to practice homeopathy, though they can do so only under the supervision of a medical doctor. In addition, members of the general public are learning how to treat common ailments and injuries.

Independent authorities say that if you decide to try homeopathy, it's best to confine treatment to non-life-threatening illnesses. Although there may be certain risks in homeopathic health care, there are other risks in conventional medical care. By being better educated about the various options available and risks inherent in each, you will more likely make the best choice of care. ❏

Whole-Body Healing

In this hands-on approach to patient care, osteopaths rely on gentle palpation and manipulation, along with standard medical procedures, to diagnose and treat a variety of health problems.

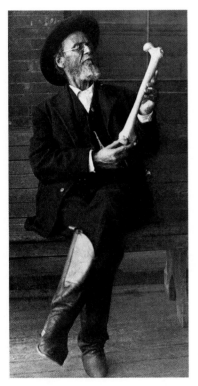

Andrew Taylor Still (1828-1917), a Civil War medic and country doctor, opened the first college of osteopathy in Kirksville, Missouri in 1892. Convinced that he'd discovered the key to illness and health, Still drafted a charter stating that the aim of the school was "…to improve our present system of surgery, obstetrics, and treatment of diseases generally…"

PERHAPS THE MOST ACCEPTED of all the alternative health care practitioners, osteopaths—doctors of osteopathy or D.O.s—are fully qualified physicians, licensed to practice in all 50 states and parts of Canada. Like M.D.s, osteopaths diagnose diseases, prescribe drugs, refer patients to hospitals, and perform surgery. D.O.s are also represented in all of the practice specialties, including surgery, neurology, gynecology, obstetrics, and psychiatry. There are also a number of osteopathic hospitals, ranging in size from small community facilities to large academic medical centers.

What distinguishes osteopaths from M.D.s is their approach to the human body. In general, M.D.s are trained to think of the body as a number of discrete systems conveniently packaged within the human frame. In contrast, D.O.s view the body as an interrelated whole, with each system and organ in constant contact. The body's proper structure and function are maintained by an intricate and complex "conversation" between brain and body. Health, therefore, is a matter of shifting balance, and any adverse changes in one part of the body will impair the functioning of other systems or organs.

Healing Thyself. D.O.s stress that the human body has a tremendous capacity to maintain and heal itself—a philosophy shared by many involved in the healing arts—but that sometimes it needs a little intervention and support to reachieve harmony. While trained in the use of standard medications and therapies, D.O.s also use a battery of manual techniques to diagnose and treat any number of medical problems, from asthma to angina. Focusing on the neuro-musculoskeletal system (the bones, muscles, tendons, tissues, nerves, spinal column, and brain), which comprises some 60 percent of the body's mass, D.O.s evaluate patients—often using a combination of gentle hands-on techniques, including palpation and manipulation.

But, rather than simply treating specific symptoms, D.O.s are more concerned with determining what is causing an imbalance and why. It is their belief that once the underlying causes have been diagnosed and treated, the body is then free to repair itself or to respond to other appropriate therapies.

For example, a patient who comes in complaining of back pain and headaches could be treated manually, given a pain reliever, relaxation exercises, and sent on his way. However, if an ulcer or some other underlying problem is causing these symptoms, then whatever relief the patient experiences will be short-lived. So, while the osteopath will certainly try to ease symptoms, he or she will also do a more comprehensive evaluation to determine the root of the problem and so provide appropriate treatment.

Where It All Started. Osteopathy was founded in the late 19th century by Andrew Taylor Still, a conventionally trained itinerant American physician. After losing three of his own children to spinal meningitis, Still began to question the efficacy of orthodox medicine, which at that time was based on the haphazard use of questionable drugs, dangerous surgeries, and other therapies.

Still believed that the human body possessed an innate ability to heal itself—a philosophy shared by Hippocrates, the teacher and scientist who is considered the father of Western medicine. As he explored alternatives, Still concentrated upon the ways in which a physician could support the body's own internal healing mechanism.

Over time, Still became convinced that health and illness were largely dependent upon the soundness and mechanical functioning of the body's structures. Based on this idea, in 1874 he formulated a new medical science, which he ultimately named osteopathy from the Greek words *osteo*, or bone, and *pathos*, which means suffering or diseases. While Still did not completely discard his previous medical training, he became primarily interested in the ways in which biomechanical dysfunction causes disease.

In 1892, Still opened the American School of Osteopathy in Missouri, and in 1897 the American Osteopathic Association was founded to promote and oversee the profession. But it was many years before osteopathy gained acceptance as a reputable health-care practice. Rejecting Still's theories and clinical successes, the orthodox medical community complained that colleges of osteopathy lagged behind medical colleges in their standard of training. However, beginning in the late 1930s, the level of training was upgraded, and eventually licenses were granted in all 50 states. Today, many osteopaths contend that they are better prepared to treat patients than most M.D.s since, in addition to their conventional medical training, they are more proficient with hands-on diagnosis and care.

Modern Osteopathy. Still's methods have survived and evolved to become part of modern health care. But just as many D.O.s have inched closer to their orthodox colleagues, so too have M.D.s come to embrace many principles put forward by osteopathy. For example, D.O.s specializing in manipulation receive referrals from orthopedic surgeons and other specialists. In addition, D.O.s commonly treat patients in hospitals as part of an overall treatment plan for those recov-

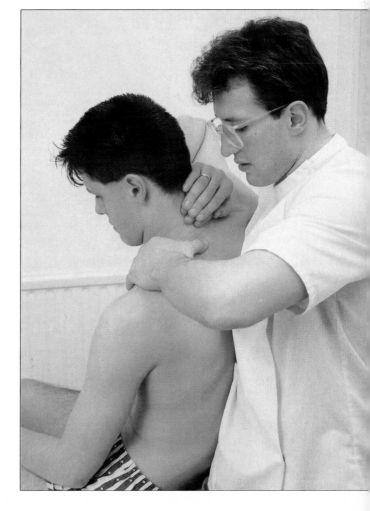

An osteopath's hands are his most valuable diagnostic and therapeutic tools. They not only help him to determine the nature of a patient's problem, but they also offer information on the best way to treat it. Here, an osteopath applies gentle manipulative treatment to restore proper function to a patient's stiff neck. Complete relief may take more than one treatment, and follow-up care will likely involve teaching the patient ways of modifying his habits to prevent further problems.

ering from heart attacks and surgery. And just as Still believed in treating the whole person, acknowledging the emotional component in physical illness, many orthodox physicians are now conceding that stress and certain psychological problems can have a profound influence on health and healing.

Osteopaths do not reject the "germ theory" of disease, they simply believe that the healthy person is less likely to succumb to infection than is the person who eats poorly, has faulty posture, or who is under considerable stress. And as medical science discovers more about the immune system, and its intricate links with the mind and body, Still's theories seem more and more sound.

There is considerable diversity today in the treatment methods used by osteopathic physicians. Many in fact practice conventional medicine and are almost indistinguishable from M.D.s. Others practice general medicine, but follow a more holistic approach to health care, combin-

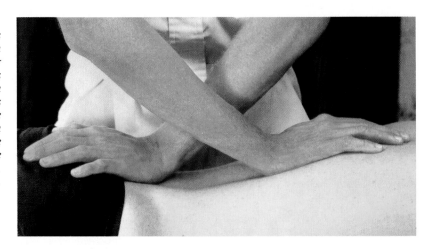

Back pain suffers often seek help from osteopaths. After evaluating the patient's condition, the osteopath in this picture applies moderate pressure to the patient's back in an effort to gently stretch the tissues, relaxing sore muscles and, in time, restoring mobility.

ing such preventive measures as consultation on fitness and nutrition, along with manipulation. A minority of osteopaths practice "pure" or "classical" osteopathy, relying on prescription drugs and surgery only when absolutely necessary. They argue that too much of the art of osteopathy has been lost in the drive by the profession to gain acceptance by the medical establishment.

Some osteopaths, particularly those of the "classical" school, refer to underlying structural problems as osteopathic lesions—a term coined by Still. But as the practice of osteopathy has evolved, other practitioners have expanded their ideas, focusing more on the whole body. In their view, too much emphasis is placed on musculoskeletal problems (to the exclusion of all other factors), thereby minimizing the complex interaction of the mind and body in health and healing.

What to Expect. Patients who chose an osteopath as their general physician are often surprised at how much time their D.O. devotes to each appointment. In addition to the standard questions directly related to the patient's health, most D.O.s also spend considerable time discussing lifestyle issues (such as exercise, diet, job, family life, stress, and others), as well as conducting the physical exam (which may include blood work, urine analysis, or X-rays as necessary).

During the physical, the D.O. takes note of the patient's posture, observing the manner of walking, sitting, and how the patient holds his or her head. In addition, the osteopath will look for any significant differences in leg length, shoulder height, and check for any curvature of the spine. According to practitioners, any of these factors could have a direct influence on the patient's health.

Next, the D.O. will lightly palpate the patient's body, a hands-on diagnostic technique that helps uncover such symptoms as tenderness, stiff muscles, swelling and inflammation, and signs of immobility. If the doctor finds it necessary, X-rays or blood work may be ordered.

If the patient is there for a specific injury, say a lower back problem, the D.O. may use gentle manipulation, of both soft tissue and the spine, to restore the function and structure of all of the moving parts. If necessary, the D.O. may also incorporate more forceful manipulations of joint tissue using a technique called the high-velocity thrust.

In addition, the osteopath may employ passive articulation techniques, where joints are moved while the patient remains passive, in an effort to reset the nervous system's control of that joint. Sometimes, the D.O. will combine treatment with relaxation techniques, such as meditation or breathing exercises.

To help the patient maintain joint movement and promote muscle flexibility, the osteopath may prescribe stretching and strengthening exercises to be done at home. Other adjunctive treatments might include stress management and advice on modifying the home or workplace for more body-friendly placement of such things as telephone, desks, computers, and chairs.

Back pain, knee problems, and other musculoskeletal injuries seem to respond well to osteopathy. However, it is also reported useful for treating a wide variety of health complaints, including indigestion; respiratory problems, such as asthma, bronchitis, or emphysema; circulatory problems; migraines; sinusitis; and cerebral palsy.

Practitioners claim that osteopathic manipulation can even help in cases of infectious disease. After prescribing the proper antibiotic, some osteopaths use certain manipulative techniques that are designed to improve circulation and stimulate the immune system. Some claim these techniques promote the flow of lymph through the body. This

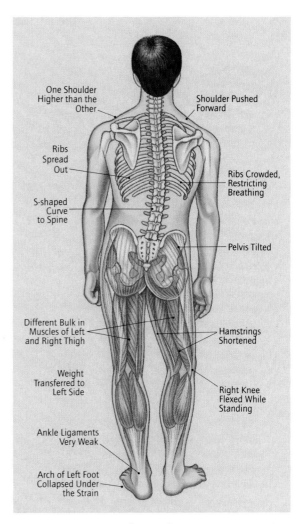

One Shoulder Higher than the Other

Shoulder Pushed Forward

Ribs Spread Out

Ribs Crowded, Restricting Breathing

S-shaped Curve to Spine

Pelvis Tilted

Different Bulk in Muscles of Left and Right Thigh

Hamstrings Shortened

Weight Transferred to Left Side

Right Knee Flexed While Standing

Ankle Ligaments Very Weak

Arch of Left Foot Collapsed Under the Strain

A thorough posture assessment is an important part of an osteopath's physical exam. This drawing highlights some fairly obvious problems, which are the product of both heredity and habit. In assembling a profile of a patient's physical condition, the osteopath will take into account such things as a lopsided stance, tilted pelvis, and collapsing feet.

liquid carries antigens, which stimulate the body to produce antibodies. Antibodies, in turn, help fight infection.

Cranial Osteopathy. This specialized diagnostic and therapeutic concept emphasizes the subtle movement of the bones of the skull, the brain, and the flow of cerebrospinal fluid around the brain and spinal column. Cranial osteopathy was developed by Dr. W.G. Sutherland, a student of Dr. Still's. Sutherland theorized that if the bones of the skull are not

---

CASE HISTORY

A WIDER VIEW OF OSTEOPATHY

The woman described here was suffering from severe shoulder pain, but during an exam, her osteopath made a surprising discovery. This case highlights the value of whole-body analysis for proper diagnosis.

Osteopaths are often the physicians of last resort — they see lots of chronic pain patients who have not been helped by standard medical treatments. For any physician, referred pain presents a particular challenge, since it often masks other problems. But an osteopath's hands are sensitive instruments, trained to uncover underlying disease.

"Paula M. was referred to me by her internist," reports Steven J. Weiss, a Manhattan D.O. specializing in pain cases. "A 37 year-old female executive, she had been experiencing severe pain in her right shoulder for several weeks, which she had first noticed while vacationing in the tropics.

"Her internist initially sent her to an orthopedic surgeon, who treated her with a series of injections, but Paula experienced no relief. At this point she was sent to me.

"My initial examination revealed extraordinary spasm and inflammation, not only involving her right shoulder, but the entire upper back, neck, and chest. Gentle palpation was extremely painful throughout these regions; indeed her whole body felt inflamed. Examination of the right shoulder joint revealed a generalized restriction in range of motion with pain, but I could find no specific shoulder injury.

"Evaluation of the rib cage and chest wall revealed marked spasm in her diaphragm, as well as a general rigidity that restricted the entire chest wall and rib cage as the patient breathed. Finally, an abdominal examination revealed an enlarged, extremely tender liver, which when palpated produced the severe pain in her right shoulder.

"Based on the physical exam and the pattern of pain, I began to suspect that the patient's problem had nothing to do with a musculoskeletal injury of the shoulder. Instead, she seemed to be suffering from disease of the internal organs, specifically of the liver and intestines.

"I sent the patient back to her internist for a thorough medical workup, with specific attention to the liver. When the tests were complete, the results revealed a parasitic infection, which had attacked the liver and was beginning to form an abscess.

"Paula was started on medication for the parasitic infection, and in a short while the pain in her right shoulder began to subside. But since some discomfort and stiffness lingered, she returned to my care. With the underlying infection gone, her body was now able to respond swiftly to osteopathic treatment. Gentle manipulation eased the pain and rigidity in her shoulder, upper back, and chest wall."

fused, then changes in their normal arrangement and motion will affect the brain and cerebrospinal fluid pressure—often causing serious, sometimes body-wide problems.

Cranial osteopaths are highly trained physicians who use refined, hands-on techniques to detect and treat subtle disturbances in motion patterns in the skull. According to practitioners, these disturbances may be symptomatic of certain disorders. Cranial osteopaths report that their methods are particularly effective for ear infections in children.

Fighting Wear and Tear. From aching feet to sore neck and shoulder muscles, many people experience some degree of discomfort every single day. The pain may be caused by injury, stress, or even gravity, but unless it becomes intolerable, most people are apt to ignore it, accepting it as an inevitable part of aging.

Osteopaths point out that chronic pain is neither normal nor inevitable. In fact, sometimes it is the result of bad postural habits that have subtly thrown the body out of alignment. But no matter what causes the discomfort, the net result is wear and tear on the neuro-musculoskeletal system, which, if left untreated, may lead to further pain, numbness, and other problems.

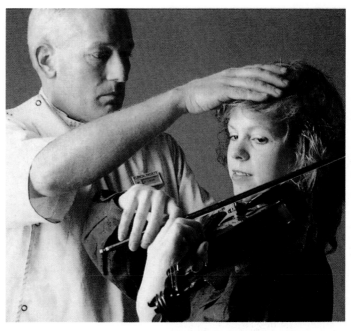

Violinists often develop chronic neck strain from poor playing posture and the stress of performing. But whether they are working with musicians or mechanics, osteopaths take into account all facets of a patient's life when designing a suitable treatment plan.

A patient's body often provides a map of his or her professional and recreational activities. For instance, office workers who spend hours on the telephone are prone to neck and shoulder problems, while typists and computer workers frequently complain of arm and wrist numbness and pain. Osteopathic treatment usually offers immediate relief, but continued improvement may depend upon the patient's willingness to make changes.

Whether the sport is downhill skiing or bowling, weekend and professional athletes are frequently sidelined by injuries—the result, oftentimes, of improper form. And while we tend to think of traumatic injuries, such as sprained ankles, as accidental, osteopaths suggest that even these may be caused by postural problems, differences in limb length, or years of misuse.

For instance, a runner with problem feet is apt to strain his calf muscles. To compensate and ease the discomfort, he may change his stride, only to find that he now has pain in his hip. In this case, an osteopath will first tend to the injured tissues, and then analyze the underlying mechanical problems, assessing leg length, and other factors that may have led to the tear. Finally, an overall treatment plan will be designed around preventing future problems. ❏

Making a Healthy Adjustment

Spurred by a desire to find a single cause for disease, Daniel David Palmer created a system based on manipulating spinal vertebrae. A century later, chiropractic provides relief for back, neck, head, and joint pain.

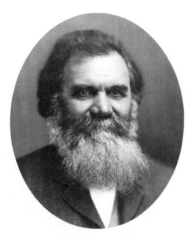

Searching for a cure *for all illness, Daniel David Palmer (1845-1913) developed the theory of chiropractic, which is based chiefly on the manipulation of spinal vertebrae. His son Bartlett Joshua Palmer, a trained practitioner and the better businessman, reorganized and expanded the school of chiropractic that his father had founded in Davenport, Iowa. Today chiropractic is probably the most popular form of alternative healing in the U.S.*

THE SYSTEM OF CHIROPRACTIC (the name comes from the Greek words *cheiro* and *prakrikos,* meaning "done by hand") was devised by Daniel David Palmer in the last decade of the 19th century. A self-taught healer, Palmer built up a healing practice in Davenport, Iowa, mainly using the laying on of hands. It was Palmer's objective to find a cure for disease and illness that did not rely on drugs, which he considered harmful. Meanwhile, he learned all he could about the structure of the spine and the ancient practice of manipulation.

In 1895 a decisive event occurred in Palmer's career. Harvey Lillard, a local janitor, had lost his hearing many years earlier. Lillard reported that the deafness occurred quite abruptly when he was performing heavy labor in a stooped position. At that time, he remembered feeling something give way in his back and he had been deaf ever since. Examining Lillard, Palmer discovered a lump on his back, which he attributed to a displaced vertebra. Palmer applied firm pressure to Lillard's dorsal vertebra and the bone slipped into place. Shortly thereafter, Lillard's hearing was completely restored. In a second instance, Palmer claimed he was able to alleviate a patient's heart condition using spinal manipulation. On the basis of these two cases, Palmer concluded that most disease is the direct result of misalignment of the spine.

Gaining a Foothold. Before long, many other people were coming to him for similar treatments, and soon Palmer further refined the basic theory behind chiropractic: that disease is caused by vertebrae impinging on the spinal nerves. He believed that the brain sends energy to every organ of the body along nerves that run through the spinal cord, and that displaced vertebrae of the spinal column can cause physical blockage and interfere with normal nerve transmission. He named the interferences that cause disease "subluxations." According to Palmer, the way to cure disease and restore normal function to organs, muscles, joints, and other tissues was to remove these interferences with quick thrusts known as adjustments. Free of these blockages, Palmer concluded, the body would once again be able to exercise its innate recuperative powers.

An adjustment or manipulation involves moving the spinal vertebrae back to their normal positions. In some cases, manipulation of the head and extremities (elbows, knees, ankles, etc.) is also practiced. Although some mechanical devices have been developed, most adjustments are done by hand.

Like an orthodox physician, the chiropractor takes a medical history and then performs an examination. Many of today's chiropractors use computers to help identify sev-

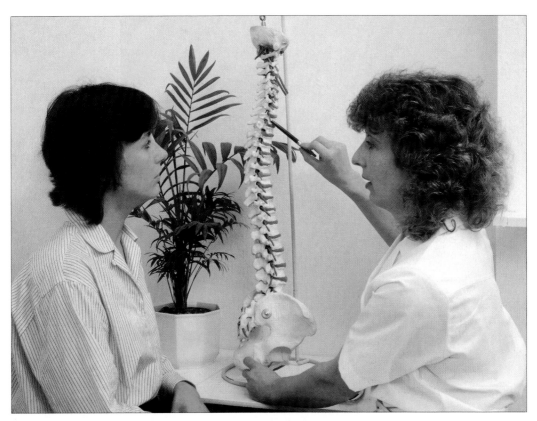

Many patients find relief from back pain through spinal manipulation. Here, a patient learns about the structure of the spine, which consists of bones, or vertebrae, that extend from the base of the skull to the coccyx. Between the vertebrae are cartilage discs, which act as shock absorbers for the spine.

eral problems associated with the "vertebral subluxation complex." With machines, by touching, or by visual analysis, chiropractors try to determine the nature of the patient's problem. The focus is on detecting muscle strength or weakness, the range of spinal motion, any structural deformities, or incorrect posture. In some instances, the electrical activity of nerves and muscles may be evaluated. In future visits, these observations can be used to document the patient's progress.

Following the examination, X-rays of the spine are usually taken in order to locate vertebral misalignments and areas of spinal stress. The X-rays are also examined for evidence of pathology, such as tumors or fractures, which would require referral to other health-care specialists.

Some orthodox physicians question whether chiropractors use X-rays excessively for diagnosis; however, chiropractors respond that the newer equipment provides adequate protection against radiation. If you have an X-ray as part of a chiropractic examination or any other medical diagnosis, be sure that the equipment used is up to date.

Adjustments are the principal treatment used by chiropractors and may be performed during the first visit. The two most common adjustment techniques are the high-velocity, low-force "recoil" thrust and the "rotational" thrust. In the first, the patient lies face down on a specially

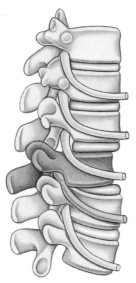

Spinal misalignment, indicated by the shaded vertebra, can cause a disc to press on a nerve and produce pain. Chiropractors call such misalignments subluxations and treat them with adjustments.

designed table that is divided into several sections, which drop or move slightly downward as the adjustments are made. The chiropractor presses a hand tightly against the skin of the spine and then performs a quick, controlled thrusting movement.

For the rotational thrust, the patient lies with the upper body twisted counter to the pelvis; rotating the spine to the limit of its normal movement, the chiropractor applies a short, fast thrust to the spine. The force of a thrust will depend on the individual chiropractor.

Two Kinds of Chiropractors. Today practitioners are likely to fall into one of two categories. The so-called "straight" chiropractors adhere strictly to D.D. Palmer's philosophy of adjustments: locating and eliminating subluxations. "Mixer" is a term that applies to practitioners who combine spinal adjustments with such adjunct therapies as exercise, heat treatment, and nutritional counsel-

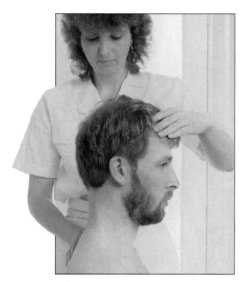

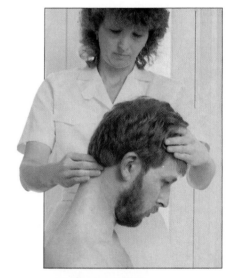

The physical examination often begins by testing the extent of spinal mobility. Starting in the neutral position, above, a patient tilts his head forward and backward, then rotates it in circles, first in one direction, then the other, as the chiropractor gently follows along. A chiropractor will assess the dynamics of spinal movement before deciding on suitable therapy. (For adjustments to the back, a patient lies on a specially designed table.)

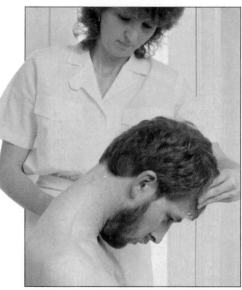

ing. The majority of chiropractors practicing today fall into the latter category, often making use of new technology and scientific data to locate and eliminate subluxations.

Head-to-Toe Therapy. The majority of all visits to chiropractors relate to back pain. However, they are also called on to treat migraines and other headaches (which are often traced to problems with neck vertebrae), sciatica, shoulder pain, tennis and golfer's elbow, leg and foot pain, and hand and wrist pain.

Some patients have also found chiropractic helpful in treating allergies, asthma, stomach disorders, and menstrual problems. Some research has shown chiropractic to be effective in lowering blood pressure and easing infantile colic. One study indicated that removal of blockage from the nervous system significantly enhanced athletes' agility, power, balance, and speed. Some professional sports teams employ chiropractors as well as team physicians.

Despite the continuing doubts of many orthodox physicians, chiropractic has a devoted following. Many patients who tried in vain to get pain relief elsewhere have sought chiropractic treatment, and now swear by it.

Once dismissed by the American Medical Association as members of an "unscientific cult," chiropractors are now licensed to practice in all 50 states and throughout Canada. Chiropractic treatment is covered by government health insurance and many private health insurance plans in both countries. ❑

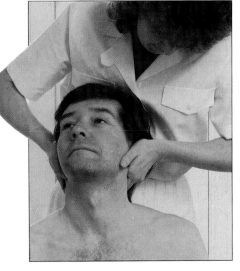

Preparing to realign vertebrae in the neck (which is also referred to as the cervical spine), a practitioner tests the patient's range of motion, then applies quick movements of relatively low amplitude, or force. Treatments may help restore joint mobility, reduce neck muscle spasms, and alleviate pain. Those who suffer from migraine and other types of headache sometimes find that adjustments to the neck lessen the frequency of headaches. Chiropractors often suggest stretching for recurring back and neck pain.

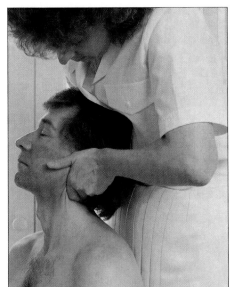

When Nature Is the Healer

Convinced that nature's ability to restore health is vastly underrated, naturopathic doctors emphasize preventive strategies for maintaining wellness and an interdisciplinary approach to treating illness.

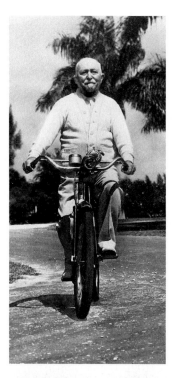

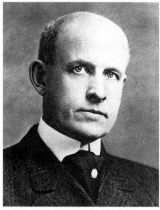

The Kellogg brothers, John (top) and Will, and C.W. Post (above) used their cereals and other food products to tout the virtues of a healthful diet. The Kelloggs helped popularize vegetarianism, which may have set the stage for the acceptance of naturopathy's whole-food diet.

DOCTORS OF NATUROPATHY are general practitioners whose training encompasses a broad spectrum of natural therapies, as well as the standard health sciences. Graduates of the two accredited colleges of naturopathy in the United States, which are graduate schools that require four years of study and clinical experience, earn the title Naturopathic Doctor, or N.D. The curriculum includes nutrition, botanical medicine, psychology, homeopathy, traditional Chinese medicine, and several types of physical medicine, such as hydrotherapy, physiotherapy, minor surgery, and manipulative therapies. Without medical degrees, naturopathic practitioners cannot deliver babies in hospitals.

Naturopathy can be seen as an umbrella medical system that embraces a multitude of healing approaches, all of them based on the body's intrinsic healing powers. It appeals to those who want to avoid relying on prescription drugs and who are interested in preventive medicine.

Naturopathic doctors encourage patients to take active roles in maintaining the body's natural state of balance. They help patients to overcome their self-image as "flawed" or diseased, and to regain the power that lies within themselves. Naturopathic doctors describe this approach as giving patients permission to be healthy. Practitioners also aim to educate patients so that they can avoid many illnesses that afflict millions of people. They believe that proper diet and a health-conscious lifestyle can help ward off atherosclerosis, osteoporosis, and other chronic degenerative diseases.

Similarities and Differences. Sometimes the therapeutic approaches of naturopathic doctors and orthodox physicians coincide. Certainly both agree on the value of exercise, a low-fat, high-fiber diet, and the importance of stress reduction. But there are also wide divergences. For example, in treating precancerous changes in the cervix, a naturopath might recommend nutrition therapy and herbal preparations rather than surgery or cauterization.

When appropriate, naturopaths refer patients to orthodox physicians, who can admit them to hospitals, prescribe drugs, and perform surgery. But naturopathic doctors feel that drugs are prescribed far too frequently and often are overpriced. They encourage their patients to rely primarily on natural medicine therapies. These include acupuncture (which is discussed in detail on pages 42-51 in this book), hydrotherapy (see pages 206-211), homeopathy (see pages 60-65), massage (see pages 156-163), vitamin and mineral therapy (see pages 282-287), shiatsu (see pages 164-167) and other types of bodywork, as well as Chinese herbal medicine (see pages 42-51) and Western herbal medicine (see pages 288-327).

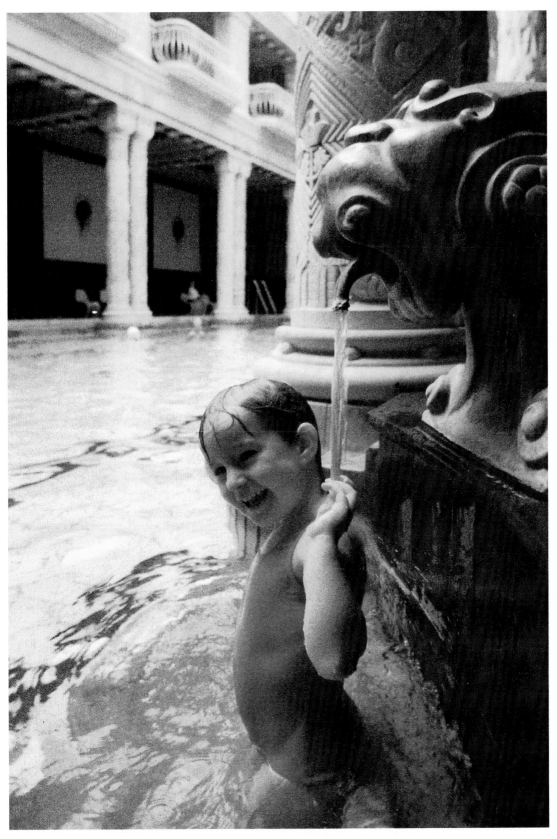

Europeans have for centuries patronized *thermal spas like the elegant Gellert baths of Budapest, Hungary. The water cure—hydrotherapy— is an important therapy in naturopathic medicine.*

A Continental Import. One branch of naturopathy developed out of the water cures that had for centuries flourished in Europe. The water cure was not just a matter of going to thermal springs, drinking the water, and bathing, but also taking cold baths, walking barefoot in the grass, and undergoing mineral-water fasts. Father Sebastian Kneipp (1821-1897), an Austrian priest, treated his own serious lung condition by plunging into ice-cold water every day for several months. Cured of his illness, Kneipp founded a water-cure clinic. Benedict Lust, a German-born physician and disciple of Kneipp, went to the United States in 1892 to teach Kneipp's methods of hydrotherapy.

Drawing from a melting pot of emigrants with diverse medical interests, a movement began to develop in the U.S. A coalition of Kneipp practitioners met in 1900 to incorporate many forms of natural medicine into one discipline, including herbal remedies, homeopathy, nutritional therapy, and massage. They adopted a new term: naturopathy. Shortly thereafter, Benedict Lust established the American School of Naturopathy in New York City.

A Commercial Offshoot. The early naturopaths attached great importance to a natural, healthy diet. So did many of their contemporaries. Will Kellogg, founder of the cereal manufacturing firm that bears his name, and his brother John helped popularize concepts of healthy eating, which coincided with naturopathic ideas. The Kelloggs, both members of the Seventh-Day Adventist Church, were vegetarians who also avoided coffee, alcohol, and tobacco.

In 1876, John Kellogg, then a medical doctor, became superintendent of a sanitarium in Battle Creek, Michigan, which had been founded by the Adventists to promote healthy living and natural remedies. As John Kellogg defined it, the sanitarium was "a place where people learned to stay well." Dr. Kellogg gained a national reputation for his views, which included a vegetarian diet, correct posture, sensible clothing, regular exercise, and exposure to fresh air and sunshine. He discouraged the use of dairy products and refined sugars.

The Kelloggs set up a laboratory at the sanitarium to develop healthy foods for patients. C.W. Post, a former patient, realized the commercial potential of health foods; he marketed a wheat-flake cereal and a coffee substitute. Will Kellogg then set up a business to mass-produce corn flakes: the Battle Creek Toasted Corn Flake Company. The name Battle Creek became synonymous with healthy eating.

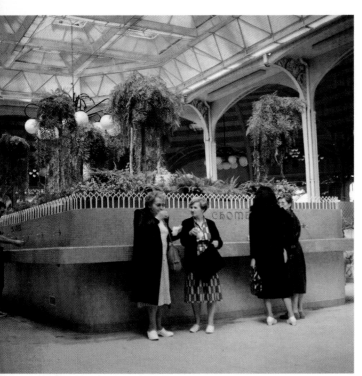

Among the world's most famous therapeutic spas is this one in Vichy, France, whose alkaline springs have been an attraction since the 17th century. It's not necessary, however, to travel great distances for hydrotherapy. Exercising in a pool may enable those with muscle and joint problems to regain partial or complete use of their limbs.

Many other people found naturopathy appealing, but this system never gained the popularity of osteopathy and chiropractic. Naturopathy was also overshadowed by the advances in orthodox medicine, including the discovery of antibiotics and the improvement in surgical techniques. The American Medical Association lumped naturopathy in with all other alternative systems, called them "quackery," and worked tirelessly to suppress them. Lacking accreditation as medical schools, many institutions that trained naturopaths

CASE HISTORY

A DIFFERENT WAY OF HEALING

A doctor of naturopathy takes a broad, holistic approach to diagnosis. Victoria Moran describes what happened when she took her five-year-old daughter to a naturopathic physician.

"Taking responsibility for my own health put me in the alternatives business. It meant replacing white flour with whole-wheat flour, beef with beans, and TV with work-outs at the gym. I also discovered alternative health-care providers and often availed myself of the services of a chiropractor, massage therapist, or acupuncturist. But when it came to medical attention for my child, I was as conservative as a three-piece suit. That's why, when my five-year-old daughter, Rachael, developed a tender lump in her chest one-and-a-half years ago, I took her to the best pediatrician I could find. He examined her and said, 'We need to watch this. Bring her back in two weeks.'

"Telling a mother to wait is as good as telling her to worry. Not being one to fret idly, I decided to use the two weeks to provide my little girl with what the natural way might have to offer. A friend suggested a doctor of naturopathy, a physician trained in using natural methods to help the body heal itself.

"The naturopath's first move was to take such a thorough history that I was relieved Rachael was only five — if she'd had any more history than that, we could have been in the doctor's office all day. After he did a standard exam, he made his recommendations: Make raw fruits and vegetables the bulk of her diet for the next 14 days; use poultices made from the herbs mullein and comfrey on the lump twice a day; and give her the herb echinacea, a purported immune enhancer, orally.

"All these instructions seemed reasonable. But when he said, 'If she were my child, I'd look into changing her school situation,' I was taken aback. I knew that the naturopathic approach deals holistically with people and seeks to address causes as well as alleviate symptoms, but switching kindergartens was a lot to ask. Nonetheless, his gentle questioning during the history had brought lengthy descriptions from Rachael of the painful teasing she'd been getting from the other children at school.

"I decided to follow all of the naturopath's recommendations, including a change in Rachael's school, effective immediately. Within a few days, the lump — which I understood to be lymphatic swelling — began to decrease in size. When we made our return visit to the pediatrician, all he said was, 'Obviously, it's gone.' Subsequent examinations bore that out, and the condition has not recurred."

Excerpted from "The Natural Doc" by Victoria Moran, *Vegetarian Times*, August 1990.

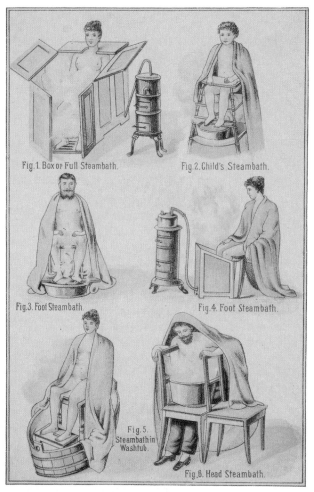

Fig.1. Box or Full Steambath.

Fig.2. Child's Steambath.

Fig.3. Foot Steambath.

Fig.4. Foot Steambath.

Fig.5. Steambath in Washtub.

Fig.6. Head Steambath.

Steam treatments *were valued as a cure-all for a multitude of diseases in the Victorian age. Too often, though, the hot, damp climate of a steam bath would help to spread germs, rather than kill them. Today's naturopaths and other natural medicine practitioners recommend steam for alleviating bronchial congestion and other problems.*

closed their doors. The resurgence of interest in natural medicine in the last two decades has focused renewed attention on the practice of naturopathy.

Partners in Prevention. Teaching the patient how to live healthfully is among a naturopathic doctor's primary goals. During office visits, time is devoted to explaining the best diet, habits, and attitudes to prevent disease.

The doctor-patient relationship begins with a thorough medical history and discussion aimed at getting a detailed picture of a patient's lifestyle. Stressing the importance of good nutrition as the basis for building and maintaining a healthy body, naturopaths urge patients to consume whole foods, which are largely unprocessed or unrefined, and to avoid those that are relatively high in fat and sugar, and low in fiber. Although these guidelines apply across a wide spectrum, a naturopathic doctor will take care to customize a diet program to suit each patient.

If needed, the practitioner will perform standard diagnostic procedures, including a physical exam and blood and urine analyses. Afterward, the doctor and patient work together to establish a treatment program. Dietary strategies are often emphasized for prevention, as well as to combat such disorders as acne, arthritis, asthma, atherosclerosis, eczema, gout, high blood pressure, and irritable bowel syndrome.

Purifying the Body. In order to keep toxins to a minimum, a naturopathic diet should contain limited amounts of animal products. In fact, such foods may be excluded altogether, thereby avoiding saturated fats. A high value is placed on foods from plants, such as fruits, vegetables, grains, beans, nuts, and seeds. They provide the adequate levels of nutrients and high amounts of dietary fiber. Salt, sugar, and food additives should be excluded when possible. The preferred drink is purified or distilled water, about eight glasses daily.

Clean living is among the foremost goals of naturopathy, and some practitioners believe that the greatest health hazards come from toxic substances that accumulate in the body. They are especially wary of heavy metals, toxic chemicals, alcohol, drugs, and food additives. According to naturopathy, there are various methods for ridding the body of toxins, including water sprays to cleanse the colon, massage to cleanse the skin, and deep-breathing exercises for the lungs.

Fasting. To promote detoxification, naturopaths are likely to suggest periodic short fasts of three to five days, during which the patient drinks water and possibly herbal teas but eats nothing. A decision to fast should be made jointly by a trained health-care practitioner and the patient.

Fasting has long been practiced for reasons that have nothing to do with health. People as diverse as Native Americans, Hindus, and ancient Greeks have fasted for religious reasons, as a rite of initiation or of mourning, or as a spiritual practice.

Those who fast for health cite many benefits of fasting: rest for internal organs; improved digestion and circulation; greater mental and spiritual clarity and energy; elimination of drug cravings; improved sleep; weight loss. Adherents say that fasting can relieve symptoms of emotional depression and anxiety and foster a feeling of well-being. Advocates of fasting during illness believe that this restraint aids healing; eating, they believe, taps energy for digestion that could be better used for recovery. In addition, some claim that fasting may release a hormone that stimulates the body's immune system in its fight against disease.

Among the most popular and least dangerous of fasts is the juice fast. Only fresh fruit and vegetable juices are consumed, though some programs also allow herbal teas and vegetable broth. Indeed, fresh fruit and vegetables are high in vitamins, minerals, food enzymes, amino acids, and natural sugars, and are easily assimilated by the body.

Even enthusiastic practitioners of fasting recognize that it can be dangerous, causing weakness, fatigue, anemia, and other disorders. The feeling of lightness that comes with fasting may, in fact, be a warning that the body is being deprived of minerals essential for nerve function. ❑

Naturopathy, which has gained acceptance in other countries, takes advantage of local resources. For example, here, at the Center of Naturopathy and Yogic Sciences in Bangalore, India, practitioners make use of banana leaves for a sweat wrap. This twenty-minute procedure opens the pores, softens the skin, and leaves the patient feeling refreshed and rested.

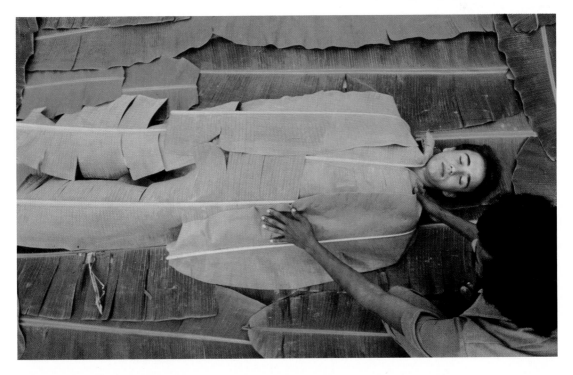

Vision Therapies and Iridology

Some optometrists say that eye exercises designed to make the eyes and mind work together more efficiently can help prevent some vision problems. Iridologists study the markings on the irises of the eyes to diagnose various ailments.

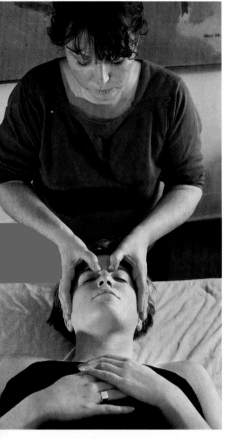

***Applying thumb pressure** can help ease eyestrain and provide relaxation. Here a practitioner of the Eastern therapy known as shiatsu gently rotates the area around the eye socket, first in one direction, then the other. The therapist starts at the top of the eye socket and moves down the side of the bridge of the nose.*

MANY PEOPLE ARE CONVINCED that poor vision is inherited, and that vision problems inevitably worsen with age, beginning at about 40. Explanations of why vision declines range from poor eating habits to insufficient exposure to sunlight, lack of physical activity, too much time spent watching television and working at computer terminals, and the accumulation of stress. According to a new theory of eye care, vision training may enable a person to get by without glasses or at least decrease wearing time or the strength of one's prescription.

Someone who wants to consult an eye specialist can choose either an ophthalmologist or an optometrist. Ophthalmologists are physicians concerned primarily with treating eye diseases like glaucoma and performing surgery. Optometrists are trained to test vision and prescribe eyeglasses and contact lenses but are not medical doctors. Today, most eye specialists who practice vision therapy are optometrists.

Improving Sight. Vision training aims not only to arrest eye problems, but to prevent them by starting at the earliest possible stage, ideally before weaknesses become entrenched. Training may improve nearsightedness (myopia), farsightedness (hyperopia), poor peripheral vision, crossed eyes (strabismus), amblyopia, which is known as "lazy eye," and other weaknesses. According to some optometrists, performing eye exercises and wearing glasses may slow the progression of myopia or stop it entirely.

Athletes find that vision training may improve their hand-eye coordination and peripheral vision. Airline pilots have used it with good results to sharpen their depth perception and focusing skills. Yet many ophthalmologists question the effectiveness of such therapy and the validity of studies on which the therapy is based.

A Coordinated Effort. Those who advocate vision training believe that the eye and brain can be made to work together more efficiently. Therapy sessions in an optometric clinic or office may require special equipment—for example, an exercise that involves walking across a balance beam with a patch over one eye. But most training involves fairly simple exercises that can be done anywhere and at any time, with no equipment. Proponents say that daily exercises can help your eyes relax and adapt better to changes in light and focus. The exercises may also help you get rid of mental blocks to seeing.

Those who call themselves behavioral or developmental optometrists often work with children, who are still developing visual habits. These optometrists say that when training succeeds, children who might otherwise wear prescription glasses for their entire lives can often avoid them.

It All Started with Bates. Dr. William Bates (1881–1931), an American ophthalmologist, was the founder and leading proponent of an eye-care philosophy that flew in the face of the orthodox approach. In 1920, Bates took issue with his own profession in his book *Better Eyesight Without Glasses.* Having examined thousands of patients over a period of several years, Bates argued against the accepted theory that wearing glasses is the only way to correct nearsightedness, farsightedness, blurred vision, and other problems.

Bates taught that poor vision is caused by weakness of the six sets of muscles that control each eye. When these muscles are healthy and well toned, he claimed, they would adjust the shape of the eyeball to achieve proper focus.

A Two-Pronged Approach. The Bates method is based on a combination of relaxation and exercise, and it considers the mental aspect of the therapy as important as the physical exertion. According to *The New Holistic Health Handbook,* compiled by the Berkeley, California, Holistic Health Center, "At a time when it was considered quackery to heal the body by means of the mind, Bates worked on the eyes by encouraging the systematic use of the memory and the imagination. His techniques resembled meditation, and anticipated certain principles of biofeedback and stress-reduction training."

Several decades later, some of Bates's original exercises plus variations on them are still being used. And practitioners trained in optometry, psychoanalysis, and other fields have expanded on Bates's fundamental belief that vision problems frequently are related to emotional stress.

Today's vision specialists in alternative medicine take into account nutrition, health, and lifestyle factors that may affect sight. Those who want to expand beyond vision training are exploring the therapeutic uses of light and color in treating learning disabilities, depression, stress disorders, sexual dysfunction, and premenstrual syndrome.

Iridology. Naturopathic doctors and other natural medicine practitioners who want to avoid X-rays and invasive procedures may use iridology as a diagnostic tool. Iridology is a system that correlates changes in the color and texture of the iris, the colored part of the eye, with physical and mental disorders. Its proponents say that iridology can

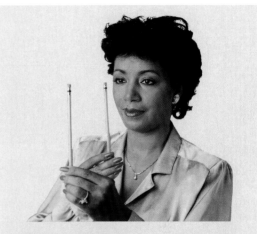

Bates Eye Exercises

An American eye doctor, William H. Bates, devised a series of exercises to relax and strengthen the eyes. Shown here is the exercise to improve focusing. Hold one pencil about three inches away from your face. Hold another pencil at arm's length. Focus first on one with both eyes, blink, then focus on the other. Repeat several times. Other exercises are:

- *Blinking.* Blink once or twice every 10 seconds to lubricate your eyes.
- *Palming.* Sit relaxed at a table or desk. Close your eyes. Place your elbows on a cushion on your lap or on the table. Keep your head level and neck straight. Without touching them, cover your eyes with your cupped hands. Perform palming twice a day for about 10 minutes at a time.
- *Shifting.* Avoid staring at objects. Instead, shift your sight constantly.
- *Swinging.* Stand with your feet far enough apart so that you are comfortably balanced. Swing easily from side to side, allowing your eyes to swing with your body's motion.
- *Splashing.* When you awaken, splash warm water on your closed eyes 20 times, then splash them 20 times with cold water. Repeat the process when you prepare for bed, but reverse the warm and cold sequence.

also be used to identify dietary deficiencies and the accumulation of toxic chemicals in the body. Natural medicine practitioners may call on iridologists to confirm or expand on a diagnosis from another source. They follow a system devised originally by Ignatz von Peczely, a Hungarian physician, in the 19th century and adapted in the 1950s by Bernard Jensen, an American chiropractor. Jensen based his practice on detailed diagrams of the left and right irises. He assigned every organ, many body parts, and bodi-

---

CASE HISTORY

LEARNING TO SEE

The English novelist and essayist Aldous Huxley (1894-1963), author of some of the most widely read books of this century, wrote of his experience with the Bates Method.

When he was 16 years old, Aldous Huxley suffered from a serious inflammation of the cornea, which left him nearly blind. "My doctors advised me to do my reading with the aid of a powerful hand magnifying glass. But later on I was promoted to spectacles. True, a measure of strain and fatigue was always present, and there were occasions when I was overcome by the sense of complete physical and mental exhaustion which only eye strain can produce. Still, I was grateful to be able to see as well as I could.

"Things went on in this way until the year 1939, when in spite of greatly strengthened glasses I found the task of reading increasingly difficult and fatiguing. There could be no doubt of it: my capacity to see was steadily and quite rapidly failing."

It was then that Huxley heard about the Bates Method of visual re-education. "Since optical glass," he wrote, "was no longer doing me any good, I decided to take the plunge."

He spent three hours, six days a week, at the oculist, learning the practices of the Bates Method. After one month, his wife reported to her sister, "We have definite improvement, though nothing spectacular as yet; what is certain is that even the right pupil is

clearing up. It moves me to see Aldous *looking at me.*"

Huxley's vision continued to improve. Although his eyesight would always remain defective, Huxley was convinced that the Bates Method had saved him from complete blindness and he became its strong champion.

"What I claimed for the Bates Method," he wrote to a doctor who had attacked the method, "was simply this…that it shows people how to make the best possible use of such visual powers as they possess.

"To the poor seer he [Bates] was saying, in effect, what the golf pro says to the poor golfer: 'Be active, and yet remain relaxed; don't strain and yet do your damndest; stop trying so hard and let the deep-seated intelligence of your body and the subconscious mind do the work as it ought to be done.' The Bates Method is not a branch of medicine, either orthodox or unorthodox. It is a method of education, fundamentally similar to the methods of education devised and successfully used by all the teachers of psycho-physical skills for the last several thousand years."

Based on *The Art of Seeing* by Aldous Huxley, *Aldous Huxley* by Sybille Bedford, and *This Timeless Moment* by Laura Archera Huxley.

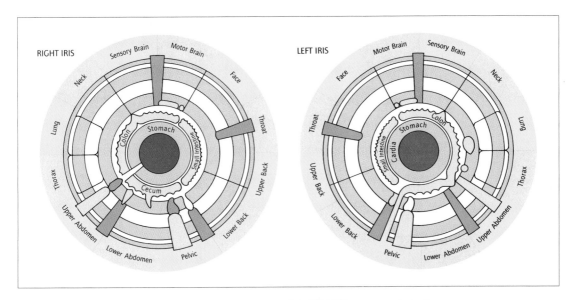

ly functions a specific location on one or both of the irises.

Concentric Circles. According to Dr. Jensen, the iris can be divided into six zones or rings related to the body's systems. The innermost zone relates to the stomach, the next to the intestines, the third to the blood and lymph systems, the fourth to organs and glands, the fifth to the muscles and skeleton, and the sixth to the skin and elimination. In general, the upper half of the iris corresponds to the top half of the body, including the brain, face, neck, lungs, and throat; the lower half corresponds to the lower half of the body.

Iridologists say that degrees of light and darkness in the iris give clues to a person's health. A dark rim encircling the iris may indicate problems in the system of waste elimination that affect the skin; white marks may signify stress, overstim-

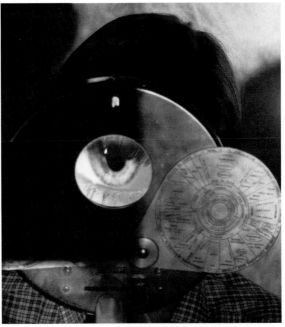

An iridologist uses a chart similar to the one at top to diagnose ailments or identify potential problems. Each area on the iris corresponds to a body part or function. A specially equipped camera provides a clear view of a patient's iris.

ulation, or inflammation; and dark marks may indicate that nutrients are low, circulation is sluggish, and other problems. Iridologists also examine the texture of the fibers in the iris. A fine-grained pattern of fibers is said to indicate a strong constitution, while a loosely woven pattern indicates a weak constitution.

Orthodox physicians typically examine the eyes for diagnostic purposes, recognizing that eye abnormalities can sometimes signal health problems. Certain patterns, such as a light gray or yellow ring around the rim of the iris, may be interpreted as a sign of heart disease. However, by and large, orthodox physicians reject the theory that the iris provides extensive information on illness or disease. They object to iridology when it discourages a patient with a serious disorder from getting proper medical diagnosis. ❑

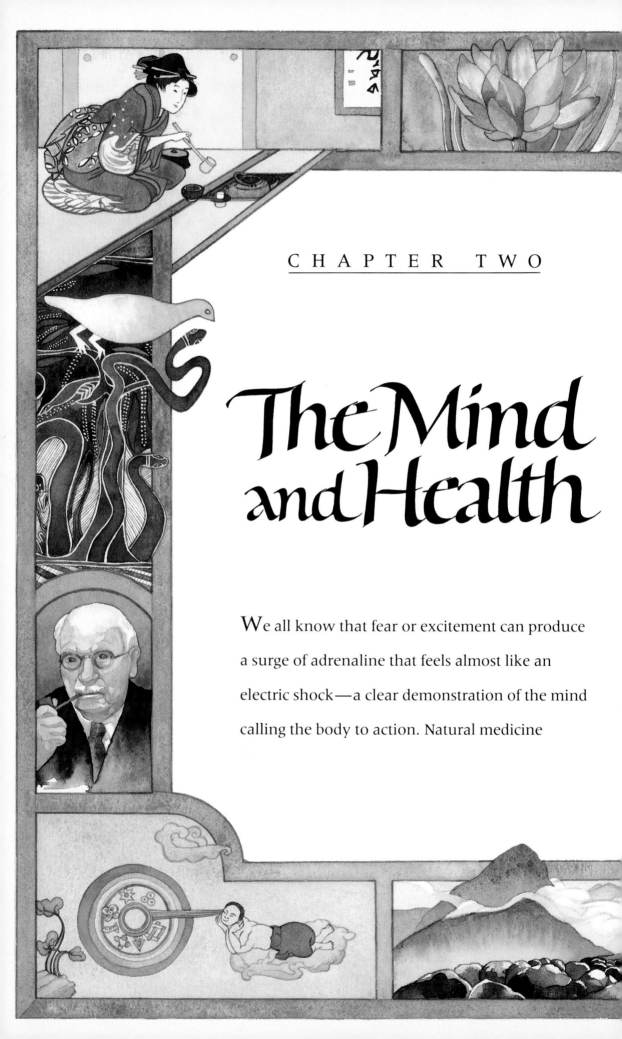

CHAPTER TWO

The Mind and Health

We all know that fear or excitement can produce a surge of adrenaline that feels almost like an electric shock—a clear demonstration of the mind calling the body to action. Natural medicine

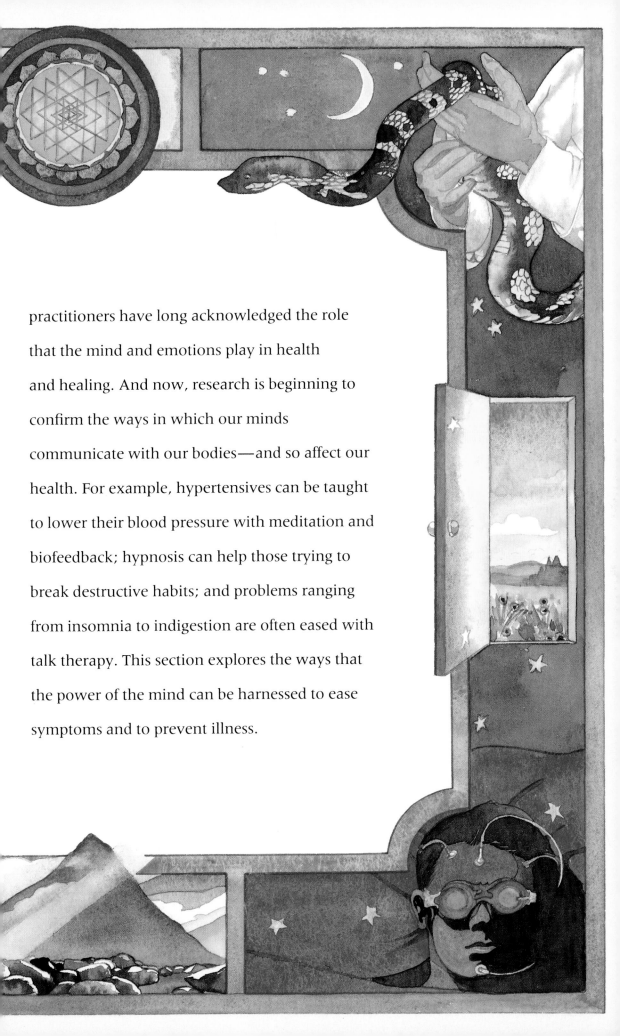

practitioners have long acknowledged the role that the mind and emotions play in health and healing. And now, research is beginning to confirm the ways in which our minds communicate with our bodies—and so affect our health. For example, hypertensives can be taught to lower their blood pressure with meditation and biofeedback; hypnosis can help those trying to break destructive habits; and problems ranging from insomnia to indigestion are often eased with talk therapy. This section explores the ways that the power of the mind can be harnessed to ease symptoms and to prevent illness.

The Mind-Body Connection

Practitioners of natural medicine have always acknowledged the role that the mind and emotions play in health. Now exciting new research gives a tantalizing glimpse into the possible mechanisms.

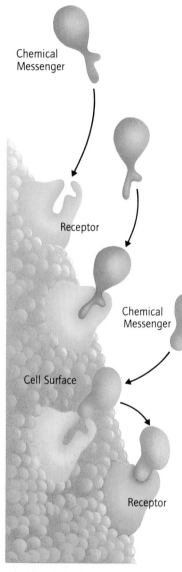

Chemical Messenger

Receptor

Chemical Messenger

Cell Surface

Receptor

Unlocking a Cell's Receptor Sites

Cells communicate via molecular messengers, whose shape determines their destination. Once dispatched they head toward a cell whose receptors are shaped to receive them. Just as a key opens a specific lock, each molecular messenger binds to a specific receptor.

IS IT POSSIBLE FOR INDIVIDUALS to learn to influence their own immune systems—that is, the system that protects our bodies from a constant bombardment of viruses, bacteria, and poisons? New discoveries suggest that the answer may be yes. Scientists from a variety of disciplines are exploring the links between the brain, endocrine, and immune systems, in part to determine to what extent our emotions may affect our health. A new discipline known as psychoneuroimmunology, or PNI, is on the cutting edge of this research.

Until fairly recently medical science accepted without much question the notion that the body and mind were separate entities, operating independently of one another. Medical science, which has focused on the strictly physical aspects of illness, has reinforced this dualism with a whole raft of successful technologies, including laser surgery, CAT scans, powerful medications, and other medical advances.

Recent research in the field of PNI has shown that the brain, endocrine, and immune systems are interconnected by a series of neural pathways. These pathways may form a communications network that enables mind and body to influence each other. But does this network actually function, and if so, how does it work? This is what PNI researchers are currently exploring.

The Mystery of Immunity. It was once assumed that the immune system was independent of the brain. If certain immune cells were placed in a petri dish infected with microbes, they would launch an attack. This seemed to imply that these cells needed no direction from the brain in order to carry out their assigned tasks.

But the immune system is an amazingly intricate and elusive defense network which scientists still do not completely understand. Whereas the circulatory system is powered by the heart, the nervous system by the brain, the immune system has no particular organ as its focal point. The lymph nodes, bone marrow, thymus, spleen, tonsils, and appendix all produce or store a variety of specialized immune cells, which are deployed as needed.

White blood cells are the front-line defenders in the molecular warfare waged by the immune system. They attach themselves to microbial intruders, and most produce antibodies which neutralize or destroy them. While the immune system makes many types of defense cells, white blood cells (T cells and others) are the keystone of immune function.

We know that the brain makes hormones and other molecular messengers that carry signals from cell to cell throughout the body. In fact, most cells have receptor sites (which are themselves specialized molecules) shaped to receive specific

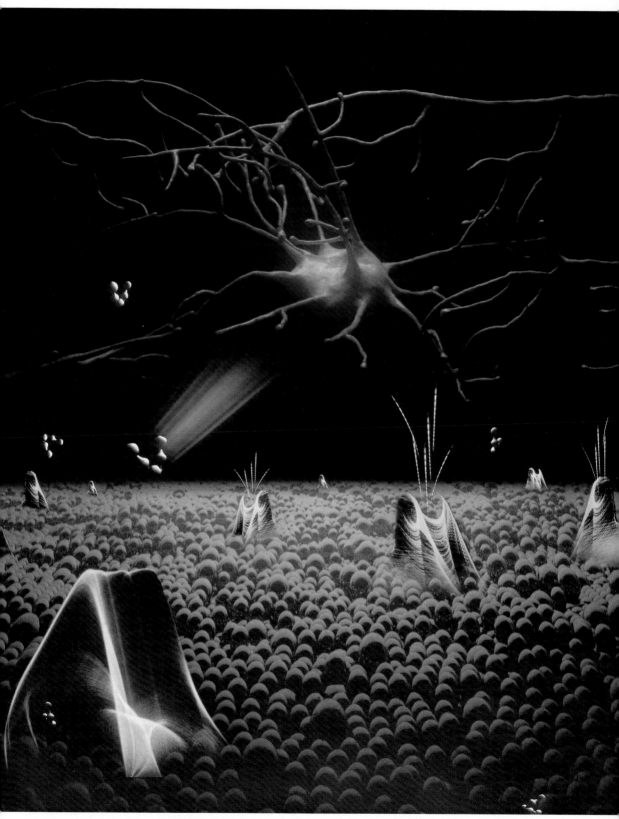

In this artist's rendition, *molecular messengers (the flying V's), are whizzing toward receptors on the surface of a brain cell. Once a receptor is unlocked, its shape changes (as represented by the cones and streaks) and further reactions can take place. The branching structure above the surface is a distant brain cell.*

messengers, just as a lock is built to receive a particular key. Some hormones made by the brain fit receptors on certain immune cells.

PNI scientists have found that white blood cells also make hormones that fit the receptors of certain brain cells. On this basis, some believe that white blood cells may have a much broader function than previously thought. As one PNI researcher puts it, white blood cells may serve as "bits of brain floating around the body."

CASE HISTORY

ONE BODY WITH MANY MINDS

Patients with multiple personalities offer dramatic evidence of the mind-body link. Amazingly, their diseases may actually change when their personalities do.

In the late 1970s, a young woman, who will be known here as Harriet to protect her privacy, checked into the psychiatric unit of a Chicago hospital. Overweight and diabetic, Harriet was also suffering from headaches, followed by blackouts lasting several hours. Once at the hospital, she was diagnosed as having a multiple personality disorder, an emotional condition in which the patient has two or more distinct personalities that alternately emerge and take control of the person's behavior.

Harriet was treated by Dr. Bennett Braun, one of the foremost experts on the disorder. Using hypnosis, Dr. Braun found four separate personalities living within his patient's body. Harriet, the host personality, was a subdued but pleasant young woman.

But with each change in identity came a distinct change in facial expressions, mannerisms, speech patterns, and other traits. The alter personalities were Judy, a withdrawn and clumsy five-year-old, Sally, an aggressive and sullen 16-year-old, and Kitty, an agreeable and well-mannered teenager.

Until recently, some members of the medical profession suspected that patients with multiple personalities were faking. Physiological evidence has now offered convincing proof that the condition is genuine: brain waves vary distinctly from one personality to another.

During one of Harriet's therapy sessions Kitty suddenly emerged. She, like Harriet, was seriously diabetic. But later, when Sally appeared, something unexpected happened — after one hour, all signs of diabetes had disappeared. The level of Sally's blood sugar was completely normal and as long as Sally was present, Harriet's body remained free of the symptoms of diabetes.

Harriet's case is not the only one to demonstrate the strange power that the mind seems to wield over the body. In another case, a young man suffered from an allergy to citrus fruit which came and went as his secondary personalities emerged. And in still another, an adult patient with apparently normal eyesight developed a "walleye" whenever a young alter personality appeared.

What causes multiple personality disorder? As the patient undergoes treatment, a chilling portrait of extreme and horrifying child abuse usually emerges. Apparently, the alternate personalities are created as a defense from emotional and physical pain that is so intense it overwhelms the person's ability to cope. These unfortunate people give us an intriguing glimpse into the incredible interplay of mind and body.

Some PNI researchers have envisioned the immune system as part of the brain. Perhaps it is the brain's sixth sense, the sense that detects viruses and other invaders. According to this theory, the immune system converts information about invaders into hormones. These powerful biochemicals are then sent to the brain where they may influence the mind by altering mood and behavior. By the same token, immune function may be enhanced or depressed by fluctuations in emotions.

But back to the original question: is it possible for us to gain conscious control over our own biochemistry? To some degree, yes. There is no doubt, for example, that people can learn constructive ways of dealing with stress. Studies have shown that during periods of significant stress, the adrenal glands step up production of chemical messengers (corticosteroids) which may depress immune function, making us more vulnerable to illness. Using meditation, biofeedback, and other techniques, many people have learned how to listen to their bodies in an effort to mitigate their response to stress. In turn, some researchers believe that by controlling our reactions to stress we are also strengthening our immune systems.

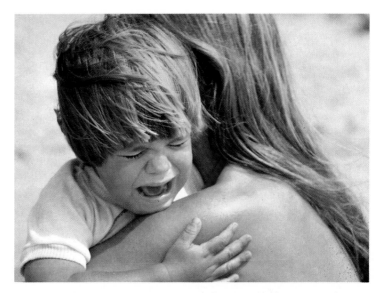

Mothers everywhere respond to their children's scrapes and bumps with a tender, "Let Mama kiss it and make it better." And though the tears may continue for a little while, most children are generally quite ready to be comforted. The mother knows that the child's pain will fade rapidly, and that her kiss provides not a cure but soft reassurance. This loving exercise, probably as old as humankind, helps to take the fear out of injuries—both physical and emotional. And because Mama says it will be better, it most certainly will.

As additional information is gathered on how mind and body interact, we may one day be able to do even more for ourselves. Like the brain, the immune system has a kind of memory, for its specialized cells recall previous encounters with viruses and other infections. Already attempts are being made to exploit this memory and the communication loop that exists between the immune system and the mind with such techniques as visualization, guided imagery, and self-hypnosis. Some PNI scientists even believe that one day we may be able to condition the immune system to prevent illness from ever occurring.

The Placebo Response. As interest has grown about how the mind affects the body, the whole question of the healing power of placebos has gained considerable momentum. Placebos are any of a variety of substances given in place of drugs. Most people have heard of them, even if they think they've never taken one. Most often, placebos are used in double-blind drug experiments, where neither the patient nor the physician knows whether the participant is getting a dummy drug or the real thing. The aim of these tests is to determine if a certain drug is any more useful in treating a specific disease than a placebo. Curiously, whether the placebo is administered deliberately by a doctor (as is sometimes the case), or by chance in a double-blind test, it often eases the patient's symptoms.

The Riddle of Vanishing Warts

It seems that only people who are afflicted with warts give them serious thought. But Dr. Andrew Weil wonders if warts might not offer a new way to investigate healing.

Miraculous cures of cutaneous warts are as commonplace as they are curious. Ask about them in any group of people, and you will easily collect typical stories.

The methods used to get rid of them range from the straightforward to the outright peculiar, with no consistency. Techniques that have treated warts successfully include: being touched by a neighborhood wart healer, applying some curative plant to the wart, rubbing the wart with a cut potato and burying the potato under a particular kind of tree during a particular phase of the moon.

Cutaneous warts are not functional problems. They are real, discrete, physical organic growths, made up of abnormal tissue infected with viruses. Nevertheless, they are susceptible to virtually instant healing brought about by belief in treatments that cannot have significant direct effects on the viruses or the abnormal tissue.

One doctor told me he had once treated a man who had lived for years with cutaneous warts over most of his body. The standard methods of removing them had only multiplied their numbers. Finally, on a whim, the doctor told the patient he would try out a new, experimental form of radiation that was somewhat risky but so powerful that it might knock out the problem. He and a radiologist colleague had the man remove his clothes and stand in a darkened X-ray room. Then they made the machines hum loudly without actually emitting any X-rays. The next day, all the warts fell off. They did not grow back.

Warts on the sole of the foot are much more stubborn than warts on the hands. One plantar wart sufferer asked how he could make his wart go away. He pressed me for a specific technique. On an intuitive impulse I told him to try rubbing the wart with a piece of dry ice before going to sleep one night. I suggested that each night and morning he spend a few minutes in visualizing white light flowing from his head to his foot along a specific route, keeping in mind the idea that this light would help his body eliminate the wart.

Six months later, I got a letter from the man. After a week, he could notice a change in the wart—it was slightly smaller. Elated, he continued his efforts and the shrinking accelerated. After a month, the wart was gone for good.

My reasons for stressing the mechanism of wart cures are several. First, it is the objective, researchable aspect of the problem. Once its components come to light, doctors will be able to see the reality and importance of this example of mind-mediated healing. Second, the same mechanism may underlie other mind-body events, such as placebo responses, faith healings, spontaneous remissions of cancer, and so forth. Third, it may provide a key to elucidating the ways that mind and body impinge on each other. Fourth, understanding the mechanism of wart cures may enable people to activate it voluntarily in themselves or others and direct it toward more serious medical problems.

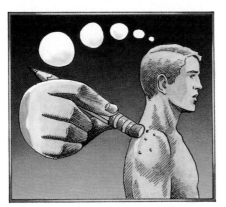

Curing warts: a case of mind over matter.

Excerpted from Health and Healing *by Dr. Andrew Weil.*

Until recently, science has paid little attention to how placebos work their seeming magic. Patients who reported being helped were often dismissed as being suggestible. Doctors concluded that they had been imagining their symptoms all along. The fact remains that placebos have been used successfully to treat a whole range of illness, from warts to heart disease.

Great Expectations. Since placebos are inert, their power must lie elsewhere. Most likely it lies in the expectations of the patient. Under the right circumstances, a placebo seems to trigger immune response, allowing the body to begin healing itself. How and why this works is still largely a mystery, but it suggests a strong but subtle link between the mind and the body.

There is a variation on the placebo response which has negative rather than positive effects. It is observed when people strongly but mistakenly believe that they have been injured, poisoned, or even hexed. For example, dozens of employees at a midwestern electronics factory became faint and nauseous after hearing a rumor that they had inhaled noxious fumes. While their symptoms were real, repeated inspections found no evidence of fumes in the factory.

Similarly, around the world, numerous instances of so-called voodoo death have been reported. In these cases, the victim is cursed by someone whom they believe has great power, and shortly thereafter dies. One theory holds that the victim's strong belief somehow affects the branch of the autonomic nervous system that controls heartbeat, causing the heart to fail.

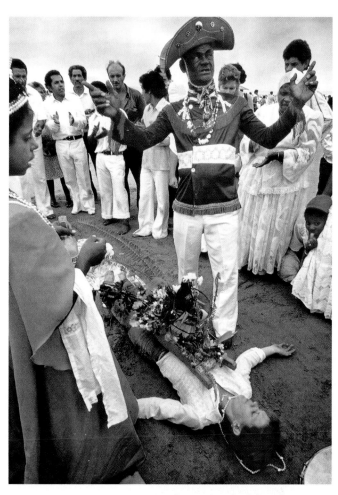

During a ritual celebration honoring the goddess of the seawaters, mediums from the Umbanda religious cult of Brazil conduct a group healing. Thousands of worshipers gather on the beach at São Paulo, bringing gifts for the goddess. Originating in Rio de Janeiro in the 1920s, the cult is an amalgamation of Catholicism and African spiritual beliefs.

The Link Between Patient and Practitioner. What's to be learned from bizarre occurrences like outbreaks of imagined illness or voodoo death? For one thing, they offer dramatic testimony to the importance of belief and expectation. Just as the victim fervently believed in the power of the hexer, so, too, do many people believe in the power of their physician, acupuncturist, or other practitioner. Whatever the direct physical effect of a particular treatment, it may also work by eliciting a mind-controlled healing response. In short, the patient's faith in both the practitioner and the therapy, and the practitioner's belief in the remedy, may determine how well a treatment works. ❏

The Healing Touch

The laying on of hands, a practice far older than Western medicine, still flourishes in the modern world. By their very nature, the cures wrought by faith healing are beyond explanation.

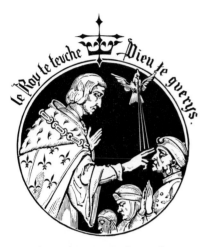

The King Touches Thee, God Cures Thee

King Louis IX of France (above), canonized sometime after his death in 1270, was celebrated for his healing powers. But he was not the only holy royal healer. In medieval times, when disease was rife and doctors scarce, kings were often called upon to heal the sick. Since royal succession was considered a divine right, kings often claimed other divine attributes as well — such as the ability to heal through touch. The royal touch was considered especially effective for treating scrofula, a disease of the lymph glands caused by contaminated milk.

ALSO CALLED SPIRITUAL OR DIVINE HEALING, faith healing relies upon summoning a higher power to help treat illness. It is accomplished through prayer, the laying on of hands, rituals, and a variety of other means. Scientific thinkers tend to believe that the faith itself is a psychological process that somehow triggers a healing response in the body, especially during healing ceremonies or rites when emotions may reach a high pitch. But whether cure is inspired by divine intervention or emotional responsiveness, an openness to the whole notion of faith healing seems to have a positive effect on almost any course of treatment.

The Key to Faith Healing Is Belief. A few healers claim to be able to cure people who do not share their beliefs, but in most cases a patient's trust is essential. Faith healing is an intensely emotional commitment, which draws on the innermost spiritual and psychological resources of patients. It is often bound up with strong religious beliefs as well as cultural values and assumptions shared by healer and patient alike. Someone brought up in the traditions of orthodox medicine, for instance, is less likely to respond to the ministrations of a Mexican village *curandero* or of a tribal shaman than someone familiar with these systems. Failure of a treatment is often attributed to lack of faith.

The earliest faith healers were shamans, priests, and medicine men who used chants and other rituals to influence spirits that were causing a particular disease. Ancient peoples apparently did not make distinctions between physical and spiritual illness; rather, they took a view of health that nowadays would be called holistic.

However, the healing arts were not uniformly practiced. Some ancient Greeks took bodily afflictions to be a sign of divine displeasure—and hence to be endured. The ancient Israelites, too, were inclined to accept illness as a punishment from on high. But early Christians viewed disease not as punishment from God, but as the result of evil operating in human life. Jesus battled evil by healing lepers, restoring sight to the blind, and causing the lame to walk. The Apostles continued this healing tradition in the name of Jesus.

Faith Healing Today. Under a variety of different names, medicine men still function in many parts of the world. In Borneo, for instance, the healer is called a *manang;* among the Alaskan Eskimos, the healer is known as an *angakok.* The sick in many such societies are treated with traditional rituals whose purpose is to exorcise hostile spirits, or to rid the victim of a curse inflicted by an enemy. Sometimes, the patient's own transgressions must be purged before healing can occur.

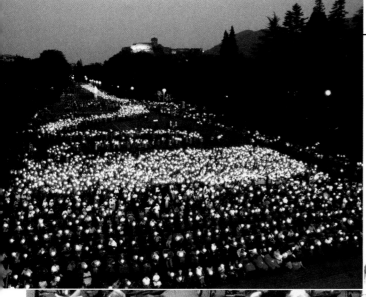

In search of a miracle, each year
hundreds of thousands of pilgrims
come to worship at the shrine near
Lourdes, France. There, in 1858,
a 14-year-old peasant girl named
Bernadette Soubirous had a vision.
The Virgin Mary appeared to her
and showed her the location of a
healing spring. A century later, the
Catholic Church instituted a system
of investigation to verify claims of
medical miracles. About 100 cures
have been authenticated.

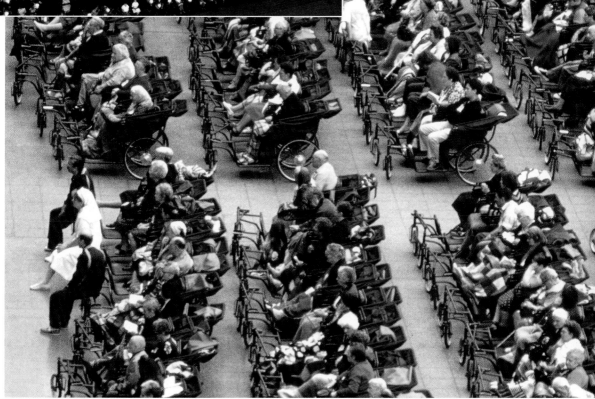

In the United States, among the best-known proponents of faith healing are Christian Scientists. They believe
that illness is an illusion based on erroneous thoughts and
that all disease can be cured by correct thinking. In the
words of Mary Baker Eddy (1821-1910), founder of Christian Science, "The mind governs the body, not partially but
wholly."

The practice of healing remains a part of many Christian ministries, but is usually expressed with prayers and
blessings. In fact, many mainstream religions offer prayer
services to alleviate the suffering of the sick, providing
emotional and spiritual support. In a somewhat different
vein, television evangelists practice faith healing before an
audience of millions.

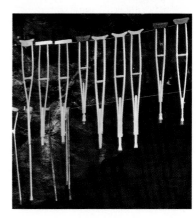

Abandoned crutches at Lourdes
testify to the power of faith.

The Laying on of Hands. The sense of touch is vital to communication and comfort. It transmits a silent assurance of loving care. Indeed, there is strong evidence to suggest that infants have died from lack of holding and cuddling. So it is not surprising that many healers rely on touch to cure illness.

Today, touch (sometimes in the form of massage) plays an important role in many natural therapies. But unlike religious faith healers, most secular practitioners believe that a universal energy supplies the healing force. This notion is derived from Eastern cultures, where the flow of energy through the body has long been looked upon as a measure of health. If the flow is unbalanced, a person may become ill. The healer's touch is meant to transfer positive energy into the patient and balance the flow.

Therapeutic Touch. Developed at the New York University Division of Nursing by Dolores Krieger, Ph.D., R.N., Therapeutic Touch combines traditional laying-on-of-hands with certain Eastern-inspired theories of energy flow. This healing technique is based on the belief that each human body projects a field of energy, which, when blocked, creates pain or disease. Practitioners of the treatment state that Therapeutic Touch allows them to detect and correct these blockages, thereby easing a client's pain and improving health. Many people have experienced relief from backache, tension, headache, or other symptoms after a few sessions of treatment. Those individuals suffering from chronic disease benefit from the tension-relieving aspects of Therapeutic Touch, although their illness will not necessarily be cured.

Becoming Sensitive to Energy Flow. According to Krieger, most people can train their hands to become sensitive to radiant energy from the body. And, once taught, anyone can administer Therapeutic Touch.

To get a sense of the human energy field, sit comfortably with both feet on the floor. Then, with your elbows out, slowly bring your palms together as close as you can without actually touching. Next, slowly move your palms about two inches apart and bring them back to the original (almost touching) position. Move your palms four inches apart, then six inches, returning after each move to the original position. Then, move your palms about eight inches apart; stop for a moment. Narrow the gap to six inches, four inches, then two inches, stopping for a moment after each move. Finally, bring the palms together again without quite touching and for a full minute concentrate on what you sense—you may feel heat, cold, tingling, pulsation, or some other sensation that is your subjective cue to your own energetic state.

The healer should be healthy and strongly motivated to heal. Before the session begins, the healer meditates for a few minutes in order to visualize the client as a healthy human being. The next step is to assess the client's energy field. To do this, the healer holds his or her open hands a

---

Stimulating Self-Worth

The healing relationship is potentially present whenever one person comes to another for healing. It is invoked by the magic ritual of shamans and by the psychotherapist.

The healing relationship communicates the love and concern of others that gives us strength and reason to heal. It communicates our worth as an individual. It communicates the irrational, just as love is irrational, and gives us hope that everything is possible through love. The healing relationship communicates high expectations for ourselves, our bodies, minds, and spirits.

We need the healing relationship — the loving touch, the positive expectancy, the sense of self-worth, even a bit of magic. Healers in all traditions hold the power to evoke this healing relationship. It is the golden thread of healing.
— **Excerpted from "The Healing Relationship" by Jerry Solfvin**

few inches above the body, and then with sweeping motions, follows the body's contours. Krieger says that your hands will feel unusual pressure or heat at those spots where the energy is blocked. The healer then tries to "unruffle" the energy, distributing the excess energy to other points along the client's body.

How Does Therapeutic Touch Work? While the scientific basis for Therapeutic Touch has not been firmly established, Dolores Krieger says that there is nothing psychic or mysterious about the treatment. In fact, she believes that the energy fields are somehow involved in blood hemoglobin levels—the part of blood that transports oxygen throughout the body.

In a series of experiments, Krieger found a significant rise in hemoglobin levels among patients treated with a laying-on-of-hands technique. As Krieger interprets these results, through touch, the healer supplies the energy to boost the client's hemoglobin levels, and thereby enhances the person's vitality.

But increased hemoglobin levels are only one way the treatment works. Krieger and other nurses who have used the method say that Therapeutic Touch helps clients to relax and eases their anxiety—which may be one reason why it is effective in reducing pain.

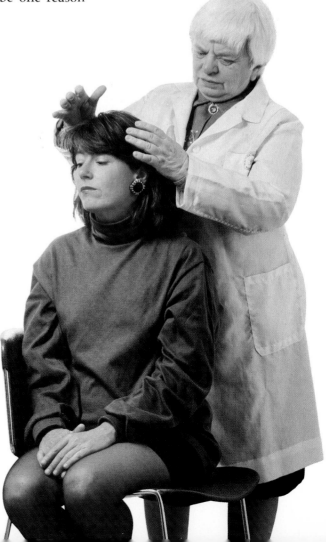

Hands-on healing is the "natural potential in all human beings," claims Dolores Krieger, first lady of Therapeutic Touch. Krieger, shown conducting a session, has taught thousands of health professionals to tap their own healing powers.

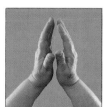 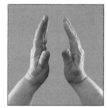

To train your hands, *begin with palms nearly together. Move them two inches apart.*

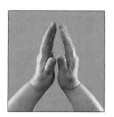 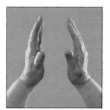

Return to original position. Repeat sequence twice, separating hands by four, then six inches.

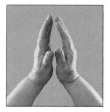 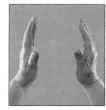

Finally, move hands eight inches apart. As hands come together, pause every two inches.

Out of Touch

*The gentle touch and probing of a patient's body used to be
a doctor's primary diagnostic tool. Today, writes Dr. Lewis Thomas,
machinery has replaced this age-old laying on of hands.*

Part of the dismay in being very sick is the lack of close human contact. Ordinary people, even close friends, even family members, tend to stay away from the very sick, touching them as infrequently as possible for fear of interfering, or catching the illness, or just for fear of bad luck. The doctor's oldest skill in trade was to place his hands on the patient.

Over the centuries, the skill became more specialized and refined, the hands learned other things to do beyond mere contact. They probed to feel the pulse at the wrist, the tip of the spleen, or the edge of the liver, thumped to elicit resonant or dull sounds over the lungs, spread ointments over the skin, nicked veins for bleeding, but at the same time touched, caressed, and at the end held on to the patient's fingers.

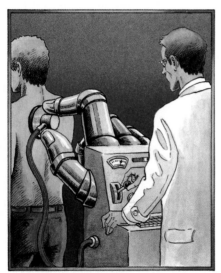

A hands-off approach to medicine.

Most of the men who practiced this laying on of hands must have possessed, to begin with, the gift of affection. There are, certainly, some people who do not like other people much, and they would have been likely to stay away from an occupation requiring touching. If, by mistake, they found themselves apprenticed for medicine, they probably backed off or, if not, turned into unsuccessful doctors.

Touching with the naked ear was one of the great advances in the history of medicine. Once it was learned that the heart and lungs made sounds of their own, and that the sounds were sometimes useful for diagnosis, physicians placed an ear over the heart, and over areas on the front and back of the chest, and listened. It is hard to imagine a friendlier human gesture, a more intimate signal of personal concern and affection, than these close bowed heads affixed to the skin. The stethoscope was invented in the nineteenth century, vastly enhancing the acoustics of the thorax, but removing the physician a certain distance from his patient. It was the earliest device of many still to come, one new technology after another, designed to increase that distance.

Today, the doctor can perform a great many of his most essential tasks from his office in another building without ever seeing the patient. Instead of spending forty-five minutes listening to the chest and palpating the abdomen, the doctor can sign a slip which sends the patient off to the department for a CAT scan, with the expectation of seeing within the hour, in exquisite detail, all the body's internal organs which he formerly had to make guesses about with his fingers and ears.

The doctor can set himself, if he likes, at a distance, remote from the patient and the family, never touching anyone beyond a perfunctory handshake as the first and only contact. Medicine is no longer the laying on of hands, it is more like the reading of signals from machines.

Excerpted from The Youngest Science
by Dr. Lewis Thomas

Reiki: Healing Through Energy Transfer. Reiki is a hands-on healing art based on the belief that there is a Universal Life Energy, present everywhere. When channeled properly, this energy promotes healing. The method was discovered—or, perhaps more accurately, rediscovered—by a Japanese theologian in the mid-1800s. While searching for an understanding of touch healing, Dr. Mikao Usui came upon some ancient Sanskrit manuscripts. Within the texts he found the principles for what later became the art of Reiki. The name, bestowed by Dr. Usui, and pronounced *ray-key*, is from the Japanese words *rei*, meaning universal, and *ki*, meaning vital force.

Relieving Congestion. According to practitioners, Reiki works to relieve energy blockages in the body, whether caused by physical, emotional, or spiritual ills. Practitioners believe that their healing method can help relieve a range of ailments, from arthritis to stress. Of course the treatment is not recommended for broken bones, acute pain, or other conditions requiring immediate medical attention.

When a Reiki healer is trained, he or she is initiated with a series of *attunements*. This process consists of the instructor, or Reiki Master, tracing ancient energizing symbols on the person's head, and then on 12 other places along the body, known in Ayurvedic medicine as *chakra*.

The therapeutic effect of Reiki is not dependent on how the hands are held or on the skills of the Reiki practitioner; what is important is the transfer of energy from one being to another. In every case, the flow of vibrations or radiant energy is reciprocal, with the practitioner and client each giving and receiving. During a healing session, the client may feel warmth from the practitioner's hands, tingling, or a sense of relaxation.

Reiki practitioners do not offer a scientific explanation of how their treatments work. But there is general agreement that one must learn this healing art through a Reiki Master. In seminars taught by Reiki Masters, students practice on one another and also learn to project life energy.

What Do Auras Reveal? According to some practitioners, we all radiate luminous energy fields that create colorful auras around our bodies. Most scientists and medical professionals doubt their existence, but for believers, auras are the outward manifestation of our mental, physical, and emotional condition.

Believers claim that changes in the character and color of our auras reflect changes in mood, energy level, or health. For this reason, some practitioners use them as a guide to diagnosis and treatment. For example, pink or white auras may denote happiness and good health, while certain shades of red may indicate suppressed anger; and gray or brown could signal an emotional or physical problem. According to Barbara Ann Brennan, author of *Hands of Light*, a person who abuses alcohol or drugs will have a dirty green aura. ❏

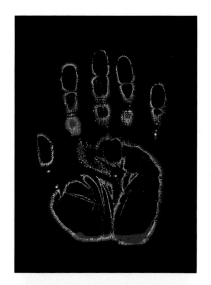

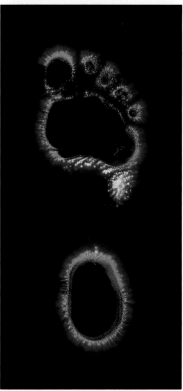

The "camera" used to take these Kirlian photographs was an electric current applied to a special photographic plate on which this hand and foot rested. While dismissed by many scientists, Kirlian photography is claimed to record the auras of living things.

Meditation East and West

Practitioners claim that meditation lets them tap into deeper levels of awareness, and enhances their daily lives. Many meditators speak of richer sensory experiences, greater alertness, and increased mental efficiency.

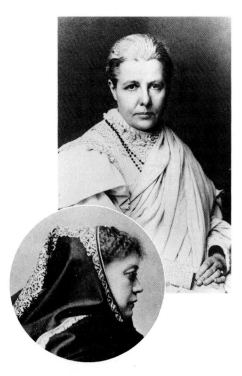

Western Pioneers of Eastern Wisdom

Helena Petrovna Blavatsky (inset) and Annie Besant (above) helped to introduce meditation and Eastern philosophy to the West through their work in the Theosophical Society. Founded in 1875, one of the Society's aims was to promote the brotherhood of humankind through an understanding of philosophy, science, and religion.

MANY PEOPLE TROUBLED by the stresses of modern life and disillusioned by materialism have turned to age-old methods of meditation to help them cope with anxiety and seek a deeper understanding of life. The concept is elusive to many of us. Meditation is not a logical process of thinking about a problem and solving it, as popular usage suggests; nor is it daydreaming, another common misperception.

To serious practitioners, meditation is a mental exercise aimed at training the mind itself. Buddhists, who have used meditation for centuries to find inner peace, have an apt saying: "An untrained mind is like a drunken monkey stung by a bee." Psychologist Robert Ornstein describes it as "a technique for turning down . . . conscious thought . . . so that more subtle sources of information can be perceived."

Meditation takes many forms, but four elements are common to most systems. First, one must find a quiet environment, in order to avoid mundane distractions. Second, a formal posture, usually a comfortably erect sitting position that keeps you relaxed yet alert.

Third, an object to focus upon. Meditation has been defined as anything "that keeps the attention pleasantly anchored in the present moment." You may focus on an object, or on a sound, word, or phrase, repeated either silently or aloud. Zen monks often ponder an unanswerable question, such as, "What is the sound of one hand clapping?" Known as a *koan*, this is not a test of logic but a device to free you from the limits of rational thought. Your focus may also be on an action, or on your own breathing.

The fourth element is a passive, receptive attitude. Concentration is not forced; if your mind wanders, you simply remind yourself to come back into focus. Saint Francis of Assisi compared the wayward thoughts that distracted Christian monks during meditation to birds flying about in the air. You can't suppress them entirely, he said, but you can calmly watch them fly by without becoming involved with them and letting them "nest in your hair."

The Ancient Roots of Meditation. Meditation has been practiced since ancient times in many parts of the world. Some early peoples probably used meditation in magical ceremonies: a shaman would meditate when seeking guidance from the spirit world.

More recently, meditation has been an aid to spiritual enlightenment in all the world's great religions, including Christianity and Judaism. But its practice is even more ancient in the Far East than in the West. Yoga, perhaps the most elaborate Eastern system of mental, physical, and spiritual training, began in India long before the Christian era and over the centuries mingled with native traditions in China, Tibet, Japan, and elsewhere. The result of this cross-fertilization has been a great variety of forms of meditation, which play an important part in Eastern cultures. Among the most familiar in the West, besides Yoga, is Zen, as developed by Japanese Buddhists.

Most Oriental traditions of meditation emphasize techniques of mental control, similar to some of the newer approaches to psychotherapy. One story tells of a pupil ask-

"Do less, accomplish more," advises Maharishi Mahesh Yogi, the founder of Transcendental Meditation. As the late summer sun casts a golden halo around him, the Maharishi enjoys a moment of silence. From the TM headquarters in Holland, he broadcasts his message of world peace: that meditation, not diplomacy or military force, will ease global tensions.

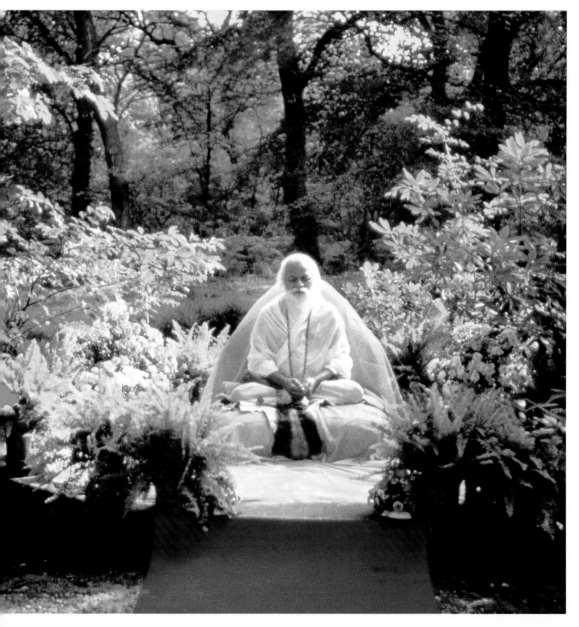

ing his master to explain the ultimate purpose of a Zen exercise. The master wrote one word: "Attention." Still mystified, the student asked more questions. The master simply wrote: "Attention. Attention." The moral, says one practitioner, is that the meaning of life can be found only through a process, not in any text.

Although their methods are usually not as formalized as those of the Zen monks or other practitioners, artists and poets have often used meditation techniques to open their minds to inspiration. William Wordsworth, for instance, wrote of his search for a "happy stillness of the mind."

The Rewards of Meditation. Meditation has a wide range of benefits. The physiological effects have been documented by scientific studies of Indian yogis, Zen monks, and other practitioners of meditation. The mechanism that produces these changes is not fully understood, but meditation seems to relieve stress and ease tension. The beneficial effects are not caused simply by keeping still; for one thing, the brain-wave patterns recorded during meditation have been shown to differ from those seen during sleep.

Among the other reactions observed are lowered oxygen consumption and heart rate and, after habitual practice, a drop in blood pressure. Physicians treating people with mild hypertension have recommended meditation (combined with dietary and other changes) before they prescribe drugs.

Meditation has been shown to decrease the levels of lactic acid in the blood. And because lactic acid is thought to be associated with anxiety, this effect is of paramount importance for most people. Indeed, some psychotherapists now use meditation to help patients deal with emotionally charged issues.

Over the years, even those seeking practical benefits have cherished the spiritual rewards of meditation. Many people say that during meditation they reach a mystical sense of oneness with God or with the universe. And although we think of mystics as dreamy and otherworldly, many spiritual sages emphasize that their ultimate aim is not isolation but greater involvement with others.

Paths to Inner Change. If you decide to try meditation, you may want to experiment with different methods in order to find one that best suits your personality and goals. The choice is wide. Meditation methods can be divided into two basic types: those that emphasize focusing on an object, and those that attempt to "empty the mind" in order to make it more accessible to new perceptions.

Lawrence LeShan, a psychotherapist who has studied meditation extensively, identifies four paths to meditation. The two that are most familiar to Westerners are the paths through the in-

Tips for Meditation and Relaxation

Most forms of meditation and relaxation require certain procedures for achieving thorough repose. The following basic elements may help you reach your goals.

- Isolated environment. Eliminate as many distractions as you can.
- Focused attention. Concentrate on a word, picture, or sound.
- Passive attitude. Don't try to make it happen.
- Comfortable position. Free yourself of tension. Wear loose clothing.
- Regular practice.

You can overdo deep relaxation exercises to the point of becoming lethargic or withdrawn. Be wary of using them in situations that require quick action.

Psychoanalyst Carl Jung was fascinated with elements of Eastern religion, particularly the mandalas, *or sacred circles. He believed that if he drew versions of these ancient symbols his designs would reveal ideas and traits hidden deep in his unconscious.*

Buddhists often use mandalas *to focus their concentration during meditation. A common* mandala *configuration is a spiraling circle protected by a square with four points, and enclosed within a larger circle. The 18th-century design from Tibet, shown below, illustrates the ideal spiritual state. The Buddhas and female counterparts in the inner circle are painted in colors corresponding to the elements. Seated in the clouds is the Buddha Vajrasattva, representing perfection and purity of the mind.*

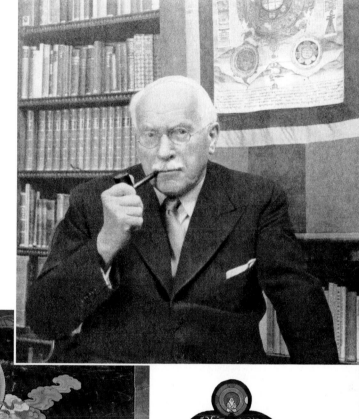

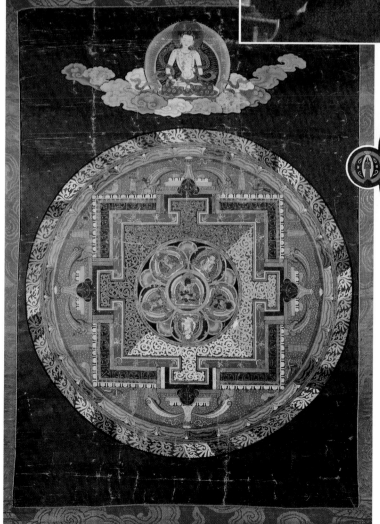

Jung drew *the vivid colors and geometric designs in this* mandala *to illustrate aspects of the creative and life force; the "masculine and feminine souls" are at the four exterior points.*

tellect (tapping different levels of awareness) and the emotions (meditations focused on feelings such as love).

The third, the path through the body, involves total absorption in bodily movements, such as is practiced in Hatha Yoga and T'ai Chi exercises. The fourth, the path of action, applies the principles of meditation to learning a skill or performing a task. Zen masters use this approach in teaching flower arranging or archery, for example. German philosopher Eugen Herrigel apprenticed himself to a Japanese master of archery, and describes his journey toward a state in which he was concerned not with hitting the target, but, in a sense, with becoming one with it, "simultaneously the aimer and the aim, the hitter and the hit."

The path of action can also mean simply going through everyday activities with total concentration. Unmon, a Zen master, urged: "If you walk, just walk. If you sit, just sit. But whatever you do, don't wobble."

Although you can probably learn some techniques, such as simple breathing exercises, by yourself, many experts advise that you find a teacher to guide you in the discipline you choose. But the aim of meditation is self-fulfillment and it is well to remember that a teacher who requires uncritical obedience is probably best avoided.

Once you choose a meditation program, stay with it. Usually at least 20 minutes a day are recommended, and, as in learning a sport, mastery may take months or years of practice. But there should be no concern about competition, or undue stress on doing the exercise well. Even people who have devoted much of their lives to meditation do not reach total concentration in each session. Saint Bernard of Clairvaux, a 12th-century monk, asked how often he was fully involved in his meditation, replied, "Oh, how rare the hour and how brief its duration."

Eastern Meditation in a Western Package. Perhaps the best known form of meditation in the West is Transcendental Meditation (TM), which came to prominence in the 1960s when it was espoused by the Beatles and other celebrities. TM's founder, Maharishi Mahesh Yogi, studied physics in his native India before turning to the study of meditation. His methods are an adaptation of an Indian system that traces its roots to sacred Hindu texts first written some three thousand years ago. But the exercises and the underlying philosophy have been simplified to make the program more accessible to Westerners.

TM is relatively easy to learn, requiring only a few short sessions. Its central feature is the chanting of a secret mantra, (a Sanskrit word that traditionally refers to an excerpt from a sacred Hindu text or hymn). A mantra is often a single syllable word, such as "Om," which in Sanskrit has a meaning similar to "the Word" in Christian theology.

Scientific studies have demonstrated physiological benefits from the practice of TM, but they are evidently not unique to this particular technique. Those who become deeply involved in TM, however, profess higher goals—namely enlightenment and world peace. ❑

The Path to Serenity

In the practice of tea, a sanctuary is created where one can take solace in the tranquility of spirit. The utensils are carefully selected, and, like the tearoom and garden path, they are cleaned; the writing of a man of virtue is hung in the *tokonoma* [alcove] and flowers picked that very morning are placed beneath it. The light is natural, but dim and diffused, casting no shadow, and the kettle simmers over the glowing charcoal embers. The setting thus created is conducive to reflection and introspection. Making tea for oneself in such a setting is sublime. Here man, nature and the spirit are brought together through the preparation and drinking of tea.

— Chado, The Japanese
Way of Tea
by Soshitsu Sen

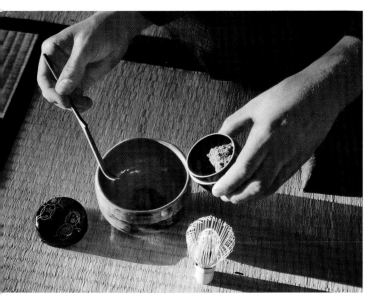

The simple act of placing the tea into a bowl with a bamboo scoop is informed by ancient tradition.

The Choreography of an Ancient Ritual

Tea ceremonies are perfectly orchestrated from the moment the host greets his guests to the final bow of departure. Developed by Zen Buddhists a thousand years ago, the rules of procedure are designed to bring harmony and spiritual tranquility to everyone involved. Each step is precisely ordained, from the simple design of the utensils to the method of preparing the tea. Even conversation is ritualized.

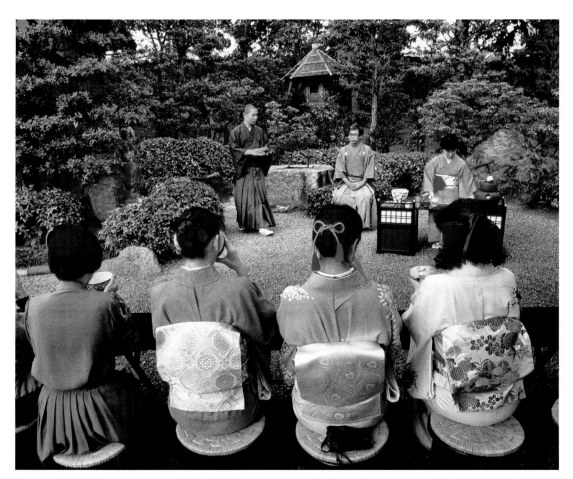

In this Kyoto tea garden, guests and hosts, arrayed in traditional finery, demonstrate the rituals of a formalized tea ceremony. Originally imported from China in the first century A.D., tea gradually assumed spiritual and aesthetic importance in certain Japanese social circles.

The Art and Science of Relaxation

We often tell people under stress to "just relax." Now researchers are discovering just how valid that prescription may be. Relaxation is no longer considered a luxury—it is essential for good health.

MOST OF US THINK OF STRESS as something that is imposed on us from the outside world. Specialists, however, define it differently: it is not simply an event outside ourselves, but our way of reacting to it. The cause of the stress, known as the stressor, may be external, such as a natural disaster or an act of war, or internal, such as a feeling of anger or anxiety. It may be physical (injury or infection), economic (getting fired), or emotional (marital problems). It may be a one-time crisis or an ongoing condition.

Whatever the cause, chronic stress has a range of unpleasant effects. It can produce or contribute to muscle strain, fatigue, headaches, ulcers, asthma, back pain, digestive disorders, high blood pressure, and heart-rhythm abnormalities. What's worse, some investigators believe that stress affects immune function, and perhaps is a factor in certain types of cancer.

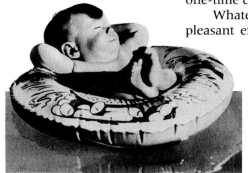

Looking utterly relaxed, *this eight-month-old child seems in little need of biofeedback, meditation, or any other modern-day, stress-reduction technique. However, while we may think of children as being immune to the symptoms of stress and tension that afflict adults, they are not. In fact, even very young children at times show such common signs of stress as sweaty palms and pounding hearts. Fortunately, for young and old alike, a quiet float aboard an inner tube can offer a relaxing way of dealing with an overdose of stress.*

In a well-known study, Drs. Thomas H. Holmes and Richard H. Rahe of the University of Washington drew up a scale of stressful events that appeared to make people more susceptible to illness. The death of a spouse was found to be the most traumatic. But the severity of the reaction to most events varied from culture to culture. For instance, a jail sentence rated second for the Japanese, but only fourth for Americans.

Some researchers believe, moreover, that such everyday hassles as traffic jams, noise, or family conflict may, over time, be even more harmful than sudden disasters. And one person's trauma—a job interview or a parachute jump—may be another's exciting challenge. In fact, while the University of Washington study found that many people fell sick after a major life change, it also found that many (about 30 percent) did not.

Fight or Flight. Whether your stress comes from an overload of major stressors or a chronic over-reaction to relatively minor ones, its immediate effects may include: rapid breathing, racing pulse, sweaty palms, nausea, and tension. In his landmark book *The Wisdom of the Body,* Harvard physiologist Walter B. Cannon described these and other related physiological reactions as the "fight-or-flight" response.

This response evolved in animals and humans living in the wild to help them cope with emergencies—such as fending off or fleeing from predators. It creates a powerful range of effects by activating the sympathetic nervous system, increasing the heart rate, dilating the pupils to let in more light, and arousing and energizing the body.

The fight-or-flight response was vital to our ancestors

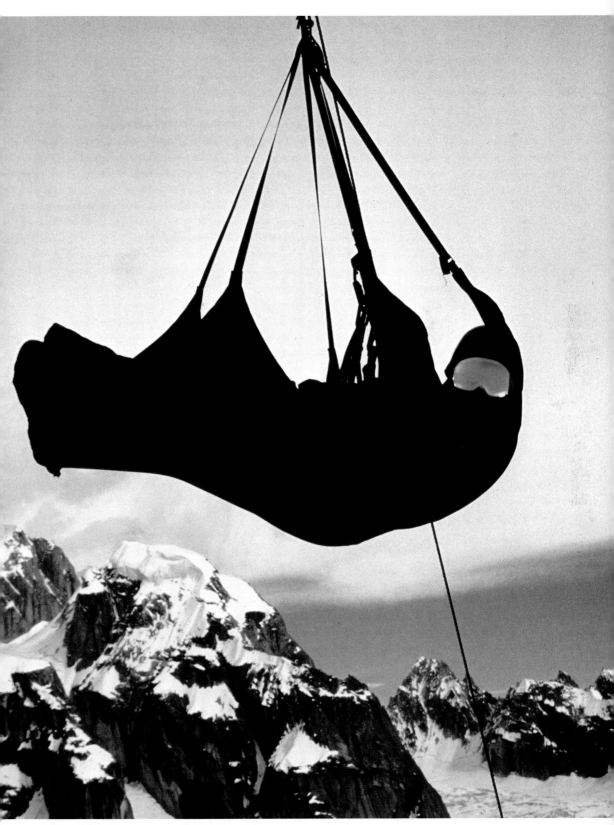

Hanging loose. *Most of us would have trouble sleeping in a hammock suspended thousands of feet above a snow-covered precipice. But not so this climber on Alaska's Mount Barrille. To counteract altitude-induced insomnia, he wears special goggles that bathe his eyes in a blue light, and he relaxes to the recorded sounds of a waterfall.*

in the wild, when quick reactions could save them from a marauding tiger or a falling tree. It can still help a pedestrian dodge a speeding car, or a cop chasing a thief. But more often it is triggered by psychological rather than physical stressors, and the subsequent reactions are often inappropriate, or even harmful. We may not even have a full fight-or-flight response every time something disturbing happens; instead we control our reaction to stress by tensing our muscles or grinding our teeth, thereby producing another set of symptoms. The result is fatigue, muscle tension, and any number of physical and mental ills.

Managing Stress with Relaxation. Just as we have an innate stress response, we also have the ability to relax. So whatever the level of stress in your life, you can gain some control over it. It may be within your power to lessen emotional strain, ease neck or back pain, deal with a variety of psychosomatic complaints, and perhaps even reduce your risk of heart attack or stroke. As science writer Daniel Goleman puts it, "Though you may not be able to stress-proof your life, you can stress-guard your mind and body."

Of course, symptoms of heart disease, cancer, or other serious diseases call for consultation with your doctor. But if you are concerned about ordinary, everyday stress, some simple tips may be of help. Start by making a list of things or situations that you find particularly stressful. If possible, avoid them. Make every effort to have relaxing sit-down meals, rather than grabbing food on the run. Many people find relief by cutting out unhealthy foods or cutting back on caffeine and alcohol. And since resentment and hostility

Have you ever noticed how a baby's abdomen rises and falls with each breath? If you're like most adults, you probably only fill your upper chest when you breathe, so you're missing some of the benefits of deep, natural breathing: increased oxygen intake, reduced tension, and improved mental alertness.

Shallow, improper breathing pushes the chest out.

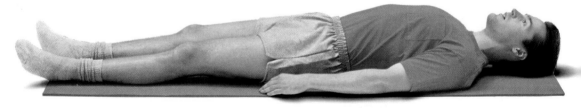

Deep, natural breathing from the diaphragm expands the abdomen.

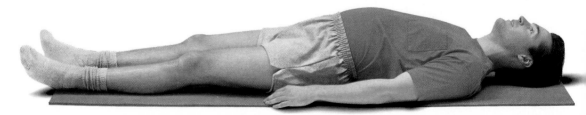

contribute to stress, try to work out conflicts with others before you reach the boiling point.

In addition, some simple relaxation aids may be helpful. Many experts recommend deep breathing or warm baths (preferable to hot baths, which can sap your energy). Relax with a hobby or exercise: playing or listening to music, reading, knitting, carpentry, handicrafts, dancing, or sports that don't produce too much competitive tension. If you feel drained in the middle of the afternoon, take a brisk ten-minute walk instead of gobbling a candy bar. The sugar may give you a quick burst of energy, but exercise will help you feel more energized and more relaxed for far longer.

The Relaxation Response. Harvard cardiologist Herbert Benson coined the term Relaxation Response in his popular 1975 book of the same name. In the book Benson analyzes the effects of various relaxation methods. While Western researchers have recently rediscovered the relaxation response, it has long formed the basis of many meditation traditions. "We claim no innovation," Benson writes, "but simply a scientific validation of age-old wisdom."

Benson began studying stress because of its apparent role in high blood pressure and heart disease. He reasoned that if the fight-or-flight response raised the heart rate and the blood pressure, then the opposite response (relaxing) could lower them.

Inspired by reports that yogis and Zen masters could control heart rate and other bodily functions that had long been considered involuntary, he tried to produce the same effects by using their methods. His earliest relaxation subjects used Transcendental Meditation (TM), in which the practitioner silently repeats a single word or phrase called a mantra. The results were impressive, and further research confirmed that other techniques can induce the same response.

In the relaxation method now used in Benson's laboratory, patients sit in a comfortable position, maintain a passive attitude, and focus on a repeated word or phrase. To avoid the mystical associations of TM, Benson originally suggested focusing on a neutral word or meaningless syllable, but later found the method even more effective if each individual chose an inspirational phrase or prayer.

Benson believes that the method can be used to enhance intellectual and creative abilities. As outlined in his book *Your Maximum Mind,* this is a two-step process: first use the relaxation response to open yourself to new ideas, then "re-program" your mind by meditating on a saying or observation related to the area in which you hope to excel.

Taking a Deep Breath

You can improve your breathing technique with simple exercises such as this one.

- Sit upright or lie supine in a relaxed position with your spine straight.
- Breathe in slowly through your nose and imagine that you are pushing that air deep into your abdomen.
- Note how your abdomen expands and rises as the lungs fill with air.
- Breathe out slowly through your nose, contracting your abdominal muscles to press the diaphragm up and push the air out of your lungs.
- Continue breathing in this way, watching how your abdomen rises and falls.

A stimulating variation:

- Inhale, following the technique described above. Hold that breath a few seconds.
- Pretend you have a straw between your lips, and blow out a small amount of air with force. Then pause.
- Continue to blow small bursts of air until you have exhaled completely.

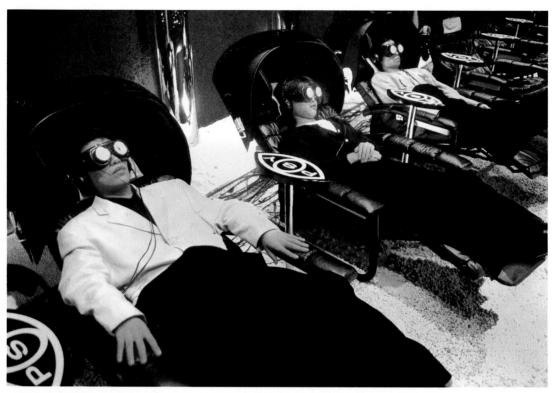

Overworked and strung out,
*stressed Japanese businessmen drop
in to the Brain Mind Gym in Tokyo
for a quick mental pick-me-up. After
stretching out on reclining chairs,
clients don special goggles and
headphones that emit pulses of light
and sound that are said to alter
brain waves, inducing deep
relaxation comfortably and quickly.*

Tanks for Relaxation. "Imagine yourself floating in a dark, virtually soundproof capsule. . . .floating as effortlessly as a child's bath toy. . .floating on water that feels neither warm nor cold." That's how some describe their experience in a relaxation tank.

These tanks, also known as isolation tanks, were developed to investigate sensory deprivation. In the 1950s and earlier, sensory deprivation was considered a form of torture, and was allegedly used to brainwash prisoners of war in Korea. At that time, many scientists believed that environmental stimulation was essential to human consciousness. Without it, the brain would "go to sleep."

But Dr. John C. Lilly, a neurophysiologist at the National Institute of Mental Health, thought otherwise. He believed that in the absence of external stimuli the human brain would maintain consciousness by producing its own stimulation. To test his theory, Lilly immersed himself in a dark, soundproof water tank. While inside, he reported feeling a state of profound relaxation, and, as he described it, "richly elaborate states of inner experience."

Lilly's work has always been eyed rather suspiciously (he was an early experimenter with LSD), but later researchers drew on his findings to perfect the flotation ("wet") tanks and isolation ("dry") chambers that are becoming increasingly popular as tools for recreation and therapy. The therapeutic technique is called *REST* (Restricted Environmental Stimulation Therapy), a term that is preferred to "isolation" or "sensory deprivation" because, as one who has tried it writes, "There *is* no such thing as sensory deprivation."

The Floating Experience. The typical flotation tank is a dark, virtually soundproof capsule or room containing a ten-inch-deep pool of water. The water is saturated with Epsom salts so that it is very dense, and is kept at exactly the same temperature as your skin—93.5°F (34°C)—so it feels neither warm nor cold.

A session in the tank usually lasts from half an hour to two hours, but you can open the tank from inside if you want to get out before your scheduled time is up. Once inside, you may feel some anxiety at first, but in a few minutes you will probably become deeply relaxed.

Studies show that floating may help lower blood pressure, decrease muscle tension, and produce other physiological changes associated with the relaxation response. In all likelihood, the lack of external stimulation will turn your attention inward. You may find yourself focusing on your heartbeat or your breathing. Or you may feel so weightless and disembodied that you register only fleeting thoughts, emotions, or images. In time, you may be able to think more calmly about troublesome problems or to direct yourself toward a desired goal. And you will probably be more open to outside suggestions; some tanks are equipped to pipe in music, taped messages, or a therapist's coaching.

Some advocates say that the relaxed state reached in a tank may be deeper than with meditation. The tank is also easier to use, needing no effort or training. It seems particularly beneficial to people who have never experienced total relaxation and do not know how it feels *not* to be tense.

Many people who have been in flotation tanks are most enthusiastic about the after-effects. When they come out, they say that their senses are sharper, they are joyfully aware of all that they see, hear, or smell, and their tensions have eased. The effects of a single session may last for several days or weeks.

"Dry" Tanks. Relaxing in a "dry" tank is similar to floating, with a few differences. You generally lie on a waterbed-like mattress (that conforms to your body shape), which is enclosed in a lightproof, soundproof chamber. In some, you can get up, move around, eat, and use a private toilet. For those who are prone to claustrophobia or anxiety, the dry tank may be less threatening than a wet tank. And perhaps because one can stay in such a tank longer without becoming uncomfortable—as long as 24 to 48 hours—it seems to help more in programs aimed at changing behavior or breaking addictions such as smoking. Floating seems to be better for general relaxation. ❏

Afloat on a sea of heavily salted water, a person relaxing in a flotation tank may drift effortlessly into a tension-free state. In fact, flotation tanks may be helpful to people who have never learned to truly relax. Shut off from the sights and sounds that normally assault the senses, many tank users emerge with a heightened appreciation for the world around them.

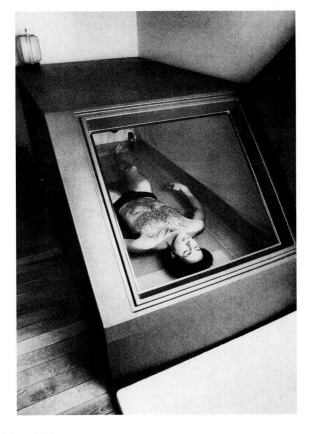

Time Out for Relaxation

The workplace can be a major source of stress and physical tension. But you don't have to stretch out on a gym mat to untie your knotty muscles. You can relax and defuse office stress without leaving your desk.

THE PHONE RINGS, jangling your nerves and interrupting work on a long overdue report. Tension has gradually pulled your shoulders up to your ears. Your eyes ache from staring at a flickering computer screen. You slump down a little further into your usual afternoon slouch, compressing your spine and squeezing hundreds of tiny nerves.

In general, office workers don't face the occupational hazards of, say, deep-sea divers, but every job has its own risks.

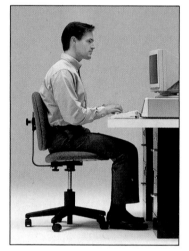

Start in a neutral position.
Your arms and legs should bend at 90° angles when you are seated. Adjust the backrest or use a cushion to support your lower back.

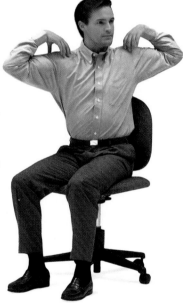

Upper-Back Stretch.
Place your hands on your shoulders and twist at the waist until you feel a stretch across your upper back. Return to center and twist the other way.

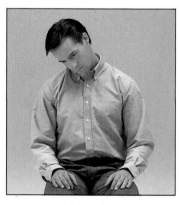
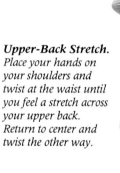

Neck Roll. *Slowly drop your head to the left and then to the right. Now drop it to your chest. Next, lift your chin as high as you can. From this position, roll your head all the way to the left. Come back to center and roll your head all the way to the right.*

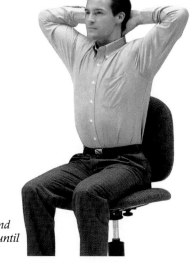

Chest Stretch. *Grasp your arms behind your neck and press your elbows back until you feel a pull across your chest.*

Long hours of sitting, deadline pressure, uncomfortable furniture, and poor posture can lead to chronic ailments.

You can prevent your office from becoming a torture chamber with a few adjustments. Position your chair at a height and distance from your desk that gives you easy access to your work surface without leaning forward. If you use a computer, adjust the screen so that you look directly at it. Turning down your office lights, or placing a hood above the terminal to shade the screen may cut down on screen glare. Frequently stand up, stretch, and walk around during the day to release tension and increase your blood flow. In addition, you can use the special "deskercises" described here to relax specific areas of tension and help you stay alert through a long stressful day at the office. ❏

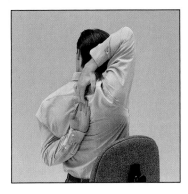

Shoulder Stretch. *Reach over your right shoulder with your right hand and from below with your left. Try to link your fingers. Repeat on the other side.*

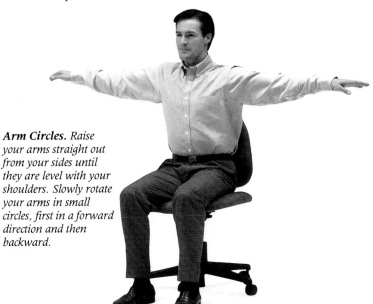

Arm Circles. *Raise your arms straight out from your sides until they are level with your shoulders. Slowly rotate your arms in small circles, first in a forward direction and then backward.*

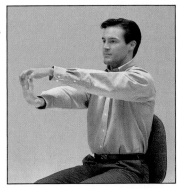

Wrist Twist. *Extend one arm in front of you. Use the other hand to bend the outstretched fingers up and back. Repeat with the opposite hand.*

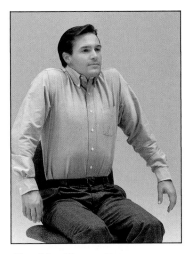

Shoulder Shrugs. *Rotate your shoulders five times in one direction, using their full range of motion. Make your rotations smooth and slow. Reverse direction.*

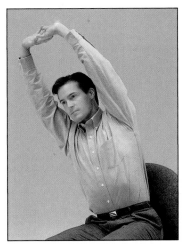

Side Stretch. *Lock your fingers and lift your arms over your head until your elbows are straight. Slowly lean to the left, then to the right.*

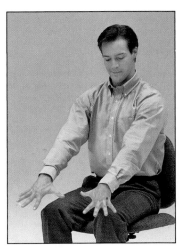

Finger Flex. *With your hands in front of you, palms down, spread your thumbs and fingers as far apart as you can. Hold for the count of five and relax.*

Biofeedback and Visualization

*The self-awareness and control to be gained through biofeedback
can be helpful in a wide variety of ills. It is a powerful technique best
learned from experts—and practiced with a specific goal in mind.*

A RELAXATION METHOD that uses state-of-the-art technology, biofeedback was developed in the 1960s by workers in fields as varied as experimental psychology and rehabilitative medicine. The term "feedback" was borrowed from electronics: in a feedback loop, information about a particular part of a working system is recorded and fed back into the system in order to adjust its operation. For example, a thermostat registers the temperature of a room, then sends a signal to turn a heater on or off until a certain temperature is reached.

In biofeedback, sensors measure muscle tension, skin temperature, or other body processes. The readings are then amplified and translated into signals that you can see or hear—or both. For example, electrodes may be placed over muscles, and you then "hear" the electrical activity through earphones; the tones you hear may vary from a low hum when your muscles are relaxed to a high whine when they are tense. A moving needle on a meter or a pattern on a screen may give you the same infor-

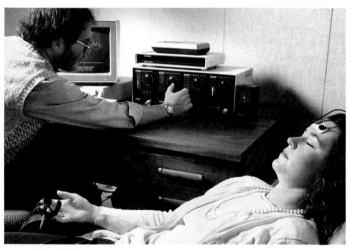

Using biofeedback, this "stressed out" woman is monitoring fluctuations in her skin temperature, and is measuring the degree of muscle tension on her temples. Eventually, as she learns to control "involuntary" responses to stress, she may be able to ease her symptoms without using biofeedback equipment.

mation visually. As you become accustomed to sensing certain of your body's processes, you can gradually gain some control over them.

A Quick Reading. Biofeedback is often used along with relaxation exercises, and proponents of the technique say that it enhances and speeds up the effects of relaxation because it lets you monitor your progress. It works best when the feedback is continuous and as nearly instantaneous as possible. Trying to control body processes, one researcher says, can be like trying to hit a dartboard while blindfolded. Biofeedback, in effect, removes the blindfold and lets you improve your performance by showing you the effect of each of your movements or thoughts. The aim is to put you in charge of your own body. As biofeedback researcher Barbara Brown, Ph.D., puts it, "The patient is no longer the object of the treatment, the patient *is* the treatment."

Methods of Biofeedback. A common technique of biofeedback uses an electromyograph (EMG). This device measures electrical activity in the muscles, and has been used to help rehabilitate patients paralyzed by stroke. Even when a person has no sensation in a paralyzed limb and cannot move it voluntarily, EMG can often detect some electrical activity in the muscles. The EMG machine amplifies the electrical sound emitting from the paralyzed limb, and as the patient becomes aware of the activity, his nervous system may stimulate more muscle activity. Eventually, new nerve endings may grow in the affected muscles and the patient may regain some mobility.

More often, EMG is used to promote relaxation in muscles that have become tense in response to stress. During treatment, sensors are placed over muscles in the forehead, back, neck, or jaw in an effort to relieve tension headache, backache, neck pain, and bruxism (unconscious grinding of the teeth). This method is also used in treating such stress-related diseases as asthma and ulcers.

Temperature Biofeedback. This device monitors skin temperature and can be helpful in certain circulatory disorders. For example, Raynaud's disease causes blood vessels to suddenly narrow upon exposure to cold or from an overload of stress, cutting off blood flow to the fingers and toes. By attaching skin-temperature sensors to the extremities, patients can learn to increase blood flow to these areas. This method may also reduce the frequency of migraine headaches, and is also used to promote relaxation.

Electrodermal Response (EDR). This biofeedback device measures electrical conductance in the skin, which is associated with activity of the sweat glands. Also known as GSR (galvanic skin response), this method (along with other techniques and devices) is used in lie detection tests. But EDR is also thought to be helpful, in combination with other therapies, in treating certain phobias, anxiety, excessive sweating, and, at times, stuttering.

Athletes, too, have used EDR in an effort to improve per-

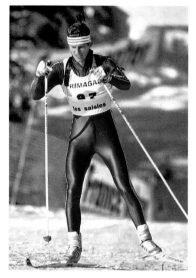

The biathalon competition pairs cross-country skiing and rifle marksmanship. Probably derived from European military training, this event demands extraordinary mental and physical control. During a race, trained athletes are able to control their heart rates so as to be calm enough and steady enough for the shooting events that are scheduled at numerous points along the course.

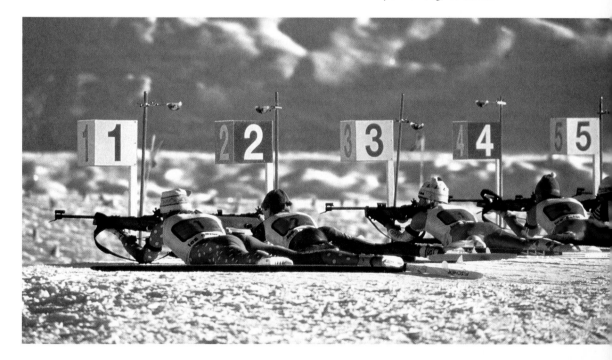

formance. Anxiety and pre-game jitters can work both for and against an athlete. While it is important to be "up" for a game, extreme anxiety can result in energy loss and may also affect concentration. By using EDR athletes try to fine-tune their level of anticipation. For instance, since the machine responds to perspiration (a common reaction to anxiety), an athlete who tends to get overly stressed before a competition might use the device to monitor anxiety, and thereby achieve the degree of calmness necessary for peak performance.

CASE HISTORY

COMBINING THERAPIES TO EASE PAIN

Biofeedback is not a medical treatment, but a learning process that helps patients develop their ability to elicit relief from symptoms. When combined with visualization, the results can be impressive.

Ellen, an overweight forty-five year-old woman, was suffering from vague, but nagging pain and other symptoms of stress. When standard medical treatment failed to relieve her distress, she turned to biofeedback in the hope of gaining some control over her body.

On Ellen's first visit to the biofeedback laboratory, the technician placed a temperature sensor on her middle finger; other sensors placed on the back of her hand and on her forehead would detect muscle tension. The temperature of the patient's hand is an indication of muscle tension, and Ellen's initial reading was 76 degrees. Since she was doing biofeedback in an effort to control stress, Ellen was instructed to relax, which would in turn dilate her blood vessels, raising the temperature of her hand.

Curiously, though she expressed an understanding of the exercise, the temperature in her hand dropped rather than rose, indicating increased muscle tension and anxiety. Her therapist, who was standing by to assist, gently urged Ellen not to try so hard — in essence her body was energizing itself for the difficult task of relaxing. He also suggested that she try visualizing something soothing — a walk on the beach, a stroll through the woods, any scenario with pleasant, relaxing connotations for the patient.

Following his advice, Ellen evoked memories of a time when her body was free of pain, and within minutes her hand temperature began to increase. Fifteen minutes later, it had jumped to almost 90 degrees.

Ellen learned two important lessons from her results. The first was that she could gain mastery over her body; and secondly, she couldn't make it happen, instead she had to let it happen. And in this case, visualization helped her break free of self-defeating thought patterns.

Even such a small success can offer a patient a tremendous boost, and throughout the rest of the biofeedback session, Ellen progressed rapidly. Keeping her mind focused on pleasant scenes, she steadily grew more relaxed.

In the last part of the session, Ellen talked with her therapist about her marriage and children, and her increasing fears about her health. As their conversation progressed, her hand temperature dropped. But with the machine recording her body's response to emotional stress, Ellen was able to see how muscle tension could produce pain.

In the next few weeks, Ellen found that a combination of biofeedback, visualization, and counseling was remarkably effective in relieving her pain and other symptoms of emotional distress.

Electroencephalograph Biofeedback (EEG). This device monitors brain-wave activity. The method is relatively imprecise, since the brain emits many electrical signals of various frequencies, only a few of which have been directly tied to specific disorders or mental states. For instance, alpha brain waves are commonly observed during relaxation. So early biofeedback researchers thought if patients could learn to increase their alpha-wave activity, they could find relief from anxiety, insomnia, and perhaps epilepsy. But further research concluded that alpha training is only useful when combined with other therapies. In newer devices, insomniacs are taught to control theta waves, and epileptics have found some relief by monitoring waves produced during seizures. As the technology advances, it may be used for other neurological diseases.

Other biofeedback devices monitor blood pressure and heartbeat to help patients control hypertension and arrythmias. And there is some optimism that biofeedback can do even more. Indeed, says Barbara Brown, "Any body function that can be measured fairly precisely and fairly continuously can be trained to come under voluntary control."

Home Practice. Biofeedback is usually taught in a professional facility by a therapist who provides advice and encouragement, along with technical expertise. But once you have learned to monitor and control your symptoms, you can sometimes attain the same results without equipment. For example, in stressful situations, you may be able to relax tense facial muscles, and so prevent a tension headache.

Hand-held, do-it-yourself biofeedback devices may even let you do some of the learning on your own. Experts warn, however, that the home equipment sold commercially varies widely in quality and price, and may not be as accurate as the instruments used by professionals. Before investing in any equipment, it is best to get professional advice. And it would make sense to talk with one or more satisfied users.

Limitations and Dangers. Biofeedback is not for everyone. As with other treatments, medical consultation is essential if you have any serious symptoms or chronic diseases. For example, biofeedback can be dangerous for diabetics and others with endocrine disorders, as it can change the need for insulin and other medications. Nor will biofeedback magically erase stress—it is best to remember that it takes time and effort to achieve the desired results.

A yogi's self-control can seem superhuman at times, as in the case of this man who appears to be quite comfortable sitting on a bed of nails. His secret? A mantra that focuses his meditative powers, perhaps distracting him from the pain. With the advent of biofeedback and other scientific gadgetry, yoga practitioners demonstrated that it was possible to control involuntary functions of the body. On an expedition to India, biofeedback experts Elmer and Alyce Green also studied yogis who could regulate their nervous systems and metabolic rates.

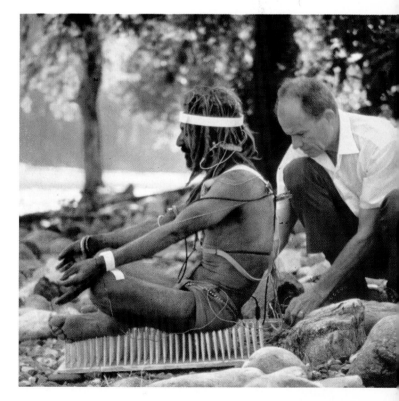

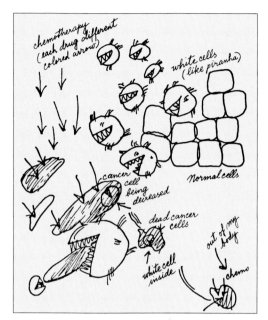

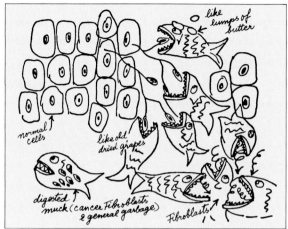

Visualization exercises *have been used to help cancer patients express their feelings about their illness. At the Simonton Cancer Center in Dallas, Texas, radiation oncologist Carl Simonton reinforces standard medical treatment with visualization exercises and other techniques. While undergoing chemotherapy for breast cancer, Betty, a patient at the Center, was asked to visualize her disease. Her first drawing (top left) showed fierce-looking white blood cells tearing into cancer cells, reflecting both her anger at being sick as well as her determination to get well. Six months later, Betty had come to terms with her anger, and in her drawing (top right) the cancer-fighting cells are still highly effective but appear less ferocious. According to Simonton, the wide eyes on the cancer-gobbling fish indicate alertness and purposeful direction, which he considers positive signs for healing.*

Visualization. Dreams, daydreams, and memories are all forms of mental imagery or visualization that provide healthy outlets for our imaginations. Recently, experts have found ways of harnessing our imaging abilities to counteract stress. Athletes, too, use visualization to enhance their performance, sometimes without realizing it. A golfer may form a mental map of the fairway, imagining precisely where he will place the ball on each shot; a high jumper may visualize every split second of his approach to and leap over the bar; a baseball pitcher may run a mental film of the ball from the time it leaves his hand until it lands in the catcher's glove.

Healing and Guided Imagery. Some of the newest and perhaps most intriguing research on visualization involves the immune system. Hans Selye found that stress depressed the body's immune response; other researchers have tried to reverse this effect, using relaxation and visualization exercises in an effort to boost immunity. A number of cancer specialists are experimenting with a similar approach against cancer.

Most visualization techniques begin with relaxation, followed by summoning up a mental image. In one simple exercise known as palming, you close your eyes, cover them with your palms, and concentrate on the color black. Try to make the color fill your whole visual field, screening out any distracting images. To reduce stress, try concentrating first on a color you associate with tension, and then mentally replace it with one that you find soothing—red changing to blue, perhaps. Or you may find it more relaxing to picture a peaceful natural scene, such as the unruffled surface of a pond, or gently rolling hills.

In a technique called guided imagery, participants visualize a goal they want to achieve, then imagine themselves going through the process of achieving it. Severely ill patients, for example, are urged to picture their internal organs and imagine them free of disease, or to picture tumors shrinking, or invading microorganisms succumbing to aggressive immune cells.

These visualization exercises have some documented health benefits. A study at Yale demonstrated that patients suffering from severe depression were helped by imagining scenes in which they were praised by people they admired— a clear boost to their self-esteem. But claims of improvements in cancer patients who used guided imagery in combination with orthodox treatment are more controversial.

Visualization and other relaxation methods may produce significant benefits, often by helping to ease pain and lift depression. Research is continuing to determine whether even more spectacular results can be achieved. ❑

PICTURING PERFECTION

Elizabeth Manley, Canada's free-style skating champion and Silver medalist in the 1988 Winter Olympics, reports on her use of visualization to perfect a difficult jump.

"I used a great deal of imagery. In learning the triple Lutz jump, for example, I would stand at the side of the boards, close my eyes, and picture myself doing the jump perfectly in my mind. Nine out of ten times I would successfully do it by preparing this way. Eventually we captured a couple of perfect jumps on videotape. I watched it over and over until it was engraved on my mind. I would actually see in my mind my entire body, the jump, and the landing position. I was then able to take that image onto the ice with me and picture myself doing the jump perfectly before it came time to perform. I would practice my imagery every night before I went to sleep. I think that training ten minutes this way was equivalent to doing a forty-five minute session on the ice. I began practicing mind/body techniques intensely two years prior to the 1988 Olympics. Besides visualization, progressive relaxation and breathing exercises helped calm me down. I believe that mind/body techniques had a lot to do with my success."

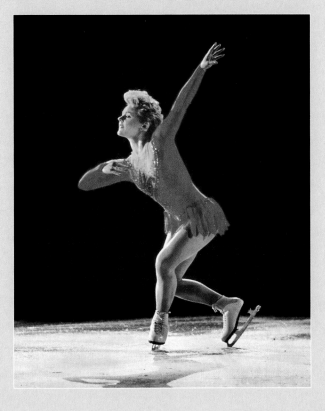

Before she steps on the ice, Manley rehearses a maneuver hundreds of times in her mind.

The Intriguing State of Hypnosis

Once dismissed as trickery, hypnosis has been found to have therapeutic uses, ranging from easing pain to conquering fear. And now, a few simple techniques may also let you benefit from hypnosis on your own.

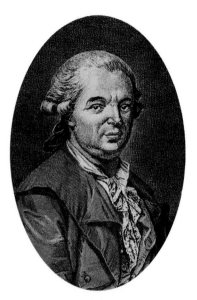

The Mesmerizing Doctor

In the late 18th century, Dr. Franz Mesmer, a charismatic Viennese physician, demonstrated seemingly miraculous cures with what he called "animal magnetism." Convinced that magnetic forces flowing through the body affected health, Mesmer used iron rods, along with soothing words and gestures, to realign the "magnetic fluids" of his patients.

While a scientific commission disproved the magnetism theory, it lent support to the principle that the power of suggestion could influence medical treatment. Mesmer's students and patients continued to cling to the idea of "animal magnetism" for a time, but the foundation for hypnotism had been laid.

NEITHER SLEEP NOR UNCONSCIOUSNESS, hypnosis is a state in which a person has shut out distractions and is free to focus intently on a particular subject, emotion, or memory. Practitioners stress how normal and commonplace the hypnotic state is. Almost everyone, they point out, experiences some form of hypnosis spontaneously—while daydreaming, reading, or even while driving long distances along a superhighway.

Such focused concentration has practical benefits, for while under hypnosis a person is more receptive to suggestions. Because of this, hypnosis has been used successfully to alleviate pain, reduce stress, overcome phobias, and break such habits as cigarette smoking, overeating, and nail-biting. In addition, chronic headache sufferers have found relief without heavy sedatives or painkillers, and people afflicted with allergies and some skin diseases have been helped as well. Often people "feel better" just by knowing that hypnosis can put them in greater control of their lives.

Hypnosis is recognized by the medical establishment; however, physicians caution that patients should get a proper diagnosis before trying it. Anyone suffering from an undiagnosed illness or who simply feels unwell should use hypnosis only under medical supervision because the treatment may mask symptoms of disease.

Easing Chronic Complaints. For those wishing to avoid drugs or surgery for certain chronic ailments, hypnosis may be an appropriate alternative. In particular, eczema and warts have been effectively treated with hypnosis, often in conjunction with counseling and medication. Allergy and asthma sufferers have also found relief using hypnosis, and some have augmented their care by using self-hypnosis to prevent flare-ups.

One recurring fear is that a hypnotist can force a subject to perform immoral, illegal, or dangerous acts. Staunch defenders of hypnotism reject this claim, arguing that the subject can "awaken" at any time and that there is no danger of loss of control. Using the services of a qualified, trained hypnotist, or practicing self-hypnosis are good ways of allaying anxiety about the treatment.

Mass Appeal. Over the years, hypnosis has come in and out of fashion. But paradoxically, as modern medicine becomes more dependent on technology and as patient care has seemed more impersonal, the appeal of hypnosis has grown for some patients. For one thing, hypnosis requires no elaborate equipment. Additionally, there is a one-on-one relationship between practitioner and subject, and the desired state of relaxation and concentration is usually induced in 15 minutes or less.

The vast majority of people can be hypnotized to some degree. The one essential element is a subject's willingness, which may largely depend upon the rapport between hypnotist and patient. Intelligent people tend to be the best subjects, and children, because they are highly suggestible, are also hypnotized fairly easily.

What You Can Expect. During a session, the hypnotist will probably ask you to concentrate on an object or on the sound of his voice. As he guides you into a state of relaxation, he will likely use permissive messages, not commands: "You may find your eyelids becoming heavy. It is all right to let your eyes close." Or the hypnotist may ask you to count backward from 20 to zero. When under hypnosis, your sense of time can be distorted so that a great deal seems to happen in a very short time.

People vary in their ability to achieve deep hypnosis. Many attain what is called a light stage. When told that their arm may feel heavy, they will have trouble lifting it. When told that their hand is anesthetized, they will feel little or no pain if pinched. A hypnotist can sometimes induce you into a deeper level with suggestions that you are descending an escalator or stairway. In this way you may then be able to achieve total anesthesia, or perhaps control various involuntary body functions like blood pressure and heartbeat.

Hypnosis may be valuable in helping a person recall long-suppressed experiences. It can also be used to help a subject recreate a time when a traumatic event occurred that still causes pain or trouble. Relief may be gained by reliving the experience under safe conditions and seeing it from an adult viewpoint.

Dispelling Fears. One persistent question about hypnosis is: "What if my hypnotist leaves—or dies—while I'm in a deep trance?" In fact, many people worry about never coming out of a hypnotic trance. But the truth is that even if a hypnotist could no longer function or merely had trouble arousing you (a rare problem), you would eventually fall into a natural sleep, and awaken shortly thereafter.

Many people also fear the effects of post-hypnotic suggestions, thinking that an unscrupulous practitioner may induce them to do things that they would never otherwise consider. The only real danger might involve suggestions that have outlived their usefulness but have not been re-

Can You Be Hypnotized?

With a little help from a friend, you can find out whether you are a good candidate for hypnosis. Noticing a correlation between hypnotizability and eye rolling, hypnosis researcher Herbert Speigel designed this simple test.

- Roll your eyes back as far as possible while slowly lowering your lids.
- When your eyes are about half closed, your friend should compare your eyes with those in the pictures below. The greater the amount of white showing, the easier it may be to hypnotize you.

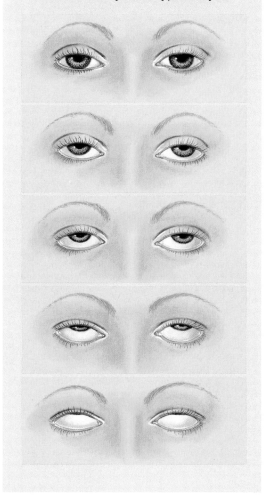

moved. For instance, one researcher anesthetized a helper's hand for a demonstration and forgot that he had done so. While the subject's hand was numb to pain for a day or two, the effect soon wore off, causing no harm. Post-hypnotic suggestion may be most helpful in inducing prolonged relief from post-operative or cancer pain. It can also be beneficial to those suffering acute emotional distress, and has been used successfully with veterans trying to cope with the extreme stress and aftermath of warfare.

Self-Hypnosis. Frequently, people who have successfully used hypnosis in overcoming stress, coping with pain, and alleviating other problems decide to learn to do it themselves. There are several reasons for doing so. Convenience is one. Instead of making regular visits to a hypnotist, some people can achieve the same results at home or at work—whenever or wherever they can find a secluded, comfortable setting.

Another motivation is self-reliance. This can apply to those who turn to hypnosis for relaxation and stress reduction, as well as those who want to break a habit like smoking or overeating. It also applies to those who use it in combination with—or, in some cases, even a substitute for—drug therapy. For instance, several studies of arthritis patients have shown that for some sufferers, hypnosis and self-hypnosis can be as effective as drug therapy. But some experts believe that to effectively reinforce treatment, self-hypnosis must first be

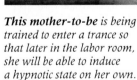

Self-hypnosis has helped many women to relax during labor.

This mother-to-be is being trained to enter a trance so that later in the labor room, she will be able to induce a hypnotic state on her own.

Women who have used self-hypnosis claim it reduces, or even eliminates, labor pains. As a result, little or no anesthesia is needed, and both baby and mother feel more alert.

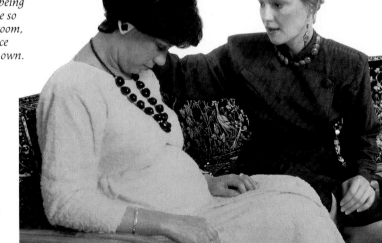

learned from a professional. After that, patients can use the technique at home to control pain or other symptoms.

Basic Techniques. There are a variety of techniques for self-hypnosis, and you may find one more effective than the others. Some people quickly learn self-hypnosis by following written or taped instructions.

All self-hypnosis begins with the subject seated in a comfortable position. You might start by relaxing your muscles and focusing your eyes on an object, a spot on the wall, or a flickering candle. As your eyes become fixated on the object, you might suggest to yourself that your eyelids are getting heavier or are blinking. Breathe deeply several times and exhale with a sigh. As you feel your eyes closing, utter a phrase such as "relax now." Alternately, you could mention your favorite color or a beautiful sight. As your eyes shut, repeat the word or words slowly. The goal is to induce hypnosis with the phrase alone—but this takes practice.

When your eyes have closed, begin relaxing your body, one muscle group at a time. Start with your forearms and biceps. Tense them, then let them relax completely. Use the same method of alternately tightening and relaxing muscles in your face, neck, shoulder, chest, stomach, lower back, buttocks, thighs, calves, and toes. As your muscles begin to relax, you should notice a heavy or wooden feeling in them.

Descending the Stairs. You might next try adding mental exercises to deepen hypnosis, like counting backward or imagining yourself descending a staircase. To confirm that you are "under," suggest to yourself that your hand is becoming numb, then pinch it hard. You should feel some pressure, but no pain. You may also wish to make an audiotape so that you can follow the same procedure each time. The repetition will help you achieve success. Just remember to speak in a calm voice and give yourself positive messages. To lose weight, for example, remind yourself how much you would enjoy being slim.

To undo the self-induction, tell yourself that by counting from 1 to 5, you will return to a stage of alertness feeling refreshed and aware. Then, with each number, you should become more and more alert.

Autogenic Training. A form of self-hypnosis, autogenic training (AT) is used, alone or with biofeedback, to produce relaxation. AT was developed in the 1930s by a

How to Hypnotize Yourself

Self-hypnosis is relatively easy to learn, and for many people the basic technique can be mastered in a few days. Some have found self-hypnosis helpful for reducing stress.

- Give yourself enough time to become completely relaxed.

- Find some small object or spot out in front of you and above your line of sight. Focus all your conscious attention to the spot or object. Continue slow, deep, satisfying breathing.

- Begin telling yourself how relaxed you feel.

- You may feel your eyes watering and blinking. Give yourself suggestions to encourage your eyes to close: *"As my eyes water and blink, it is as if the more they blink the more they are clearing away all worries, concerns, and anxieties."*

- Visualize a real or fantasy place of peacefulness and comfort — a place away from all concerns and distracting thoughts.

- Focus your attention and your images on sensations in your hands and fingers. Visualize feelings of coolness, numbness, warmth, heaviness, or lightness. When you detect one of these feelings, encourage it to expand with more suggestions.

- The change from regular waking consciousness to hypnotic consciousness can be a subtle one. You might not notice it the first time or two you try. Be patient with yourself.

Adapted from Self-Hypnosis, a Complete Manual for Health and Self-Change *by Dr. Brian M. Alman with Peter T. Lambrou.*

German psychiatrist, Johannes Schultz, who was interested in how hypnosis affected the body, brain, and nervous system. Since hypnotized people often feel that their limbs are heavy and warm, Schultz devised a system of exercises meant to evoke these sensations and so induce deep relaxation, but without the need for a hypnotist.

Autogenics and Meditation. Merging some of the auto-suggestions of hypnosis with meditative elements of yoga,

---

CASE HISTORY

USING HYPNOSIS FOR SURGERY

Instead of general anesthesia, Dr. Victor Rausch, a dental surgeon, decided to use self-hypnosis during an operation for the removal of his gallbladder. This is his account of the experience.

"The reason I chose self-hypnosis as my mode for anesthesia was a selfish one. I had a burning curiosity and desire to experience firsthand the mental changes that would have to occur within myself if the procedure was to be successful. I wanted to discover to what extent I could control my body through the use of self-hypnosis, and was prepared to take the risk.

"The night before surgery, I used progressive relaxation to achieve a very inner comfortable tranquility. Focusing on the feelings of confidence, absolute certainty of success and elation, I drifted into a very deep hypnotic sleep.

"I received no premedication. After being wheeled into the operating room, I climbed onto the operating table. I immediately sensed the tremendous tension everyone was under but still felt very calm and relaxed myself.

"The surgeon asked me if I was ready. When I said yes he felt along the line of the intended incision. Without hesitation, he drew the scalpel firmly across my abdomen.

"At the precise moment the incision was made . . . I felt an interesting flowing sensation throughout my entire body. Whatever happened, I was suddenly much more aware of my surroundings, people in the room and

bodily sensations, than I had ever been before.

"According to the operating team there was no visible tensing of the muscles, no change in breathing, no flinching of the eyelids and no change in facial expression.

"I could mentally direct the flowing sensation to any area and achieve complete control and still be totally aware of every step of the operation.

"Consciously I felt completely detached. It was as though I were an observer rather than the patient. To this point approximately three minutes had elapsed from the beginning of surgery. I felt strong and knew that the procedure would be absolutely successful.

"Throughout the procedure I perspired profusely, yet my pulse and blood pressure remained steady. After the final sutures were in place, the anesthetist asked me if I might care to walk back to my room. I enthusiastically agreed, climbed off the operating table and walked around the operating room. I felt no pain and no discomfort. I felt pure elation. The anesthetist sent for my robe and slippers. We all linked arms, walked into the hall and proceeded via the elevator to my room."

Excerpted from Cholecystectomy with Self-Hypnosis *by Dr. Victor Rausch*

AT focuses mainly on bodily sensations, and only later adds mental training. Like meditation, you should neither be so intent on achieving your goal that you become anxious, nor so passive that you fall asleep.

Before starting, choose a quiet, relaxed setting. You can perform the exercises while sitting upright in a straight-backed chair, sitting on a low stool and leaning forward, or while lying on your back.

The training consists of reciting several times one of six basic exercises or verbal formulas. While each exercise takes only a few minutes, initially it may be repeated up to 10 times a day. As you become skilled at the first exercise, you add the second, and then a third, until you can do all six in succession. Gradually, the length of a session increases to 30 or 40 minutes, and the frequency of practice decreases to twice daily. Moving at a slow but steady pace, most people are able to master the entire set of exercises within just a few months.

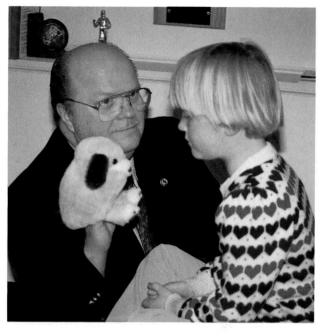

Using a hand puppet, *a therapist makes a game of hypnosis to capture and focus a child's imagination. Children, even those with short attention spans, are particularly responsive to hypnotic suggestion, perhaps because they are trusting and imaginative. The technique may help with a variety of problems, from bedwetting to coping with grief.*

Getting Started. To begin, close your eyes and repeat several times, "My right arm is heavy" (if you are right-handed). The same formula is applied to your other arm, then to both arms at once, then to each leg and both legs together. The feeling of heaviness you will experience is thought to correspond to muscle relaxation.

The second exercise is meant to produce a feeling of warmth, corresponding to dilation of the blood vessels. The trainee repeats, "My right arm is warm," and so forth, just as was prescribed in the first exercise. The third is, "My pulse is calm and regular." Then, "My breathing is deep and even," or "It breathes me." The fifth exercise is, "My abdomen (or solar plexus) is warm" (omit this if you have an abdominal disorder). Lastly the trainee repeats, "My forehead is cool."

Once you have mastered the basic exercises, you may wish to develop "intentional formulas" to change behavior patterns like smoking and overeating. For instance, you might tell yourself, "I have control of my diet. I can eat less and become more attractive." Such messages work best when they are simple and persuasive.

There is considerable debate over how autogenic training works to produce relaxation. However, studies of brain-wave changes and other physiological processes have shown that AT mitigates the body's response to acute stress, apparently by reducing the stimuli reaching areas of the brain that are linked to the autonomic nervous system. But whatever the mechanism, AT has been used for a range of emotional and physical disorders, from depression and anxiety to migraines and allergies. ❏

The Stuff of Dreams

Dream images are highly personal. For example, a dream of an old, deserted house may produce fear in one person and feelings of nostalgia in another. Your own dreams may provide clues to your inner feelings.

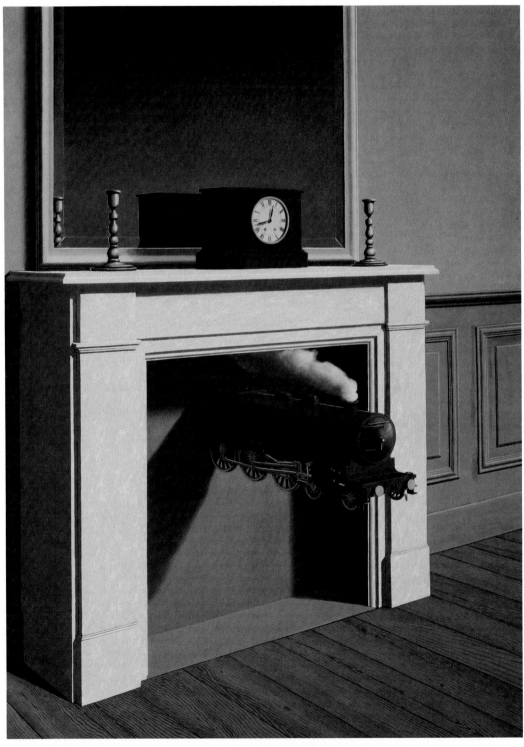

In dreams, anything can happen. *Logic and probability are suspended, and a locomotive can burst from a fireplace, as in the painting* Time Transfixed *by René Magritte. Dreams were once considered messages from the gods; now they are seen as unique reflections of personal experience and emotions.*

WHAT CAN OUR DREAMS tell us about ourselves? Do they reveal hidden or repressed desires, as some psychologists believe? Or are they simply random images, devoid of any significance or meaning? While both theories may have some validity, we are still a long way from completely understanding either the meaning or the function of dreams.

One thing we do know is that dreams are successions of images, thoughts, and emotions experienced by the mind during sleep. Sleep researchers have determined that most dreaming occurs during a stage in our sleep cycle known as REM (for rapid eye movement). EEG readings taken during the REM stage reveal brain-wave patterns that are quite close to those observed in people when awake.

During any night's sleep, a person will experience about five REM periods, lasting from 10 to 30 minutes. While laboratory studies have shown that everyone has several dreams each night, the dreams that we remember usually occur during the last REM period, just before we awaken. So, people who claim that they never dream simply cannot recall these nighttime experiences. Some sleep researchers speculate that during REM sleep our brains lack the chemicals that transfer thoughts into long-term memory; if this is true, it is not surprising that we forget our dreams so quickly.

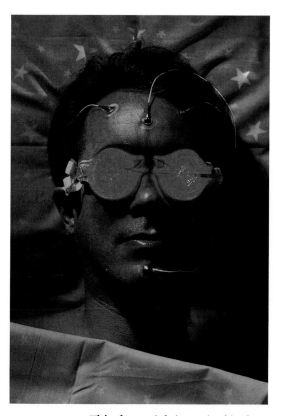

This sleeper is being trained in the art of lucid dreaming. Flashing red lights inside his mask signal the onset of REM sleep, the cycle when most dreams occur. They serve to remind him that he is asleep and that anything that happens is a dream. With practice he will be able to control the content and outcome of his dreams.

Dream Theories. Sigmund Freud was one of the first researchers in modern times to develop a comprehensive theory about dreams. According to Freud, dreams are the "royal road to the unconscious" and represent thoughts that the conscious mind has censored. As a result, dreams are highly symbolic and hard to unravel.

Freud's theory was highly regarded, but when REM sleep cycles were discovered, and dreams were found to have a biological component, many scientists and psychologists reformulated their thinking about the meaning of dreams. Some even went so far as to suggest that dreams were simply the result of random nerve activity and had no real significance. But many of these hard-liners eventually conceded that the plots or stories in dreams represent the mind's efforts to make sense of these random nerve impulses, and so may have some psychological resonance. In other words, even in sleep, our minds are filled with a lifetime of memories, desires, and ideas that could affect the content of our dreams.

The Function of Dreams. Far from being the exclusive province of human beings, animals also experience REM-like sleep and dreams. For this reason, some researchers have suggested that dreaming may have a biological function, perhaps serving as "mental house-cleaning," a time for memory processing, and for ridding the mind of un-needed information. Some dreams, particularly bizarre ones, may be material that is being "spiked" from our memory banks, or, as one researcher put it, "We dream to forget." Still other researchers suspect that dreaming may play a role in learning and brain development, noting that infants spend much more time in REM sleep than adults.

Working with Dreams. Even if we do not fully understand the function of dreams, most psychologists still believe that they can provide a key to our inner feelings and attitudes. While many people think of dreams as tools for gaining a better understanding of themselves, others have used them to help solve problems and boost creativity. For instance, Elias Howe worked for years trying to build a mechanized sewing machine, to no avail. Then one night he dreamed he was being attacked by warriors; as they raised their spears, Howe noticed that there were holes in the tips of the weapons. There was the answer to his problem: a needle with a hole in the tip instead of the shank.

In any dream work, the first step is to remember your dreams as fully as possible. Since upon awakening we tend to forget them quickly, keep a pencil and paper, or a tape recorder, at your bedside so that you can make notes. Don't neglect fleeting dream fragments; sometimes a seemingly incongruous "flash" provides an important clue to the meaning of a dream.

Although you may learn from dreams on your own, a group in which people share dreams, with or without a trained leader, may bring added benefits. A sympathetic group of people may encourage you to talk about dreams, and problems, that you previously suppressed. Also, by describing a dream aloud, you may begin to see things that you otherwise would have missed. And other people can often suggest interpretations that you would not think of by yourself.

It is important that group members not interrupt a dreamer's narrative, however, and remember that only the dreamer can tell whether a particular interpretation is right for him or her. One writer urges anyone commenting on another's dream to begin, "If it were my dream. . ." A dreamer can generally tell if an interpretation is right when all the details seem to "click" into place.

An insight may prompt a group member to see a problem in a new light, perhaps even to take action. For example, Jeremy Taylor, a minister interested in dreams, recalled a dream group in which a theological student remembered dreaming about pastel colors. Asked if he associated the words "pastel" and "pastoral," he realized that his com-

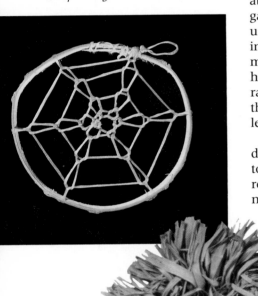

Ojibway Indians hang "dream nets" over their children every night in an effort to trap bad dreams. Good dreams are able to slip through the center hole.

During dream-guessing ceremonies, the Husk Faces, an Iroquois medicine society, wore masks woven from cornhusks. The Iroquois believed dreams to be the language of the soul, and considered illness to be an alienation between body and soul. These dream-guessing rites were part of an elaborate healing ceremony.

mitment to pastoral work was "pastel," or weak; he had entered theological school only to please his parents.

Gestalt therapists work with dream groups in a special way. "Gestalt" comes from a German word loosely translated as "pattern," and Gestalt therapy aims to help people bring conflicting areas of their lives into a harmonious pattern, or, as one practitioner puts it, to help "unfinished business become finished." Dreams can further this process because they are the dreamer's creations. Every character and every object in the dream is seen as part of the dreamer, often a part that he or she prefers not to recognize while awake. Through exercises, the dreamer acts out the dream, playing or actually becoming different characters or things, until they merge into an integrated whole.

Lucid Dreaming. Many people have had the experience of suddenly realizing during a dream that they are dreaming. Lucid dreaming is the ability to continue dreaming while at the same time observing the dream objectively, as in a movie theater. Some people can produce this effect at will. Physiologically, lucid dreaming is said to be simply a more aroused state of sleep. Subjectively, it may enable you to influence events in the dream, perhaps changing the outcome. This ability, say practitioners, can help you to confront difficult problems and gain more control over your life.

Dr. Stephen LeBerge of Stanford University, a pioneer in the field, says that many people have lucid dreams spontaneously, perhaps the same people who can set a "mental alarm" to wake them at a specified time without a clock. But others can learn the skill. You can start by closely studying your ordinary dreams. Then you might practice asking yourself several times a day whether you are dreaming or not. After a while, this question will surface during your dreams. Try to remain conscious as you fall asleep, and even as you dream. It is tricky; you may find yourself jolting awake, or slipping into a fully dreaming state.

Some people use lucid dreaming to tame nightmares and give their dreams happy endings; confronted by a terrifying dream figure, they fight and kill it. But it is better to question the demon than to destroy it, experts say. Only then can you recognize conflicts and learn to handle them constructively. Often the demon shrinks or disappears when you challenge it, or it turns into a person with whom you have had trouble— perhaps a parent or spouse; by asserting yourself in your dream, you may start an imaginary dialogue that helps you to see the other person's viewpoint. ❑

You and Your Dreams

No matter how clear dream memories appear to be on first awakening, unless the additional effort is made to record them, they almost invariably disappear from memory.

- Make a written record of your dreams, no matter what means [tape, rough notes from the middle of the night] you use to record them.

- When you record your dreams, do so in the present tense (reserving the past tense for what is experienced as memory in the dream). Make sure always to note the date and day of the week of a dream.

- Give your dreams titles when you write them down. The moment of picking a title is often a doorway to insight.

- Remember that every dream has many meanings and many levels of meaning, so don't be dazzled by [your first interpretation].

- Imagine different ways your dreams might have continued had you not awakened when you did.

- [Review] your dreams periodically. Be open to seeing new patterns and directions of development.

- Share your dreams with people you care about. Ask them about their dreams.

Excerpted from Dream Work *by Jeremy Taylor*

Dreamtime in Aboriginal Australia

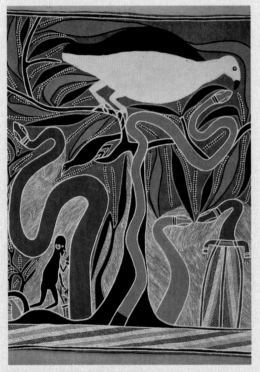

The Dreamings of Australian Aborigines are not dreams in the Western sense. Perhaps the word suggests how Aborigines bridge the physical and spiritual worlds. They believe that ancestral beings once walked the earth, shaping the land and everything in it. These beings now live on eternally in the Dreamtime, a spiritual dimension that exists simultaneously with the physical world. Dreamings are the myths that describe those ancestors and their deeds, and they provide a vast store of themes for Aboriginal art.

Painted on bark, this dreaming tells of Gurrumurringu, the artist's dreamtime ancestor, who was eaten by a snake for disobeying an aboriginal law.

As he works, a father explains his dreaming to his son. The family pet, a possum, perches on the child's head. Each clan has its own dreamings which are passed on to the next generation. To paint another's dreaming is a serious offense.

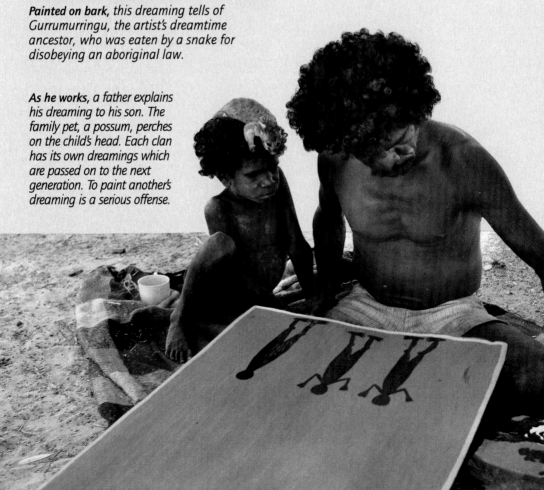

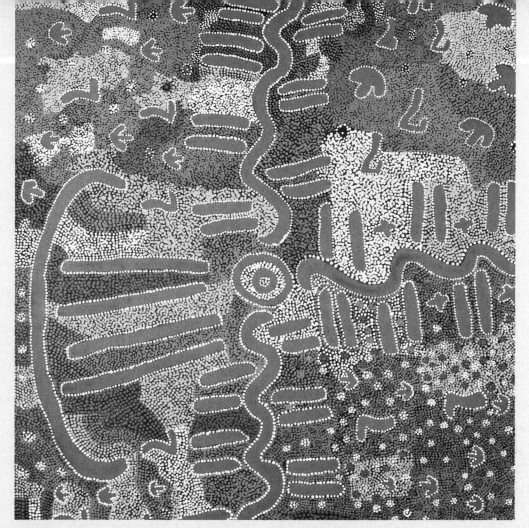

Modern acrylic paints offer a vibrant spectrum of colors. This painting, Water Dreaming at Mikanji, shows the aftermath of a storm that occurred when several dreamings met at a waterhole.

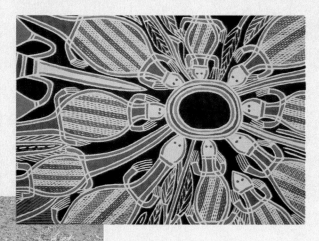

Dreamings confirm a clan's right to live in a particular area. Often an artist will describe a painting by saying, "This is my country."

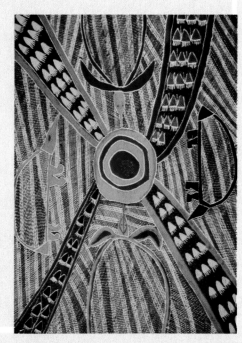

Turtles and anteaters drink from a sacred waterhole. This dreaming, like many others, has probably been painted thousands of times. Aborigines have the oldest tradition of visual art in the world: 30,000 years.

Looking Inward

By casting new light on our lives, therapy can help us tap our innate power to help ourselves. Whether you want to deal with depression, break a bad habit, or find the "real" you, there are many options to choose from.

THERE ARE SO MANY BRANDS of psychotherapy available for exploring the self or for treating emotional wounds, and the choices can be confusing. Some are geared toward probing the unconscious to get at the root of conflicts, others are designed with the idea of fixing problems through behavior modification, and still others aim to bolster the patient's self-esteem. But these are just three of many approaches.

Why choose therapy? When problems of a psychological nature arise, they often manifest themselves with physical symptoms: we can't sleep, we're fearful and short of breath, or we just feel plain blah. Frequently, we first turn to friends, family members, or our personal physician. But if symptoms persist, it might be wise to seek the help of a mental health professional.

When searching for a therapist, you should consider your own personal philosophy and therapeutic goals and try to find someone whose technique matches your needs. For instance, if you are not one for deep soul-searching, you'll probably be happiest in short-term treatment geared toward helping you with specific problems. The following is a summary of the major treatment options available.

Psychodynamic Therapies. Freudian psychoanalysis laid the groundwork for some of the newer styles of therapy now available. Sometimes referred to as the talking cure, it is probably the best-known therapy, yet it has the smallest following. For one thing, it requires a large time commit-

Freud's couch, now in the Freud Museum in London, has come to symbolize psychoanalysis. Therapeutically, the couch is meant to promote relaxation. In addition, by facing away from the therapist, the patient may feel less inhibited and more willing to say whatever comes to mind.

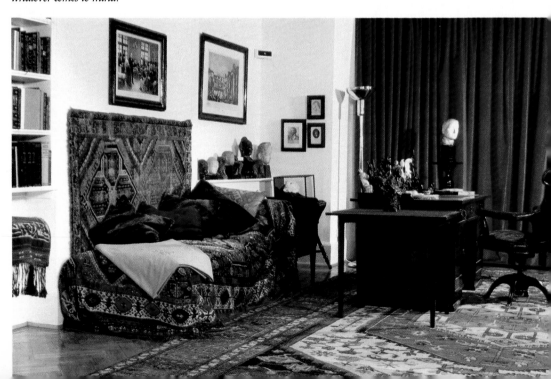

ment (up to 5 sessions per week). The treatment was developed by Sigmund Freud, who saw personality and behavior as shaped by unconscious conflicts and desires. It relies on a combination of techniques, among them free association (saying whatever comes to mind) and dream interpretation. During a session, the patient talks openly in a flow of associations. In this way, unconscious material may become conscious, and available to interpretation.

Variations on classical psychoanalysis are now widely practiced. Most require fewer sessions, and the therapist is more interactive, but the perspective toward treatment remains faithful to many (but not all) of Freud's ideas. Over the years many psychoanalytic thinkers broke with Freud, generally because they felt he put too much emphasis on sexuality as a motivator in human behavior, and not enough on other factors influencing personality development. These neo-Freudian approaches also moved toward more direct face-to-face therapy and shorter treatment. Still, the goal is to resolve neurotic symptoms or behavior by bringing unconscious internal conflicts to the surface.

During the course of treatment, a patient usually develops a strong emotional reaction to the therapist. Known as transference, the response usually mirrors the patient's relationship with a parent or other significant person in his life. The therapist's task is to help the patient interpret and understand the root of this emotional response, and in so doing, make a start at resolving some of his conflicts.

Short-term psychodynamic therapies are also available. These treatments are suitable for patients who are less interested in delving deeply into their psyches, and more concerned with solving a specific problem. Generally, sessions are once a week for a period of 12 to 25 weeks.

Changing Through Re-training. Markedly different from psychodynamic therapies, behavior therapies focus on unlearning the problem rather than probing its causes. For instance, a psychodynamic therapist might trace a client's obesity to poor self-esteem stemming from now-repressed childhood conflicts. A behaviorist would say it doesn't matter why you began to overeat. If you can learn to lose weight now, the results will make you feel better.

According to the late behaviorist B.F. Skinner, people act as they do because throughout their lives certain behaviors have been reinforced. Therefore, we can change destructive patterns using the same principle. Skinner's ideas gave rise to behavior modification, an approach based on the notion that almost any human behavior can be altered by manipulating its consequences—desired actions

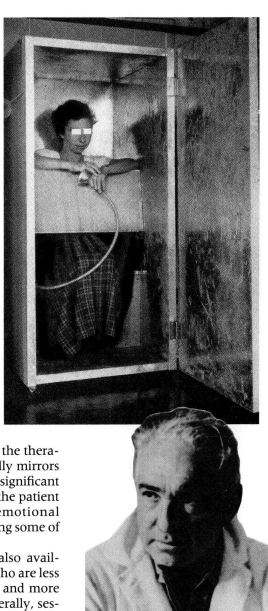

Wilhelm Reich, *shown above with his controversial "orgone box," was the first of Freud's students to treat body as well as mind. Reich claimed to have discovered the biological basis of the emotions, which existed in a universal energy that he called "orgone." His box was designed to accumulate and concentrate this energy for therapeutic treatment. Together with medical techniques, the orgone box helped patients to overcome muscle and character rigidity.*

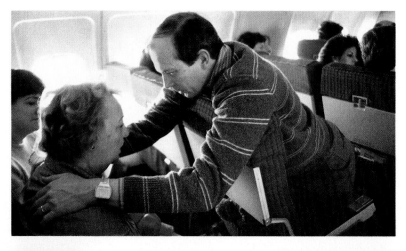

Aboard their flight home, recovering aerophobics accept congratulations from their group leader. Before stepping onto this 747, the group toured the cockpit of the plane and did conditioning exercises to help them overcome their fear of flying.

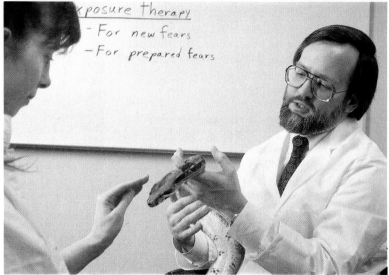

Ophidiophobia, the excessive fear of snakes, can be mastered. At the University of Michigan's Anxiety Disorders Program, Dr. Randolph Nesse (right) helps patients gradually overcome their phobias by repeated voluntary exposure.

are rewarded, while unwanted behaviors are discouraged.

In another version of behavioral therapy, Joseph Wolpe developed a method to help patients overcome fears and phobias by training them to approach stressful situations gradually in a relaxed state. Known as systematic desensitization, the method has helped many people overcome their fear of flying and many other phobias.

One-on-one behavioral treatment usually takes place during weekly office sessions, though it generally requires fewer total visits than traditional psychotherapy. The nature of the problem influences which of several strategies will be selected. However, aversion techniques—punishments—are employed rarely, and only with the patient's approval. Behavior therapy appears to work best with symptoms that can be tackled step by step, such as phobias, bedwetting, and some sexual problems.

Cognitive Treatment. Quite different from either psychodynamic or behavioral therapies, cognitive therapy is based on the idea that how we perceive ourselves and our world determines how we feel and act. It was developed in the 1950s by Dr. Aaron Beck, a psychiatrist at the University of Pennsylvania. While doing research on depression, Beck observed that each of his depressed subjects had a skewed self-image, which was fostered by how they processed information. Like malfunctioning radios, they were picking up only negative signals, at deafeningly loud volumes.

What you think, Dr. Beck concluded, dictates how you feel. And a sense of self based on generally negative thoughts, or cognitions, reflects a distorted perception of reality. So retooling these faulty thought patterns can improve your mood. The reason this works, cognitivists say, is because of connections between psychological and physiological states. Changes in cognition are thought to generate a biochemical response, which may make you feel less depressed or anxious. Over a relatively short course of treatment—as brief as a dozen weekly sessions in some cases—a cognitive therapist helps the patient recognize her particular destructive thought patterns and learn how to use logic to reprogram them.

Unlike psychodynamic therapy, the focus is on the present. When you suddenly find your mood swinging, cognitive therapists suggest using an "instant replay" technique. What was crossing your mind immediately before the change? Chances are you'll discover it was one of a handful of common cognitive traps like "all-or-nothing thinking," in which you see any situation short of perfect as a complete failure. Or maybe you were doing the "binocular trick," magnifying your problems while minimizing anything positive. Cognitive therapy has proven particularly useful in treating depression. It has also worked well with phobias and, most recently, in couples therapy.

Humanistic Therapies. These methods were developed by psychologists who felt that traditional therapies were focused too much on pathology and not enough on our potential for growth. The premise is that each of us has the inner resources for healing and change, but that we subvert our own needs by doing what we think we "ought" to do.

Humanistic therapy is intended for people who want to achieve their fullest potential. As the patient expresses thoughts and feelings, the therapist is supportive and responsive, thus encouraging self-esteem. Such empathy will help the patient accept himself as a competent, worthwhile person, with potential for finding psychological health and well-being.

Programs such as EST, Insight, and Self-Actualization grew out of humanistic therapies, and all have as their goal discovering the "true self." Often individual sessions are augmented with intensive weekend "encounter" groups. ❏

Choosing a Therapist

Choosing a therapist can be as confusing as selecting a type of therapy. In fact, the term "therapist" reveals nothing about a person's training. But the following list should help you discern the differences among the many well-trained professionals.

- Psychiatrists are physicians (M.D.s) who specialize in mental disorders. As doctors, they can prescribe medication, and many are trained in talking-based psychotherapy.
- Clinical psychologists generally hold Ph.D.s and have broad training in psychological research, personality assessment, and various therapies.
- Psychoanalysts may or may not have M.D.s, but have had rigorous training in an analytic institute.
- Social workers generally have graduate degrees, and many have specific training in the practice of psychotherapy.
- Certified pastoral counselors are members of the clergy who have earned a graduate degree in some area of mental health. These therapists offer counseling with a religious component.
- Counselors in schools, prisons, or on the job offer guidance about specific problems, but are generally not qualified to give a more in-depth psychological assessment.

Sharing Professional Help

Gaining perspective about oneself is the goal of many therapies. But group therapy offers a particularly effective means of self-exploration. In addition, group interaction may actually speed the therapeutic process.

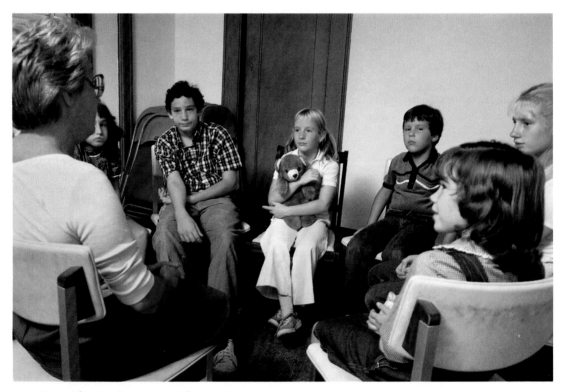

***Group therapy** is not commonly used with youngsters. But, with the help of a psychologist, these children are learning to cope with the difficulties of living with addicted parents. Children often feel responsible for their parents' behavior, but talking with fellow group members may help them to view their situation a little more realistically. Therapy also encourages them to express their feelings openly, instead of acting them out in destructive ways.*

MANY PEOPLE ENTER THERAPY feeling frightened and isolated, convinced that they are alone in their problems—that no one thinks as they do, feels as wretchedly as they feel, or has fears or fantasies like theirs. Social problems may heighten this sense of isolation. Group therapy can offer a comforting and reassuring environment for many people, but particularly for those who want to work on their social skills, who have difficulties with relationships, or who feel particularly alone.

One special advantage of group therapy is that individuals are able to see themselves from various vantage points, and in this way may gain a broader perspective than in one-on-one therapy. Although each group member must share the time and attention of the therapist, the reciprocal support of the group may actually enrich the therapeutic process. Patients not only receive advice and suggestions from other group members, but they in turn are counted on to provide support and counsel, which can provide a much-needed sense of self-worth.

Group Structure. Most groups are composed of five to twelve members, and while individuals may share similar problems or concerns, most groups bring together a mix of people. Therapy sessions generally meet once a week for an hour and a half. In a typical session, discussion begins spontaneously with one member bringing up an issue of personal concern. But as the conversation develops, the therapist or another group member may interject comments about how various members are responding and behaving toward each other. Groups vary greatly in character and tone—some are dramatic and intense with lots of challenge and confrontation, while others are quiet, supportive, and emotionally nurturing.

Groups are laboratory versions of real life—people see themselves mirrored, gauge how others react to them, re-create family constellations, and other important relationships, all through their interactions with group members. A man who has trouble relating to women, for instance, will probably find that the women in the group rebuff him, too. But, because the group is a safe and honest forum, he can ask these women for help with his problem. The other men in the group can share their experiences as well, and everyone in the group can offer emotional support. When the man is ready to make changes, the group becomes a protected space for testing new behavior.

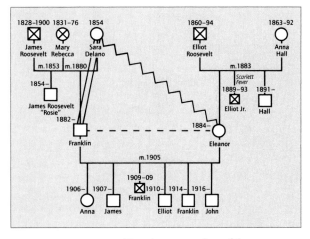

Dramatizing Behavior. One particularly useful way groups help members "rehearse" new behaviors is through psychodrama, a therapeutic technique invented in the 1920s by a Rumanian psychiatrist, J. L. Moreno. In a psychodrama, members of the group enact the roles of the people in one member's life. Starting with a description of a conflict that has significance for a group member, the scene progresses spontaneously as other group members play various parts. As the drama unfolds, often the person whose problem is being staged will gain some surprising new insight about himself.

To get an overview of the many complex interactions within a family, some therapists use genograms. Employing the symbols of genealogical charts (square = male, round = female), genograms add notations that express emotional ties. This genogram of President Franklin D. Roosevelt's family depicts a classic in-law problem. Raised as an only child, F. D. R. had close ties with his mother, Sara Delano (double line), and a strained relationship with his wife, Eleanor (dashed line). The constant competition between Eleanor and her mother-in-law is indicated by a jagged line.

A Natural Grouping. Most people in group therapy were originally referred by a therapist who thought that they might benefit from social interaction. But since the 1950s, psychologists have also begun to treat families in group therapy. Families typically come to therapy when one member—often an adolescent—develops a serious problem. This "identified patient" seems to be the source of all unhappiness, but soon enough a more complex dynamic is revealed. The goal of family therapy is to sort out roles and discover how each family member affects the others—the end result being that the troubled individual gets help, and the family unit functions more harmoniously.

Marital therapy works in much the same way, with one person in the couple initially being identified as troubled, but during treatment, a more complicated reality generally surfaces. Couples therapy, like family therapy, is most successful when each person involved truly wants to be in therapy, and is motivated to make the changes necessary to ensure that the relationship is sustained. ❑

The Magic of Creative Therapies

The creative arts can often play a significant role in the treatment of physical and mental illness—succeeding sometimes where other methods have failed. A sense of accomplishment may work wonders.

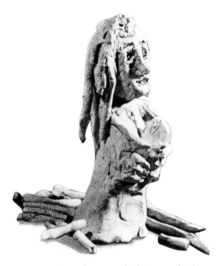

Creation can bring revelation. *This clay figure was made by a woman who intended to portray someone "able to cope and look nice." Although initially displeased with her efforts, she eventually accepted the figure's untidy hair, clumsy hands, and dreary demeanor. In doing so, she came to understand something about herself—that she had a difficult time coping with her time on Sundays, "I only realized what Sunday was like and what it meant after making her—and that is what you don't understand unless you have yourself painted or modelled."*

IN AN ART THERAPY SESSION at a psychiatric hospital, 18-year-old Henry paints a picture of a house with two distinct and disparate sides. Guided by an art therapist, he tries to relate his paintings to his difficulties in school. Like the house, Henry feels he has two sides. One is calm and in control. The other, the side he shows at school, is disorganized and "very, very, anxious." Prompted by Henry's painting, other patients in the group are able to admit that they, too, have feelings of being divided in this way.

In the hands of experienced art therapists, clay, watercolors, charcoal, and oil paints can become effective therapeutic tools. Painting, for instance, may help a patient express painful memories that have been locked inside. As the therapist helps the painter interpret images on the canvas, an underlying problem may come to light.

In addition to visual arts like painting and sculpture, dance, drama, music, and journal writing are all used therapeutically for a wide range of conditions, including psychiatric illnesses such as schizophrenia and autism; mental and physical disabilities; learning disorders; emotional problems like depression and anxiety; and addictions of many kinds.

Sometimes referred to as creative arts or expressive therapies, these treatments emphasize doing. The simple act of creating can produce a sense of achievement and confidence that in itself may have positive effects on health. Artistic talent is not a requirement because the goal is to involve the patient and not to produce beautiful art. The success of a therapy is measured solely by a patient's physical and emotional improvement.

Give and Take. Another objective of creative arts therapies is interaction. By taking a role in a drama or playing the drums in a musical ensemble, for instance, patients learn to cooperate and communicate with other people. Often dance, sculpture, and other forms of artistic expression can free patients to share thoughts and emotions that are sometimes difficult for them to reveal in words.

Have you ever experienced a

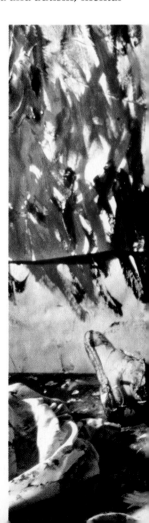

burst of energy when a fast, upbeat song came on the radio? Or felt calm after hearing a particularly soothing passage of classical music? Just as mood and attitude can be affected by music, so can physiological functions such as respiration and heart rate. In hospitals, relaxing music has been shown to decrease blood pressure in coronary patients. Interestingly, the most relaxing music seems to have a tempo about 70 to 80 beats per minute—the average resting pulse rate.

Typically used with the physically and mentally disabled, music therapy seeks to break down the barriers that can isolate them from the rest of the world. Through music, children with impaired hearing or speech difficulties may discover new ways to communicate. And it can also help introverted or withdrawn patients become more confident and outgoing. In addition, music therapists frequently work with schizophrenics and autistics to try to draw them out of their private worlds.

The Joy of Movement. Nine-year-old Meredith, a child with cerebral palsy, moves uncertainly around the dance floor. Her movement therapist offers a word of encouragement and a steadying hand when she stumbles or wobbles. The little girl laughs excitedly when she, her therapist, and another child form a choo-choo train and weave around

Joy and triumph radiate from the face of this young psychiatric patient, whose hands and overalls are now splattered with as many colors as the canvas. The very act of creating a painting may provide the key to healing. Through art, the patient is able to express thoughts and emotions that may not come through in words.

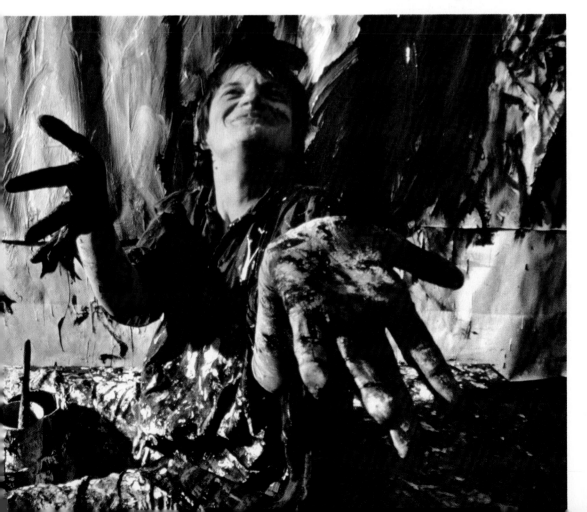

the room. At the end of the session Meredith sprawls over a huge rubber ball and happily reaches out to clasp her therapist's hands. They exchange a hug before Meredith goes home with her mother.

Dance therapy has given Meredith better balance and a more active sense of rhythm. It lets her touch others, enjoy music, and do something pleasurable with her body, free from the fear of failure. On a purely physical level, dance therapy has helped Meredith improve her strength, coordination, and range of movement. But dance is also applied effectively to a wide variety of psychiatric and emotional problems, ranging from addiction to depression. For example, dance therapy helped one woman, a victim of child abuse, find a way of dealing with her anger and shame. Another patient, whose inability to express her feelings was interfering with her relationships, said she felt "stuck" in therapy until she tried dance. For some people, the combination of touch, movement, and rhythm opens doors that "talk" therapy doesn't.

Drama as Therapy. Acting comes naturally to most of us. In childhood, we experiment with adult roles by pretending to be nurses, firemen, and astronauts. In drama therapy, the world of make-believe becomes the means of exploring real-life social and psychological problems. Some of the techniques used in drama therapy, "role-playing," for example, are also found in more traditional kinds of psychotherapy, such as Gestalt and psychodrama. But drama therapy puts greater emphasis on the theatricality of drama, incorporating masks, puppets, props, actual performances, and written scripts. Drama therapists are generally proficient in the techniques of the theater—directing, acting, costumes, sets, and stagecraft—as well as in those of psychotherapy and psychology.

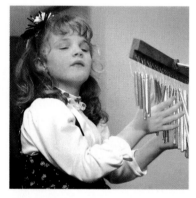

Through music therapy, *a blind child is given a new way of connecting with the world. Devices as simple as wind chimes can be effective therapeutic tools.*

Drama therapy has produced some remarkable results in institutional settings. As an adjunct to special education programs, it helps mentally disabled children improve their language and motor skills. Techniques such as improvisation and role-playing have been effective in preparing prison inmates for life outside prison walls.

The method seems to be very effective with emotionally and developmentally disturbed children and adults—people who have difficulty establishing relationships with others. Through drama, patients have the chance to "try on" different emotions, thoughts, and behaviors in a non-threatening situation. By playing fictional characters, patients sometimes can act out

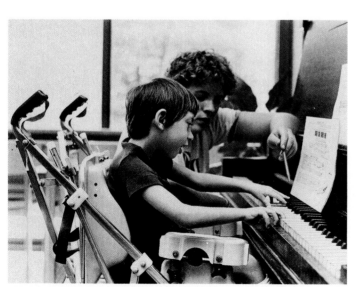

Creative expression, *whether through piano lessons or painting, may give disabled children a special sense of accomplishment.*

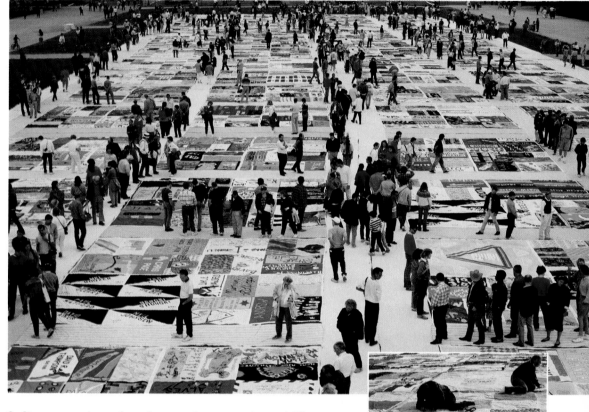

feelings or actions that they can't express in real life. One technique commonly used with disturbed patients is story-telling. Typically, the therapist selects a familiar and simple story that is related to the patient's problem. Fables and folk-tales often feature situations and characters that reflect the real world. For example, someone who feels let down by a parent might identify with the fairy tale *Hansel and Gretel*. Members of a therapy group would assume characters and act out the story. How people choose to interpret their roles often reveals a great deal about themselves. The therapist helps patients identify the links between their characters' actions and their own lives. In a similar fashion, nursing home residents are able to recapture a sense of purpose and self-worth in life when they share their "oral histories" with others.

Writing From the Heart. Journal writing has helped many people release frustrations and sort out problems. And it may actually keep you healthy. Certain studies indicate that people who write about important issues in their lives are healthier than those who keep feelings bottled up inside.

As a form of therapy, writing is more than simply keeping a record of daily activities. Writing therapists agree that the feelings connected with a problem are just as important as the facts. You may wish to start by choosing an issue that has been bothering you lately. Describe the situation or event thoroughly, recording what you were feeling at the time and how you are feeling now. Your reflections may help put the past in perspective. Even if you think you have nothing to say on a given day, keep to the schedule you've fixed for writing in your journal. ❑

The AIDS Memorial Quilt, laid out in front of the Capitol in Washington, D.C., creates a stunning panorama. Each three-by-six-foot quilt piece commemorates one AIDS victim. The work of grieving relatives and friends, these panels range from highly artistic to simple and intimate. Sometimes, handwritten messages were added even as the quilt was displayed. Making a piece of the quilt was, in the words of a survivor, "part of a healing process."

Out-of-Control Habits

Many people now use the term addiction to describe not just physical dependence, but almost any kind of compulsive and self-destructive behavior. Treatment options have broadened greatly in recent years.

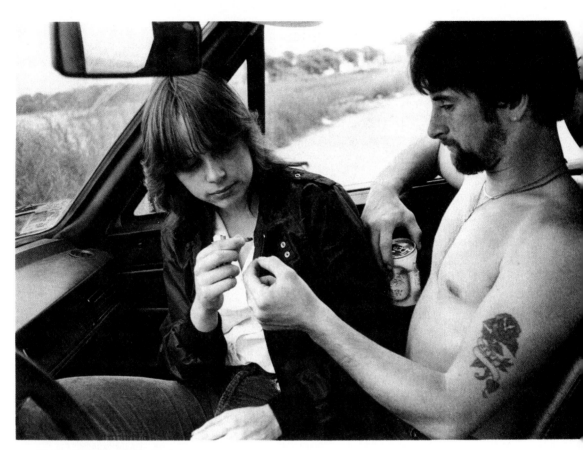

Teenagers often fall prey to peer pressure, and like adults, use alcohol or drugs to cope in social situations, or as a way of dealing with emotional pain. Of course not all kids who experiment end up addicted, but alcohol and drug abuse can seriously interfere with normal social and emotional development. Addiction is a complex problem at any age, and most recovery programs are designed to help addicts cope, as well as helping them to kick the habit.

TODAY, ADDICTION AND COMPULSIVE BEHAVIOR of all kinds seem rampant. Many people are concerned not only with losing control over their use of alcohol and drugs, but over food, smoking, gambling, and even shopping. But what is the nature of addiction, and how do we explain its hold over certain individuals? Smoking-related illnesses, for example, kill more than 100 people a day in Canada, yet though warned of the hazards of smoking, nicotine addicts are frequently unable to kick the habit—despite numerous attempts. Or consider the alcoholics who trade away family and career rather than quit drinking.

Chocolate, exercise, coffee, work, sex, indeed almost everything these days has been labeled as being addictive. But when and how does a simple experiment or indulgence spiral into a full-blown addiction?

The Nature of Addiction. One theory is that some addicts have abnormally low levels of some of the body's naturally occurring neurochemicals, such as endorphins. These neurochemicals affect mood and behavior, and when the balance is tipped, an addicted person may try to compensate by ingesting a substance that produces the same, or a far more intense, feeling. In this light, addiction seems to stem from an effort to self-medicate. A user's first attempts to medicate himself with drugs or other substances usually lies within his control. Gradually, however, he loses control, and choice becomes compulsion.

A Disease? How does compulsive shopping, gambling, or other non-chemical addictions fit the self-medication model of addiction? Some experts believe that every addiction is a search for wholeness or inner peace, and compulsive behavior is yet another misguided attempt to fill an internal void. If this is true, then any effort to conquer an addiction must be accompanied by an exploration of what has created this feeling of incompleteness in the first place.

But Alcoholics Anonymous and other self-help groups

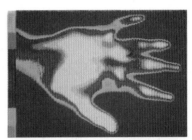
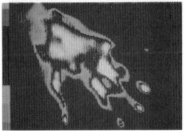
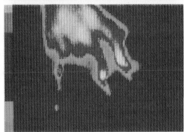

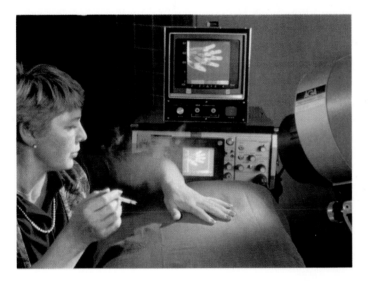

with a similar approach argue that the substance itself creates the need. The important thing is absolute avoidance— a goal achieved through the group support of people with the same addictions, along with recognition of self-destructive behavior patterns, and assistance in overcoming them.

In fact, Alcoholics Anonymous (as well as many medical experts) consider addiction to be a disease. The disease concept of alcoholism is an old one, the idea being that the individual is powerless over his or her drinking due to a biological vulnerability. This theory is now applied very broadly not just to alcoholism, but to every conceivable form of addictive or compulsive behavior.

While she smokes, the woman at the left can actually see how nicotine affects her blood circulation. At the start (top), a heat-sensitive camera displays her entire hand as nearly white, which indicates warmth. But as she absorbs more nicotine (middle), her blood vessels constrict, reducing the flow of blood to her fingers. After just a few puffs (bottom), her hand radiates so little heat that her fingers seem to vanish.

Who Gets Hooked? Clearly not everyone who has a drink, eats chocolate, shops too much, or plays the slots becomes an addict. So why do some people succumb while others, whose difficulties in life may be just as great, do not? For one thing, many experts feel that most addicts share an important characteristic, a feeling of insecurity or incompleteness, no matter how successful their lives may appear to others. Without alcohol, drugs, or other substance or compulsive behavior of choice, addicts feel uncomfortable, and lack a feeling of wholeness. However, in the view of many specialists, there is most likely no single cause for addiction.

Contrary to popular mythology, no genetic basis for addiction has been firmly established. Scientists have yet to turn up an "alcoholism gene," for instance. But some studies do suggest a genetic predisposition to addiction. For example, children of alcoholics have been shown to be more prone to developing drinking problems.

Overwhelmed by Outside Forces. Some experts support the view that addiction is influenced by external factors—that family environment plays a part, as do cultural norms, peer pressure, and other factors. Another view is that the proliferation of addictive behavior reflects larger social problems—for instance, the rising divorce rate. And still another group suggests that our over-reliance on drugs and medical technology to cure everything from bad breath to bad moods has made us too ready to try to "fix" every twinge and unpleasant feeling we experience.

But whatever the cause, there is no arguing the fact that addictive and compulsive behaviors have all contributed a great deal of misery, taking a toll not just on individuals, but on their families as well. Fortunately, many treatment options provide hope for those who recognize the fact that they have lost control of their lives.

Some are able to stop their addictive behavior either on their own, or with the encouragement of family and friends. Many turn to support groups, such as Alcoholics Anonymous, or seek professional help from a therapist or physician. For others, enrolling in an out-patient treatment program, or entering an in-patient facility, is the only way to make a clean break from addiction or other forms of compulsive behavior.

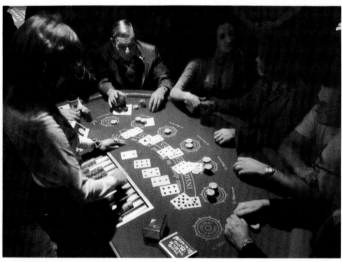

Compulsive gamblers know that the odds always favor the house. But even after losing thousands of dollars and plunging deeply into debt, the hope of a big win spurs them on. Therapists are now treating compulsive gambling like any other addiction, and recommend psychotherapy, support groups, and behavior modification to help gamblers overcome their habits.

Innovative techniques to curb addictions and compulsions are also available. Hypnosis and autogenics have been used successfully by some overeaters. Those who wish to stop smoking have had good results using hypnosis and acupuncture. And acupuncture, visualization, and psychodrama have all been used to treat alcohol and drug addiction, with varying degrees of success.

Most experts agree that addicts need to do more than just kick their habits. For lasting recovery, they need to think about rebuilding their lives, to find meaning and motivation to move ahead. And all addicts need to learn how to enjoy life without their substance of choice. ❏

The Search for Gratification

Addictions, writes Dr. Andrew Weil, can fool us into thinking we feel better. But this is only temporarily true and what we are really doing is giving our addictions power over our inner selves.

Addiction is a basic human problem that all men and women experience in some form. I reject the concept of "addictive personality" unless it includes everyone. The only reason we do not see the universality of this problem is that some kinds of addictive behavior, such as making money, drinking coffee, falling in love, exercising, and working compulsively, are socially acceptable and do not attract attention.

Addiction is not a psychological or pharmacological problem and cannot be solved by methods of psychology and pharmacology. It [addiction] is at root a spiritual concern because it represents a misdirected attempt to achieve wholeness, to experience inner completeness and satisfaction.

Why do we think that we need something to make us feel content: another slice of pizza, a piece of chocolate, a cigarette, a drink, a snort, a lover, another possession? Is there a way to feel complete and whole in ourselves without reaching for an external source of satisfaction?

Since the roots of addiction penetrate deeply into the very essence of our humanness, changing addictive behavior is not easy. For some of us it may be the work of a lifetime. A basic strategy for wellness is to be free of harmful habits. If we cannot easily change our addictive nature, we can try to be aware of our addictions and work to move them in directions that are less harmful. For example, a cigarette addict who stops smoking and becomes an exercise addict is no less an addict but is a much healthier one.

We all come into the world with wounds; they come with human birth, no matter what kind of family we grow up in, no matter what kind of society we live in. Much of our human seeking is a search for healing. We long for a sense of completeness and wholeness and for an end to craving. Most often we look for satisfaction outside of ourselves. That is the root of addiction.

Ironically, whatever satisfaction we gain from food, drugs, sex, money, and other "sources" of pleasure really comes from inside us. We project our power onto external substances and

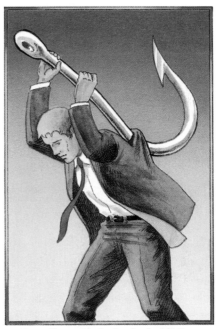

Grappling with the hook of addiction.

activities, allowing them to make us feel better temporarily. This is a strange sort of magic. We give our power away in order to achieve a transient sense of wholeness, then suffer because the objects of our craving seem to have power over us. Addiction can be cured only when we consciously experience this process, reclaim our power, and realize that wounds must be healed from within. Suffering and craving goad us into action, forcing us to discover who we are, to identify with our true selves.

Excerpted from Natural Health, Natural Medicine *by Andrew Weil, M.D.*

"We're All in the Same Boat"

Self-help groups provide a wellspring of support for millions of people, whether their problems are physical or emotional. Many are modeled after the twelve-step program created by Alcoholics Anonymous.

WHETHER YOUR PROBLEM IS a craving for cocaine or for love, there is probably a group of people with similar experiences who can provide help and support. Therapeutic self-help groups are the most popular, and seem to be among the most successful ways of treating a whole range of difficulties. Such groups do not provide the medical attention that chronic alcoholics, drug addicts, and compulsive overeaters may require, but they do provide unwavering (but not uncritical) emotional support. Many self-help groups are modeled on Alcoholics Anonymous (AA), the oldest and possibly most successful of them all.

Dr. Robert Smith, an Akron physician, and Bill Wilson, a New York stockbroker, founded AA in 1935 after helping each other stop drinking. AA sees alcohol addiction as a disease of the mind, the body, and the spirit. Recovery can be achieved through a twelve-step process, beginning with the alcoholic's admission that he is powerless over alcohol. The addict acknowledges that he must accept the help of other members of the group and from a "Higher Power."

Everyone Is Welcome. Anyone who thinks he or she has a drinking problem and wants to stop drinking can join AA. "It takes a drunk to understand a drunk," AA says. At AA meetings, members get up and offer testimony about their drinking and tell how their lives have changed since recovery. Feelings and experiences, good and bad, are shared among the group, whose collective aim is to maintain sobriety "one day at a time." All AA members are assured of anonymity.

Newcomers to AA are encouraged to find a sponsor within the group, a more experienced member who can be called upon day or night for counsel. This is important at the start, when the new member must avoid old drinking companions. The last of the twelve steps of Alcoholics Anonymous is carrying the message of recovery to other alcoholics. In assisting others, many alcoholics are able to change lifelong patterns of self-centeredness.

A Growing Movement. It is estimated that some 200 twelve-step programs now exist. These include groups for smokers, gamblers, workaholics, and even for sex and shopping "addicts." Self-help groups are also available for non-addicts, for instance the families of alcoholics, survivors of incest or child abuse, the hearing-impaired, victims

---

THE TWELVE STEPS

1 We admitted we were powerless over alcohol—that our lives had become unmanageable.

2 Came to believe that a Power greater than ourselves could restore us to sanity.

3 Made a decision to turn our will and our lives over to the care of God *as we understood Him.*

4 Made a searching and fearless moral inventory of ourselves.

5 Admitted to God, to ourselves and to another human being the exact nature of our wrongs.

6 Were entirely ready to have God remove all these defects of character.

7 Humbly asked Him to remove our short-comings.

8 Made a list of all persons we had harmed, and became willing to make amends to them all.

9 Made direct amends to such people wherever possible, except when to do so would injure them or others.

10 Continued to take personal inventory and when we were wrong, promptly admitted it.

11 Sought through prayer and meditation to improve our conscious contact with God *as we understood Him,* praying only for knowledge of His will for us and the power to carry that out.

12 Having had a spiritual awakening as the result of these steps, we tried to carry this message to alcoholics, and to practice these principles in all our affairs.

The Twelve-Step approach of Alcoholics Anonymous has helped thousands of problem drinkers stay sober. While many self-help groups have developed individual creeds for coping with addictive or compulsive behavior, most are based on AA's original principles.

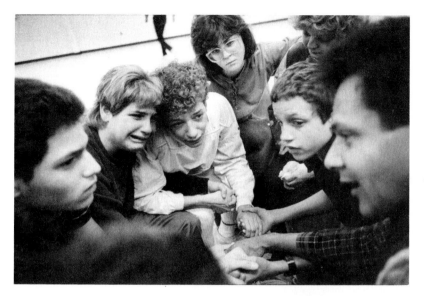

At an alcohol and drug treatment center for adolescents, patients help one another through the pain and turmoil of recovery. Many of the counselors are graduates of the program, and are aware of the difficulties of staying sober.

During treatment, addicts are encouraged to vent their feelings, no matter how unpleasant or disturbing. Since the first step toward full recovery is admitting the problem, the patients force each other to tell the truth about who they are, how they feel, and what they have done. Many addicts have long gotten away with lying to themselves as well as to others, a ploy that fools no one who has done the same.

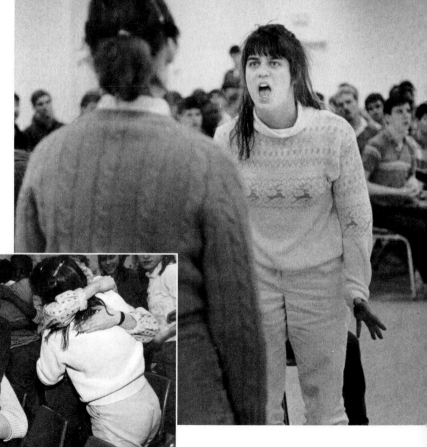

Group support ensures that nobody is alone. A warm, friendly hug makes it easier to get over the rough spots on the road to recovery.

of lupus, caretakers of the chronically ill, and many more.

Unlike group therapy sessions, which are lead by trained professionals, self-help groups are made up entirely of individuals who share a common problem. The goal of these groups is to help members gain control over their lives, and the vehicle is mutual aid and support. By talking and listening to fellow sufferers, individuals seem to find the solace and encouragement necessary to make changes or come to terms with their difficulties.

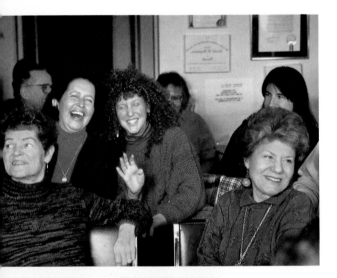

Taking the Step. In the past several years, support groups have gained larger and more enthusiastic followings. What is it about this approach that appeals to so many people? Part of the answer probably lies in the feeling of fellowship and camaraderie that self-help groups engender. Many individuals who join are comforted to find out that others know just what they are going through—because they have gone through it themselves. In addition, support groups are non-judgmental by their very nature, and people find that they can reveal their deepest fears and secrets without shame or embarrassment. And in doing so, many who have long felt isolated in their pain, or who have felt locked into destructive patterns, have found the strength to make changes in their lives.

Some therapists point out that self-help groups offer a structured and non-threatening approach to solving problems or overcoming addictions. Maintaining abstinence can be terribly difficult, and regular meetings and group support can help the newly sober (and others) stay on track toward full recovery.

Others feel that self-help groups may be filling a void. As society becomes more and more complex, these groups may help some individuals regain the sense of warmth, kinship, and support traditionally supplied by family, church, or community. For many, self-help groups seem to provide a safe haven and a sense of belonging. And as members share their pain, they also share the hope that change and growth are possible for everyone.

When should you seek the help of a support group? Probably when you are feeling overwhelmed by a problem, or feel isolated in your misery. And you need to be truly ready to accept the assistance of others. It is also important to make a commitment, at least initially, to attend meetings regularly. Unless you live in an extremely remote area, finding a self-help group that addresses your particular problem or need should not be difficult. You can start by contacting the social service agencies in your community.

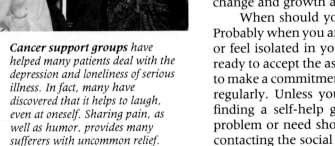

Cancer support groups have helped many patients deal with the depression and loneliness of serious illness. In fact, many have discovered that it helps to laugh, even at oneself. Sharing pain, as well as humor, provides many sufferers with uncommon relief.

An Immune Booster? A number of support groups are available for cancer victims, and studies indicate that patients who attend not only show psychological improvement, but they tend to live longer than patients who go it alone. Although some researchers are skeptical, others believe that positive changes in attitude and mood result in boosting immune function.

Like the twelve-step programs for addicts, many of the groups for cancer sufferers emphasize taking life "one day at a time." By doing so, patients are more likely to enjoy the small pleasures of life and less likely to be overwhelmed by depression and feelings of hopelessness. ❑

OVEREATERS ANONYMOUS

Compulsive eating is as hard to control as any other addiction. It leads to ill health and often to social isolation. As this story illustrates, support groups can make a difference.

"My mother prepared me well for the role of fat person. Being overweight herself, she knew how my life would run. She told me how people treated you: the jokes, the rejections, the cruelty. 'Develop your mind,' she told me. 'That's something they can never take away from you.' I got married the day after I graduated from high school. I didn't fit into my wife role. I stayed home and got bored and depressed. I ate. I gained weight slowly, eight or nine pounds each year. I put a lot of time and thought into special recipes. Supper became a grand occasion.

"I handled the money. We got behind in our bills. I could not stand to be a failure at managing money. That was when the shoplifting began, and it was emotional dynamite right from the start. The stealing soon became focused on food. Not once did I consider myself a thief. I was just trying to cope. My husband insisted I get out of the house and get a job. My desk drawer at work always had three or four candy bars in it. I ate in the car, I ate in the middle of the night. At five feet in height, I weighed 232 pounds and was getting heavier. I couldn't tie my shoelaces. My feet swelled and my legs ached; I had to buy ankle braces.

"Then I saw an ad in the paper for Overeaters Anonymous. I cut out the address and time of the meeting and put it in a kitchen drawer and left it there for four months.

"But the ad said help was available. I still had doubts. A fat club was insulting. And I knew I wouldn't mesh well with other people. Still, I went. There wasn't any answer for me anywhere else. They had me pegged, I knew I was home. I went on the program the next day at 220 pounds.

"I would like to be able to say that once I found the program all my problems vanished and I have had perfect abstinence and life has been wonderful. But that has not been my experience. I wanted the program and I knew it was right for me. But at times I've wanted it my way — and this is one program you don't manipulate.

"So my experience has been up and down. Always growing. Sometimes it's easy; I'm like a kite in the breeze. Sometimes I resist. Then I bog down and sometimes I break abstinence. But I just go back on.

"It has been a year now. I've lost 80 pounds. Twelve inches off my waist. Instead of a 24½ dress I wear a 13. I'm aware of how sick I've been, of how far I have to go. But that's OK. I know the way."

Excerpted from Overeaters Anonymous *by Overeaters Anonymous, Inc.*

Primal Therapy and Rebirthing

These techniques aim to help adults come to terms with their problems by letting them relive what they believe to be their earliest experiences. For some people, this means re-creating the trauma of birth.

DEVELOPED BY ARTHUR JANOV, a psychologist who trained as a Freudian analyst, primal therapy is meant to help clients find and liberate the wounded child within themselves. According to Janov, neurotic troubles are primal, that is, they begin in childhood when a baby senses that its basic needs are not being met. The aim of primal therapy is to help the client replay painful scenes from childhood, get at the root of the problem, and so find relief.

Janov developed the concept for primal therapy after treating a young man for neurosis. On a hunch, he urged the man to call out "Mommy! Daddy!" repeatedly. The client did so and soon began to cry like an infant. Soon thereafter, the man emitted what Janov described as "a piercing, deathlike scream that rattled the walls of my office." The client displayed evident improvement after this— and primal therapy was born.

Neurosis begins, according to Janov, when the client ignores the primal pain because he can't believe the reality of it. Primal therapy helps the client dredge up this pain, and scream out the rage of it. And according to the theory, clients who purge themselves of the miseries of childhood can rid themselves of adult emotional problems.

During primal therapy the client generally lies on a mat reliving the worst experiences of childhood, such as the denial of love, sibling envy, and physical mistreatment.

At the start of a rebirthing session, the client lies down on a mat and tries to achieve a state of deep relaxation. Then, with encouragement from the rebirther, the client practices connected breathing, meaning that she inhales and exhales without pause.

Some clients claim to have relived childbirth. They are encouraged to make as much noise as they like: screams, shouts, sobs, baby talk. Success, the emptying out of what Janov calls "the inner reservoir of primal pain," comes in a shuddering surge of pain, screams, sobs, and heavy breathing—a process which may take weeks or months.

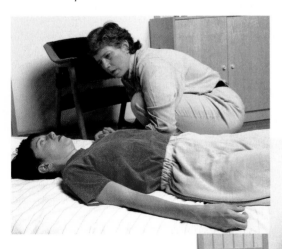

The client's outstretched arms are considered to be a sign that she is struggling with the rebirthing process, just as a baby struggles through delivery. This stage of rebirthing is often the most difficult.

Rebirthing. Practitioners of rebirthing believe that many adult conflicts begin at birth from the simple trauma of the natal process. In their opinion, the shock of the birth experience, or of other traumatic experiences in early childhood, may inhibit breathing mechanisms. This in turn lowers the quality of life in adulthood. During rebirthing, traumatic moments are relived in order to deal with their negative effects. Enthusiasts say that rebirthing may also help identify other unconscious dilemmas that are causing problems.

Rebirthing was started in the 1970s by Leonard Orr, a staff member of EST (Erhard Seminar Training). During long baths, Orr began experimenting with prolonged relaxation and various breathing rhythms, and ultimately found that he could enter into an altered state of consciousness. According to Orr, these experiments led him to relive his birth trauma and to focus on the very first breath he took outside the womb, an effect he found liberating and therapeutic.

A New Beginning. From his experiences, Orr refined rebirthing, putting strong emphasis on a focused breathing technique known as conscious connected breathing. In a typical session, the client relaxes on a bed or in a tub of warm water, while the rebirther directs him or her through various breathing patterns—deep, shallow, rapid, slow—which often produce a variety of sensations, from dizziness to exhilaration. Known as the resistance phase, the client is encouraged to breathe through these physical reactions, which may take from five to thirty minutes. According to rebirthers, once this is accomplished, the client will feel deeply relaxed, euphoric, and may experience profound insight. In addition, rebirthers claim that the breathing training promotes circulation and boosts energy through the release of tension. After a number of private rebirthing sessions, a client may be able to go through the process alone. ❏

Feeling totally relaxed, and yet buzzing with energy, the client rests after finishing the rebirthing session. In this state of relaxation, many people feel charged with clarity and insight about themselves, and are eager to try rebirthing again. Advocates say that with each session, clients reach deeper levels of awareness, and release greater amounts of emotional tension.

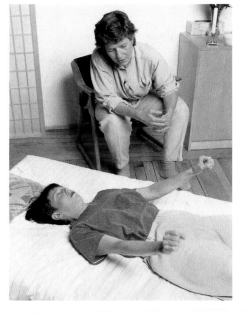

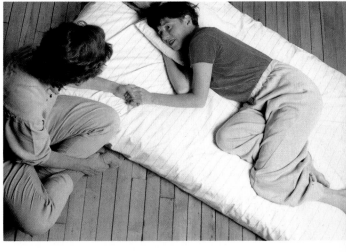

To break through the resistance phase, the client is encouraged to "breathe through" the experience, which may take from five to thirty minutes.

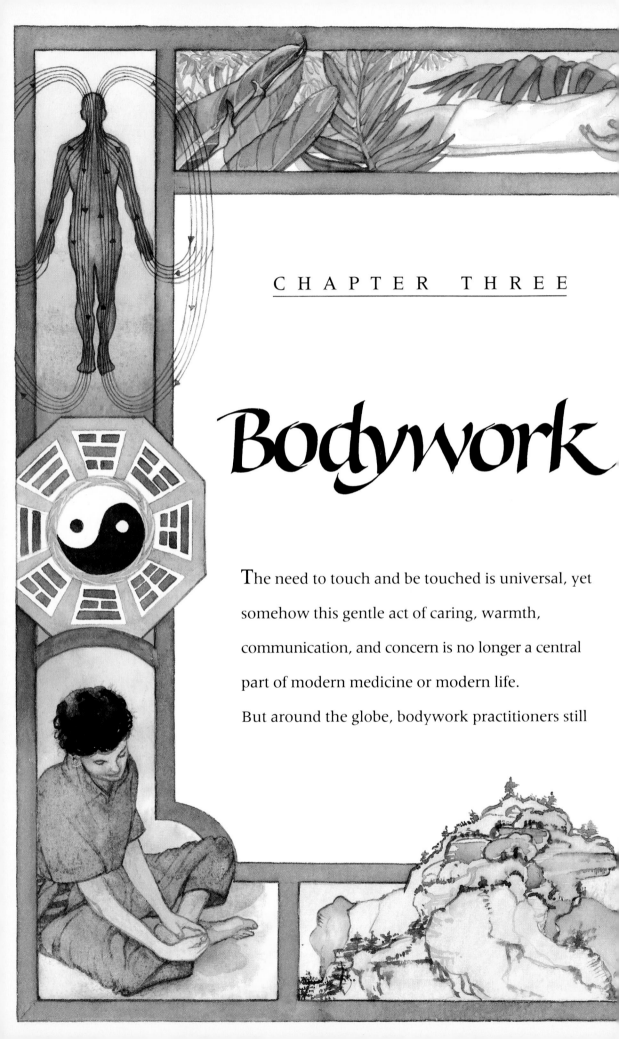

CHAPTER THREE

Bodywork

The need to touch and be touched is universal, yet somehow this gentle act of caring, warmth, communication, and concern is no longer a central part of modern medicine or modern life.

But around the globe, bodywork practitioners still

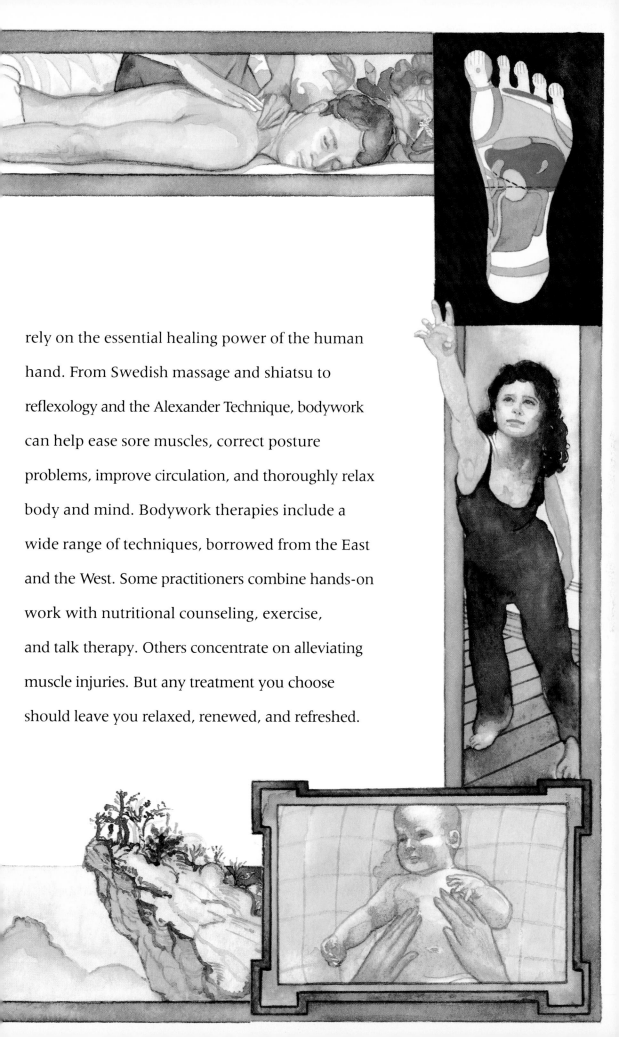

rely on the essential healing power of the human hand. From Swedish massage and shiatsu to reflexology and the Alexander Technique, bodywork can help ease sore muscles, correct posture problems, improve circulation, and thoroughly relax body and mind. Bodywork therapies include a wide range of techniques, borrowed from the East and the West. Some practitioners combine hands-on work with nutritional counseling, exercise, and talk therapy. Others concentrate on alleviating muscle injuries. But any treatment you choose should leave you relaxed, renewed, and refreshed.

The Art of Bodywork

Almost all bodywork therapies aim to release tension, which is thought to accumulate in the body because of stress or emotional trauma. These treatments often provide clients with a heightened sense of well-being.

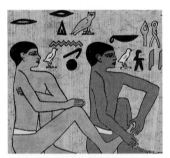

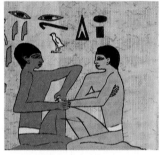

Bodywork in Antiquity

Found in the "physician's tomb" of Ankhmahor in Saqqara, Egypt, these pictures show a physician (the darker figure) massaging a patient's foot, and then his hand. The manipulations being performed bear striking resemblance to modern bodywork practices — especially reflexology. The inscription reports their dialogue: "Do not hurt me," says the patient. To this the physician replies, "I shall act in such a way that you will praise me."

BODYWORK IS AN OVER-ALL TERM for a wide range of massage-like therapies. Some utilize techniques of massage to treat specific ailments or to help improve muscle tone and circulation. Others teach more efficient use of the body, and some focus primarily on improving posture.

Today, there are a tremendous number of different treatments to choose from—ranging from deep manipulation of muscles and ligaments to gentle stroking of the skin. However, most bodywork treatments fall into one of four basic categories: pressure-point therapies; movement re-education; deep-tissue manipulation; and any combination of the three treatment styles.

Pressure-Point Therapies. Shiatsu, reflexology, and polarity borrow from traditional Chinese or Ayurvedic medicine, and aim at releasing energy blockages by manipulating specific pressure points on the body. Practitioners of shiatsu apply pressure to points all over the body, while reflexologists focus primarily on the feet. In polarity, the therapist uses hand placement to balance the body's flow of electromagnetic energy.

Movement Re-education. One of the best-known disciplines is the Alexander technique. Through discussion, example, and light body manipulation, this therapy teaches clients to improve posture and breathing, discard bad habits of movement, and use their bodies with greater ease.

Deep-Tissue Manipulation. Rolfing and Hellerwork are among the therapies that manipulate the fascia, the fibrous connective tissue that binds muscles together. The aim is to bring the body into proper alignment with gravity and to relieve chronic stress.

Bodywork Combinations. Many practitioners of bodywork therapies are proficient in more than one technique, and may combine a few approaches to achieve better results. In addition, meditation, diet, talk therapy, and certain exercises may also be incorporated into an over-all treatment plan. For example, Aston-Patterning derives from Rolfing, and also involves massage, movement re-education, and counseling.

Choosing a therapy and finding a practitioner can be confusing. Probably the best course is to ask around and go with the recommendation of a physician or physical therapist, or perhaps a friend who has had experience with a particular treatment. The major forms of bodywork are represented by institutions or associations that provide training and certification. These associations seek to maintain standards of practice, and may be able to recommend a local practitioner. ❏

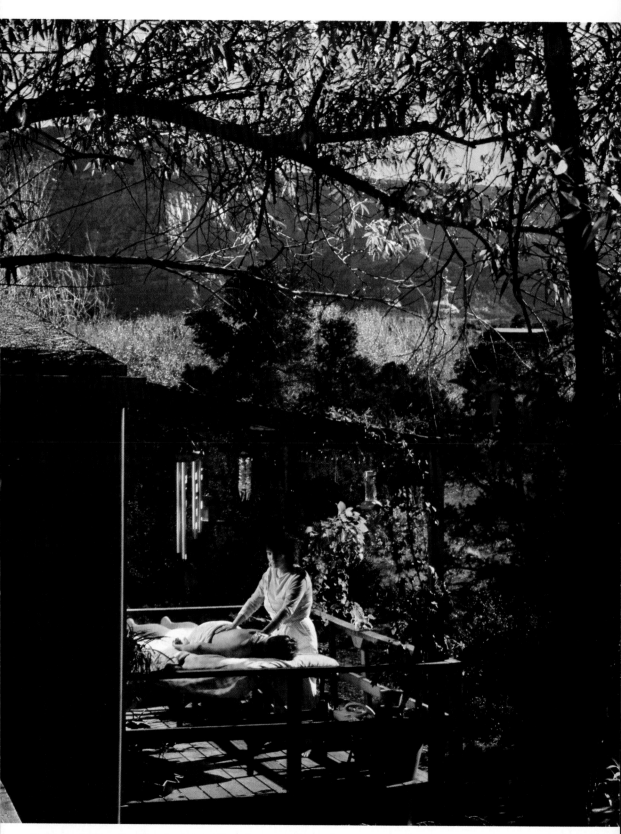

A massage given in a lovely, tranquil setting can enhance the soothing effects of the treatment. And while bodywork practitioners rarely offer the kind of luxurious surroundings pictured here, they frequently try to put clients at ease with comfortable furnishings, soft lighting, and quiet background music.

The Many Benefits of Massage

If you've never been massaged by a skilled practitioner, you're in for a treat. There are many types of massage: some can soothe aching muscles, others may ease stress, and all aim to give you a sense of well-being.

"THE PHYSICIAN MUST BE EXPERIENCED IN MANY THINGS," wrote Hippocrates, the father of Western medicine, in the 5th century B. C., "but assuredly in rubbing . . . for rubbing can bind a joint that is too loose, and loosen a joint that is too rigid." Indeed, rubbing—better known as massage—has long been known to have a great many beneficial effects, physical as well as mental.

In Eastern cultures, massage has been practiced continually since ancient times. A Chinese book from 2,700 B.C., *The*

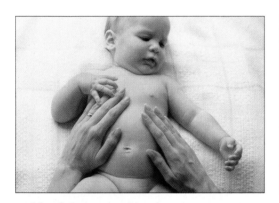 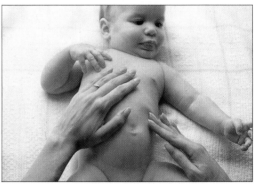

Babies thrive on touch, *and massage can provide parents with a special way of comforting a tiny, new presence. Regular massage may help babies sleep better, and some parents have used it to relieve colic. Before starting, make sure the room is very warm; then, with the baby lying face up, slowly and gently rub a little vegetable oil all over the body, moving your palms in light, rhythmic circles. When massaging the abdomen, always move in a clockwise direction.*

Yellow Emperor's Classic of Internal Medicine, recommends "breathing exercises, massage of skin and flesh, and exercises of hands and feet" as the appropriate treatment for "complete paralysis, chills, and fever." Swedish massage, the method most familiar to Westerners, was developed in the 19th century by a Swedish doctor, poet, and educator named Per Henrik Ling. His system was based on a study of gymnastics and physiology, and on techniques borrowed from China, Egypt, Greece, and Rome.

Different Strokes. Out of both the Eastern and Western traditions, a great many forms of massage have developed. Although the philosophies and styles differ, they share the common intention of mobilizing the natural healing properties of the body in order to help maintain or restore optimal health. The Eastern styles, such as shiatsu, focus on balancing the body's vital energy (qi) as it flows in pathways known as zones or meridians.

The Western styles, such as Swedish massage, work primarily to affect the muscles, connective tisssues (including tendons and ligaments), and cardiovascular system. A variety of gliding, kneading, and percussive strokes are used, along with deep circular movements and vibrations, in order to relax the muscles, improve circulation, and increase mobility. The strokes can be varied in depth and rhythm: where relaxation is the primary goal, they may be lighter and more flowing. Where stretching or tissue work is the intention, the strokes may be deeper.

A Reputation Restored. Massage has long been tainted by two widespread misconceptions: first, that it is something shady practiced in dimly lit parlors; and secondly, that it is a self-indulgence for the rich and famous. As these myths have faded, massage has once again gained recognition for its healing and relaxation potential. Recipients often report sleeping better, having greater energy, fewer aches and pains, and an over-all sense of well-being.

Increasingly, doctors, chiropractors, and physical therapists are hiring massage therapists to work with patients recovering from a wide range of conditions, including joint injuries, chronic back and neck pain, arthritis, sciatica, and migraine headaches. Professional and weekend athletes alike are discovering the benefits of massage to help prevent injuries, improve performance, and reduce soreness after exercise. For example, Bill Rodgers, the Olympic medal winner and veteran marathon runner, used self-massage to relieve painful muscle spasms, which allowed him to finish the New York City marathon. Professional dance companies have also employed massage therapists.

How Does It Work? A host of physiological and psychological effects have been attributed to massage, which may explain its range of benefits. When muscles are chronically tense or overworked, waste products such as lactic acid can accumulate in them, causing soreness, stiffness, and even muscle spasm. By improving the circulation into and out of the muscles, massage helps speed the elimination of these toxins, easing discomfort. At the same time, the increase in blood flow brings fresh fuel and oxygen to body tissues, which can enhance the healing process after injury or speed recuperation from disease.

In addition, overly contracted, tight muscles may compress blood vessels and restrict blood flow, or they may entrap nerves, causing pain and loss of function. Massage can help relax and stretch tight muscles, improving circulation, freeing trapped nerves, and alleviating pain. And beyond the physical effects, many recipients of massage also report enormous psychological benefits. For some, a massage in a peaceful environment provides time to let go of stress, and the opportunity to give in to one of life's simple pleasures.

What to Expect. A typical massage session lasts an hour. The client, either partially or fully undressed, is wrapped in a sheet or towel, and lies on a massage

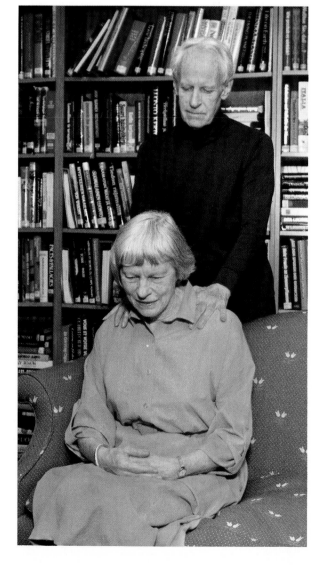

People of all ages can enjoy the many benefits of massage. Older people may prefer to receive massage while sitting up in a chair, particularly if their joints are stiff. Combined with good diet and regular exercise, massage can help ease many problems associated with age, including high blood pressure and muscular aches and pains.

table or other firm surface. Only those parts of the body being massaged are exposed. Since a relaxed environment enhances the experience, the room should be warm and peaceful and the lighting low. Before beginning, it's best for the client to tell the massage therapist about any injuries or discomfort. Most massage therapists apply a light oil to their hands to make the massage movements smoother.

Basic Techniques of Swedish Massage. Traditional Swedish Massage uses five main strokes, and many variations, to achieve its relaxing and healing effects. Many therapists use a variety of techniques, and they will ask you to tell them if any strokes feel uncomfortable.

Effleurage is a long, gliding stroke, done with the whole hand or the thumb pads. When done on the limbs, all strokes

Back Massage Tips

- **Keep the room warm**, and except for the back, keep your partner covered.
- **Work at a table** positioned at a height that is comfortable for your back. Or work on a pad on the floor, kneeling next to your partner. A bed, even with a firm mattress, is too soft.
- **If your partner** is uncomfortable, try putting a pillow under the ankles and/or abdomen.
- **Use a natural vegetable** oil as a lubricant. Warm it by applying it to your own hands first.
- **To add pressure to your** strokes, lean in and use your body weight — don't rely on the strength of your arms and hands alone.

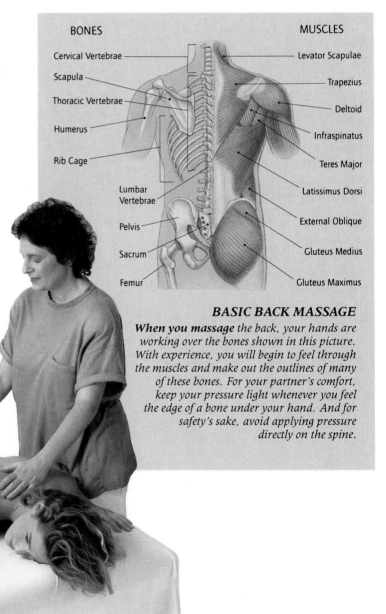

BONES

Cervical Vertebrae
Scapula
Thoracic Vertebrae
Humerus
Rib Cage
Lumbar Vertebrae
Pelvis
Sacrum
Femur

MUSCLES

Levator Scapulae
Trapezius
Deltoid
Infraspinatus
Teres Major
Latissimus Dorsi
External Oblique
Gluteus Medius
Gluteus Maximus

BASIC BACK MASSAGE

When you massage the back, your hands are working over the bones shown in this picture. With experience, you will begin to feel through the muscles and make out the outlines of many of these bones. For your partner's comfort, keep your pressure light whenever you feel the edge of a bone under your hand. And for safety's sake, avoid applying pressure directly on the spine.

WHOLE HAND EFFLEURAGE

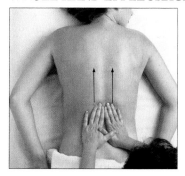

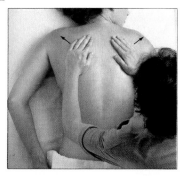

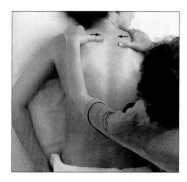

Place one hand on each side of the lower spine. Slide your hands toward the neck, following the contours of the back. Pressure should come from leaning your weight into your hands.

Two-thirds up the back, start sliding your hands sideways and up toward the shoulders. Lighten pressure as you go over edges of the shoulder blades; otherwise keep pressure even and your hands in contact with the back.

At the shoulders, slide your hands back toward the neck, across the tops of the shoulders. Wrap your fingers lightly over the edge of the shoulder and sink your palms into the muscles as you glide.

THUMB EFFLEURAGE

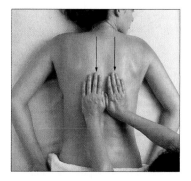

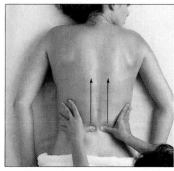

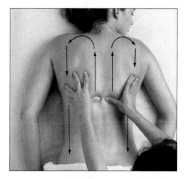

When your hands meet at the base of the neck, slide them down the back to the beginning point. Use lighter pressure on the return stroke to rest your hands. Repeat this sequence three or four times.

This stroke is similar to the first, but more focused. Using your thumbs, glide up the back, staying in the furrows along either side of the spine. Keep your other fingers flat on the back.

Continue until thumbs approach the base of the neck. Finish by gliding your hands across the tops of the shoulders, and return by sliding hands down the rib cage. Repeat, starting farther from the spine.

FANNING OUT

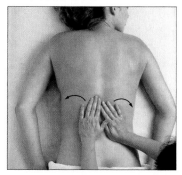

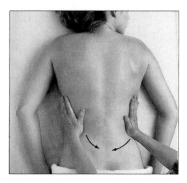

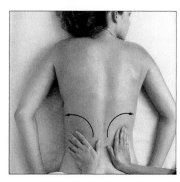

Start with hands flat on the lower back. Spread your hands apart from each other, drawing a half circle with each hand, toward the sides of the body. Think of spreading the back muscles wider.

Continue the circles down the sides of the ribs until your pinkies touch the table. Now pull up through the waist with firm contact. Keep your hands curved to the shape of the body.

Finish by bringing your hands back to starting position, applying pressure with the heels of your hands. Repeat the stroke several times, each time starting higher on the back, until you've covered the whole back.

are toward the heart to aid blood and lymphatic flow. *Petrissage* generally involves kneading and compression motions—rolling, squeezing, or pressing the muscles to enhance deeper circulation.

Friction is the most penetrating of the strokes, and consists of deep circular or transverse movements made with the thumb pads or fingertips. *Tapotement* consists of a series of briskly applied percussive movements, using the hands alter-

KNEADING PETRISSAGE

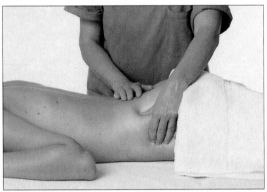

Begin on the buttocks, *working the side opposite you. Pick up as much muscle as you can between the thumb and fingers of one hand, and squeeze or "milk" the muscles toward the surface.*

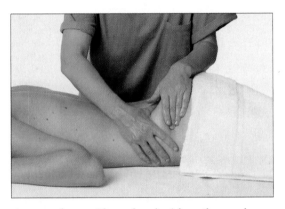

As you release *with one hand, pick up the muscles with the other hand. Keep handing the muscles back and forth, scooping and kneading with a circular movement. Maintain a steady rhythm.*

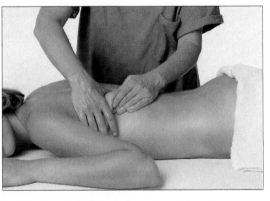

Once you establish *a rhythm, start to knead up the outer edge of the back toward the shoulder. Move slowly, inch by inch, giving each muscle area attention, until you reach the armpit.*

Finish by kneading *the shoulder area, picking up as much muscle as possible with each hand. Don't pinch or squeeze the muscles in a painful way. Repeat on opposite side.*

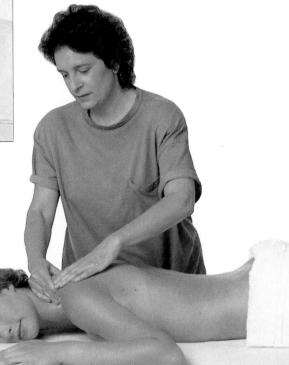

nately to strike or tap the muscles for an invigorating effect. There are many variations on this stroke. *Vibration* involves applying a very fine, rapid shaking movement.

A proper massage is generally safe for most people, but a massage improperly performed, or on someone who has suffered an injury or illness, can cause damage. So it's very important to choose a qualified massage therapist. The American Massage Therapy Association, the oldest and largest

ROLLING STROKE

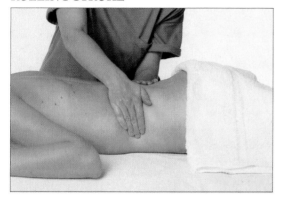

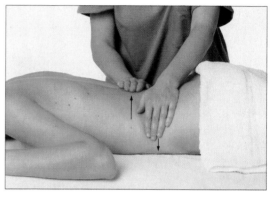

Place hands *on opposite sides of the lower back with fingers pointing away from you. Bring hands together, one pulling, the other pushing toward the middle of the back until hands meet and pass lightly over the spine.*

Continue in same direction *until hands have exchanged starting positions, making a complete ring across the back. Repeat, moving up a few inches. Keep pressure firm on the sides, light across the spine.*

EFFLEURAGE FROM THE HEAD

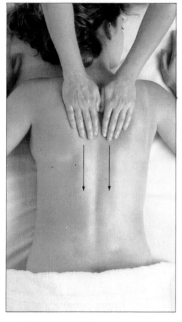

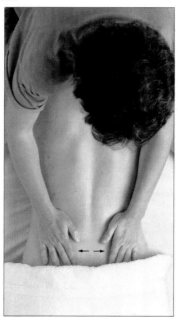

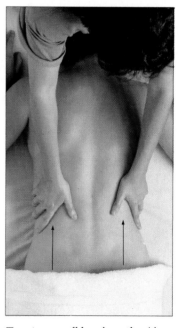

Position yourself *at the top of your partner's head with one hand on each side of the spine, just below the neck. Glide your hands to the base of spine, keeping fingers together. Lean into this stroke.*

When you reach *the base of your partner's spine, separate your hands and glide them firmly across the top of the buttocks. Maintain a steady pressure, giving a nice stretch across the lower back.*

To return, *pull hands up the sides of the ribs, and back to the starting position. Repeat this stroke three or four times. You can return to this effleurage between any of the following strokes.*

THUMB CIRCLES

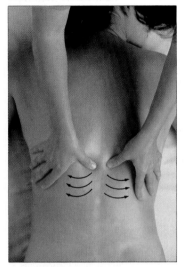
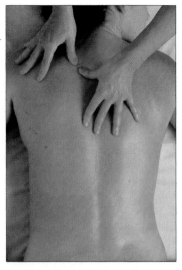
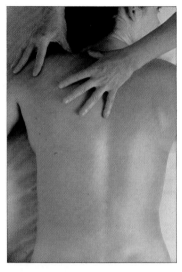

Place a thumb on either side of the spine and slowly work down, making circles with each thumb. Apply pressure during the first half of each circle, pushing away from the spine.

Now place thumbs on one side of back. Make alternating circles: second thumb starts a circle as the first thumb finishes. Work the area between the spine and the shoulder blade.

Use the same stroke to work across the top of one shoulder. Make circles slowly, and try to feel any tight spots in the muscles. Give those spots extra attention. Repeat on opposite side.

FRICTION ALONG THE SHOULDER BLADE

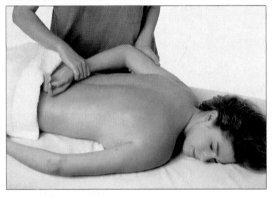
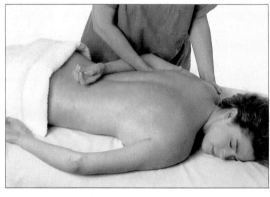

To work the shoulder area more thoroughly, take your partner's forearm, and gently place it behind her back. The edge of the shoulder blade will stand out. (Don't attempt this if it causes any discomfort.)

Place your hand under the front of your partner's shoulder and slide so that your partner's shoulder rests on your hand. Keep your hand there for support as you perform the next stroke with your other hand.

With your free hand, use the flat tips of your fingers to make slow circles along the shoulder blade. For a penetrating effect, try making circles which move the skin over the muscles rather than circling your fingers over the skin. Return arm to side and repeat sequence on opposite side.

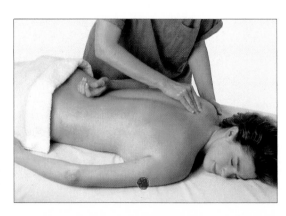

massage organization, requires 500 hours of study, including courses in anatomy, physiology, and the processes of injury and disease, before a therapist can join. Such massage therapists are trained to identify contraindications, and to refer you to other health professionals when necessary.

Massage should be avoided when any of these conditions are present: fever, acute inflammation, infection or illness, phlebitis, thrombosis, malignancy, jaundice. Massage should also be avoided directly over the site of a recent injury, or over bruises, burns, varicose veins, skin rashes or eruptions. Massage may be helpful for persons with chronic conditions such as heart disease or arthritis, but should be performed only with a doctor's okay. Pregnant women should consult a doctor before having a massage. ❏

STRETCHING THE BACK MUSCLES

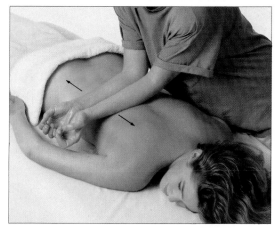 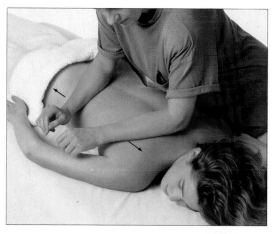

To give a nice stretch to the long muscles of the back, place your forearms next to each other in the center of the opposite side of the back with palms facing up. Slowly, and with pressure, begin to slide your arms apart.

As you spread out, your arms should rotate so that your palms will be facing the floor. Repeat this stroke a few times on the side opposite you, then on the side closer to you. You can end the massage with this soothing stroke, or . . .

TAPOTEMENT

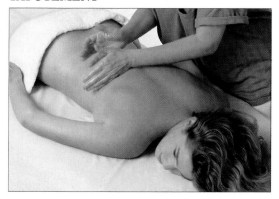 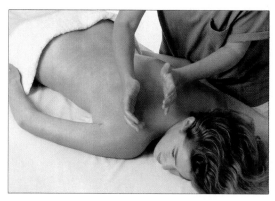

If you want to finish on a more invigorating note, use this version of tapotement called hacking. Tapotement is a brisk percussive movement, done with loose wrists and relaxed hands. Raise your hands above the back with the palms facing each other.

Let the edge of your hands alternately strike the back, with a rapid, regular rhythm. Concentrate on keeping wrists loose, and on pulling hands off the back as soon as they hit, so the effect is light, not pounding. Avoid kidneys (above waist) and spine.

Pressure-Point Massage

By applying pressure at points along the body, shiatsu and acupressure practitioners attempt to unblock the body's energy pathways. In doing so, they are also helping to summon our natural healing response.

SHIATSU, FROM A JAPANESE word meaning "finger pressure," is a form of massage that uses manual pressure to stimulate and free energy pathways within the body. Like many aspects of Japanese culture, shiatsu has its roots in China, and grew out of the ancient Chinese philosophy of health and medicine that includes massage, acupuncture, and herbal remedies. By combining acupuncture with traditional massage, the Japanese developed a bodywork therapy that aims to maintain or restore the body's balance of energy.

Life Energy. Unlike Western massage, which is based on physiological principles, shiatsu is based on the Eastern concept of qi, or "life energy," which is believed to flow through the body along channels called meridians. According to this theory, the human body has 12 major meridians, most named for the organ to which they correspond. Situated along these meridians are places where the qi tends to gather. In traditional Chinese medicine these are known as acupuncture points, but the Japanese refer to them as tsubos. Stress, injury, disease, poor diet, and other factors can impair the functioning of these points, trapping energy. Shiatsu practitioners aim to release this blocked energy by putting pressure on the tsubos. In doing so, energy is released to circulate freely, and the body is better able to heal itself.

In addition to clearing energy blockages, shiatsu practitioners also attempt to balance the two forms of energy within the body: the yin energy, which is quiet and deep, and the yang energy, which is active and on the surface. A client who showed signs of fatigue or depression, for example, would be diagnosed as being in a yin state. To ease the symptoms, the shiatsu practitioner would try to stimulate the yang energy. Conversely, a client with such yang symptoms as irritability or tension would need a yin treatment to calm him.

The Five Elements. Another aim of this bodywork therapy is to restore the balance within the Five Elements. According to traditional Chinese medicine, the universe is composed of five elements—Fire, Earth, Metal, Water, and Wood. The human body is considered a microcosm of the universe, and so is also composed of these

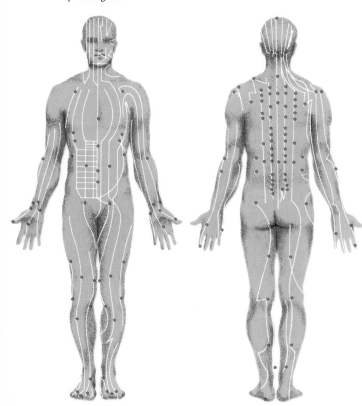

Tsubos are the points along the meridians where the body's qi often accumulates. Most lie fairly close to the surface of the skin, along the front and back of the body. The goal of the shiatsu practitioner is to free trapped energy from these points. According to practitioners, anyone can learn to find at least some of these points; you may feel a twinge or tingle upon pressing one.

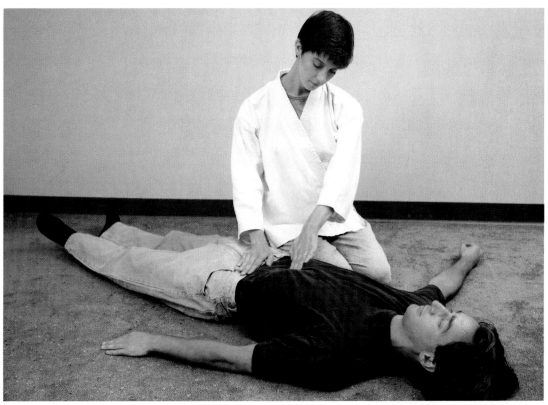

Five Elements. Each element is associated with different organs, meridians, and characteristics. For example, the Wood element is connected with anger, and a hostile person would be diagnosed as having an imbalance within that element. To alleviate the anger, appropriate meridians would be treated to restore balance.

Shiatsu differs from Western massage in technique as well as in theory. While Swedish massage therapists use long, flowing hand movements to knead muscles, shiatsu practitioners apply rhythmic and gradual pressure to the meridians and tsubos. Although the pressure is applied primarily with the fingers, practitioners will also use the knees, elbows, toes, heels of the hands and feet, and the pad of the foot. While the amount of pressure applied varies, at no time should there be sudden or severe pain.

What to Expect. A shiatsu massage usually takes 45 to 60 minutes. Unlike Swedish massage, no oil is used and the client remains fully clothed. While shiatsu can be given in almost any environment, the best place is on a carpeted floor in a warm, airy room. The firmness of the floor helps the practitioner bring the weight of his body into the tsubos being pressed. Shiatsu experts say that it is important that the practitioner approach his work in an aware and sensitive state, and that his own body be relaxed and centered.

The session begins with the client lying on his back. The practitioner first treats the Hara, the area between the rib cage and pelvic bone which is considered the central storehouse for the body's qi. Next he moves to the front of

A basic shiatsu session begins and ends with work on the Hara, the area between the ribs and the pelvis. The Hara is said to be the storehouse of our body's strength and vital energy; it is often used diagnostically as a measure of general health. Pressure to this area should be smooth and gradual, with hands moving in a clockwise direction.

Acupressure Tips

According to the experts, successful acupressure depends on technique. Before treating yourself, or anyone else, read these few tips.

- Place fingertip on the acupuncture point, making sure it is at a right angle to the body.
- Begin stimulating the point by pressing with a circular motion, gradually increasing the force until a deep, constant pressure is achieved.
- Press each point for no more than four minutes.
- Do not use acupressure directly over cuts, infections, or scar tissue.

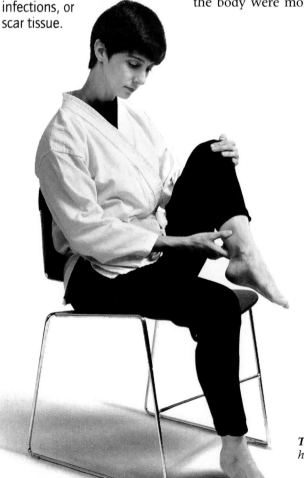

the legs, arms, neck, head, and face. The client is usually encouraged to breathe slowly and rhythmically to aid relaxation, and pressure is applied only during exhalation.

Shiatsu is considered most effective as a way of maintaining the body's health and stamina. Although primarily a preventive technique, advocates also claim successful results in treating certain ailments, such as constipation. But shiatsu should be performed with caution on people with contagious diseases, bone fractures, disorders of the heart, liver, kidneys, or lungs, cancer, or infectious skin diseases. Of course, a physician should always be consulted in the case of serious illness.

Acupressure. Shiatsu and acupressure are often thought of as being different names for the same massage technique. While they share the same philosophy, shiatsu is a relatively new treatment primarily used as a preventive therapy, and to keep the body operating at top form. Acupressure, on the other hand, is an age-old therapeutic technique, which, like acupuncture, was probably developed to treat specific symptoms or disorders.

Both acupressure and acupuncture most likely grew out of our natural instinct to touch or rub an injury. Thousands of years ago the Chinese observed that some areas of the body were more sensitive than others. Furthermore,

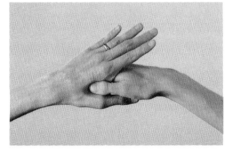

For headache relief, *press the point in web of flesh between thumb and forefinger.*

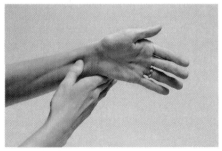

To relieve nausea, *press thumb into area two inches above crease in the wrist.*

To ease menstrual cramps, *measure a hand width from the inner ankle, and press.*

pressure on these areas seemed to have some effect on other, apparently unrelated parts of the body. This realization led to the development of Chinese medicine's intricate network of points and meridians. Originally, pressure to the points was probably applied with the fingers. Only later did the Chinese begin to stimulate the points with needles.

Nowadays, acupressure is thought of as a first-aid technique, and may be used to treat such common disorders as headache or backache. ❏

FREEING ENERGY BLOCKAGES

Gina Martin, a licensed massage therapist, practices shiatsu. Here she tells the story of a desperate client who found relief from chronic itchiness after years of suffering.

"Ever since she was a child, Margaret, a woman in her late 20s, had been suffering from intermittent bouts of itchy skin, which were often so severe that she was unable to sleep. Many a night she would lie awake fighting a desperate urge to scratch, finally dropping off into an exhausted sleep as dawn approached.

"Over the years, her bouts of itchiness had grown more frequent and more severe. All of her attempts to have the problem diagnosed and treated had been unsuccessful. She had been tested for allergies, but none were found; she'd had cortisone treatments, which provided no relief. Some physicians, finding no obvious rash or other outward symptoms, prescribed tranquilizers and suggested that her problem might be 'nerves.' But Margaret felt strongly that the problem was not just 'in her head.' Finally, on the recommendation of a friend, she came to see me for shiatsu treatments.

"During the first session, Margaret lay on her back while I checked the energy areas of her abdomen. Because there exists an important connection between the skin and the bowel, I asked her about her regularity. I also asked her questions about her life style, job, stress level, diet, exercise, medical history, and emotional state. Gradually a pattern began to emerge.

"An important clue was that Margaret was also suffering from chronic constipation — a problem, like her itchiness, that she'd had since childhood. She'd lived with constipation for so long she almost didn't think to mention it. Fortunately she did. According to Chinese medicine, this pattern of itchiness and constipation pointed to an imbalance in the Metal element, one of the Five Elements that make up the body. A blockage of energy in one area, the large intestine, would affect another area, the skin. In other words, Margaret's constipation was causing her itchy skin.

"I treated Margaret by applying pressure along the energy pathways of the body called meridians. Using both hands, I paid special attention to the points used for treating constipation. The pressure removes the blockages and allows the energy to flow freely. It simply opens the body up and, unlike drugs, has no side effects. I also taught her self massage techniques to use on her own to relieve the constipation. Over the course of three weeks, Margaret came to see me for three one-hour sessions, and both her itchiness and constipation totally disappeared.

"As Margaret discovered, the body wants to be in balance. Sometimes it just needs a little help."

Discovering Reflexology

This is a 20th-century version of an ancient healing and relaxation technique, which focuses on certain parts of the body. By applying gentle pressure to the feet, reflexologists attempt to ease pain, relieve tension, and restore energy.

A HEALING ART GENERALLY used to promote relaxation and to improve health, reflexology is a technique of applying pressure to specific points on the feet, hands, or ears. The method is most commonly used on the feet, largely because they have so many nerve endings and so are quite sensitive. Reflexologists believe that the foot functions as a microcosm of the entire body, and that reference points or reflex areas in the foot correspond to all the major organs, glands, and parts of the body.

The toes, for example, correspond to the head and

RELAXATION SEQUENCE

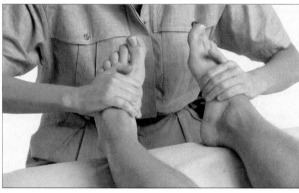

Warm-up: *A typical session begins with the practitioner "greeting" the feet, starting on the top.*

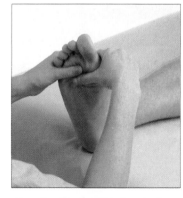

Pressing firmly, *slide thumbs from either edge of the foot, across the sole, and back. Work the entire sole.*

Reflexology *is a soothing way of easing tension. With the client lying comfortably, the session begins with a series of warm-up exercises.*

neck; the ball of the foot to the chest and lungs; the arch to the internal organs; the heel to the sciatic nerve and the pelvic area; and the bone along the curving arch of the foot to the spine. Furthermore, the right side of the body is reflected in the right foot, the left side in the left foot, and the various reflex points extend from the top of the foot to the bottom.

Proponents believe that applying pressure to a specific area of the foot spurs the movement of energy along channels in the body to the corresponding area—a process which promotes better health by reducing stress, improving circulation, eliminating toxins, speeding healing, and generally balancing and energizing the body. Reflexologists recommend the therapy for alleviating or controlling simple chronic conditions such as asthma, headaches, migraines, constipation, sinus trouble, bowel irritation, and kidney stones. Some practitioners also cite clients who

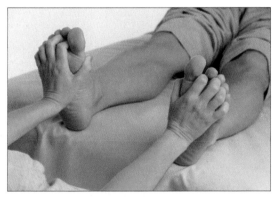

Continuing the warm-up, *the reflexologist grasps the bottoms of the feet and presses into them.*

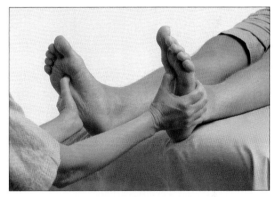

Press a thumb *into the solar plexus point on each foot, release, then rotate the thumb on the point.*

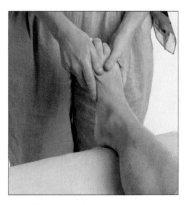

The thumb rotations *continue on the top of the foot, working down from the toes to the ankles.*

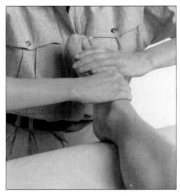

Wringing. *Twist the hands in opposite directions, as if wringing out a towel; continue up the foot.*

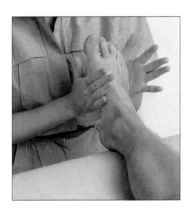

Foot boogie. *"Saw" the hands back and forth so each foot is lightly slapped from side to side.*

have lost weight or who have experienced a burst of creativity as a result of a reflexology session.

Origins. As a healing technique, reflexology is probably as old or older than acupuncture, with which it has many similarities. Variations of reflexology have long been practiced in Egypt, India, Africa, China, and Japan. Like most Eastern healing arts, it is based on the concept of a life energy (the Chinese qi, the Indian prana) flowing through

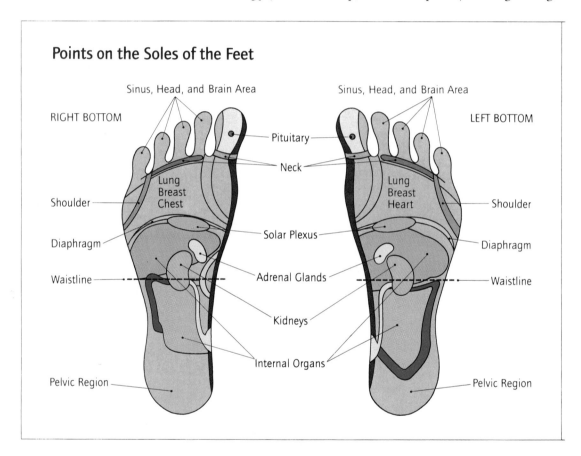

Points on the Soles of the Feet

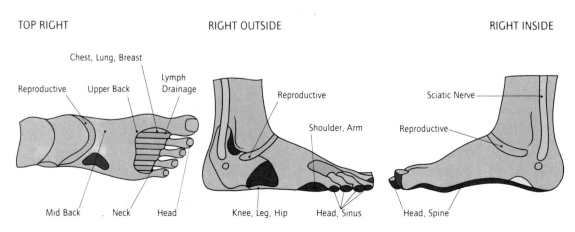

Points on the Top and Sides of the Foot

the body along pathways called zones or meridians. According to the theory, illness results if the energy flow becomes blocked or otherwise impeded. A reflexology session works to free the flow.

20th-Century Reflexology. Western reflexology dates from the early years of this century when Dr. William Fitzgerald, an American ear, nose, and throat specialist, devised a theory of "zone therapy." He divided the body into ten vertical zones of communication, five on a side, each of which extended from the head to the fingertips and toes. By applying pressure to various parts of the body—most commonly the hands and feet—he claimed that the functioning of different organs could be improved and pain eased. A colleague, Dr. Edwin Bowers, demonstrated the theory by showing he could stick a pin into a volunteer's face without causing him any pain if pressure was first applied to the corresponding reference point on another part of the body.

Fitzgerald's theory was further refined in the 1930s by Eunice Ingham, a physical therapist, who discovered that the ten zones could be best accessed through the feet. She then worked out a detailed map showing which areas of the feet corresponded to which organs and parts of the body. After publishing her findings in a book in 1938, Ingham established a reflexology institute and continued to teach and lecture widely. Many of today's reflexologists use the Ingham method. Other practitioners use the Laura Norman method, a training program taught in hospitals, universities, and other institutions.

The Mystery of How It Works. While practitioners agree that the technique relieves tension and clears blockages in the body's flow of vital energy, there are different theories as to how this occurs. According to one, reflexology stimulates sensory receptors in the nerve fibers of the foot. This produces energy that quickly travels to the spinal cord, where it is dispersed throughout the entire nervous system. Another theory postulates that the treatment relaxes the body, thereby reducing any constriction of the blood vessels and improving circulation.

Reflexology is also said to produce its beneficial effects by breaking up and dissolving crystal deposits (caused by an excess of uric acid in the body) that have settled in the feet. Still another theory contends that during the treatment, a group of pain-blocking chemicals called endorphins are released into the bloodstream, easing pain or producing a feeling of well-being.

Other advocates assert that reflexology may be more effective than other forms of massage because it is less intrusive. Many people are more comfortable about having their feet worked on than they would be about having their entire bodies massaged.

What to Expect. Reflexologists say any treatment can be beneficial for most people, with the exception of those suffering from serious illness or injury. For general relax-

Points on the Palms

LEFT PALM UP

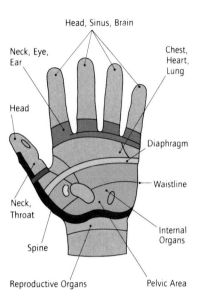

RIGHT PALM UP

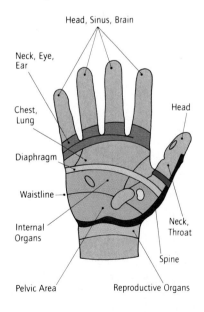

SEVEN BASIC TECHNIQUES

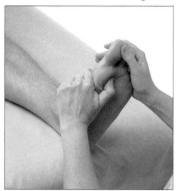

Thumb walking. *Press your thumb into the sole; inch it up by bending and unbending it.*

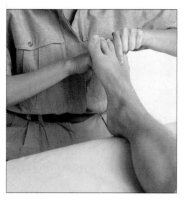

Finger walking. *Inch your index finger forward by flexing and unflexing the first joint.*

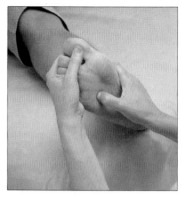

Rotating on a point. *Press your thumb lightly beneath ball of foot, and gently rotate the foot.*

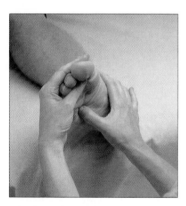

Flexing on a point. *Press your thumb into an area on the sole, and flex the foot several times.*

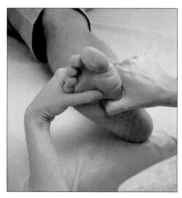

Pivoting on a point. *As you thumb-walk across the sole, use the other hand to pivot the foot.*

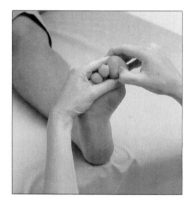

Hook and back-up. *Press firmly with the outside of your thumb and push the skin back.*

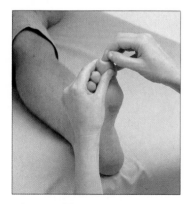

Finger rolling. *Applying light pressure, roll the end of your index finger across the top of each toe.*

ation, a 30 minute to 1 hour session once a week should be sufficient. For a specific problem, two or three sessions a week may be recommended. Some people are said to notice a change in their condition immediately; for others, it may require several sessions.

During a typical session, the client lies on a massage table with head slightly elevated, and bare feet facing the reflexologist. Since relaxation is crucial to the treatment's effectiveness, the client is instructed to breathe easily; many practitioners also try to encourage relaxation with soft lighting and quiet background music.

A session begins with a gentle massage of the feet. Then, using his or her thumbs and index fingers, the reflexologist applies sustained pressure to each foot in turn, with special attention being paid to sore or tender areas. While the client may feel considerable pressure during the session, there should be no pain. Often there will be a tingling sensation in the body part that corresponds to the reflex area of the foot. During a prolonged course of treatment, a client may exhibit such symptoms as aching joints, sore throat, diarrhea, or increased urination. Reflexologists say these symptoms are a result of the body's normal detoxifying process and are not dangerous. If these symptoms occur, the client is encouraged to eat sparingly and drink a lot of liquids to help speed the process along. Many clients report immediate positive effects after a session, including a decrease in stress, increased energy, and a feeling of vibrancy and well-being.

Doing It Yourself. You can also try reflexology on yourself or on a companion, but you should do so only as a relaxation technique, not as a cure for illness. If you are working on someone else, have the person sit or lie comfortably, with spine straight. A bed, reclining chair, or massage table is ideal.

Start by gently massaging each foot separately and then, beginning with the left foot, apply a steady, even pressure on the solar plexus reflex area, which is just below the ball of the foot. Move the pressure slowly forward in a caterpillar-like motion up to the toes, then work back down the foot. Massage the bone that forms the arch, and when you reach the heel, begin moving forward again. Finally, massage the top of the foot, ending with a gentle stroke up the ankle and lower calf. For best results, each foot should be massaged twice. If an area feels especially tender, try coming back to it later, but be careful not to overdo it or to cause any discomfort.

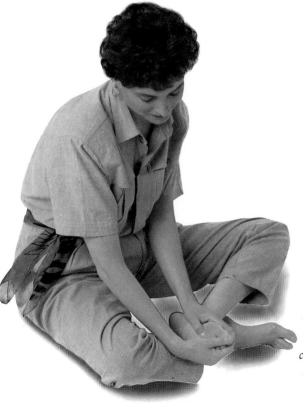

Self-reflexology may ease stress. Think about where you're feeling the most tension, and find the corresponding reflex point on your foot. Work the area until you relax.

Developing the Proper Technique

Thumb-walking, an important reflexology technique, may require a little practice.

- Applying steady pressure, walk the thumb forward by slightly bending and unbending at the first joint.
- Don't straighten the thumb completely; you'll cover an area too quickly and miss reflex points.
- Remember, it may take time to build strength in your thumb, so you may feel a little soreness at first.

LUNGS AND CHEST

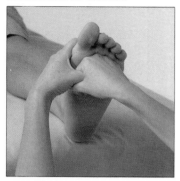

Lung Press. *Push the knuckles of your fist against the base of the toes and the ball of the foot.*

Foot Treatment Sequence. Once you've studied the map of the foot and learned the basic techniques, you may wish to try giving reflexology to a friend. On these pages is a routine for basic relaxation.

To get yourself ready and to put your partner at ease, start with the relaxation exercises shown on page 168. Relax each foot separately, and end with a thumb press on the solar plexus points. Before working the points outlined in these photographs, thumb-walk up the zones of each foot. Remember, reflexology is meant to be soothing and relaxing, so watch for blisters, calluses, and other tender spots.

The session should last between 20 to 30 minutes, or until either of you becomes tired. Beginning with the left foot, work each point suggested here, then switch to the right foot. Finish the session with the relaxation techniques. ❑

SHOULDER

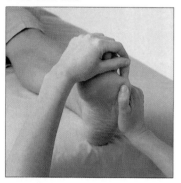

Using the thumb walk, *move your hand up the outside of the foot, toward the little toe.*

NECK

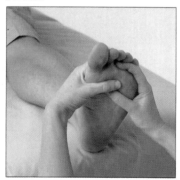

Following the line *at the base of the toes, thumb- and finger-walk around the entire foot.*

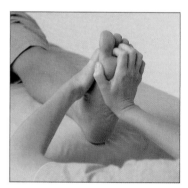

Grip your fingers *around the "toe ridge" at the base of toes and pull down toward the heel.*

NECK AND HEAD

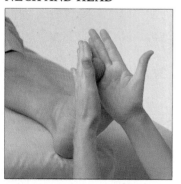

Toe Boogie. *Hold toe between your hands and "saw" back and forth, rocking toe from side to side.*

SINUS AND EYES

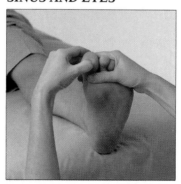

Holding the foot *with one hand, thumb-walk the bottom of each toe, starting from the top downward.*

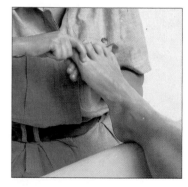

Now finger-walk *the toes of each foot, moving down along the front of the toes.*

PITUITARY

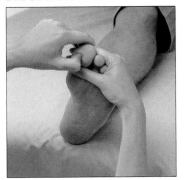

Use the hook and back-up on the very center of the large toe; push toward the outside of the foot.

SPINE

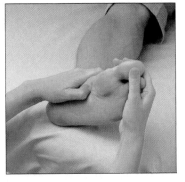

Thumb-walk up the outside of the arch, from the heel to the middle of the big toe.

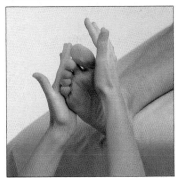

While pressing the top of your hand against the bottom of the foot, thumb-walk down the same area.

KIDNEYS

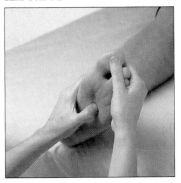

As you press the kidney point, in the center of the foot, rotate the entire foot toward the inside.

ADRENALS

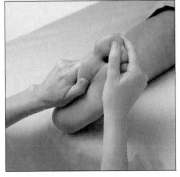

Press the adrenals point, slightly above and inside of the kidney point, while rotating the foot.

ENTIRE FOOT

To relax the entire body, use the foot boogie; rock the foot back and forth between your hands.

SOLAR PLEXUS

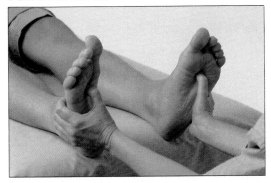

Press your thumbs into the solar plexus points—the fleshy part just below the balls of both feet.

BREEZE STROKE

End the session with breeze strokes to both feet. Lightly stroke the top of each foot from the ankle toward the toes.

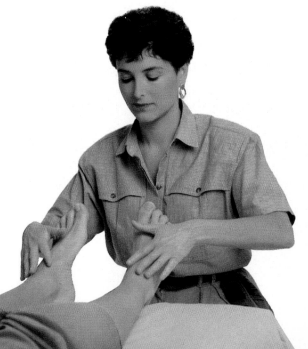

Energy in Motion

Polarity therapy is aimed at both relaxing and recharging the body.
By combining gentle manipulation techniques with diet and exercise,
polarity practitioners offer clients a more balanced approach to life.

POLARITY THERAPY is a method of mind/body healing based on the concept that life energy permeates every muscle, bone, organ, and cell of the human body. This energy is said to circulate within and around the body in specific currents and patterns, much as electrical energy flows through a power cable. As long as the flow of energy remains unimpeded, we remain mentally and physically balanced—and in peak health.

Developed by Dr. Randolph Stone, an osteopath, naturopath, and chiropractor, polarity combines four interrelated aspects: gentle hands-on manipulation, yogic stretching and exercise, dietary counseling, and the creation of a positive attitude and life-style. Stone's concept of energy is borrowed from both the Chinese and Ayurvedic traditions of medicine; the principle aim of the therapy is to redirect energy by the gentle touching of specific sites.

Charging the Body. According to Stone's "Polarity Principle," movement of energy within the body is the result of two opposing fields, one positive and one negative. This is true for any kind of energy flow, from electricity to atomic fission. In the case of the human body (which is bipolar), the head has a positive charge, while the feet have a negative charge. So too, the right side carries a positive charge, and the left side is negative. When our body poles are in dynamic balance, we are in a state of harmony or well-being. Proponents of the therapy believe that this state is achieved when the life energy is able to flow freely throughout the body. As a result, we are re-

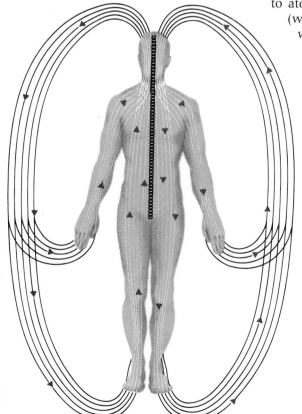

Polarity practitioners believe that life energy circulates around and through the human body, energizing everything in its path. According to the theory, the energy channels may become blocked due to stress, illness, or other factors. Polarity therapy works to redirect the energy along its natural pathways.

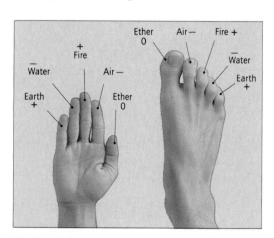

Each energy current carries a charge and flows from the body through a specific finger or toe. The currents are named for one of the five elements of the Ayurvedic system of medicine.

laxed and our powers of self-healing are in top form. But various agents, from stress to toxins, can cause the energy flow to become misdirected or blocked, and so impair our natural healing abilities.

Polarity therapy aims to get the energy currents moving freely again and back in balance. In doing so, practitioners claim, polarity therapy recharges and revitalizes major organs, bolsters the nervous system, and promotes emotional and mental stability. "The better our energy currents flow, the better we're able to attract what we need to be healthy human beings," says one polarity practitioner.

The Five Elements in Dynamic Balance. To reestablish the balance, polarity therapists target five long vertical currents flowing up and down the left side of the body, and five flowing up and down the right side, front and back. Each of these currents relates to one of the five elements of Ayurvedic medicine—Ether, Air, Fire, Water, or Earth. Each is also associated with a particular energy center or "chakra" on the body, and each chakra governs a particular system within the body.

The Ether chakra is located in the throat area and governs the voice, hearing, and joints of the body. Next comes the Air chakra, which controls respiration, circulation, and the nervous system. The Fire chakra, located just above the navel, governs digestion and metabolism; the Water chakra controls the reproductive and lymphatic systems, as well as body fluids. And finally, the lowest energy center in the body is the Earth chakra, which governs waste, elimination, and the skeletal system.

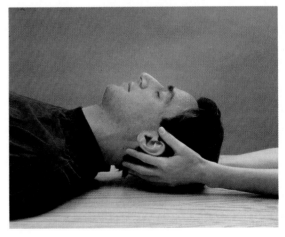

*A **polarity** energy balancing session usually begins with a head cradle. With the fingers on the neck and thumbs by the ears, the practitioner gently cradles the client's head, applying no pressure. This position may be held for as long as is comfortable for practitioner and client. Energy balancing sessions are meant to recharge the life force, helping the client to relax and release emotional and physical pain.*

In a typical session, the client lies on a massage table while the practitioner seeks out areas of tension or blockage. Most polarity manipulations are very simple and gentle, and are meant to encourage the client to enter a deeper state of relaxation. The practitioner usually places both hands on the body, which is said to set up a polarity relationship of positive and negative charge. In this way the flow of life energy is stimulated; as the amount of available energy increases (by combining the practitioner's energy with the client's), areas of pain or blockage are revitalized and clogged energy is released. Often, the balance is restored in just one session, and many clients report a deep sense of well-being. However, practitioners say that long-standing or severe conditions may require a series of sessions, and improvement will be more gradual.

The Role of Diet, Exercise, and Counseling. Nutritional counseling, also based upon the Five Elements concept, is another important component of polarity. Through diet, clients are urged to rid the body of toxins and to develop better eating habits. Some initiates may begin with a dietary cleansing program highlighted by a "liver flush," a

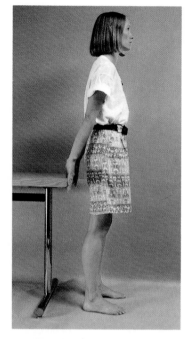

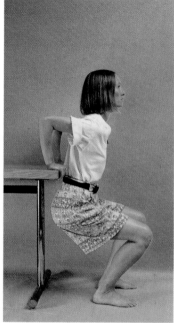

The cliffhanger works on the chest and shoulder blade areas. Standing with your back to a table, position your feet shoulder-width apart, and place your palms on the table edge for support. Take a deep breath and, as you exhale, slowly lower your body, keeping your spine straight. Make sounds to help you release tensions. Stay down for about 30 seconds, then slowly rise.

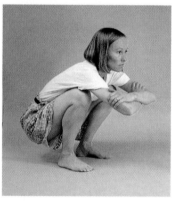

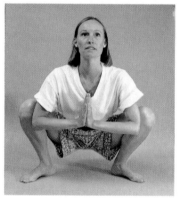

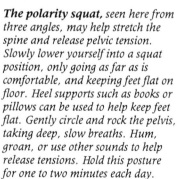

The polarity squat, seen here from three angles, may help stretch the spine and release pelvic tension. Slowly lower yourself into a squat position, only going as far as is comfortable, and keeping feet flat on floor. Heel supports such as books or pillows can be used to help keep feet flat. Gently circle and rock the pelvis, taking deep, slow breaths. Hum, groan, or use other sounds to help release tensions. Hold this posture for one to two minutes each day.

tonic of lemon juice, olive oil, grapefruit or orange juice, and garlic. This may be followed by a regimen of vegetarian food, but not everyone embarks on this diet.

Polarity yoga exercises and counseling play supporting roles, too. The exercises combine rhythmic movements and deep breathing, and most are easily learned for home practice. Counseling is also integral, because most polarity practitioners believe that a positive state of mind is essential to good health. During sessions, the polarity therapist works with the client to help work out and resolve highly charged negative emotions, such as anger or sadness.

Polarity therapy is not designed as a primary treatment for serious illness, but many people find it extremely relaxing and comforting. It is used by some as preventive therapy, in the hope the body will never get so out of balance that we become ill. In addition, some have found it useful in relieving certain types of pain, including headache, backache, and muscle cramps. Others have found it effective in relieving indigestion, constipation, and the general discomforts of everyday stress and anxiety. ❑

Attaining a Healthy Self-Awareness

The goal of bodywork, writes Deane Juhan, is to bring the mind and the body together into one harmonious whole. These treatments do not cure directly but are there to point the way.

Bodywork is a kind of sensorimotor education, rather than a treatment or a procedure in the sense common to modern medicine. Nothing material is added or taken away, so there are no dosages to be strictly adhered to, no statistical rates of success for particular manipulations.

If a student is having learning difficulties in school, I cannot effectively tutor him by simply pouring into his eyes and ears the information that will appear on the exam. The very nature of his problem is that he is not assimilating these things as he should. I must first find out something about what he does know, and then I must find what stops him from acquiring the things that he does not. I must enter into an active relationship with him, discover what forms information must take before he can successfully absorb it and apply it appropriately.

This process is partly objective and partly subjective, and the effective tutor is the one who knows how to find the balance between the two. This is the manner in which bodywork proceeds, first finding the reflex patterns of response that are presently active, and then searching for the quality of sensory input that will begin to alter those patterns for the better.

A point worth remembering here is that in this educational experience it is not the bodyworker who is "fixing" the client. The bodyworker is not attacking a localized problem with specialized tools, confident of achieving certain results. Instead, he or she is carefully generating a flow of sensory information to the mind of the client, information that is not being generated by the client's own limited repertoire of movements—new information that the mind can use to fill in the gaps and missing links in its appraisal of the body's physiological processes. It is then the mind of the client that does the "fixing"—the appropriate adjustment of postures, the fuller and more flexible relationship between neural and muscular responses.

The bodyworker is not an interventionist; he is a diplomatic intermediary between physiological processes that have lost track of one another's proper functions and goals, between a mind that has forgotten what it needs to know in order to exert harmonious control and a body politic which increasingly utilizes disruptive demonstrations and even the threat of all-out civil war to regain its governor's attention.

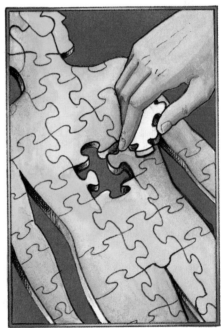

Bodywork: The sum of many parts

Touching hands are not like pharmaceuticals or scalpels. They are like flashlights in a darkened room. The medicine they administer is self-awareness. And for many of our painful conditions, this is the aid that is most urgently needed.

Excerpted from Job's Body: A Handbook for Bodywork *by Deane Juhan*

The Alexander Technique

Long appreciated by dancers and actors, this technique has helped many people discover how to use their bodies with greater efficiency. Better posture is both the key to and the reward of the Alexander technique.

The Man Behind the Method: Alexander

With his years of experience on the Australian stage, F.M. Alexander was well-equipped to take his technique public. By 1904, doctors were referring patients to Alexander; encouraged, he set off for London with his brother to recruit a wider audience. In a short time, their clients included some of the leading actors of the day.

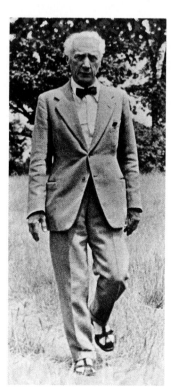

THE ALEXANDER TECHNIQUE is a method of adjusting body posture to relieve chronic pain or muscle tension, and to increase range of motion. Through gentle physical and verbal instruction, clients learn how to eliminate such common problems as slouching, hunching, and the habitual (and harmful) tensing and twisting of the spine. Many of us develop these habits in response to stress, strain, and even gravity, and, over time, experience an unhappy combination of tension, pain, fatigue, and stiffness. According to proponents, Alexander training teaches better use of the body, and so can largely reverse these conditions.

The Alexander technique is widely used in the rehabilitation of injured muscles and joints. Practitioners claim it can be effective in alleviating such chronic conditions as back and neck pain, asthma, headache, ulcers, spastic colon, and TMJ (a painful jaw affliction). However, adherents feel that anyone can benefit from learning the technique, since it promotes better all-around physical and mental health. It has long been popular with singers, dancers, musicians, and actors who wish to improve performance skills and avoid injury. More recently, professional athletes have been using it for the same reasons.

Taking a Closer Look. Around the turn of the century, F. Matthias Alexander, an Australian actor, began to suffer from bouts of voice loss while performing. His doctor prescribed medication and rest, but his symptoms persisted. It wasn't until Alexander began to study himself in a three-way mirror that he discovered the source of his problem. He found that when he started to recite, he tensed his muscles and pulled his head back and down, depressing his larynx. As a result, his breathing was labored and his voice strained. These habits were so firmly ingrained that Alexander was totally unaware of them until he observed himself in the mirror.

Gradually, Alexander found that he could learn to eliminate his bad habits, and in doing so, his tension eased and his voice problem disappeared. He was so successful that other people came to him for help, among them such notables as George Bernard Shaw and Aldous Huxley. In the 1930s, Alexander started a program to train others to teach his method, and today it is taught worldwide.

Replacing Bad Habits with Good Ones. Much of the Alexander technique is conveyed through the hands-on guidance of the teacher. It was Alexander's contention that incorrect positioning of the head with relation to the neck and torso could result in misplaced muscular effort and unnecessary tension. Once the head-neck-torso unit is brought into proper alignment, proponents say, the rest of

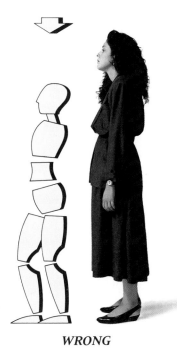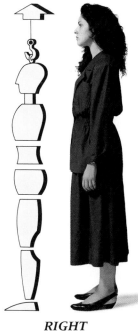

WRONG   RIGHT

Perfect posture, *Alexander reasoned, is a matter of mechanics, but most people must first relearn how to stand. When the spine is out of alignment (left), the lower back curves unnaturally. Alexander suggested that his clients imagine a hook pulling the spine into proper alignment (right). This lengthens the torso, giving the lower back the support it needs.*

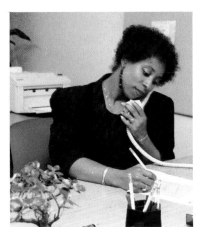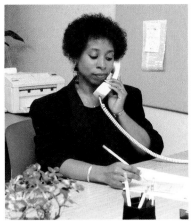

WRONG   RIGHT

When talking *on the telephone, do not prop the receiver between your head and shoulder. According to Alexander practitioners, this posture wrenches your head, neck, and shoulders out of alignment. Instead, keep shoulders straight and hold the phone to your ear.*

the body will follow suit, easing pain, tension, and other problems. With this in mind, the student is given verbal instructions to repeat silently while the teacher uses his or her hands to gently guide the student into carrying them out. For example, the tendency to pull the head down and compress the spine is countered with the thought, "Let the head ease up off the spine so the spine can lengthen." The habit of tensing and rounding the shoulders is corrected with the thought, "Let the shoulders release out to the sides."

Alexander exercises help students become aware of their bodies and so make conscious changes. But no Alexander teacher will ever tell a student to "stand up straight" or "hold your shoulders back." Instead, students are taught to *release* muscles, not tense them. Released muscles are those that are working efficiently for the task at hand, not straining in any way. Ironically, many bad postural habits

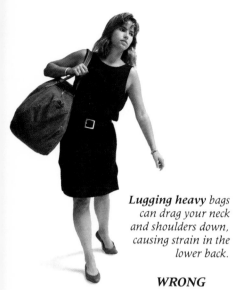

Lugging heavy bags can drag your neck and shoulders down, causing strain in the lower back.

WRONG

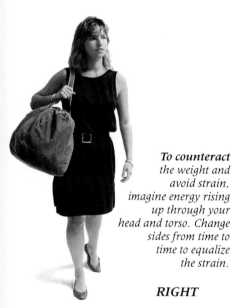

To counteract the weight and avoid strain, imagine energy rising up through your head and torso. Change sides from time to time to equalize the strain.

RIGHT

feel correct because we have grown used to them over the years. So one goal of the technique is to get clients to give up what feels "right" by replacing it with what, at least initially, may feel "wrong" or awkward.

Promoting Relaxation. To reinforce the techniques used in class, students are told to keep their instructions in mind while they go about their daily activities. With time, the new beneficial movement patterns will gradually and automatically replace the harmful ones. In addition, some students find it beneficial to lie down for 15 to 20 minutes and visualize their Alexander instructions. Like meditation, this practice is a good way to relax mentally and physically, particularly at the end of a busy day. There are a number of visualization techniques designed to increase body awareness and improve posture. In one very simple exercise, the student is told to imagine a gold string attached to the crown of his or her head, pulling the torso upward, lengthening the spine and freeing the body from the pull of gravity.

Another exercise, which can be performed under the guidance of a practitioner or on one's own, is done while lying on the floor with knees bent and head slightly elevated in what is known as the semi-supine position. The goal of this exercise is to release and strengthen all the muscles of the body from head to toe, not through movement, but through visualization. For example, if the student feels tension in the legs, he or she can imagine relaxing the muscles from the hip joints to the knees. In a short time, the student may actually feel the legs totally relax as the knees open out from the hips. The rest of the body can be de-stressed in a similar fashion.

Many people practice the Alexander technique not only to promote better health and posture, but to generally improve the quality of their lives. And by learning a more relaxed, natural posture and pattern of movement, many have been freed from years of chronic pain. ❑

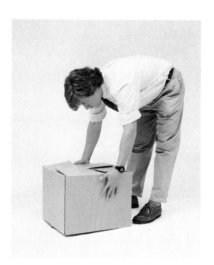

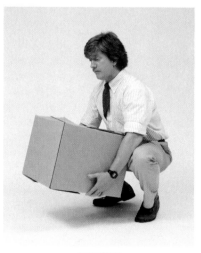

When lifting, never bend from the waist (left). By doing so, you risk injuring your back. Instead, bend from your knees and keep your back lengthened (right). Also, stand close to the object you are lifting.

WRONG   **RIGHT**

A Life Transformed

*In the letter that follows, a writer describes the benefits he derived
from the Alexander technique. The letter was written to
Lulie Westfeldt, who pioneered this therapy in the United States.*

The work of F.M. Alexander first came to my notice in 1938. As the years passed my curiosity continued, and by 1955 I needed Alexander treatment badly, for I was worried by frequent and prolonged numbness in my left leg which had become so troublesome that at times it would make me stumble. Fortunately, in November of this year I met a pupil of yours, and made arrangements to see you for lessons the following January.

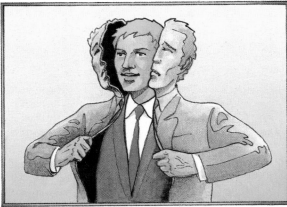

Shedding the bad habits of a lifetime

To be specific, the trouble in my left leg disappeared and has only returned on two or three occasions when I was particularly tired, and then yielded at once to some Alexander work. Apart from this, I have had a marked increase in physical well-being, and have been free from the periods of exhaustion and nervous weariness which used to follow intense work.

My work (which is that of a writer and editor) forces me to spend long hours—ten hours a day is by no means uncommon—sitting at a desk, writing or reading. Only those who have done it for 20 years know how physically wearisome and demanding such immobility can be; in fact, it is not physical immobility at all, but a routine of twists, fidgets, and jumps caused by thwarted muscles and nerves.

Lessons with you, and daily practice along the lines you point out, have made a most welcome change in this physical misery. I still sit at a desk all day and part of the night but I sit in quite a different way; walking has taken on a new quality of pleasure; because I am not nervously exacerbated, I plan my work better, and actually get more work done with less trouble.

I know that you discourage your pupils from talking about psychological changes which follow work on Alexander's lines, and I appreciate the fact that cranks and featherweight messiahs must be discouraged. Nevertheless, I must add that during 30 months of Alexander work I have found new powers of endurance which are not solely physical.

Everybody in their forties is trying to get his second wind for the second and hardest lap in the race of life; some people find it one way and some another, and a sad number do not find it at all, and seem to shrivel as the years pass. Whether I have found it in the Alexander lessons and their application I cannot, with complete confidence, say, but certainly they pointed the way to a development for which I had hoped, and could not have reached unaided. As you yourself have said, the work emphasizes and discloses what the pupil essentially *is*, and in my own case I regard it as a means of self-exploration, as well as a technique of physical retraining.

Excerpted from F. Matthias Alexander:
The Man and His Work *by Lulie Westfeldt.*

New Directions in Bodywork

A number of long-time practitioners of bodywork have developed their own distinctive techniques. Although their methods have much in common, each has something unique to offer.

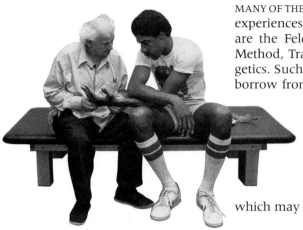

Basketball star *Julius Erving consulted Feldenkrais when tendon problems threatened to sideline him.*

MANY OF THE NEWER bodywork methods reflect the personal experiences of their founders, and among the best known are the Feldenkrais method, Rubenfeld Synergy, Rosen Method, Trager Psychophysical Integration, and bioenergetics. Such techniques develop as practitioners blend and borrow from other methods, while formulating a system that is uniquely their own.

Almost all bodywork methods go on the assumption that emotional stresses can affect the body, and result in chronic pain, tension, and other physical symptoms. On this basis, most bodywork techniques introduce people to new ways of handling tension and stress, which may help them feel better and function better.

Movement Awareness. An extremely painful chronic knee problem prompted Russian-born Israeli physicist Moshe Feldenkrais to develop his own rehabilitation

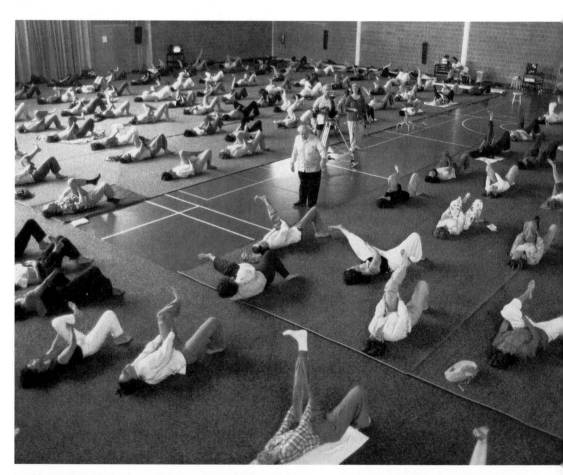

Led by *Moshe Feldenkrais, pupils in an Awareness Through Movement class learn new ways of using body and mind.*

method in the 1940s. Wary of surgery, he embarked on a program to teach himself how to walk again—painlessly. According to Feldenkrais, the key to his recovery was learning to work *with* gravity instead of against it.

The goal of the Feldenkrais method is to help clients become aware of, and correct, poor physical habits that are putting undo strain on the joints and muscles. From this awareness, clients are then able to learn ways of using the body that are less damaging.

In one-on-one sessions, known as Functional Integration, the therapist uses touch to gently guide the client through various motions. In this slow, relaxed manner, the client is able to register the small changes in feeling that accompany each movement. In group workshops, called Awareness Through Movement, students practice everyday motions—such as sitting or standing—and concentrate on what gives them the greatest ease of movement, with the least amount of effort or strain.

Releasing Tension. Developed by Ilana Rubenfeld, a former musician and conductor, Rubenfeld Synergy is a blend of bodywork and psychotherapy. Rubenfeld was dissatisfied with therapies that relied just on touch or just on talk, so she melded the two approaches to form her own eclectic therapy. Drawing on her training in the Alexander technique, the Feldenkrais method, and Gestalt therapy, she combined the gentle touch and subtle movement adjustments of the first two with the emotional release of the third.

Rubenfeld Synergy is conducted in one-on-one sessions or in groups. During treatment, synergists, as practitioners are called, gently move their hands around the client's body to find tense areas or other problem spots. But rather than trying to massage the trouble away, synergists encourage clients to talk about emotional issues that may be producing tension or pain. As Ilana Rubenfeld puts it, the method helps clients to "consciously let go of whatever they are holding in their bodies."

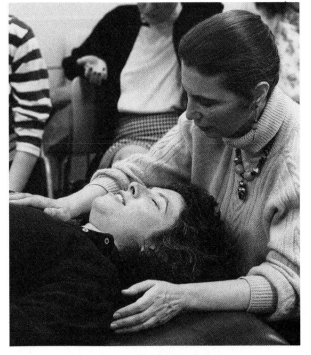

Ilana Rubenfeld, founder of the Rubenfeld Synergy method, uses touch and her caring presence to help clients release tensions, tap long-repressed memories, and express deep feelings.

Rosen Method: Letting Go. Like most of the newer bodywork techniques, Rosen Method treats the mind and the body as one. The method was created by Marion Rosen, a physical therapist who noticed that those clients who talked about their condition during sessions improved more quickly than those who did not. According to Rosen, chronic muscular tension is primarily caused by repressed emotional conflicts.

During treatment, the Rosen practitioner targets tense areas with gentle but deep pressure, which is intended to help the client relax. At the same time, the practitioner comments on what he or she is feeling in the client's body—tense spots, for example—and encourages the client to be open about what he or she is experiencing. And because emotions are believed to evoke bodily responses, the practitioner feels for changes in muscle tension or in the client's breathing rhythm. For instance, as the practitioner probes with gentle questions, he may notice that the client's back slightly arches or that a tense muscle suddenly

CASE HISTORY

RELEARNING BODY-AWARENESS

In his book The Case of Nora, *Moshe Feldenkrais describes how he helped a stroke patient regain mastery over her own body. Like a developing infant, Nora made slow, but remarkable progress.*

In the early 1970s Moshe Feldenkrais was in Zürich, Switzerland giving a series of radio talks, when he was contacted by the family of a woman named Nora. She was an intelligent and well-educated woman who had suffered a stroke a year earlier. According to Feldenkrais, "She could no longer write her own name . . . she could not locate doors and she often bumped into furniture. In spite of all this, her intelligence was almost unimpaired."

After an initial examination, Feldenkrais decided it would take a year or more of daily lessons for Nora to make any worthwhile progress.

"Awareness is learned. We have to learn that there is a sense of right and left which we carry with us. Nora's body-awareness had failed her and she had regressed to an earlier state," Feldenkrais wrote. Children, he theorized, learn awareness gradually as they grow. "One can imagine, or actually watch, how a baby is helped and helps himself to become aware of his nose, eyes, and the rest of himself. I personally believe that the baby lying in his mother's arms to be fed has no experiences other than sensory changes . . . these changes register in his nervous system. They form his awareness." In Nora's case, he found that she had regressed to a point at which she could not put her feet into

shoes correctly, could not turn over while lying down, and could not guide her body towards the seat of a chair.

Feldenkrais began by reducing the tension in Nora's muscles using a variety of hands-on techniques. He found that her body responded with only faint movements. The first step was to help Nora relearn the difference between the right and left sides of her body, a process which, with many regressions, took nearly two months.

When the time came to teach Nora to read and write again, Feldenkrais tested her eyes and found that, physiologically, they had suffered no impairment. Once that fact was established, he taught her to read and then to write her own name. At the end of about three months, Nora could hold a pen in a proper writing position. One day she wrote "Nora" fifty times. Gradually, Nora achieved mastery over her body as well as her reading and writing.

A year after her last treatment, Feldenkrais was in Zürich again. There, to his surprise, he ran into Nora strolling through the city on her weekly shopping trip. "A pleasant surprise," Feldenkrais remembered, "and no questions asked. The usual commonplace greeting, 'Ah, nice to see you,' concluded our common/uncommon adventure."

softens. Then as the client is made aware of these changes, he or she may recall a long repressed memory, which, according to Rosen, is now being held in the body in the form of muscle tension. By dealing with repressed feelings, some clients experience relief from chronic tension and other symptoms.

The Light Touch of Tragerwork. The innovation of Milton Trager, M.D., Trager Psychophysical Integration focuses on the subconscious roots of muscle tension. The treatment involves a variety of movements that are meant to promote relaxation and to increase range of motion and flexibility.

According to Trager, we all develop mental and physical patterns that may limit our movements or contribute to pain and tension. These restrictive patterns may be the result of the stress of day-to-day living or they may develop after an injury or other trauma. During a typical session, the practitioner gently and rhythmically rocks, cradles, and moves the client's body so as to encourage the client to see that freedom of movement and relaxation are entirely possible. The aim of the treatment is not to manipulate or massage specific joints, but to promote a feeling of lightness, limberness, and well-being.

Clients are also taught a series of exercises to do at home. Called Mentastics, these simple, dance-like movements are designed to help clients maintain and enhance the feelings of flexibility they may have experienced during their sessions. According to Betty Fuller, co-founder of the Trager Institute, Psychophysical Integration and Mentastics offer "a learning approach to using yourself well . . .to having all your pieces and parts well integrated and coordinated."

Bioenergetics. Developed by Alexander Lowen, a psychiatrist who trained under Wilhelm Reich, bioenergetics also combines psychotherapy with bodywork. Reich theorized that tension and rigidity in the body caused psychological problems, and vice versa. Lowen agreed, but expanded Reich's ideas to create his bodywork system.

According to Lowen, repressed emotions create chronic muscular tensions, which he (and Reich) called "armoring." The energy used for "armoring" saps the strength we need to cope with everyday life. In a typical session, the client assumes a variety of positions that help the therapist spot areas of tension. Then, through a combination of deep breathing, talk therapy, bioenergetic exercises, and occasional massage, the client and practitioner work on relieving tension and releasing bottled emotions. When appropriate, the clients may also be encouraged to scream, cry, kick, and lash out (by hitting a bed with their fists or a tennis racket). Clients are also taught a number of simple, tension-relieving exercises that can be performed at home. ❑

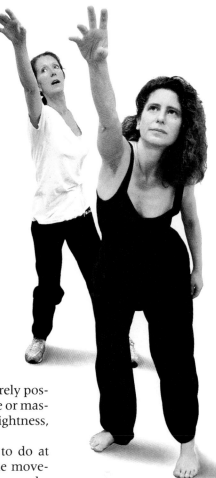

In addition to doing hands-on bodywork, Rosen Method practitioners also teach a number of lively, dance-like exercises that are designed to increase range of motion. In classes or individually, clients perform a series of gentle stretching, swinging, and jumping movements. According to Marion Rosen, the exercises encourage people to have fun while rediscovering the joy of movement.

More Than Skin-Deep

Practitioners of "deep tissue" therapies attempt to strip away tension and stiffness by massaging deep into the body's network of connective tissue. In doing so, they aim to restore flexibility and ease of movement.

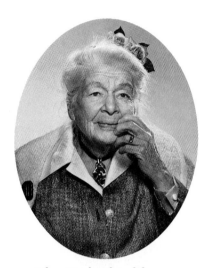

The Redoubtable "Dr. Elbow": Ida P. Rolf

Ida P. Rolf's unconventional method of working out knots deep in her clients' fascia gave rise to the affectionate nickname of "Dr. Elbow." Rolf discovered that by using her elbows and knees she was able to give a much deeper massage than if she'd just used her hands. In the 1960s, Fritz Perls, founder of Gestalt therapy, invited Rolf to demonstrate her technique at the Esalen Institute in California. It was Perls who instilled in Rolf an appreciation for the strong connection between mind and body.

ROLFING, THE BEST KNOWN of the deep tissue therapies, is a method of strengthening and realigning the body through vigorous massage. Also called Structural Integration, it was developed by Ida Rolf, a biochemist with interests in osteopathy, chiropractic, yoga, and Alexander technique. Unlike other bodywork practitioners, Rolf focused not on the spine or muscles, but on the fascia, the elastic sheathing network that helps support the body.

Fascia is the connective tissue that binds muscle fibers together, links muscles and bones, and covers the organs, nerves, and blood vessels. Its job is to shape and support the body, and hold the bones in place. However, according to Rolfers, the fascia can be damaged by physical injury, emotional trauma, and bad postural habits. The result is that the skeleton is thrown out of alignment, causing physical problems and pain. Rolfers attempt to bring the body back into balance in order to restore efficiency of movement and increase mobility.

The Stackable Column. Rolfers conceive of the human body as a stack of blocks—head, shoulders, torso, pelvis, and legs—held in place by the fascia. Gravity exerts an even vertical pull on each block in the column, so that when these blocks are balanced and aligned, the stack is stable. But if one is nudged out of place, the others shift to compensate, weakening the entire structure. Instead of working *with* the body, gravity now works *against* it, hindering movement and requiring extra energy for every task.

By stretching and lengthening the fascia, Rolfers aim to restore its natural form and pliability. In doing so, they are also realigning the major sections of the body. Instead of being a wobbly tower, they claim, the body will again be a strong, well-balanced column. However, Rolfing is not just a bodywork treatment. Ida Rolf also acknowledged a strong connection between emotions and physical health. In her view, chronic tension could harden the fascia and pull the body out of alignment. Rolfing practitioners report that clients frequently recall painful or traumatic memories as specific parts of their bodies are being worked on.

Working Layer by Layer. A Rolfing treatment consists of ten sessions, each lasting between 60 and 90 minutes. After taking a medical and psychological history, the practitioner makes a visual evaluation of the client. Then "before" photographs are taken so that changes in the client's body can be evaluated later.

Rolfing is sequential, and in the first session the practitioner concentrates on the outermost layer of fascia that underlies the skin. To achieve their aim, Rolfers use fingertips, knuckles, and even elbows to knead the muscle and tissue layers like bread dough. With each subsequent treatment, the massage gets deeper, and many clients find Rolfing somewhat painful—although the pain stops as soon as the treatment ends.

Why Get Rolfed? While Rolfers make no claims to cure illness, they do say that the treatment can improve posture and respiration, reduce stress, and generally give a person more energy. Adherents say that just about anyone, from athletes to elderly people, can be Rolfed. The goal is to restore the body's resilience, efficiency, and vitality. And for those who tap reservoirs of inner pain, it may provide a means of resolving emotional conflicts.

Other Deep Tissue Treatments. Rolfing has given rise to several related disciplines, such as Aston Patterning and Connective Tissue Polarity. Perhaps the best known is Hellerwork, a method devised in the 1970s by a former aerospace engineer, Joseph Heller. At one time Heller was president of the Rolf Institute in Colorado, but split off to create his own form of deep tissue manipulation.

Like Rolfing, Hellerwork focuses on massaging the fascia. But Hellerwork practitioners also believe that manipulation alone is inadequate for long-lasting improvement. To maintain alignment and mobility, clients are given movement exercises designed to eliminate their bad habits and to teach them how to stand, walk, sit, and move most efficiently. In this way, Hellerwork can be used preventively as a way of avoiding pain and stiffness, and generally improving health. In addition, sessions also incorporate talk therapy to deal with emotional issues that may surface during the course of treatment.

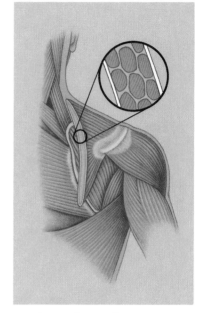

Fascia envelops and protects the muscles, but it is also subject to injuries, stresses, and strains.

A full Hellerwork treatment consists of eleven 90-minute sessions. As in Rolfing, Hellerwork starts from the outer layers of fascia and works in, like "peeling an onion," Heller says. ❑

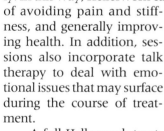

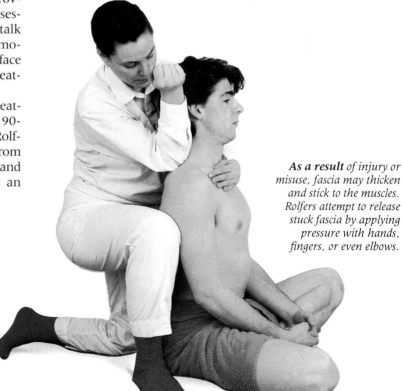

As a result of injury or misuse, fascia may thicken and stick to the muscles. Rolfers attempt to release stuck fascia by applying pressure with hands, fingers, or even elbows.

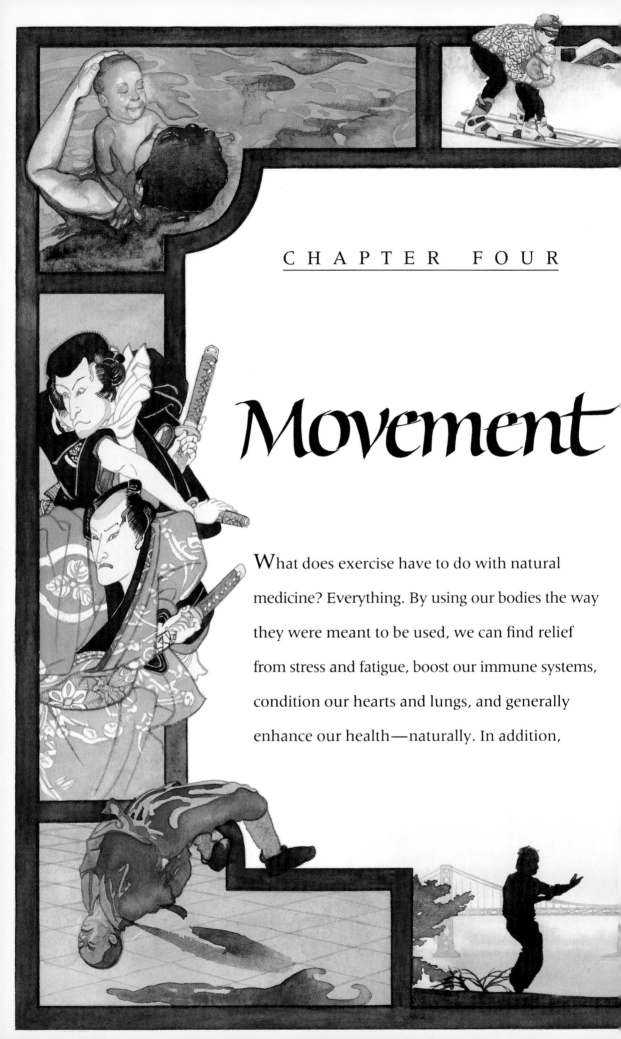

CHAPTER FOUR

Movement

What does exercise have to do with natural medicine? Everything. By using our bodies the way they were meant to be used, we can find relief from stress and fatigue, boost our immune systems, condition our hearts and lungs, and generally enhance our health—naturally. In addition,

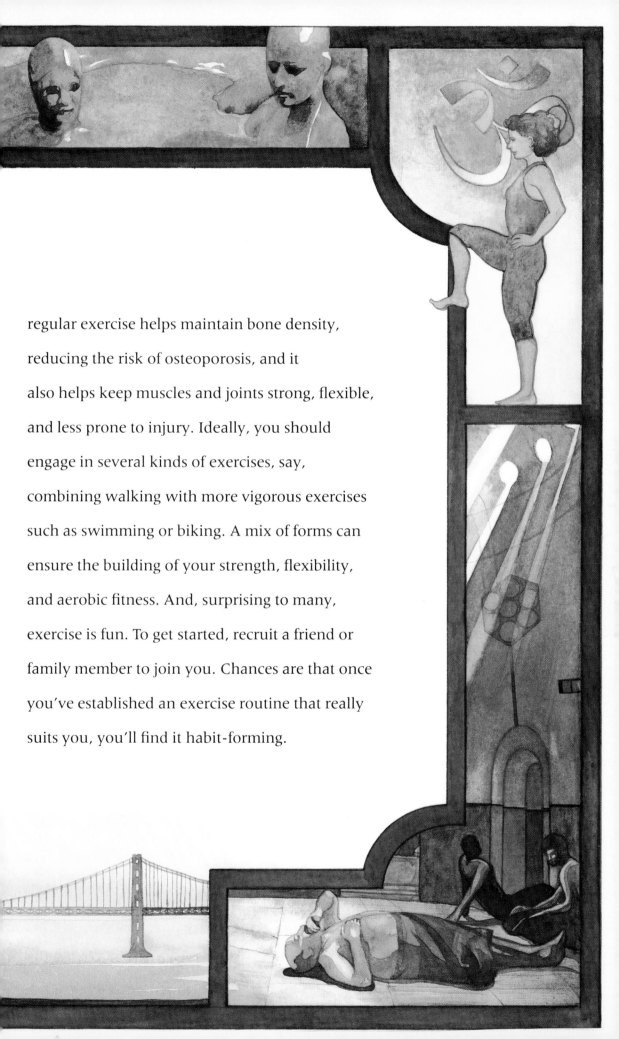

regular exercise helps maintain bone density,
reducing the risk of osteoporosis, and it
also helps keep muscles and joints strong, flexible,
and less prone to injury. Ideally, you should
engage in several kinds of exercises, say,
combining walking with more vigorous exercises
such as swimming or biking. A mix of forms can
ensure the building of your strength, flexibility,
and aerobic fitness. And, surprising to many,
exercise is fun. To get started, recruit a friend or
family member to join you. Chances are that once
you've established an exercise routine that really
suits you, you'll find it habit-forming.

Why You Should Exercise

The benefits of an active life are so numerous that it is hard to understand why everyone doesn't make physical fitness a top priority. In fact, through physical fitness many have found the proverbial fountain of youth.

EVERY SYSTEM IN YOUR BODY—circulatory, respiratory, digestive, nervous, skeletal, and muscular—works at top efficiency only when you have regular exercise. Though any physical activity may qualify as exercise (walking to work, going up and down stairs, doing housework, mowing the lawn), the question is how much time you are active as compared with the amount of time you spend sitting, riding in a car, or lying down. The more active you are, the better your chances of staying healthy.

Patients in hospitals are now routinely rousted out of bed at the earliest possible moment because we know that bedridden patients are at risk of developing pneumonia, blood clots, and urinary tract infections. But it was not until recently that we discovered yet another hazard of the sedentary state: bone loss. After returning from space, astronauts were found to have suffered small but significant loss of bone density. While in orbit, their bodies were not subject to the effects of gravity. The absence of a gravitational pull dramatically revealed that when bones have no resistance to work against, they weaken. However, the pull of gravity alone isn't enough. For strong bones and healthy bodies, we also need exercise.

Our Bodies Are Designed for Work. At one time our survival depended both on an ability to escape from danger and a capacity for hard work. Physical conditioning was the natural result of such a life. But modern conveniences have changed the way we use our bodies. Instead of toiling in the fields or chasing down dinner, many of us spend all day at a desk and our evenings in front of a television set. Elevators have replaced staircases, vacuum cleaners have replaced rug beating. The automobile has become so much a part of our lives that in some areas anyone seen walking on the sidewalk is viewed with suspicion. So if our daily routine does not provide the necessary movement to keep us fit, we owe it to ourselves to find another way.

Using our bodies as they were meant to be used is an essential part of living a healthy life. Dr. James Rippe of the University of Massachusetts Medical School has observed, "We have scientific evidence to support what has always seemed true: regular exercise helps prevent many diseases, lengthens life span, and improves quality of life."

Our risk of developing one of the "illnesses of civilization" can be decreased by regular exercise. For some time now it has been known that exercising can reduce blood pressure, lower cholesterol levels, improve the ratio of lean muscle to fat, and strengthen and increase the heart's efficiency. All of these effects decrease the chance of death due to cardiovascular disease. More recently, scientists have noted a possible connection between certain types of can-

---

The Most Dangerous Sport

We are constantly being warned to check with our physicians before beginning athletics. What we are not told are the risks of not beginning athletics — that the most dangerous sport of all is watching it from the stands.

"The weakest among us can become some kind of athlete, but only the strongest can survive as spectators. Only the hardiest can withstand the perils of inertia, inactivity, and immobility. Man was not made to remain at rest."

— Excerpted from "Dr. Sheehan on Running" by G.A.Sheehan, M.D.

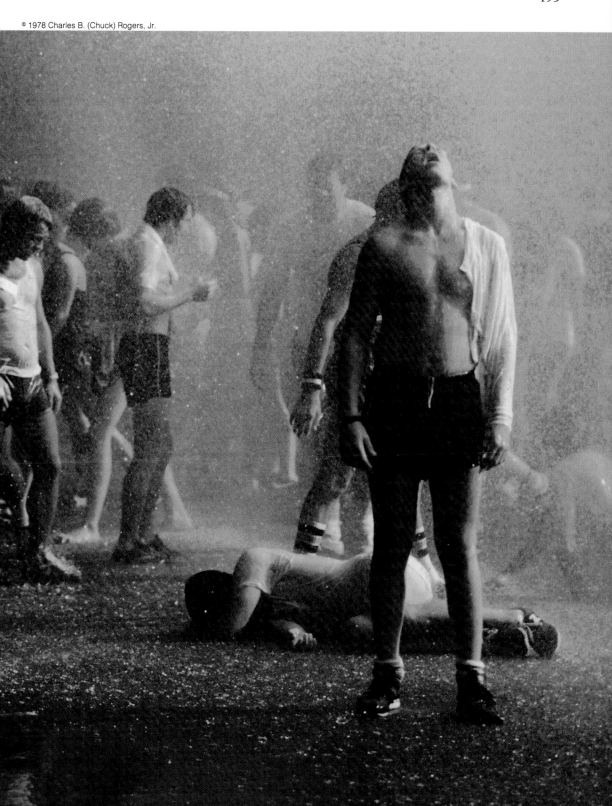

Hot and exhausted *after an Atlanta road race, runners pause to recover as steam rises from the pavement. Viewed from the sidelines, road racing, particularly on a sweltering day, looks downright crazy. But the number of runners seen on today's streets attests to the popularity of the sport. The urge to compete undoubtedly spurs some runners on, but many more derive satisfaction from simply being fit and active.*

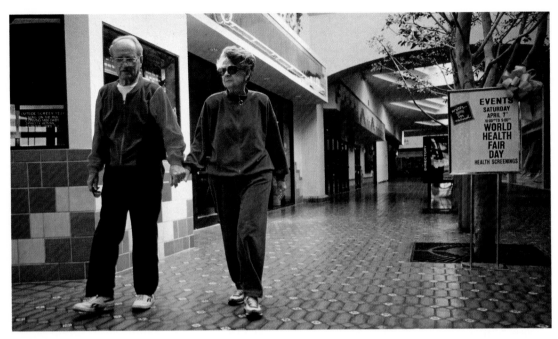

Many people *have discovered that shopping malls are safe and social places for walking workouts. In these climate-controlled environments, weather need never deter the fitness enthusiast. And for many, the sights and sounds of a mall provide welcome distraction and help keep their sport from becoming a chore. While it will never be an Olympic sport, mall walking may give rise to legions of new health and fitness buffs.*

cer and inactivity. And finally, exercise, combined with a sensible diet, has been found to be effective in combatting obesity.

Women benefit from regular exercise in another important way—exercise reduces the risk of osteoporosis by increasing bone formation and delaying bone loss. For women who already have the condition, exercise can help stop the progression of the disease. And because regular exercise reduces glucose-stimulated insulin secretion, it is helpful in controlling diabetes, as well as in reducing the risk of adult-onset diabetes. Exercise also stimulates the secretion of other kinds of hormones that have been linked to decreases in clinical symptoms of anxiety, and depression.

In addition, by improving circulation and nourishing tissues, exercise increases the range of movement of body joints, reduces the effects of stress and tension, and decreases or even cures insomnia. Of course there is some risk of injury with any kind of exercise. But the improved strength, balance, and coordination that comes from regular exercise greatly reduces the risk of all kinds of injuries.

Planning a Fitness Program. Many activities can improve physical fitness, but some may be more suitable for you than others. A well-rounded fitness program should incorporate three basic components: cardiovascular endurance, muscular strength, and flexibility. Following this guideline, any program you select should include exercises that increase heart and lung capacity, stretch tight muscle groups and strengthen weak ones.

Cardiorespiratory fitness refers to how well the lungs deliver oxygen to the blood, and how well the heart and circulatory system send blood and its nutrients throughout the body. Programs that develop heart and lung capacity are often referred to as being aerobic, and they accomplish their goal by elevating the heart rate for a sustained period. Aerobic exercise typically serves as the foundation for any fitness program since a healthy heart and lungs are essential to the safe and skillful performance of almost all activities and sports.

Depending upon your level of fitness and what you hope to achieve, most experts recommend a minimum of 20 minutes of aerobic exercise three to five days a week. You may choose any activity that uses large muscle groups, that can be maintained continuously, and that is cardiorespiratory in nature. Examples include brisk walking, swimming, jogging, running, bicycling, cross-country skiing, skating, stair-climbing, hiking, dancing, basketball, soccer, and racketball. Intensity, or the speed of the workout, is crucial and is measured by how fast the heart is made to beat. Usually the goal is to reach 65 to 90 percent of the exerciser's highest possible heart rate and sustain this rate for some length of time.

Muscular strength and endurance exercises use progressive resistance to increase the size and strength of muscle fi-

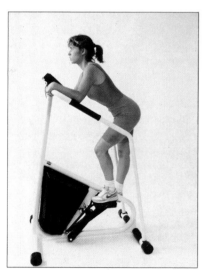
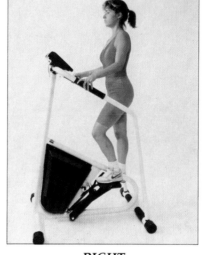

WRONG   **RIGHT**

Stair machines are a good choice for an aerobic workout, provided you don't have knee problems. But don't cheat yourself out of an efficient workout by slouching and leaning on your forearms (left). Stand straight and let your legs do the work (right).

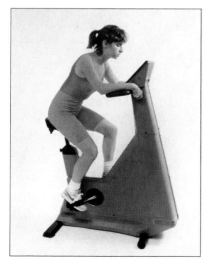
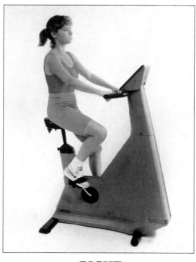

WRONG   **RIGHT**

When using a stationary bicycle, avoid the common pitfalls of inexperience (left). To get the most out of your workout, make sure the seat is set at the right height and that you are sitting up comfortably and without straining.

bers, resulting in a greater physical ability to perform work. Weight-lifting machines, such as Nautilus, are typical of the types of resistance equipment used in building strength. Push-ups, chin-ups, and curls produce similar results, but require no special equipment since they utilize the body's own weight as the source of resistance. Despite popular conceptions, strength and endurance training is not just for weight-lifters, boxers, and body-builders, but is an effective way of improving general fitness, converting fat to muscle, and increasing metabolic rate.

CASE HISTORY

SETTING THE CLOCK BACK

At the age of 52, Elliott Galloway, once a high school athlete, was overweight and sedentary. He took up running and gradually got back in shape, erasing 20 years in the process.

"I've watched a young boy without much obvious talent work his way to become one of the nation's top collegiate distance runners. I've seen housewives become world-class marathoners and old friend Frank Shorter, an Olympic champion. But the person who has inspired me the most isn't an Olympian, a world recordholder, or a national champion. Instead it's a man who started to run when he was 52.

"At that age, Elliott realized that over half of his high school football teammates had died of degenerative diseases. At 200 pounds, he was a heavy fat eater and non-exerciser whose doctor had told him he had to exercise if he was to survive. This former high school all-state football player just knew that 30 years of inactivity shouldn't prevent him from running circles around the slow joggers he saw in the park. Reality, however, was harsh; when he began his exercise program, he couldn't make it to the first telephone pole.

"Each day Elliott pushed himself to that next telephone pole. After 4 to 5 months, he could run a mile or so. Running helped the weight come off and as it melted, running became easier. At first, walking was rough on his ego, but he found that interspersing the running with walks helped increase his endurance with reduced stress.

"He kept up with his telephone pole course and soon found he could run a 5-kilometer (race), then a 10-kilometer. As he learned to run efficiently, he realized that his 8-minute miles felt similar to the 5-minute miles of his college track days.

"Slowly his body remembered how to run. In 1978 he qualified for the Boston Marathon, 45 pounds lighter than when he'd started. Then a few days before his 59th birthday, Elliott ran the Callaway Gardens (Georgia) Marathon in 2:59!

"This is an exciting story for me, for Elliott Galloway is my dad. What's inspired me most is the daily discipline and positive health style, which has made Dad younger than he was 20 years ago. The odds are that my dad will continue to inspire me as he runs into the next century. In the process, my son can get to know him, and better know himself.

"There are thousands of stories like my dad's, each a significant act of courage. Each person that's done it now has a psychological edge in the battle of passing years. You don't have to just sit there and let things get worse. The choice is yours."

Excerpted from Galloway's Book on Running *by Jeff Galloway*

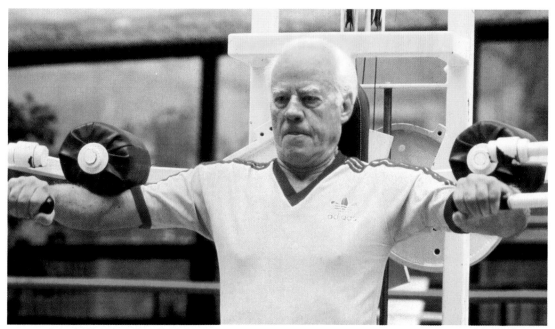

Flexibility training is an aspect of fitness that is often neglected. Many people choose activities that focus on strength and cardiorespiratory fitness, partly because there is so much documented scientific evidence in support of both, but little in support of flexibility. However, most physical fitness professionals consider it a key element in achieving top physical performance. Some people are naturally less limber than others; to avoid strain or injury, the safest flexibility exercise is a slow, sustained stretch.

Increasing range of motion around a joint is what flexibility training is all about. Many things determine a joint's flexibility, including the structure of the joint and the resilience of the attached muscles and connective tissue (fascia, ligaments, and tendons). As muscles become stronger through exercise, they also become tighter—unless flexibility training is done. On this basis, gentle stretching can be used preventively. Done regularly, it may reduce the tightening effect of strength training, running, and other endurance activities, and reduce the risk of injury.

Moving For the Fun of It. All the technical information about the benefits of exercise tends to overlook one important aspect of fitness: the simple joy of moving well and feeling fit. Starting any new activity or exercise program takes some patience and hard work, but many people soon find that they actually like it! Many enjoy the cosmetic benefits that come from improved circulation and muscle tone; others like the social aspect of joining a group for an exercise class. And still others are thrilled to discover that they have more energy than ever before.

Walking is a particularly good way to start getting in shape—and it doesn't require special equipment or entail learning a new skill. Start easy, say, walking at a good pace for 15 minutes or so, then gradually increasing both speed and

Staying fit well into old age has become a priority for increasing numbers of older people. According to most experts, regular exercise and good habits can help stave off many of the physical problems associated with aging. For instance, many aches and pains attributed to arthritis are the result of weakening muscles, a problem that can be successfully countered with strength training and other exercise.

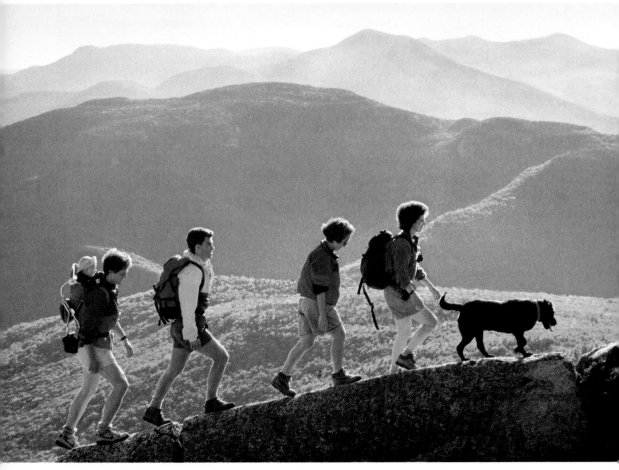

A day hike is one way for the whole family to combine fun with exercise. Small mountains with well-marked trails require no special training, but be sure to wear sturdy shoes and carry enough water.

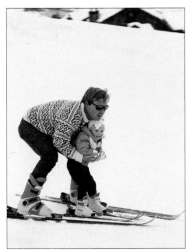

Skiing is *an exhilarating sport that the whole family can enjoy. Children are eager to try the activities that their parents like. Start them early, and they are more apt to develop a lifetime of good fitness habits.*

distance as you begin feeling more fit. Add stretching and strength training for a more complete workout.

Weighing the Risks. Even though regular exercise is essential to good health, there are risks involved in each kind of activity. No one over the age of 40 should begin a vigorous fitness program without a stress test, to check for coronary artery disease, and a thorough physical exam. Those who engage in aerobic activities, where the heart rate and lung capacity are pushed to near capacity levels, and who do not check with a doctor first, risk serious consequences if undetected health problems do exist.

Many people start exercise programs with enthusiasm, thinking that if a little is good, then more must be better. Injury is often the consequence of such rashness. No matter what activity you choose, start slowly and use the proper equipment. Certain aerobic activities, such as tennis and jumping rope, can be hard on the joints and may cause injury. Shoes that give ample support and adequate cushioning will help, but more important are good posture and strong abdominal muscles. When doing muscular strength and endurance training, begin slowly, and add weight or repetitions gradually. If strength training is rushed, the end result will most likely be very painful—and slow healing—pulled muscles. And flexibility exercises can cause pain and perhaps even permanent damage to the connective tissues if they are stretched beyond a certain point.

Don't Go It Alone. Even though more and more people are starting exercise programs, studies have found that 50 percent drop out within the first six to 12 months. Many give up because they are bored or discouraged. Since fitness gains can only be maintained through regular and frequent activity, motivation to continue an exercise program is essential. For this reason, many join health clubs or studios where exercise classes are available. Others persuade family, friends, or coworkers to join them in activities such as partner stretches, mall walking, and outdoor cycling. Most find that exercising with someone else makes sticking to their fitness goals easier.

Results are surely a strong motivator, but success is much more likely if you select fitness activities that you truly enjoy. Many experts advise choosing a number of different exercises or sports so that you can vary your routine, an approach often referred to as cross training. A diverse group of activities will make your fitness program much more interesting, and lessen the odds that it will become routine and boring. Additionally, no single activity fulfills all the elements—aerobic, strength, and flexibility—that build physical fitness. For instance, while running develops aerobic fitness, it tends to decrease flexibility. Variety also reduces the risk of certain overuse injuries, such as tendinitis, that may develop if one activity is pursued exclusively.

To get the most out of exercise, many people are turning to personal trainers. These physical fitness pros are trained to custom-design exercise programs to suit the individual, taking any weaknesses into account. In addition, many personal trainers have a thorough knowledge of anatomy, physiology, kinesiology, injury prevention, and various exercise methods and so can ensure that each person has the opportunity to attain the desired level of fitness in the safest possible way. To find a trainer, contact a health club or sports medicine clinic. ❏

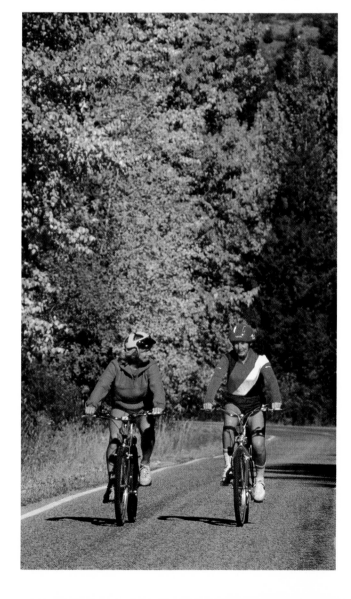

Cycling is an excellent aerobic activity, and one that is easily enjoyed with a companion. Experts advise choosing a bike with at least 10 speeds so that you can more efficiently climb hills. Be sure to wear a cycling helmet to prevent a head injury in the event of a fall.

A Basic Exercise Routine

These exercises are designed to improve strength and flexibility, and, combined with aerobic activity, to give you a good, all-around workout. The goal is to feel invigorated, not exhausted, so go at your own pace.

DONE REGULARLY, the exercises on these pages will help increase strength and flexibility. However, they will not develop aerobic fitness. For a complete and well-rounded fitness program, alternate three days of aerobic activity with three days of strength and flexibility training.

Target Heart Rate. How do you know if you're performing an aerobic activity at the right intensity? One method is by determining your target heart rate. This can be calculated by subtracting your age from 220, and multiplying the result by 65% and 90%. During aerobic exercise, you should try to maintain a heart rate that falls between the two. For instance, if you are 50 years old, your target heart rate is between 111 and 153 (220 - 50 x .65 and 220 - 50 x .90) beats per minute. So, if during your workout your pulse drops below 111, you are not working hard enough, but if it rises above 153, you're pushing too hard.

Getting Started. Warm-up exercises are an essential part of any workout, for they give the body time to adjust to increased energy demands. Also, by limbering up the muscles, you'll prevent fatigue and injury. The *upper body stretch, head and shoulder isolations,* and *roll down* are warm-up exercises

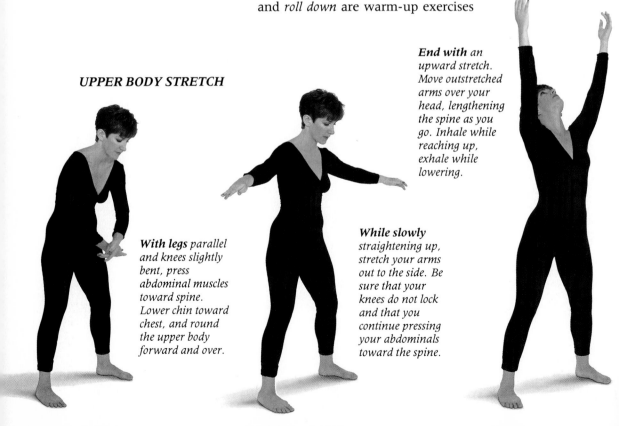

UPPER BODY STRETCH

End with *an upward stretch. Move outstretched arms over your head, lengthening the spine as you go. Inhale while reaching up, exhale while lowering.*

With legs *parallel and knees slightly bent, press abdominal muscles toward spine. Lower chin toward chest, and round the upper body forward and over.*

While slowly *straightening up, stretch your arms out to the side. Be sure that your knees do not lock and that you continue pressing your abdominals toward the spine.*

HEAD AND SHOULDER ISOLATION

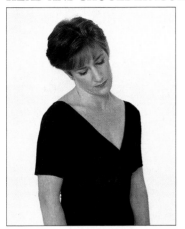
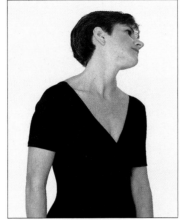

Standing with legs parallel and abdominals pulled in, slowly rotate head in a circle, keeping shoulders down as you stretch the neck muscles. Reverse direction; repeat several times.

Standing as shown, bring shoulders forward, up, back, and down in one continuous, rolling motion. Move slowly, using your full range of motion. Repeat 4 times in each direction.

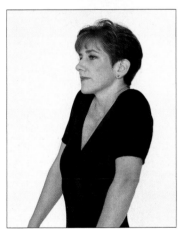
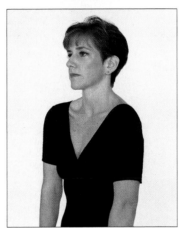
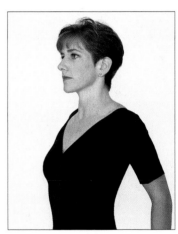

ROLL DOWN

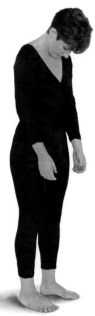

With knees slightly bent, hang for 30 seconds, breathing deeply to relax. Roll up one vertebra at a time, shoulders and head last.

Standing with legs parallel, start the roll down by bringing chin into the neck. Keep your abdominals tucked in close to your spine.

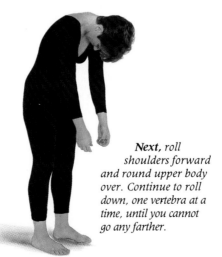

Next, roll shoulders forward and round upper body over. Continue to roll down, one vertebra at a time, until you cannot go any farther.

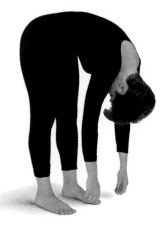

SIDE STRETCH

To stretch your right side, lie flat with knees bent and arms extended over head. Grasp your right wrist with your left hand, and exhale as you gently stretch.

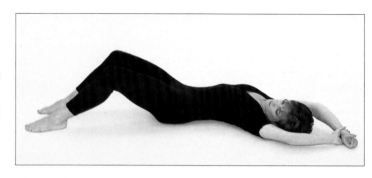

For a left side stretch, simply switch your hands, grasping the left wrist with the right hand. Be sure abdominal muscles are pulled in toward the spine.

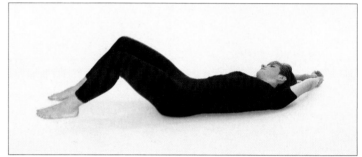

UPPER ABDOMINAL CURL

Lying with knees bent, feet flat, and hands behind head, use your abdominal muscles to lift upper body off the floor, holding chin toward chest. Exhale as you curl up, and inhale as you slowly uncurl. Start with 15, and work up.

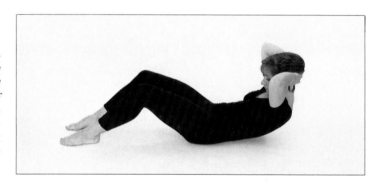

LOWER BACK RELEASER

Lie on floor with knees bent, feet flat. Grasp legs under thighs with forearms, and pull knees toward chest. Keep back flat against floor, and try to relax muscles in hip sockets.

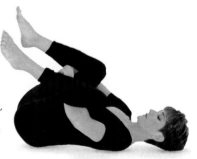

Extend left leg while continuing to hold the right. Pull right knee in and make several small circles. Repeat on the other side.

that are also marvelous tension relievers; enhance the effect by breathing deeply and rhythmically.

Working Out. Once you are warmed up, you can move on to an aerobic workout or to the floor exercises illustrated here. If you do an aerobic activity, be sure to cool down at the end of your session by gradually decreasing the pace of your workout for 5 to 10 minutes. Or cool down with any five of the floor exercises.

For a strength and flexibility workout, allow yourself at least 30 minutes for the floor exercises. Many back problems are the result of weak abdominal muscles; the *abdominal curls* and *leg changes* are both excellent exercises for strengthening these muscles. *Lower back releasers* help back problems by stretching tight back muscles. When doing exercises on your back, keep the abdominals pulled in, which keeps your lower back pressed against the floor.

Hamstring stretches and *leg circles* are good toning, stretching, and strengthening exercises for the hips and buttocks. The *hamstring stretch* should be done gradually, but do not force the leg if it is painful. As you are doing the *leg circles*, concentrate on lengthening your stretch and be sure to press your arms, shoulders, and lower back to the floor. And once you've mastered small circles, challenge your strength and flexibility with larger ones—the larger the circle, the harder the exercise.

Swimming may also help prevent back problems. Exe-

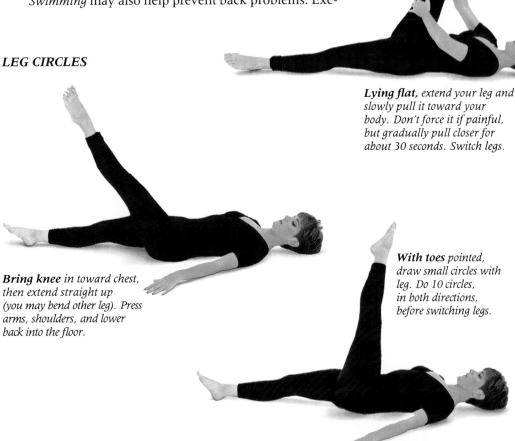

HAMSTRING STRETCH

Lying flat, *extend your leg and slowly pull it toward your body. Don't force it if painful, but gradually pull closer for about 30 seconds. Switch legs.*

LEG CIRCLES

Bring knee *in toward chest, then extend straight up (you may bend other leg). Press arms, shoulders, and lower back into the floor.*

With toes *pointed, draw small circles with leg. Do 10 circles, in both directions, before switching legs.*

LEG CHANGES

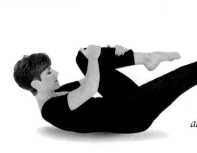

With right hand on ankle and left on knee, bend right leg and pull towards chest. Tuck chin into chest, raise other leg to a 45-degree angle.

Pull bent leg in with arms, then switch legs, alternating from right to left for up to 20 repetitions. Be sure abdominals press lower back to floor.

SWIMMING

Lie on stomach with arms and legs extended. Then raise head, and begin by reaching out and up with right arm and left leg.

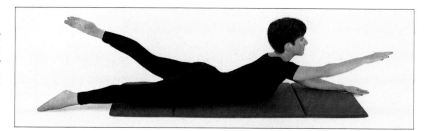

Hold the position, then lower your limbs, and repeat on the other side. Do 10 on each side, moving slowly.

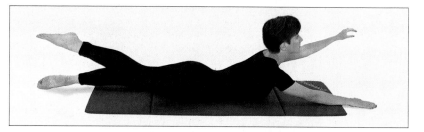

Keeping head and chin up, lift both arms and both legs. Paddle opposite arms and legs, but much faster than above.

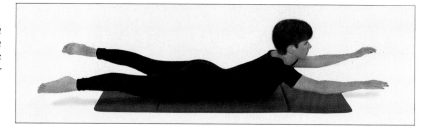

REST POSITION

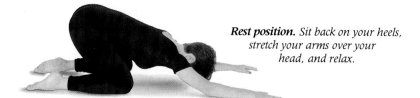

Rest position. Sit back on your heels, stretch your arms over your head, and relax.

cute each move slowly with the goal of reaching and stretching farther. But if you have lower back problems, place a pillow under the hips.

Partner Stretches. Start off with the warm-up exercises described on the previous pages. The *leg pull* and *side stretch* should be done in sequence; don't switch places until one partner has completed both. Repeat the *leg pull* five times and the *side stretch* four times on each side. The *hip circle* and *hamstring stretch* should also be done in sequence before you switch places. When doing the *hip circles,* gentle, full circles will help increase range of motion in the hips. End the routine with the *inner thigh stretch*, pulling slowly and gently until your partner says to stop; hold the position for 30 seconds. While you're being pulled, try to relax your head, spine, and leg muscles by breathing deeply. ❏

PARTNER STRETCHES

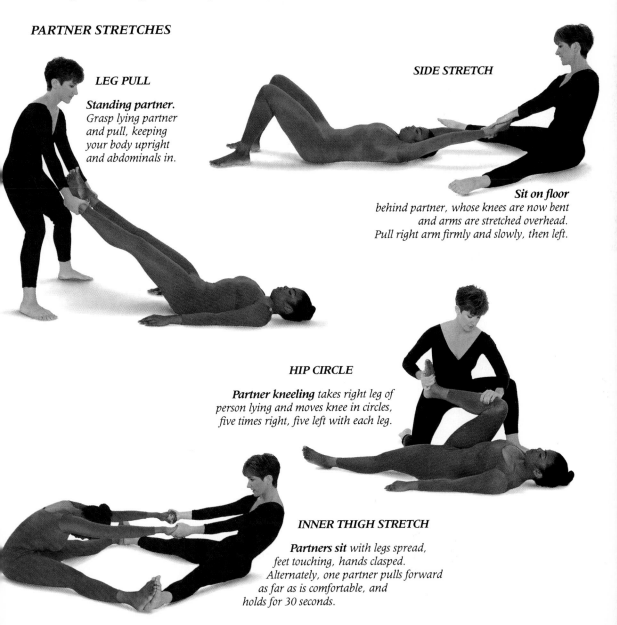

LEG PULL

Standing partner.
*Grasp lying partner
and pull, keeping
your body upright
and abdominals in.*

SIDE STRETCH

Sit on floor
*behind partner, whose knees are now bent
and arms are stretched overhead.
Pull right arm firmly and slowly, then left.*

HIP CIRCLE

Partner kneeling *takes right leg of
person lying and moves knee in circles,
five times right, five left with each leg.*

INNER THIGH STRETCH

Partners sit *with legs spread,
feet touching, hands clasped.
Alternately, one partner pulls forward
as far as is comfortable, and
holds for 30 seconds.*

Water, Water Everywhere

Used internally or externally, cold, hot, or tepid water has an amazing range of therapeutic uses. And while its density challenges the muscles of swimmers and water-walkers, its buoyancy facilitates exercise therapy.

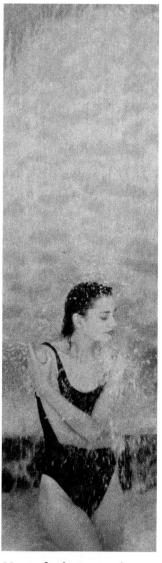

Many of today's spas rely on technology to recreate the gifts usually supplied by nature. Here a woman gets a soothing massage under a cascade of volcanic water shipped in from a centuries-old European spa.

THE IDEA OF USING WATER TO CURE ILLNESS and preserve health is probably as old as civilization itself. In the 5th century B.C., the Greek physician Hippocrates recommended natural spring water for its salubrious effects. The Romans were devotees of the bath, building huge, handsome public structures for their elaborate bathing rituals. There, daily, Roman citizens might swim or exercise. Afterwards, they would have sweat and dirt scraped from their bodies by means of a special instrument called a strigil, and then probably have a massage before entering a succession of rooms with either steam or hot, warm, or cold water tanks.

The Romans appreciated the relationship of water to cleanliness, relaxation, and general good health. Aqueducts brought water to numerous public bathhouses throughout Rome. One of the more spectacular works—the Baths of Caracalla—covered 28 acres. The Romans considered their bathing rituals so important that they carried the custom throughout their empire. The bathhouse was one of the first buildings constructed at each new settlement; the remains of these structures can still be visited today in places such as Bath, England. The mineral springs of Spa, Belgium, were also well known to the Romans, and it is from this village that the name spa is derived.

Taking the Waters. Mineral springs are the focal point of many spas, ancient and modern. Water from these springs was widely believed to have medicinal properties. Seeking cures for everything from acne to anxiety, people travelled to drink and bathe. The 1800s and early 1900s were the Golden Age of spas such as Saratoga Springs, New York, where the wealthy came to see and be seen. Nowadays, spas cater to people who seek an invigorating yet relaxing routine. This usually includes massage, mud packs, fresh air, exercise, healthy food, and lovely scenery.

Using water to treat illness has always been a part of folk medicine, but during the era of spas and water cures such treatment came to be known as hydrotherapy. Although the notion that mineral water has medicinal properties is no longer commonly held, using water of varying temperatures and pressures is recognized as an effective course of treatment for a variety of health problems.

Thalassotherapy. A variation on the mineral spring is the seaside spa where the visitor may experience thalassotherapy (the word is derived from the Greek word *thalassa*, meaning sea). The same properties attributed to mineral water have frequently been claimed for seawater. During a typical treatment, clients are massaged while partially submerged in seawater. They may also be sprayed with jets of seawater, covered with packs of seaweed,

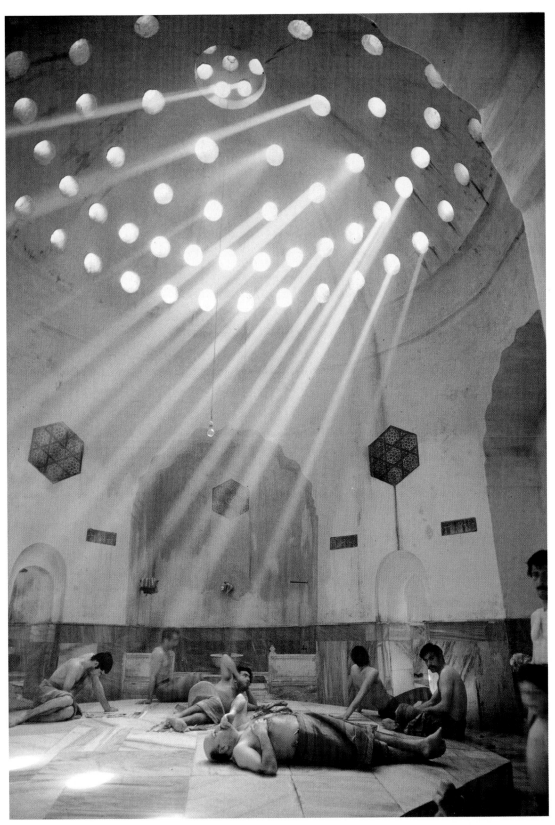

The sun's golden rays pour into a Turkish bath in Istanbul where towel-wrapped bathers relax.
Traditionally, bathers enter a cool room, then move into progressively warmer rooms, where temperatures may reach 150° Fahrenheit (65.6° Celsius). Next follows a vigorous massage, and finally a refreshing cold rinse.

cleansed, and wrapped in hot towels. While this is no doubt pleasant, so far there is no evidence that seawater has healing properties beyond providing feelings of well-being.

How Heat and Cold Affect the Body. Heat dilates blood vessels, increasing the circulation. This is why some find that a hot footbath actually helps unclog congested nasal passages. As the blood supply is drawn to one place, it decreases elsewhere. Thus when the blood vessels in the feet and legs dilate, the swelling in the nasal passages may be reduced, allowing more air to pass. Heat also relaxes muscles, eases stiffness in the joints, and relieves aches and pains.

Because heat treatments increase the heart rate, anyone with high blood pressure, a heart condition, or diabetes should consult their doctor before using heat, as should anyone on medication. And heat therapies should not be used on infants or the elderly because of their extreme sensitivity to temperature. Pregnant women, too, should steer clear of these treatments.

Cold, on the other hand, causes blood vessels to contract, reducing blood flow, swelling, and inflammation. It can also reduce fevers and act as a local anesthetic. Ice packs are an effective treatment for headaches, nosebleeds, muscle spasms, bruises, contusions, and sprains.

Hydrotherapy commonly uses either full or partial baths to warm or cool the body. Wet packs or compresses are also used. These are most effective for ailments that are limited to a specific area of the body, but they also provide an alternative to water baths if bathing is not possible.

Running from a hot room to a cold bath may sound

Water exercise is an ideal way for women to stay in shape during pregnancy. Many find it easier to stay cool and relaxed since the buoyancy of the water bears the weight of their expanding bodies. In addition, the support of the water eliminates stress on the joints, making stretching and toning exercises safe even in the last trimester of pregnancy.

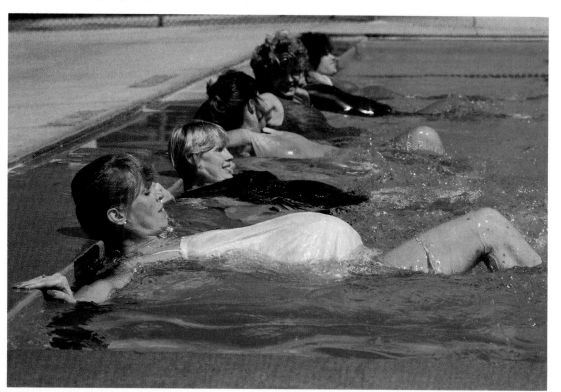

like torture, but it is actually quite exhilarating. In Finland, bathers sit in hot, dry saunas for 20 minutes or so, then race outdoors and either roll in snow or jump into an icy lake. Turkish baths, like saunas, are usually hot and dry (it is the Russian bath that uses steam), but all end with a cold shower or plunge. In the United States, Native Americans have long practiced their own version, using a sweat lodge that is constructed for this purpose. There, steam is retained when cold water is poured over heated stones. As the temperature rises in the lodge, those inside begin to sweat profusely. Like the Finns, Native Americans often end their sessions with a dip in a stream if one is nearby.

Contrast as Therapy. As bathers go from a hot water to a cold water bath, their blood vessels first dilate, then contract, which invigorates the circulatory system. But beyond being stimulating, improved circulation also relieves muscle cramps, reduces inflammation of tissues, and may help the body fight infections and heal more quickly.

The sitz bath is a variation on this technique and is used to treat abdominal ailments and injuries. Those being treated sit in a tub of warm, hip-level water, while their feet remain outside the tub. Sometimes the feet are placed in another tub of cold water. In this case, the positions are reversed after a few minutes, and the routine is repeated several times.

Soothing and Social. Although many people tend to think of a long soak in hot water as the ideal way to relax, in fact, water that is either hotter or colder than the skin will be stimulating rather than calming. If the purpose of bathing is to relax, the water should be tepid, that is, approximately the same temperature as the skin. In Japan, the ritual of daily bathing has significance above and beyond cleanliness. For centuries, the Japanese have appreciated water's soothing effect on mind and body, and public bathing has long been popular. Upon entering a bathhouse, the bathers first thoroughly soap themselves and rinse off. Once clean, they enter a tub and sit down to relax in neck-deep water, and perhaps chat with friends and neighbors.

The American version of the Japanese bath is the hot tub, which many enjoy as a way to unwind at the end of a stressful day. Others enjoy relaxing in baths equipped with whirlpools or underwater jets to benefit from another type of hydrotherapy—hydromassage. Using water pressure to massage all or part of the body is a technique long favored by rehabilitation experts. With water supporting most of

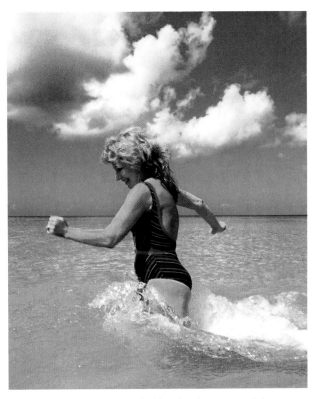

Whether in the ocean, a lake, or a pool, water-walking in thigh-deep water is great for building strength and burning calories. Not only that, but it provides an excellent aerobic workout without stressing the knees or other joints. For years, professional athletes have worked out in water while recovering from injuries. But lately, recreational joggers and others have discovered the many benefits of exercising while partially submerged.

the body's weight, muscles are more relaxed and a more intense massage is possible. The gentle swirl of the whirlpool bath is quite effective in relaxing stiff or injured muscles and joints, and easing pain. And soaking in naturally aerated water, which is found in some mineral water springs, feels refreshing against the skin and probably explains in part why bathing in mineral springs was such a popular activity in the heyday of spas.

Even without massage, water is a wonderful medium for physical rehabilitation. Water's natural buoyancy supports weakened bodies or limbs, allowing the injured or disabled to move more freely and safely than they can out of the water. In water, those suffering from joint or muscle ailments can exercise and regain strength without running the risk of putting too much strain on the injury. For the disabled, water allows the body freedom of movement, which is almost as important as the physical benefits gained from water exercises.

A Cushion for the Baby. Many pregnant women have discovered that it is easy and comfortable for them to exercise in water. Like everyone else, pregnant women need to exercise. Many also want to prepare for the physical demands of childbirth. But with a steadily increasing midsection and a shifting center of gravity, the usual modes of exercise can suddenly become difficult, or even risky. In water the problems of circulatory stress and loss of balance are eliminated.

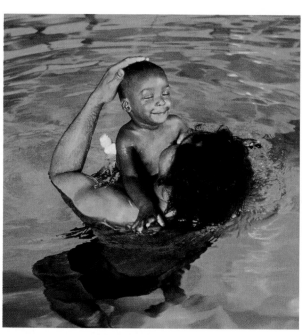

Hydrotherapy in combination with other treatments has enabled this 20-month-old child to overcome some of the afflictions of cerebral palsy. Not only is he able to enjoy the pleasures of water play, but he has actually begun to walk as well.

In fact, water exercises of all kinds are becoming increasingly popular for everyone. Swimming has always had its devotees. It is considered an ideal exercise because, unlike many other activities, there are very few injuries associated with it. At the same time, swimming forces muscles to work against water, which is 12 times as resistant as air. With each stroke, muscles are lengthened and strengthened. Depending on how forcefully you swim, the exertion required of the heart and lungs can make swimming a good aerobic activity.

However, water exercise is no longer confined to swimming laps. Synchronized swimming, while not an aerobic activity, is a good way to increase stamina and breath control, and tone and strengthen the entire body, especially the shoulder, leg, and abdominal muscles. Aquatic exercise routines are a new option for working out. A water workout can be geared toward flexibility, strength, or aerobic fitness—different results are achieved depending on the kind of strokes used.

Even walkers and runners have taken to the water. Originally a rehabilitative exercise, walking and running in water are now used in training programs for healthy athletes. Fitness buffs have also taken to the activity in part because it is simple and, if you have access to a beach or public pool, relatively inexpensive. Like walking on land, water-walking requires no special ability. Due to water resistance, you may walk slower in thigh-deep water than on land, but still burn the same number of calories. And for many, it is an especially enjoyable activity because it can be done in the company of others. ❏

A SUDDEN CURE

After Oliver Sacks broke his leg, he spent some weeks in a convalescent home. When he left there, he had not yet regained full control of the leg and went to a specialist for advice.

"I phoned Mr. W.R. of Harley Street, who said he would see me the next day.

" 'Now, as regards your walking. You walk as if you still had the cast. Yet you have 15 degrees of flexion already. Enough to walk normally if only you used it. Why do you walk as if there were no knee? It is partly habit, I think, because you have "forgotten" your knee.'

" 'I know,' I said. 'I feel that myself.'

" 'What do you like doing?' he continued. 'What comes naturally? What is your favorite physical activity?'

" 'Swimming,' I answered.

" 'Good,' he said. 'I have an idea.' There was a half-smile on his face. 'I think your best plan is to go for a swim. Will you excuse me for a minute?' He came back in a minute, the smile more pronounced. 'A taxi will be here in five minutes. It will take you to a pool.'

"The taxi arrived and took me to the Baths. I rented a towel and trunks, and advanced tremblingly to the side. There was a young lifeguard, lounging by the diving board. 'I've been told I ought to take a swim,' I said. The lifeguard unwound himself languidly, looked mischievous, and suddenly said, 'Race you!', at the same time taking my stick with his right hand and pushing me in with his left.

"I was in the water, outraged, before I knew what had happened — and the impertinence, the provocation, had their effect. I am a good swimmer. I felt challenged by the lifeguard. He stayed just a little in front of me, but I kept up a fast crawl, and only stopped because he yelled 'Enough!'

"I got out of the pool — and found I walked normally. The knee was working; it had 'come back' completely.

"When I saw Mr. W.R., he gave a big laugh and said 'Splendid!'

"I realized then that the whole scene, the scenario, was his doing, his suggestion. I burst out laughing too."

" 'It always seems to work. What one needs is spontaneity, to be tricked into action. It's the same with a dog. It happened with mine — Yorkshire terrier, sweet bitch, broke her silly leg. It healed perfectly, but she'd only walk on three legs. It went on for two months. So I took her to Bognor, and waded out to sea. I took her out as far I could, and then dumped her in. She swam back with a strong symmetrical paddle, and then scampered off along the beach on all four legs. Same therapy in both cases — unexpectedness, spontaneity, somehow evoking a natural action.' "

Excerpted from A Leg to Stand On *by Oliver Sacks, M.D.*

Cleansing with Mud, Sand, and Sweat

Using soap and water is not the only way to cleanse the body. Many people are going back to the ancient ways — bathing in mineral springs, being buried in sand, covering themselves with mud, and steaming their bodies to induce heavy perspiration.

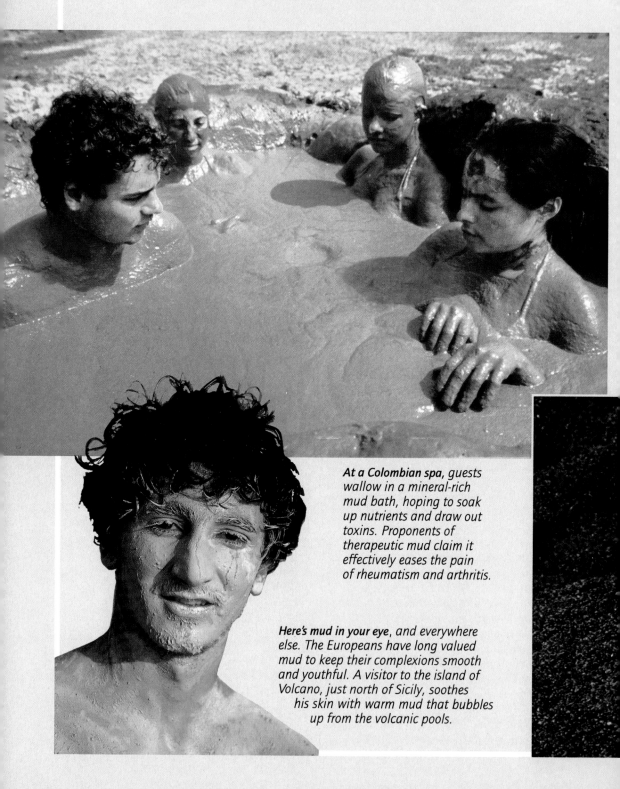

At a Colombian spa, guests wallow in a mineral-rich mud bath, hoping to soak up nutrients and draw out toxins. Proponents of therapeutic mud claim it effectively eases the pain of rheumatism and arthritis.

Here's mud in your eye, and everywhere else. The Europeans have long valued mud to keep their complexions smooth and youthful. A visitor to the island of Volcano, just north of Sicily, soothes his skin with warm mud that bubbles up from the volcanic pools.

A young Navajo eases his cold symptoms in a sweat lodge. Blankets or skins are stretched taut across an oval-shaped frame to make the hut airtight. Water is then poured over hot rocks to produce steam.

Native Americans believe that spiritual and physical health are closely connected. The warm, moist air relieves congestion, but at the same time it purifies the youth's soul and mind. The sweat house serves as more than a medical treatment in village life. Warriors preparing for battle used to purify themselves in a sweating ceremony. It is still used as a part of other religious rituals. Then, too, the sweat house may simply be a gathering place for the men of the tribe.

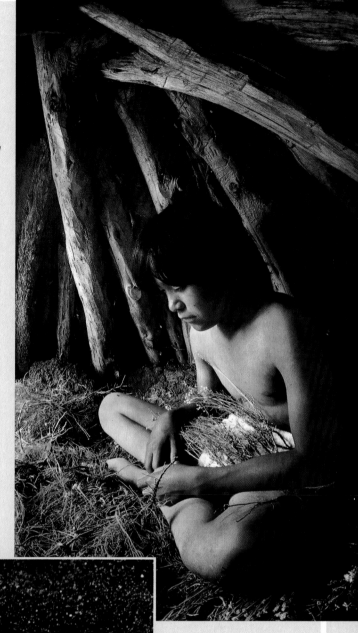

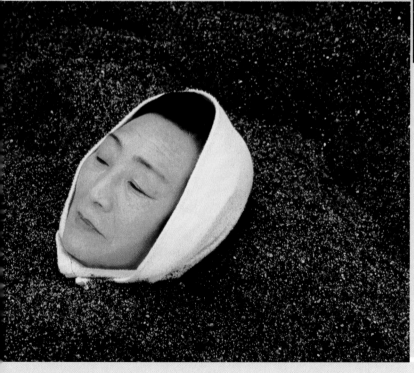

Buried in hot black sand, a woman at Japan's Surigahama sand baths serenely absorbs the penetrating heat. The temperature of the volcanic sand is too hot for most people to remain for more than 20 minutes. Treatments like this are popular in Japan, where they are used by many to improve circulation, ease pain, and stimulate perspiration.

The Ancient Practice of Yoga

This Eastern approach to health and well-being has attracted many devoted Western followers. Regular practice of yoga increases fitness, but it may also reduce stress and improve concentration.

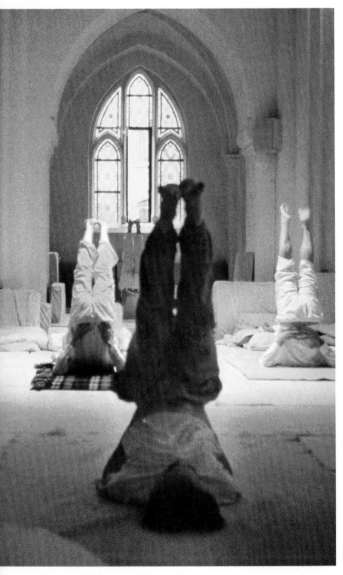

***Meditation adds** another dimension to the practice of yoga. Here, advanced students perform a yoga posture known as the shoulder stand. Yoga can enhance the total physical relaxation needed to achieve a deep meditative state.*

YOGA IS AN ANCIENT PHILOSOPHY as well as a system of exercises for physical and mental self-discipline. As an exercise, it combines stylized poses with deep breathing and meditation. Yoga was developed in India some 5000 years ago, and the word itself derives from a Sanskrit term meaning to yoke or join together. The ultimate aim in yoga is to unite the human soul with the universal spirit.

While this goal may sound lofty, many have discovered that yoga's simple exercises are excellent for relieving stress and improving overall physical condition. Yoga is often portrayed as a stretching form of exercise only. Correctly done, yoga develops strength as well as flexibility, yet is so gentle it can be practiced by anyone at any age. When yoga's special breathing techniques are mastered, yoga becomes a powerful method of managing stress.

Ancient Practices. There is evidence that some form of yoga was practiced as early as 3000 B.C. The first written description was found in the *Yoga Sutras*, a book partially attributed to Patanjali, an Indian physician and Sanskrit scholar. While its age has not been precisely determined, parts of the manuscript are thought to have been written as early as the second century B.C.

The importance of proper breathing in yoga is based on the notion that a life energy, prana, flows through and vitalizes the human body. Breathing, yoga practitioners believe, is the physical manifestation of prana. So by controlling one's breath, a person also controls his or her energy. Yoga poses are generally done with deep, diaphragmatic breathing. This, according to practitioners, increases oxygen flow to the brain and body, easing stress and fatigue, and boosting energy.

Meditation is another component of yoga, and many enthusiasts rely on yoga breathing as an aid to reaching a deep meditative state. Practiced regularly, meditation quiets the mind, and may create a profound feeling of relaxation that can carry over into the whole day. Yoga students compare meditation to a vacation for the mind, and say that daily prac-

SUN SALUTATION/WARM-UP

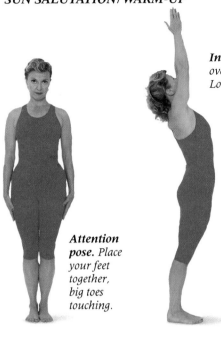

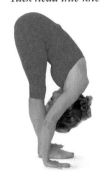

Inhale and raise arms overhead, palms touching. Look up, tighten thighs.

Exhale, bend knees, and touch palms to floor. Tuck head into knees.

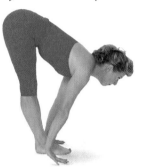

Lift head and chest after inhaling. Extend your back. Look up.

Attention pose. Place your feet together, big toes touching.

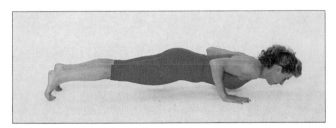

To straighten your body, inhale and walk your legs back. Drop down to push-up position.

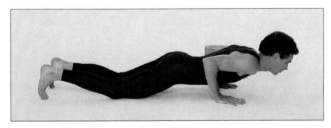

For beginners, or those with lower back pain, drop to modified push-up position, with knees touching floor.

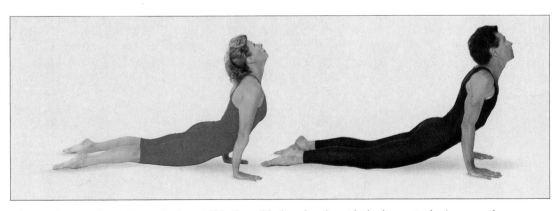

Flatten the tops of your feet on the floor. Lift body and look up but do not let back sag. For beginners or those with weak arms or lower back problems, keep knees on the floor and lift buttocks.

SUN SALUTATION (cont.)

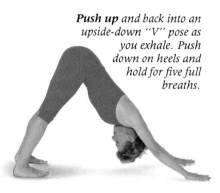

Push up *and back into an upside-down "V" pose as you exhale. Push down on heels and hold for five full breaths.*

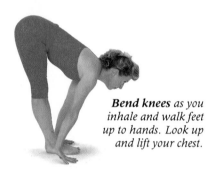

Bend knees *as you inhale and walk feet up to hands. Look up and lift your chest.*

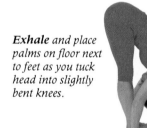

Exhale *and place palms on floor next to feet as you tuck head into slightly bent knees.*

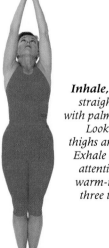

Inhale, *bring arms straight over head with palms touching. Look up, tighten thighs and buttocks. Exhale and resume attention pose. Do warm-up sequence three to ten times.*

tice can reduce feelings of anger, fear, and depression.

In traditional yoga there are eight stages in reaching a blissful state. Some of these stages have become popular forms of yoga. One of the most familiar in the West is hatha-yoga, which emphasizes poses and breathing technique. Good health is the goal in hatha-yoga.

The assumption of all systems of yoga is that the body and mind are strongly connected, and must be balanced for one to maintain a state of good health. For example, this means that one doesn't try to eliminate physical tension without also thinking about any underlying psychological factors that may be contributing to the problem. The integration of mind and body is achieved, in part, through the slow and deliberate way that the poses are performed. By concentrating on each move, the practitioner becomes more attuned to his or her body. And while regular practice helps promote relaxation, the mind is fully focused on and responsive to what is happening with the body.

Getting Started. One of the advantages of yoga is that it can be practiced almost anywhere, without special equipment, by people of all ages. All that's necessary is a warm, quiet room and a blanket, mat, or towel. It's best to wear loose or stretch clothing, such as shorts, sweat clothes, or leotards. Yoga is traditionally practiced barefoot, although some students prefer to wear socks or soft shoes.

Many students find practicing first thing in the morning is an excellent way to revitalize the mind and body, while others find practice at night helps induce deep, restful sleep. Others split their routine, performing their poses in the morning and their breathing and meditation exercises at night. Practice sessions need not be lengthy, but should be done daily. As little as 15 minutes of exercises and 15 minutes of breathing and meditation each day can yield benefits.

Sessions may begin and end with the *corpse pose.* While the name is somewhat off-putting, the practice is meant as a way of thoroughly relaxing and centering the body. To begin, lie on your back, arms at your side, palms up, and legs open. While in this position, spend a few minutes consciously relaxing each part of the body, moving from the forehead to the tips of the toes while you visualize tension leaving every muscle. This resting position may also be done during your exercise routine, to relax the body between poses.

After you're physically relaxed, do some meditation, using yoga breathing exercises, to calm your mind. Some students find that repeating a sound to themselves (such as the traditional om), or visualizing a peaceful image like a meadow or sky, can make meditation easier. For most students, 10 or 20 minutes a day of meditation is enough to create a deep feeling of calmness and relaxation. Some students also report that the practice helps release powers of intuition and creativity and improves their concentration.

Yoga exercises consist of a series of poses, or asanas, that are performed slowly and gently. A complete routine is designed to work all parts of the body, stretching and toning muscles, while also keeping joints flexible. Advanced poses

BIG TOE POSE

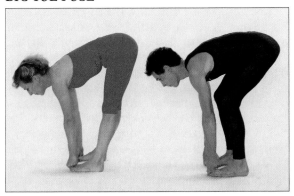

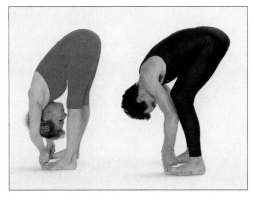

Bend over and grab big toes with first two fingers. Lift head, inhale, and look up. For beginners or those with back problems, keep knees bent.

Exhale and bend farther, pulling legs with arms. Relax head and neck, take five breaths. Inhale and look up. Slowly resume attention pose.

TRIANGLE: EXTENDED, INVERTED POSES

With feet apart (right) and left foot angled away from body, inhale and extend arms from sides. Exhale, bend at hips. Grasp left big toe with left hand. Hold for 5–8 breaths, rise on inhale, switch sides. Beginners grasp shin or ankle. Then, again standing upright (below), inhale and extend arms from sides. Exhale and rotate torso to left, with right arm touching floor near left foot, left arm outstretched. Take 5–8 breaths, rise, switch sides. Beginners may touch shin or ankle.

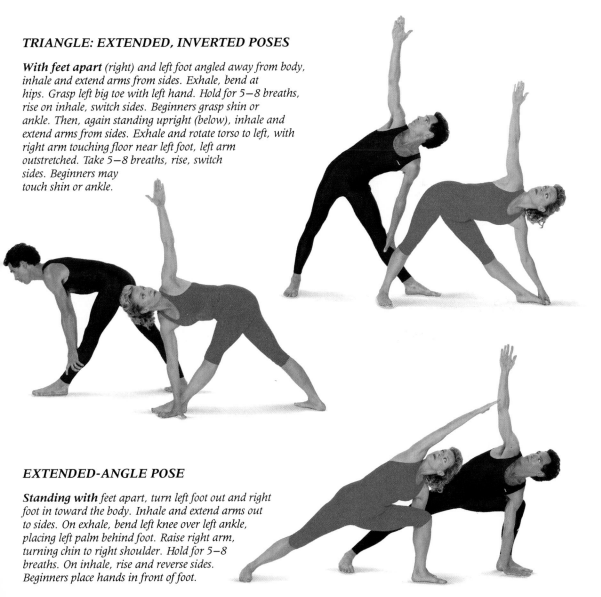

EXTENDED-ANGLE POSE

Standing with feet apart, turn left foot out and right foot in toward the body. Inhale and extend arms out to sides. On exhale, bend left knee over left ankle, placing left palm behind foot. Raise right arm, turning chin to right shoulder. Hold for 5–8 breaths. On inhale, rise and reverse sides. Beginners place hands in front of foot.

KNEE-UP POSE

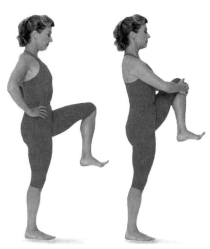

Lift *your right leg as you inhale. Flex foot, take 5–8 breaths. Exhale and release. Alternate legs. Repeat, clasping knee to pull leg toward chest.*

are also intended to massage the internal organs. Especially for beginners, it's a good idea to take yoga lessons with an experienced teacher, who can provide both encouragement and practical advice. Performing the poses incorrectly or in an extreme manner may cause muscle strain or tears.

When performing the asanas, try to concentrate on each movement—the process of moving is just as important as attaining a given position. Remember never to strain or to continue holding any posture if it causes pain. Yoga isn't a competitive sport, and the extent of the stretch is less important than the technique. Each asana may be repeated up to three times, but it's better to perform a posture once correctly than three times quickly and sloppily. Try to perform the poses in the prescribed order, since the routine is meant to help balance the different muscle groups.

Adopting a Healthy Lifestyle. Yoga practice is not a substitute for medical care. The emphasis is on prevention of illness by maintaining balance within the mind and body. Still, many practitioners believe that yoga has yielded positive physiological changes for them. For example, studies have shown that yoga practice has been credited with easing a range of complaints,

WARRIOR POSE

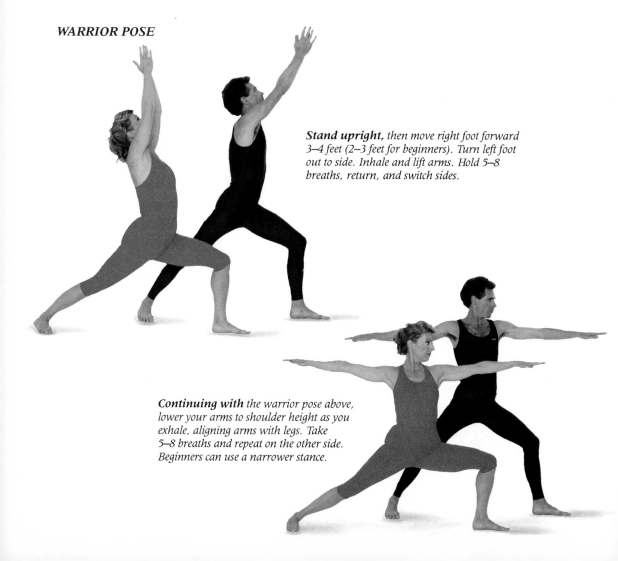

Stand upright, *then move right foot forward 3–4 feet (2–3 feet for beginners). Turn left foot out to side. Inhale and lift arms. Hold 5–8 breaths, return, and switch sides.*

Continuing with *the warrior pose above, lower your arms to shoulder height as you exhale, aligning arms with legs. Take 5–8 breaths and repeat on the other side. Beginners can use a narrower stance.*

SEATED FORWARD BEND

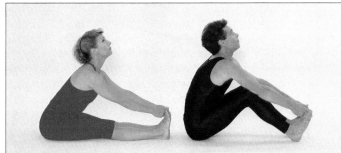

Sitting with outstretched legs, or bent knees for beginners, inhale. Grasp big toes with first two fingers of each hand. Exhale, lift chest, extend back.

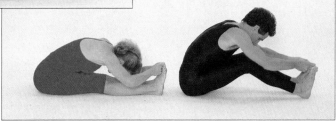

Keeping back extended and chest up, exhale. Bend at the hips with thighs and abdominals tightened. Take 5–8 breaths, inhale, lift head, then exhale.

BACK-LIFT

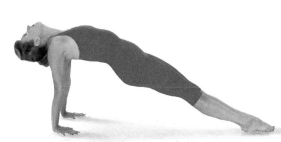

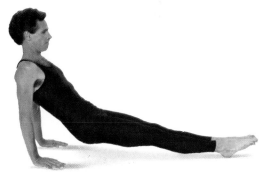

Still seated, put hands behind you. Lift body and drop head. Take 5–8 breaths, exhale, and sit up.

For beginners, keep chin tucked in and head facing forward. Lift as high as possible.

SINGLE FORWARD BEND

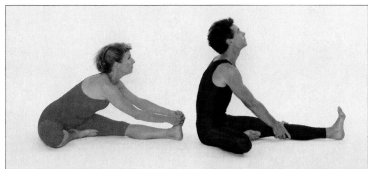

Extend left leg. Place right foot on inner left thigh. Bend over to grasp left foot. Inhale. Lift chest, extend back, look up. Beginners grasp knee or shin.

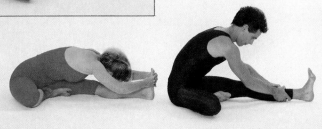

Holding leg, exhale and pull gently to bend over. Keep back straight, lift chest and look up. Take 5–8 breaths, return to upright, exhale. Switch legs and repeat.

including back pain, stress, migraine, and insomnia. In addition, some have found yoga helpful in reducing high blood pressure, pulse rates, and joint pain, and increasing range of movement. People who practice yoga regularly often cite such benefits as increased vitality, greater emotional stability, improved concentration, better muscle tone and posture, and weight loss. However, if you're overweight or suffer from high blood pressure, arthritis, or spinal disk injuries, it's a good idea to check with the doctor before trying yoga.

SPINAL-TWIST POSE

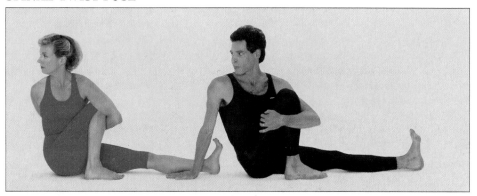

Extend left leg with foot flexed. Bend right leg so that heel aligns with buttocks. Inhale and stretch left arm into air. Exhale and twist right, bringing left forearm toward thigh. Look back over right shoulder. Keep back straight. Beginners twist as far as you can.

BOUND-ANGLE POSE

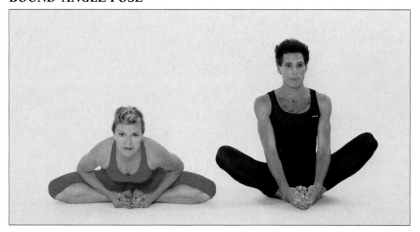

Bring soles of feet together, grab ankles, and pull heels toward groin. Inhale, lift chest, and extend your back. Exhale and bend over. Gently push thighs down by flexing inner thigh muscles. Keep back straight. Beginners bend forward carefully.

CORPSE POSE

Relax, lying absolutely still for 10–15 minutes. Allow your mind to follow your body into rest. Contemplation and meditation may follow.

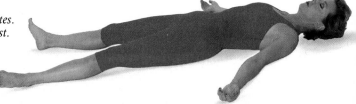

Some physicians have found that yoga can be especially helpful as an adjunct therapy. Recently, Dr. Dean Ornish, a physician and researcher concerned with coronary artery disease (CAD), conducted a study in which participants suffering from CAD combined yoga and moderate exercise with a vegetarian diet and participation in a support group. The results showed that such lifestyle changes could actually reverse the course of heart disease. ❏

THE INSIGHT OF A YOGA THERAPIST

Meditation can often guide a therapist toward an intuitive diagnosis of an illness. Here, Maureen Lockhart describes her treatment of a patient who had trouble breathing.

"In many cases, insight and intuition gained through meditation will provide the right means to help people in the right way. For example, an osteopath sent me a patient with a breathing problem. My very first impression of the man was 'barrel-chested, hard outside, soft inside.' None of this meant anything to me until I discovered that the man was a journalist with a hard-boiled exterior but a soft heart who had been the victim of a malicious prank as a small child and had nearly drowned in a barrel of water.

"For the first session I simply watched him go through some easy breathing and stretching movements and it became obvious that he could not breathe in properly. Breathing in for him meant breathing in water and drowning. Any inducement to increase his in-breath brought a panic response. I could see what his problem was quite clearly, but I didn't know if I was going to be able to help him solve it. For several days I focused on him for a few minutes in my meditation session, but nothing happened. Then, around the fourth or fifth day, he appeared in my meditation holding a beautiful long-stemmed red rose. I hadn't a clue what the meditation meant, even by the time my student arrived for his next session.

"Then it came to me. I asked if he liked flowers and when he said he did, I asked him if he'd noticed how one has to smell a flower. I explained that *trying* to smell a flower doesn't seem to work; the smell eludes one unless you become totally passive and let the fragrance come to you. I asked him to experience this with a real flower; then to imagine he was smelling a flower. Although difficult at first, he learned to breathe passively through this method, gradually deepening his breath so that he could breathe in without tension or fear. Eventually, I just had to remind him to 'smell a flower' whenever he was tense in order to see him visibly let go and relax.

"After some practice in concentration we were able to explore the original trauma. He became the little boy in the barrel, but a little boy who, although he'd had a nasty experience, was still alive and had grown up into a man who was still alive and no longer afraid of being in the barrel. It took some time to get through this block but, when we did, this very courageous, gentle man stopped carrying his barrel around with him; he lost weight, ate better, slept better and, when he telephoned me one day to tell me he didn't need me any more, *was* better."

Excerpted from The Art of Survival *by Dr. M.L.Gharote and Maureen Lockhart*

The Martial Arts

These self-defense arts are difficult to master, not because they require brute strength, but because they demand discipline and intense concentration. Among the rewards of study are impressive grace and confidence.

KNOWN PRIMARILY AS MEANS OF self-defense, the martial arts, including karate, judo, t'ai chi, and others, are also done for pure sport and to improve physical fitness. As fighting techniques, they are strictly defensive, and in most cases students are taught never to court trouble or to use their skills aggressively.

These arts, which originated in East Asia centuries ago and have spread throughout the world, share another component—the goal of study is to develop mentally and spiritually as well as physically. Through rigorous, highly disciplined—and repetitive—moves, body and mind are trained to act in concert, naturally and instinctively.

Despite the elaborate array of kicks, stances, and punches that typify many of these "combat sports," most of the martial arts in fact emphasize self-control and non-violence. Practitioners adhere to strict rules of conduct and bow to their opponents as a show of respect.

In traditional karate tournaments, for example, contestants rarely touch one another; instead they stop their blows within a centimeter or two of their opponents' bodies. In aikido, masters learn to gracefully avoid blows until their opponents weaken or are injured. And while the goal of a Western sports competition is victory, winning plays a relatively minor role in the Asian martial arts. For the practitioner, mastering the movements and forms, observing rituals (such as bowing), gaining self-discipline, and showing respect for one's teacher and opponents are all significant ends in themselves.

Tracing the Roots. There is evidence that martial arts were practiced in many parts of the world as early as 2000 B.C. Some think they developed from ancient ritual dances celebrating folk heroes, animals, and nature. Later, the movements may have been adopted by Taoist physicians to relax the body after hours of meditation, and by monks as means of self-defense.

Most likely, the martial arts of Asia originated in India and Tibet, and later spread to China, Japan, and Korea. According to legend, the Buddhist monk Bodhidarma, who founded Zen Buddhism, traveled thousands of miles from India to China some 1,500 years ago, and ended up teaching young monks at the Shaolin monastery. Find-

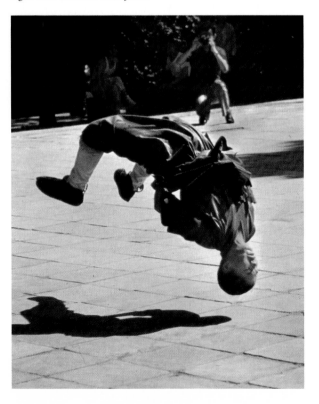

Buddhist monks *at China's Shaolin monastery, the birthplace of kung fu, endure the rigors of ascetic devotion with the help of martial arts. Here a monk prepares for long hours of meditation by doing elaborate training exercises. The monastery, founded in 496 A.D., accepts only eight new students each year.*

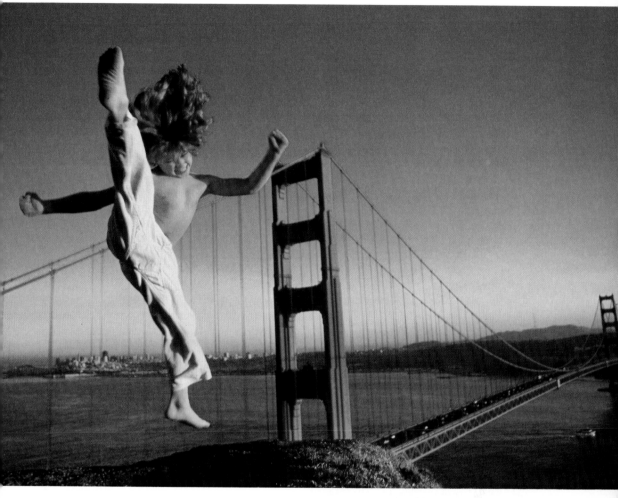

ing his students so weak from inactivity that they would fall asleep during meditation, Bodhidarma developed exercises to increase their strength and stamina. These exercises, it is said, were the basis for many of today's martial arts.

For centuries, the martial arts were practiced only in Asia. They were imported to the U.S. after World War II by American troops who had been stationed in Japan and Korea. The practice of martial arts has increased in the last 20 years, the result of a number of popular movies, concern about crime, and growth in the number of schools teaching the techniques.

A Wide Range of Disciplines. The martial arts share much in the way of philosophy, technique, and training, but over the centuries, a variety of schools and styles has evolved. The most commonly practiced styles are often classified as either "external"—referring to methods such as karate or judo that stress endurance and muscular strength—or "internal"—indicating forms, such as aikido and t'ai chi, that stress relaxation and control. But, regardless of the classification, all of the martial arts are physically demanding, and mastery requires a long period of serious training. A few widely taught methods are described here.

Many karate enthusiasts start young. Since mastery requires dedication, not strength, age is no impediment to success. Indeed, this young expert started at the age of two, and he earned a second-degree black belt by age eight.

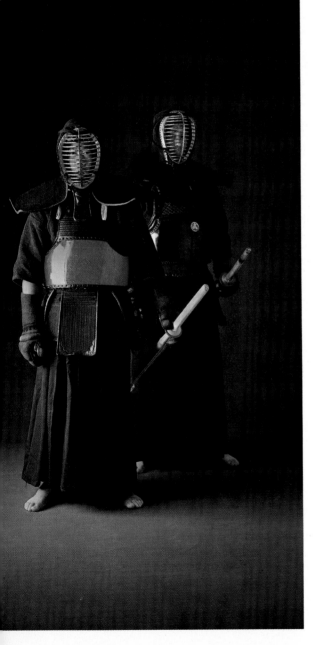

Kung Fu. Well-known but less well understood, kung fu is actually a generic term used to describe many Chinese martial arts. The Chinese have a long tradition of martial arts, developed over the centuries as a means of protection in a land frequently torn by war and conflict. In much of China, kung fu is actually called wushu, from the Mandarin dialect. Wushu was originally the formal name for many Chinese martial arts, and is still used in much of China. The name kung fu, more common throughout the West, is from the Cantonese dialect.

While kung fu's precise origins have been obscured by time, the Shaolin monastery in China was long the center of its practice. The Manchu rulers eventually succeeded in partially destroying the monastery (it was later restored), but the monks managed to escape and began quietly teaching their martial arts to farmers and villagers throughout China.

Traditional kung fu training was rigorous, with students enduring months of waiting and manual labor before being accepted to study with a master. Once accepted, they spent months practicing basic stances, only later learning sets of stylized movements. After mastering the physical aspects of the art, advanced kung fu students practiced meditation and breathing exercises to further focus their energies. Nai gung, or "inner strength," was the product—and indeed the goal—of long years of discipline and practice.

While modern-day kung fu students

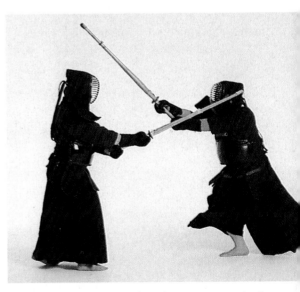

Kendo, a Japanese martial art, is an Eastern style of fencing. Dressed in protective armor and face masks, kendo students engage in ritualized swordplay, using leather-bound bamboo "weapons."

may no longer wait for admission or endure months of manual labor, the training is much the same as it was during the days of the Shaolin monks. There are dozens of styles of kung fu, but in each, stance training is still emphasized, and mastery requires years of self-discipline, concentration, and hard work.

Advanced kung fu students often continue their studies with weapons training. Varied in size, shape, and utility, weapons are used almost as an extension of the hands, with students practicing the same basic strikes and stances as they do when weaponless. Another advanced technique is known as iron palm training. Initially, students thrust their hands into a bucket of fine sand. Then, as they become accustomed to the sand, they graduate to coarser grades, from small pebbles to rocks, and finally to iron filings or ball bearings. Iron palm training should never be undertaken except under supervision of a master.

Karate. One of the best-known of the martial arts, karate, like the term kung fu, refers to a whole range of fighting styles that use hand blows and kicks as their basic techniques. It is believed to have developed on Okinawa when the island's inhabitants, prohibited by their rulers from carrying weapons, were forced to devise secret forms of unarmed combat to protect themselves from conquerors and marauding bands of pirates.

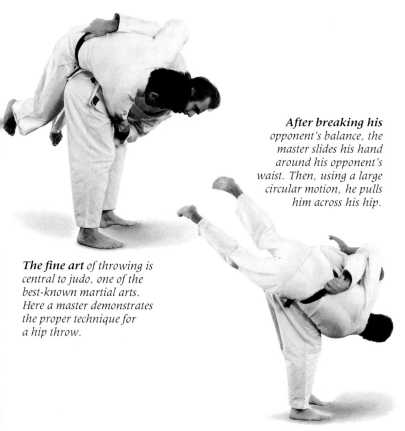

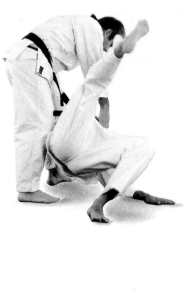

Learning how to land is another important element of judo. But contests are judged on the proficiency of the throws, not on the graceful manner in which the contestants fall.

After breaking his opponent's balance, the master slides his hand around his opponent's waist. Then, using a large circular motion, he pulls him across his hip.

The fine art of throwing is central to judo, one of the best-known martial arts. Here a master demonstrates the proper technique for a hip throw.

Karate spread to Japan in the 20th century after Crown Prince Hirohito witnessed a martial arts demonstration by a master named Gichin Funakoshi. The prince was so impressed that he invited Funakoshi to Tokyo to teach. From Japan, karate traveled to Korea, where it was modified and developed into tae kwon do, which literally means "the way of kicking and punching." While it is similar to karate, tae kwon do places more emphasis on the use of the legs, while karate relies equally on both arms and legs. Thai boxing and Okinawa-te are among the other styles that were strongly influenced by karate.

Many myths surround karate. For example, practice does not entail breaking boards or bricks. These are stunts done for demonstration. The "karate chop" hand position (correctly called "knife hand") is used less often than the fist, and flying kicks are seldom performed. Like most of the martial arts, karate practice is geared toward developing proper technique, coordinating mind and body, and the focusing of energy. A karate master's concentration can become so developed, it is reported, that simple eye contact may be enough to repel an adversary.

Karate students work out barefoot, and wear pajama-like uniforms known as gis. A student's top is tied with a belt whose color signifies rank. Before stepping onto the training area, students bow toward it as a sign of respect. Then, after lining up according to rank, class members do a few minutes of meditation to center their attention. Stretching and calisthenics are usually included in the warm-up, after which students practice basic stances, kicks, punches, strikes, and blocks.

Following the warm-up and practice of stances, students next move in unison through a variety of formal exercises known as katas, or forms. Developed centuries ago, all

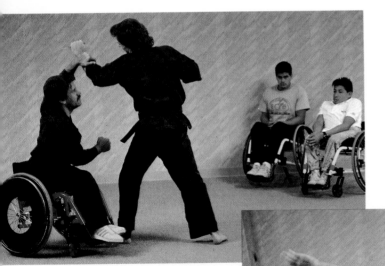

At a California rehabilitation center, paraplegics learn the ancient art of kung fu. One wheelchair-bound instructor, an eighth-degree black belt, notes that kung fu has helped him gain self-confidence. In fact, he is so accomplished that he frequently overpowers his able-bodied colleagues.

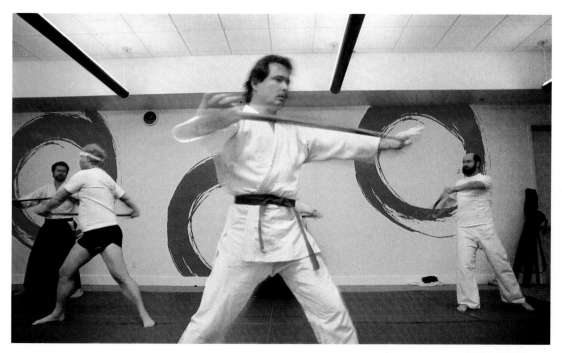

the forms are difficult to perfect and may take many years to master. Classes end with free sparring between partners. Energetic and challenging, free sparring allows students to use their repertoire of techniques and forms, but they stop their blows just short of the point of contact.

Judo. More of a competitive sport than a means of self-defense, judo emphasizes posture, balance, and good judgment. Superficially, a judo class bears resemblance to a karate class. Students wear white gis bound with colored belts denoting rank, they bow to the room and to one another, and they practice rigorous forms. However, the goal of judo is to throw an opponent and pin him or her for a certain length of time with any number of arm locks and holds. Mastering the art of throwing depends more on balance and agility than it does on strength. By learning to yield when an opponent pushes, or moving toward him when he pulls, the student places his opponent off balance, making him easier to throw.

While the goal of judo may be to throw an opponent, to avoid injury, students must also learn the fine art of falling. During ukemi (falling practice), students are taught to absorb the shock of a fall by slamming the palms of their hands into the mat.

T'ai Chi Chuan. Described in greater detail in the next few pages, t'ai chi stresses breathing and meditation along with strength and flexibility training. Fundamental to t'ai chi is the notion that a life energy circulates along channels in the body, known as meridians. T'ai chi movements circulate this energy, thereby stimulating different organs of the body. For this reason, some Chinese physicians prescribe t'ai chi to help patients recover from illness.

At one American corporation, employees are offered aikido lessons to help them unwind and release stress. After learning the basic moves, some students train with wooden staffs known as jos. Like many of the martial arts, aikido combines sport with philosophy, flowing movement with discipline.

Aikido. One of the youngest of the martial arts, aikido is a subtle, stylized technique that began in Japan in the 1920s. While students are taught to subdue opponents with hundreds of movements, holds, locks, and escapes, aikido is essentially non-competitive. Technically, it is more of a throwing art, like judo, though many of the moves resemble the fluid and dancelike techniques of t'ai chi. The goal of aikido is to harmonize one student's qi with that of his opponent, in order to disarm him both physically and emotionally.

Choosing a Method. The martial arts aren't for those looking for a quick and easy method of fitness or self-defense. Almost all methods take months or years of disciplined training with a master (a sensei in Japanese, or a Sifu in Chinese). Students attend classes as infrequently as once a week, or as often as every day, usually for one-hour sessions. A Japanese practice hall is usually called a dojo, meaning "sacred hall of learning," while a Chinese hall is known as a kwoon.

In many large cities today, there are a number of martial arts schools available. Let your own interests and temperament guide your choice. If you like competitive sports, you may wish to consider judo. If getting fit and learning some techniques of self-defense are more to your liking, consider kung fu or karate. T'ai chi and aikido are more gentle, and may even be described as forms of moving meditation. Students often describe these disciplines as having a calming effect on mind and body, and the slow, fluid movements are easy on the joints.

In Pursuit of Health and Well-being. Like any fitness program, martial arts offer health benefits if practiced regularly. Many styles are ideal for developing strength, and increasing flexibility and muscle tone, especially in the lower body, back, and abdominal areas. With their emphasis on concentration and relaxation, martial arts also offer effective ways of relieving stress.

Of course, some styles are also a means of self-defense. While this is most evident in the external arts like karate, even a relatively "soft" martial art like t'ai chi can be used defensively. But some experts emphasize that the main benefit of the martial arts may be in helping students develop enough self-confidence to feel comfortable in almost any situation.

Whatever method you choose, the martial arts do demand a basic level of health and fitness. Before starting, visit a variety of classes. Also, have a checkup or discuss any medical concerns with a physician. ❑

A martial arts master demonstrates his strength by thrusting his arm into a barrel of tightly packed dried soybeans. Neither a show of bravado nor brute force, the master's skill points to long years of mental and physical training.

Portal to the Spirit

Don Ethan Miller first studied the martial arts as a means of self-defense. But as his physical prowess increased, he discovered the spiritual dimensions of this ancient practice.

I began studying the Oriental martial arts twenty years ago, a short, overweight smart kid with glasses on the Upper West Side of Manhattan. I hated being unable to defend myself from the gangs of tough kids around whom I had to thread the most circuitous of routes to reach junior high school unscathed. Though I was motivated originally by self-defense, something else grabbed hold of me from the very first time I walked into the Downtown Dojo, a school of judo, in 1960.

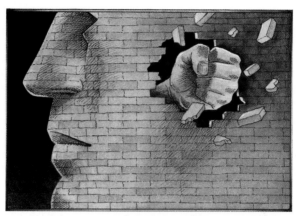

Gaining access to the powers within one's mind

I was taken by the aesthetic of the place: the huge, open, mat-covered practice hall, the shoes lined up outside the door, the neatly displayed plaques on the walls. There was a mystery there beyond the mere exoticisms of a foreign culture. After two decades, I can at least name the mystery: the martial arts have been for me a doorway into terrains of experience beyond the normal "limits," into other realms where the common assumptions about conflict and fear, effort and energy may be overturned and completely reordered.

Thus, when I now approach a stack of three two-inch cinder blocks to attempt a breaking feat, I do not set myself to summon up all my strength. Instead, I relax, sinking my awareness into my belly and legs. I breathe deeply, mentally directing the breath through my torso, legs, and arms. I imagine a line of force coming up from the ground through my legs, down one arm, and out through my palm, through the stone slabs, and down again into the ground. I am no longer a thirty-two-year-old writer in sneakers in his suburban back yard: I am a spiritual traveler, making the necessary preparations for a journey to a different world.

I do not hit the bricks; I do not break them. Rather I take a deep breath, hold it for half a second, then *release* suddenly but smoothly, focusing on the energy line and allowing my arm to express it. My palm passes right through the place where the blocks were, but they have apparently parted just before I get there, and there is no sensation of impact, no shock wave, no pain. Hours later, what remains is not a sense of destructive power but the feeling of attunement with the mysterious but very real power of life itself. Passing through the bricks is only a way of entering another realm.

The real value of martial arts study, in other words, has nothing to do with physical feats such as brick breaking; in fact, it is not even primarily concerned with fighting. Their real value lies in what the martial arts tell us about ourselves: that we can be much more than we are now; that we have no need of fear; that our capacities for energy, awareness, courage, and compassion are far greater than we have been led to believe. They tell us that all our personal limits can be transcended. Beginning with the next breath, drawn deeply.

Excerpted from an essay by Don Ethan Miller in The Overlook Martial Arts Reader, *edited by Randy F. Nelson.*

T'ai Chi: The Supreme Ultimate

The slow, relaxed movements of this martial art appeal to a wide range of students. Many practice for the sheer pleasure of exercise, others are drawn toward developing supreme self-control and concentration.

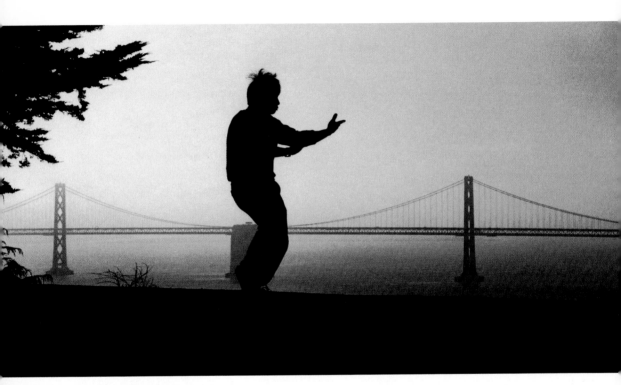

In many cities and towns it is not uncommon to see people practicing t'ai chi in parks or other scenic locales, particularly as the sun is rising. According to Chinese philosophy, nature's qi flows most strongly at dawn. For this reason, t'ai chi practitioners often assemble in large groups to greet the start of a new day.

ONE OF THE BEST-KNOWN of the martial arts, t'ai chi is both a self-defense strategy and, more commonly in the West, a gentle exercise technique. In Chinese the words t'ai chi chuan mean "supreme ultimate fist," a reference, in part, to its lofty status among the martial arts.

T'ai chi consists of a series of postures performed in sequences. Known as forms, they vary in complexity, with some involving 18 postures and others more than 100. Students move from one posture to the next in a flowing motion that resembles dance. While not as physically demanding as karate and judo, t'ai chi takes a long time to master. Movements are learned slowly and carefully, creating a state of restful action in which the mind can concentrate on every motion. But the pace of class may quicken as students acquire proficiency and agility.

Tracing T'ai Chi's Roots. The origins of t'ai chi are obscure. There are reports that it was being practiced some 5000 years ago, and ancient Chinese drawings depict monks performing movements that look similar to t'ai chi. Some accounts of its origins describe the founder as a monk and kung fu student at a monastery in China in the thirteenth century. After witnessing a fight between a bird and a snake, the man noticed that the snake managed to avoid the bird's attack using swift, but subtle movements; from these observations, he developed the art of t'ai chi. Newer theories credit a Chinese general who, in the seventeenth century, improvised t'ai chi by combining martial arts with theories of traditional Chinese medicine.

Like aikido, the Japanese martial art, t'ai chi was influenced by the idea of Tao, which means "the way" or "the path," described by the Chinese philosopher Lao-tze. His philosophy, known as Taoism, stresses that humankind must attain harmony with nature and the universe. When in perfect harmony, things function effortlessly and spontaneously, according to natural laws. So, too, the body operates by the same principles. "When people are alive," Lao wrote, "they are soft and supple. When a plant is alive, it is soft and tender." T'ai chi practitioners believe that the qualities of softness and suppleness can be developed by cultivating the life force, qi, that flows through the body.

Clarity Through Contradiction. Among the most intriguing aspects of t'ai chi are its various contradictions and seeming paradoxes. These are rooted in the Chinese notion of yin and yang, the law of complementary opposites. For instance, alert relaxation is essential to each movement. The body should remain supple and at ease, but not to the extent of going limp. Movement likewise entails opposition or contradiction. To move to the right, for example, you must first turn slightly leftward; to rise up, you must first sink slightly. The movement called push can be performed most effectively *without* the application of force: the arms and shoulders relax, the elbows hang loose, and the palms of the two partners meet without touching. All movement in t'ai chi describes circles, spirals, or arches. To achieve this effect is sometimes termed "curved seeking straightness." This refers to the necessary curvature of limbs.

Perhaps the ultimate paradox in the "supreme ultimate fist" pertains to the principle of softness. T'ai chi devotees believe that a combination of external suppleness and internal

The Solo Form

The postures on the next few pages illustrate most of the movements that are basic to t'ai chi. Let these pictures pique your interest, but proper technique must be learned from a master.

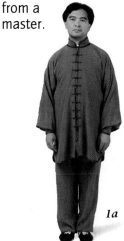

1a

Beginning *t'ai chi. Stand comfortably with hands at side and feet together.*

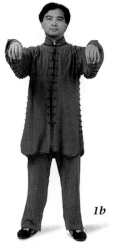

1b

With left *foot, step to the left and slowly raise arms to shoulder height.*

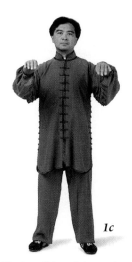

1c

Next, *pull hands toward your shoulders, in a smooth, continuous motion.*

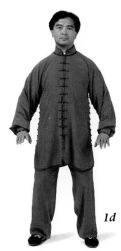

1d

Finally, *while bending your knees slightly, lower your hands to your side.*

PARTING THE HORSE'S MANE

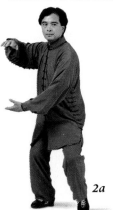

2a

With weight on right leg and left toe touching ground, "hold the ball."

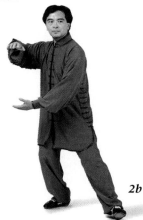

2b

Step forward, at a 45-degree angle, on left leg and place heel down.

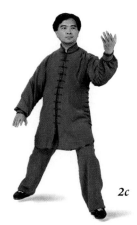

2c

Shift weight onto left leg. Raise left hand diagonally and press right palm down.

HOLDING THE BALL

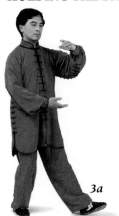

3a

With weight on back leg, "hold the ball," left hand on top, right below.

firmness can overpower brute strength. When self-defense techniques are used, t'ai chi practitioners do not try to meet force with force. Instead they yield to evade a blow, then use the momentum of the opponent's body against the attacker. As one popular t'ai chi maxim puts it, "Four ounces can topple 1,000 pounds."

Concentrated Movement. Most students learn t'ai chi in classes; the movements, once memorized, can also be practiced at home. There are no uniforms, and students generally wear loose, comfortable clothing, and practice either barefoot or in soft shoes. In most classes, t'ai chi is non-competitive. Unlike other martial arts, there are no colored belts to indicate rankings. But there is a movement to certify t'ai chi as an Olympic event, so objective standards would have to be devised and applied.

Classes generally begin with several minutes of standing meditation, designed to calm the mind and awaken energy.

GRASPING THE BIRD'S TAIL

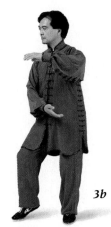

3b

Shift weight forward onto left leg, bring right toe near left foot, turn body and look right.

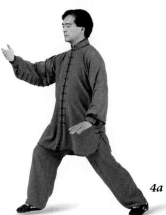

4a

Step right with right leg and push out with forearm. Press left hand downward.

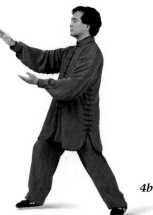

4b

Raise left hand up to meet right, and, as you do, turn right palm downward.

GRASPING THE BIRD'S TAIL *(continued)*

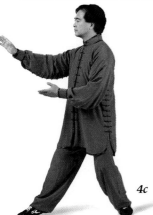

4c

Pull back; *sit back on your left leg as you pull your hands back.*

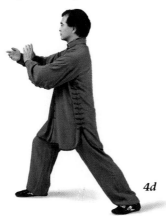

4d

Shift *weight forward to right leg. With left palm on right wrist, press forearm forward.*

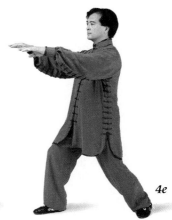

4e

Separate *your hands, while keeping your weight shifted forward on right leg.*

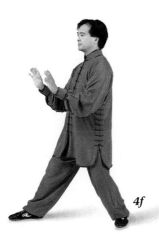

4f

Shift weight *back onto left leg, and pull your hands in toward your chest.*

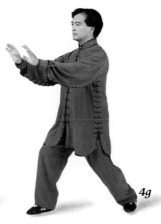

4g

Finally, *shift your weight forward while you push both palms forward.*

WAVE HANDS LIKE CLOUDS

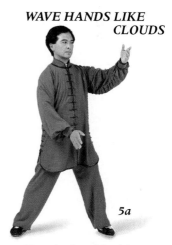

5a

Turn body *to left; right palm circles clockwise as left circles counter-clockwise.*

SINGLE WHIP

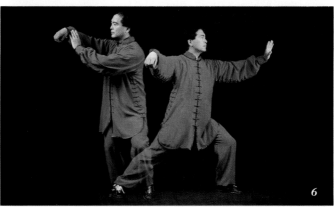

5b

Turn to *right, take half-step left with right foot. Reverse arm circles. Repeat 4 times.*

6

Make a *"bird's beak" with right hand, and place left fingers on right wrist. Step left and shift weight forward, bending knee. Stretch left arm outward, pointing fingers up.*

BRUSH KNEE AND PRESS (right and left style)

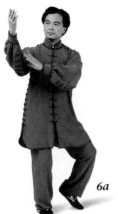 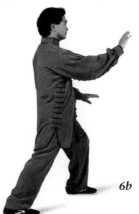 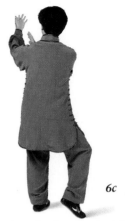

6a

Step back, raise right palm; place left palm near right elbow.

6b

Step out on left leg. Push right hand out as left palm brushes over left knee.

6c

Step back and raise left palm while placing right palm near elbow.

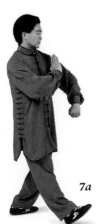

6d

Step out with right heel. As left hand presses out, right brushes across right knee.

BLOCK, PARRY, AND PUNCH

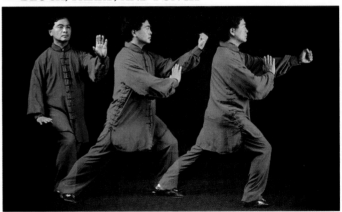

This photograph shows the sequence of motions that are described below. While postures are learned individually, they must flow together gracefully when performed.

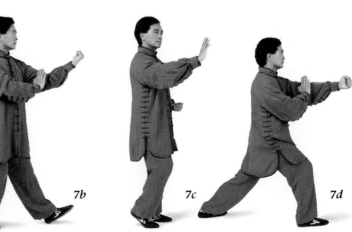

7a *7b* *7c* *7d*

Sit back on left leg, lower left fist, and place right hand near shoulder. Step up with left heel, and strike with left fist. Place right hand near left elbow.

Move right foot next to left, but push weight onto left. With left fist at waist, block with right palm. Step forward on right foot, punch with left fist.

HOLDING THE BALL

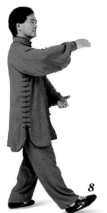

8

Sit back on left leg and "hold the ball," left hand palm up, right palm down.

GRASPING THE BIRD'S TAIL

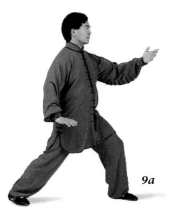

9a

Step forward with left leg, push out with left forearm, press right palm down.

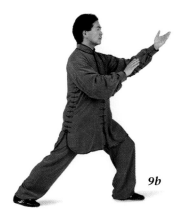

9b

Raise right palm upward to meet left hand, which rotates palm downward.

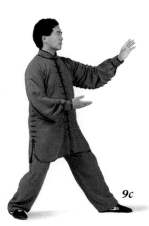

9c

Sit back on right leg, separate hands and pull them toward you.

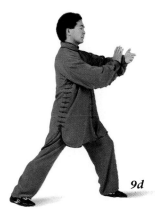

9d

Shift weight forward to left leg. Placing right palm on left wrist, press forearm forward.

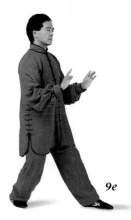

9e

Pull back both hands toward chest as you sit back on right leg.

Students then practice the forms, both to develop balance and coordination and as a kind of moving meditation. To achieve thorough relaxation of mind and body, students are taught to concentrate on a point two to three inches below the navel, a point referred to in Chinese as tan tien. This area is believed to be the storehouse of the body's qi and the point from which all energy emanates.

Concentration on the tan tien is referred to as centering. This essential principle of t'ai chi calls for both physical and mental balance. Practitioners are encouraged to "sink to gravity," using the muscles just enough to perform the movements without fighting gravity.

Many movements have names from nature, such as "snake creeps in the grass," "needle beneath the sea," and "white crane spreads its wings," reflecting t'ai chi's links to the plant and animal worlds. Movements are circular and rhythmic, and postures flow from one to the next. Each is

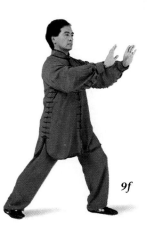

9f

Shift weight forward onto left leg, pushing forward with both palms.

WAVE HANDS LIKE CLOUDS

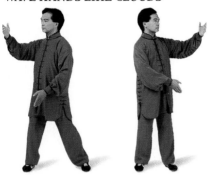

Yin and yang, the Chinese theory of opposites, extends to the performance of t'ai chi. In other words, each posture done toward the right must be countered with one toward the left, and vice versa. For this reason, the sequence on this page repeats the postures illustrated in 5a through 7d, with the moves done in the opposite direction. Complementary motion helps direct the qi to all areas of the body. When doing t'ai chi, students are encouraged to relax completely. While the process may seem painfully slow, with practice the moves become almost second nature.

SINGLE WHIP   BRUSH KNEE AND PRESS (left style)

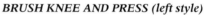
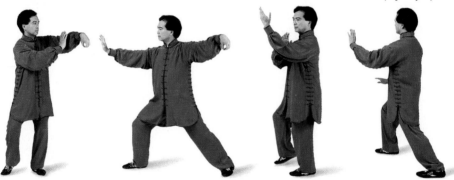

BRUSH KNEE AND PRESS (right style)

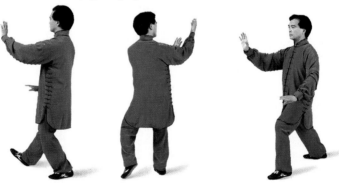

BLOCK, PARRY, AND PUNCH

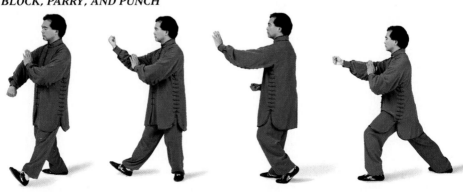

performed slowly and gracefully, with strict attention to body position and breathing techniques.

Perfecting a movement requires harmonious integration of breath and form. Students are encouraged to breathe naturally and deeply, with the mouth closed and exhalation through the nose. Respiration should come from deep within the diaphragm instead of the chest. A physiological benefit of deep breathing is to increase oxygen in the blood, which may have an energizing effect on the body.

Working with a Partner. After slow practice of the forms—each of which may last 25 minutes—students work with partners. In one practice exercise called "push hands," partners face each other with their wrists and forearms extended. Following a series of prescribed moves, the partners try to keep their arms in constant contact. As one partner pushes, the other yields. Students become sensitive to the back-and-forth pressure, while remaining balanced, alert,

RIGHT HEEL KICK

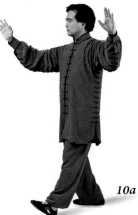

10a

Sit back *on right leg, and bring both hands upward. making a circle with arms.*

LEFT HEEL KICK

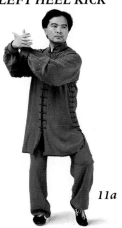

11a

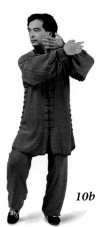

10b

Step forward *with right toe, circle arms down, cross them, move up to left ear.*

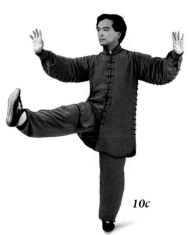

10c

Complete circle, *separating hands, raise right leg and kick outward with heel.*

Lower right *leg, turn left 180 degrees. Circle arms down; bring up to right ear.*

and relaxed. More advanced students may practice "freestyle" push hands, in which the aim is to maintain contact with the partner, but also to upset his or her balance. Students may use any moves they choose. Breaking contact gives one's opponent the upper hand.

T'ai chi practitioners say that the benefits of long-term, consistent practice include improved muscle tone, poise, flexibility, balance, and coordination. In addition, regular practice can increase agility and stamina, sharpen reflexes, and boost energy and well-being. It has been recommended for those suffering from arthritis, especially of the knees and lower back pain.

The calming, meditative effect of t'ai chi may also be effective in relieving stress. Some practitioners have found it useful as an adjunct to other therapies in treating ulcers and various digestive disorders. Followers of traditional Chinese medicine say that regular t'ai chi practice can also help balance the body's energy and prevent health problems. ❏

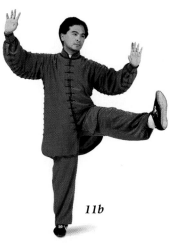

11b

Separate *hands, kick with left heel. Lower arms, and return to beginning posture.*

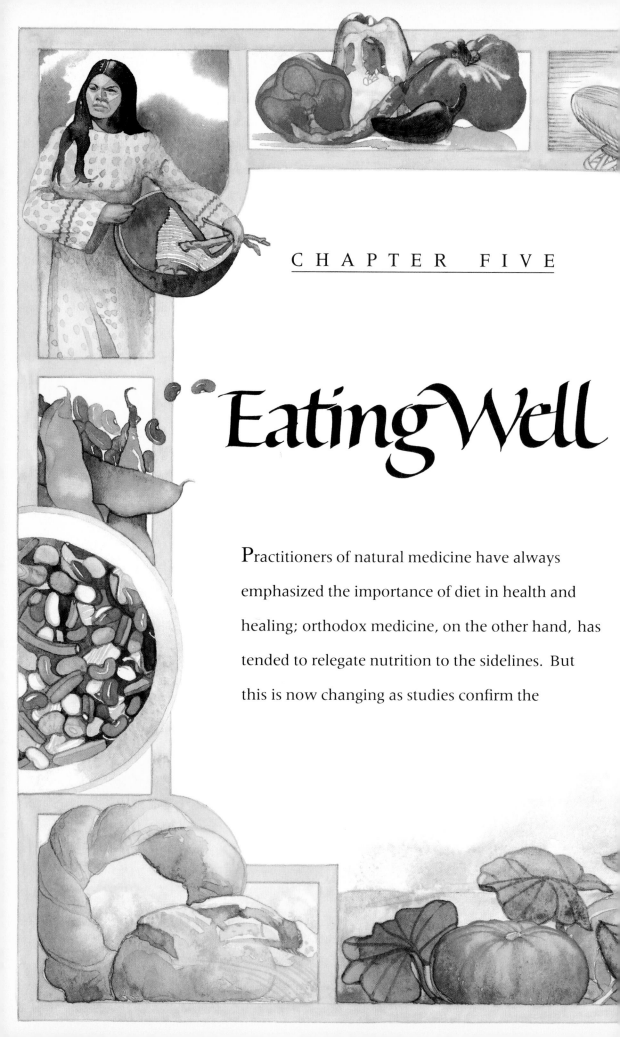

CHAPTER FIVE

Eating Well

Practitioners of natural medicine have always emphasized the importance of diet in health and healing; orthodox medicine, on the other hand, has tended to relegate nutrition to the sidelines. But this is now changing as studies confirm the

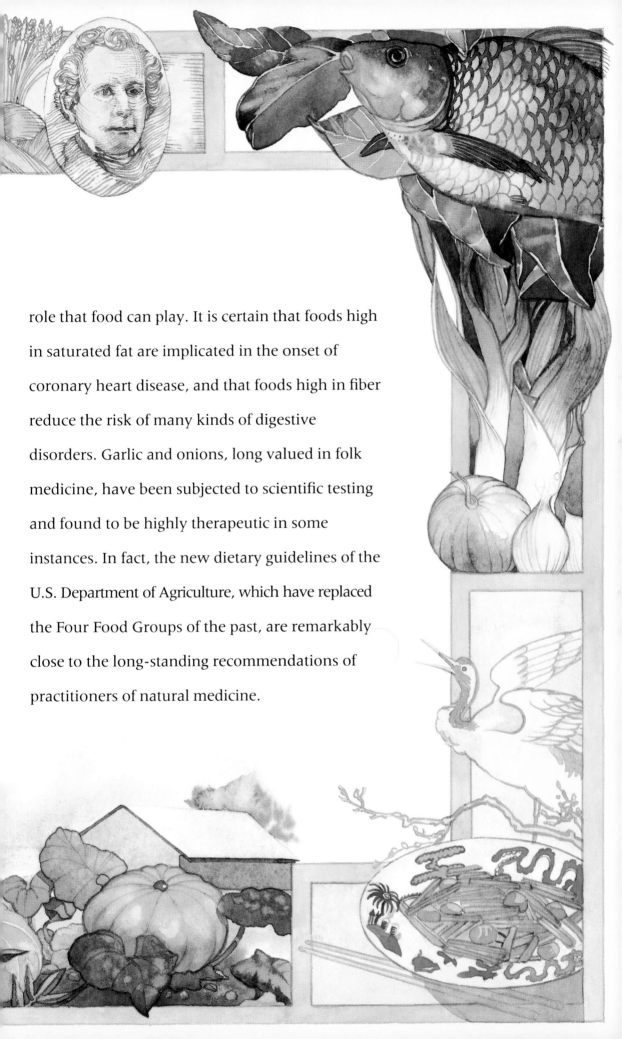

role that food can play. It is certain that foods high in saturated fat are implicated in the onset of coronary heart disease, and that foods high in fiber reduce the risk of many kinds of digestive disorders. Garlic and onions, long valued in folk medicine, have been subjected to scientific testing and found to be highly therapeutic in some instances. In fact, the new dietary guidelines of the U.S. Department of Agriculture, which have replaced the Four Food Groups of the past, are remarkably close to the long-standing recommendations of practitioners of natural medicine.

The New Nutrition

Dietary strategies offer convenience, choice, and control—possibly more of all three than any other approach to natural medicine. What's more, eating right can lower your risk of developing a chronic disease.

"YOU ARE WHAT YOU EAT" has long been the rallying cry of natural health practitioners. And now, a thoroughly researched report from the U.S. government confirms this traditional belief. *The Surgeon General's Report on Nutrition and Health* states, "For the two out of three adult Americans who do not smoke and do not drink excessively, one personal choice seems to influence long-term health prospects more than any other: what we eat."

Our genetic makeup, the environment in which we live and work, and our ability to manage stress are among the factors that determine how long we live. Natural medicine urges us to take charge of our own health, beginning with an active plan for maintaining wellness and preventing disease. And nowhere is the saying "An ounce of prevention is worth a pound of cure" truer than in the kitchen.

A Crucial Trade-off. For many of us, staying healthy no longer requires a simple shift in eating habits. It boils down to two words—fat and fiber. The problem is too much fat, too little fiber. We need to switch from the food-consumption pattern that has become standard fare in much of the Western world, trading a diet that is high in fat and low in fiber for one that is low in fat and high in fiber.

Thousands of studies worldwide indicate that excess dietary fats place us at increased risk for coronary artery disease, strokes, diabetes, high blood pressure, and breast and colon cancer. Fewer people would suffer disability and death from these diseases, say researchers, if fat intake—particularly saturated fat—declined.

A diet based on the new nutrition consists of hearty meals, with lots of whole-grain bread and pasta, plenty of fruit and vegetables, and other low-fat, high-fiber foods. Many people who switch to such eating habits lose excess weight without having to pay attention to calorie counts.

Changing Needs, Changing Policy. In the first half of the 20th century, the nutrition policy of the U.S. government focused on overcoming dietary deficits. By the second half of the century, that goal had not only been met, but for many segments of the population had been wildly exceeded. It's now time for an about-face. Too many people are eating more than they need, especially when it comes to fat.

Enjoying post-war abundance, Americans dined regularly on thick, juicy cuts of meat. The well-marbled sirloin steak or slab of roast beef sometimes got as much as 70 percent of its total calories from fat. Those who thought they were eating low-fat, high-protein meals were deceived. Lunch favorites like hot dogs and ham-and-cheese sandwiches also contributed substantially to dietary fat intake.

During this period, more Americans than ever were

Eat With Gusto, Not Guilt

"Food is fun, and sound nutrition need not diminish the pleasure. More than anything else, it's the nonsense of nutrition — unreasonable food fears and unnecessary prohibitions — that takes the joy out of eating. So no-nonsense nutrition is as much a matter of what you put in your head as what you put in your stomach, and it starts with discarding food prejudices.

"What nutrition can do for you depends very much on what it is *not* doing now. Remember, nutrition is the primary means of realizing your genetic potential. Without an adequate amount and proper balance of nutrients, you are simply not going to live as long or as healthily, look as good, or work as hard as you are genetically programmed to do. Neither will you be able to run as fast, resist infection as well, or overcome illness as easily."

— Excerpted from "The California Nutrition Book" by Paul Saltman, Ph.D., Joel Gurin, and Ira Mothner

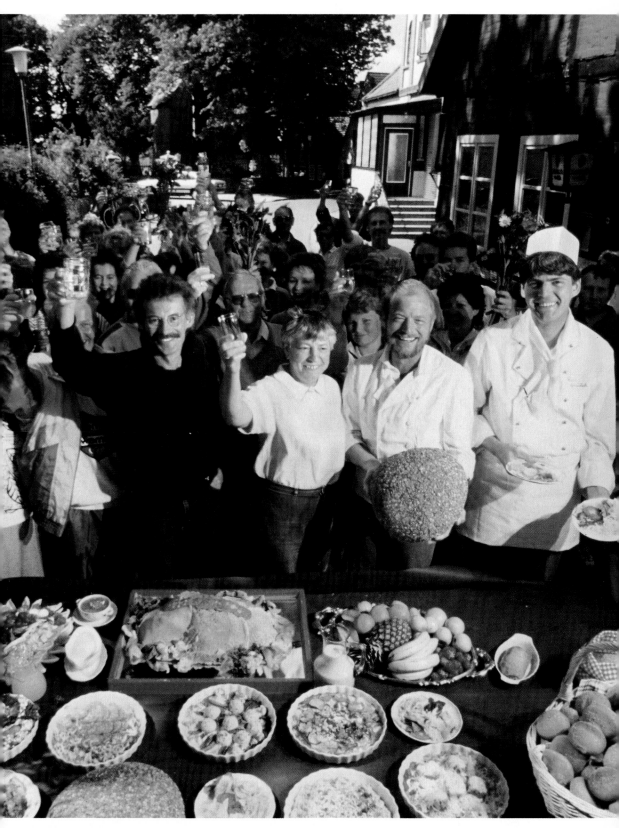

Changing dietary habits *is easier when you have friends to support you. That was the idea when the entire town of Wremen, Germany, started to take preventive measures for better health. Initiated by a local physician, the town's new dietary regimen stressed high-fiber, low-fat foods and exercise.*

suffering cardiovascular problems. Concern grew about the relationship of dietary fat to blood cholesterol levels and heart disease. Starting about 1950, researchers nationwide began to investigate dietary fat as a probable cause of coronary heart disease. This term refers to various problems caused by impaired blood circulation to the heart muscle. The most common results are angina (severe chest pain), heart attack, and sudden death.

In Praise of Variety. People who want to eat healthier diets should try to add greater variety to their meals. Many people mistakenly believe that they eat a wide selection of foods. Not so, claims William Castelli, M.D., director of the Framingham Heart Study, the nation's oldest continuous study of the cardiovascular status of a city population.

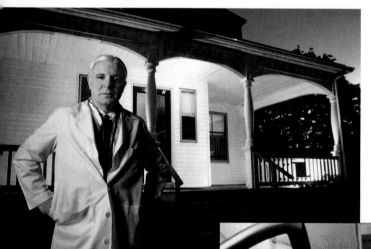

"Most American families eat from only 10 or so recipes," says Dr. Castelli. "And for three-fourths of us, the diet is too rich." In buying meat, for example, consider the advantages of the new grade Select. It has approximately one quarter as much fat as Prime cuts, according to Dr. Castelli. Rather than have us forgo many of our favorite dishes, the new nutrition urges us to update them in healthy ways.

Many of us can remember being instructed that our daily diet

Much of what we know about cholesterol and heart disease comes from sources like the Framingham Heart Study. Dr. William Castelli (above), director of this long-term, multi-generational study, measures such risk factors as family history, obesity, inactivity, and high blood pressure and cholesterol levels. At right, a fourth-generation participant has her oxygen intake and heart function measured as she runs next to her mother, grandfather, and great-grandfather.

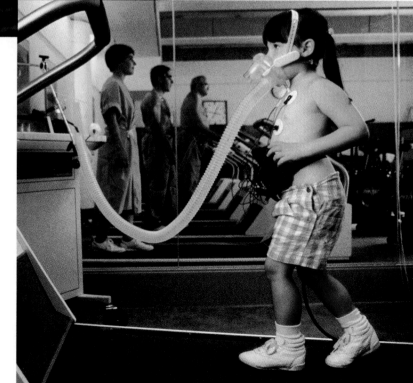

should include four kinds of food: the meat group, dairy products, fruits and vegetables, and cereal and bread. These classifications overlooked the fact that foods contain a variety of nutrients. For example, meat was represented as pure protein; in fact, meat may derive more than 50 percent of its calories from fat. American cheese, classified as "dairy," is actually three-quarters fat, one quarter protein. Eggs, which were seen as a first cousin to meat, poultry, fish, and other protein sources, contain about twice as much fat as protein: approximately 65 percent fat, 32 percent protein, and 3 percent carbohydrate.

For those people who chose their foods in the belief that particular foods contained only one kind of nutrient, the "four food group" approach was misleading. It was also incomplete. The chart made no mention of cookies,

New Priorities

These guidelines for daily eating, which the U.S. Department of Agriculture developed, can help adults with their food choices. One serving of meat, poultry, or fish is about 2 to 3 ounces. People with small frames need fewer servings than those with large frames.

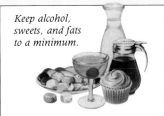

Keep alcohol, sweets, and fats to a minimum.

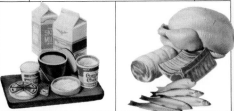

Have 2-3 servings of milk, cheese, yogurt, and other dairy products, preferably low-fat or fat-free.

Have 2-3 servings of meat, poultry, eggs, fish, or such plant proteins as nuts or dry peas or beans.

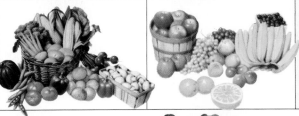

Have 3-5 servings of vegetables, with lots of dark yellow and dark green leafy varieties.

Have 2-4 servings of fruit. Serving size: a medium apple, ¼ cup dried fruit, ¾ cup juice.

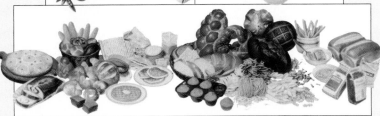

Have 6-11 servings of cereal, bread, grain, grain products.

cakes, and other calorie-laden baked snacks and desserts. And the chart gave no upper limits. "Two or more servings" of meat, poultry, and eggs daily could mean four, six, or more.

For too many people, adhering to the Basic Four tipped the dietary balance in favor of excess, particularly an excess of fat. Casting aside the old nutrition doctrines, we understand that sensible eating involves learning what's really in each kind of food. We need to be concerned not

THE PERILS OF A MODERN DIET

Until they began to eat modern Western food, the Pima Indians of the Arizona desert were a healthy tribe. Today, they suffer from the highest incidence of diabetes in the world.

For thousands of years, the Pima Indians of Arizona's Sonora Desert gathered food from the land. Here they managed to find nutrient-rich mesquite pods, the fruit of various cacti, the seeds of the chia plant, and acorns. They supplemented this diet with tepary beans and corn, which they planted during the desert's brief rainy season.

Today, however, good health is far from common among the Pimas. According to Native Seeds/Search, a genetic research group, more than 50 percent of Pimas over the age of 35 suffer from type II, adult-onset, diabetes.

"As the Pima abandoned their ancestral diets," reports John Willoughby, "in favor of a modern diet high in fat, sugar, and processed foods, the incidence of diabetes skyrocketed, and rampant obesity appeared."

Scientists have established that adult-onset diabetes is genetically determined, but is triggered by diet. The Pima carry a so-called "thrifty gene," which converts excess food into stored fat with greater than usual efficiency. This trait was crucial to survival in the feast-and-famine environment of the Pima's ancestors. Over the centuries, the Pima Indians — and other indigenous people from Hawaii to Australia — ate a low-fat, low-sugar diet, which their bodies metabolized efficiently.

But today, eating a modern diet, the Pimas' genetic advantage may have backfired. The efficiency of their thrifty gene has led to widespread obesity, contributing to adult-onset diabetes, among the Pima.

Some Pima are beginning to understand the value of their traditional foods. One of them is Adrian Hendricks. "He grows native crops in his own garden," writes Willoughby, "and sticks to a traditional low-fat, high-carbohydrate Pima diet, including squashes, tepary beans, corn, melons, and sunflower seeds. It not only helps to keep him in excellent physical shape but he also feels it generally fits better with his metabolism.

"As scientists continue to study the subtle interplay of food, genetics, and climate," says Willoughby, "they may well find that this is true for each of us. Whatever our ethnic background, a primal diet designed to fit our particular genes may one day replace blanket dietary recommendations as the most effective weapon against diabetes, heart attack, stroke, and other such 'diseases of modernity.' "

Adapted from Primal Prescription *by John Willoughby, courtesy* Eating Well.

with arbitrary food groups but with the basic components of food, starting with the macronutrients.

The Three Macronutrients. Protein, carbohydrate, and fat are known as macronutrients (macro is from the Greek *makros,* meaning big or long). Micronutrients, which include vitamins, minerals, and trace elements, are also important dietary components. A third category is non-nutritive components, which include fiber, water, additives, and a multitude of chemicals in plants and animals, some of which have yet to be identified.

Nearly all foods contain a combination of two or three of the macronutrients. The exceptions are foods like butter, oil, lard, and shortening, which are 100 percent fat, and honey and sugar, which are 100 percent carbohydrate.

Following the basic principles of moderation, variety, and balance, the ideal diet provides all the nutrients needed for life. With adequate amounts of protein, carbohydrate, fat, vitamins, and minerals, you will have nourishment for growth and replacement of bone, muscle, and other tissues. You will have enough energy for daily living and plenty left over for exercise.

Most of us eat at least twice as much protein as we need. Generally, a high-protein diet is recommended only in special circumstances, as for example when someone is recovering from illness, severe burns, or other accidents. Proteins are made up of amino acids. When dietary protein from plant or animal sources is converted to body protein, amino acids provide basic components of cells and tissues, serve as catalysts for biochemical reactions, and bolster the immune system.

Remember Starch? Not so long ago, we were urged to beware of starches. Eat the meat, but throw the hamburger bun away. Other foods to avoid were pasta and potatoes. Starches were supposed to make you fat. In fact, these foods—carbohydrates—are the body's basic source of energy. They are converted to glucose, the body's chief fuel.

Carbohydrates are usually characterized as being either simple or complex, depending upon the length of the chemical chains that form them. Simple carbohydrates, including sugar, honey, molasses, and corn syrup, often come in fat-laden packages (think of ice cream) that are high in calories, but low in vitamins and minerals. One exception to this rule is fruit, which although loaded with fructose (a simple carbohydrate) also contains a healthy store of vitamins and minerals.

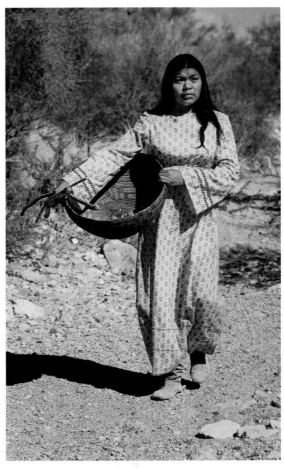

*A **Pima woman** fills her basket with native foods. A traditional Pima meal might feature cholla buds, mesquite pudding, and brown and white tepary beans. An excellent source of calcium, cholla buds also are rich in soluble fiber, which helps to regulate blood sugar. Over the years, many Pimas abandoned their traditional foods after donations of government-surplus staples, such as lard, sugar, and processed cereals, gave them a taste for more Western fare. As a result, Pimas now suffer among the highest incidence of type II, adult-onset diabetes in the world—prompting a movement to readopt the healthier foods of their past.*

The Truth About Cholesterol

Scare headlines have people worried at the mere mention of the word cholesterol; yet some cholesterol is vital to our good health. It is only a problem when there's too much of it.

Despite all the bad press, cholesterol isn't really "bad." Cholesterol forms the building block of some important hormones in the body, including sex hormones such as testosterone and estrogen. It is also an important component of cell membranes.

Your body makes all the cholesterol it needs, even if you don't eat any cholesterol in your diet and even if you reduce your saturated fat intake. In fact, three-fourths of the cholesterol in your blood is made by your body. It's the *excessive* amounts of cholesterol and saturated fat in the diet that lead to coronary heart disease.

With rare exceptions, your body makes exactly the right amount of

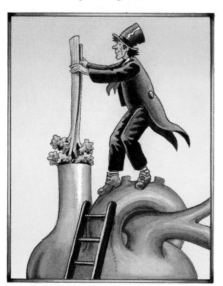

Vegetables can help unclog arteries.

cholesterol to meet your needs. You have exquisitely sensitive feedback mechanisms that tell your liver to increase or decrease the amount of cholesterol it manufactures as needed. Within limits, when you eat more cholesterol, your body makes less of it. But when you eat a large amount of cholesterol, you may overwhelm your body's ability to handle it.

Fat is not "bad" either; we just eat too much of it. The average person needs to consume less than fourteen grams of fat to meet the daily requirements of essential fatty acids, which your body needs to synthesize a variety of important substances. Unfortunately, the average American consumes at least eight times that amount. Over time, this extra fat builds up in the arteries.

All oils are 100% fat—in other words, *oils are liquid fat.* Although many people believe that adding olive oil or safflower oils to their food will lower their cholesterol levels, this is, unfortunately, simply not true. *Adding any oil to your food will raise your cholesterol.* While some oils are higher in saturated fat than others, *all oils contain some saturated fat.* So the more oil you eat the more saturated fat you consume. Canola oil is the oil lowest in saturated fat. If you use any oil, canola oil should be your choice.

In epidemiological studies, scientists observe large groups of people, often for many years, without giving them any type of treatment. What do the studies tell us? In general, the more cholesterol and saturated fat you eat, the higher will be your blood cholesterol level and your blood pressure. High blood cholesterol levels and high blood pressure increase the risk of coronary heart disease. The more cholesterol and saturated fat you eat, the greater your risk of coronary heart disease, even if your blood cholesterol level and blood pressure do not rise very much.

We have learned that people both in this country and in other parts of the world who eat a low-fat vegetarian diet have low blood pressure, low blood cholesterol levels, and low rates of heart disease.

Excerpted from Dr. Dean Ornish's Program for Reversing Heart Disease *by Dean Ornish.*

Complex carbohydrates include vegetables, legumes, pasta, cereals, and whole-grain breads. These foods are also good sources of fiber. In the ideal diet, at least 55 percent of the daily calorie intake should come from carbohydrates—and 80 percent of these should be complex carbohydrates. You may find that by cutting back on meat, and centering your meals around grains or pasta that you actually lose weight without feeling deprived. This is because these foods tend to be naturally low in calories, and provide fiber that is quite filling. However, a calorie is a calorie no matter where it comes from, and eating more than your body needs will produce a weight gain.

A Backward Glance. If we compare our grandparents' diet to our own, the differences are dramatic. Our parents' parents ate a lot more foods of plant origin, and their diet was much lower in fat. If we go back a lot farther, say, four million years, we find that our ancestors subsisted almost entirely on plants.

While it's true that fat adds a pleasing taste and texture to many foods and produces a feeling of satiety, if we overdo it, we pay dearly. Dietary fats contain a combination of three types of fatty acid: saturated, monounsaturated, and polyunsaturated. Saturated fat is metabolized differently than unsaturated fat. When saturated fatty acids are most prominent, as they are in foods of animal origin, fatty deposits can build up on the walls of arteries and lead to heart disease.

The fat we carry on our body, which can be traced to not only diet, but the build that we have inherited and other genetic factors, performs many needed functions. It's a protective barrier for organs, a concentrated form of energy, and a medium for the absorption of fat-soluble vitamins. Fat beneath the skin insulates us against the cold.

How to Monitor Dietary Fat. The American Heart Association and the American Cancer Society suggest that we limit our fat intake to 30 percent of total calories. Knowing which foods tend to be high in fat, particularly saturated fat, is important. Red meat, poultry, fish, butter, milk, eggs, and cream are among the most fatty unprocessed foods in the American diet. Processed food is often high in such saturated fats as coconut oil, palm oil, and palm kernel oil.

To find out how much fat consumption is right for each of us, we divide by two our desired weight (in pounds). A man whose desired weight is 150 pounds will want to limit his daily fat intake to 75 grams. ❏

Facts About Fats

Dietary fats are a concentrated source of food energy. They are also the source of linoleic acid, an essential nutrient, and the fat-soluble vitamins A, D, E, and K. While we all need some dietary fat each day, a tablespoon is generally sufficient. When cutting back on fats, it is helpful to know which are the worst dietary culprits.

- **Triglycerides** are fats that contain, in varying proportions, three groups of fatty acids — saturated, polyunsaturated, and monounsaturated.

- **Saturated** fats are the only fatty acids that raise blood cholesterol levels. Butter, margarine, and fats in meat and dairy products are all especially high in saturated fat.

- **Monounsaturated** and polyunsaturated fats do not raise blood cholesterol levels. Canola and olive oil contain the highest proportion of monounsaturated fat compared with other cooking oils. Highest in polyunsaturated fats are safflower and corn oil.

- **Cholesterol** is an essential fat made by the liver. Many people get additional cholesterol by eating meat and dairy products. Too much dietary intake may raise blood cholesterol levels, and lead to heart disease. Cholesterol is transported through the bloodstream by lipoproteins.

  HDLs (high-density lipoproteins) are called "good" because they move cholesterol away from artery walls and back to the liver.

  LDLs (low-density lipoproteins) are called "bad" because they keep cholesterol circulating in the blood, causing the arteries to become clogged with deposits.

Protecting Your Health Naturally

Can foods alone cure illness? Recent research suggests that some may contain powerful disease-inhibiting chemicals. But reaping the protective benefits of foods may require a lifetime of sensible eating habits.

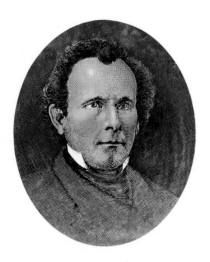

King of Wheat

An early advocate of whole grains and healthy eating, Sylvester Graham (1794-1851) is best known as the father of the graham cracker. A Presbyterian minister and fiery orator, Graham believed that the refinement of flour was contributing to the moral, spiritual, and physical ruination of society. His solution: whole grain breads, fresh fruits and vegetables, hard mattresses, and cold showers.

FOR THE ORTHODOX PHYSICIAN, it's one thing to say that we should eat enough to get the nutrients we require, but quite another to state that eating right may help prevent disease. Apart from the amused acknowledgment that yes, perhaps, chicken soup does help to alleviate the miseries of the common cold, those in the forefront of modern science tend to dismiss as folklore the notion of food as medicine or therapy. But the tide may be turning. In the not-too-distant future, hundreds of familiar foods may turn up in scientific research facilities—in the laboratory, not the cafeteria.

Promising Avenues of Research. A five-year study sponsored by the National Cancer Institute is investigating the potential disease-inhibiting power of phytochemicals, non-nutritive compounds found in plants. Phytochemicals are what give plants their flavor and odor, but many also protect plants against fungal or bacterial infections, which leads scientists to ask whether certain phytochemicals may offer similar protection to humans. "We are looking at naturally occurring anticarcinogens in foods," says Dr. Carolyn Clifford, chief of the diet and cancer branch of the National Cancer Institute. Among the foods that are receiving special attention are garlic, carrots, celery, parsley, citrus fruits, soybeans, flaxseed, and licorice root.

Some experts think the future looks bright for "designer foods" that will target specific health needs—meaning we could select foods that have been fortified with an arsenal of cancer-preventing phytochemicals. For example, researchers suspect that indoles, chemicals found in cabbage, broccoli, brussels sprouts, and other cruciferous vegetables, may offer protection against some breast cancer.

These phytochemicals may be beneficial in a number of ways. Some researchers suggest that indoles work by blocking estrogen receptor sites in breast tissue (estrogen is a female hormone that may promote tumor growth in some individuals). Another possibility is that they actually suppress the secretion of the estrogen hormone. One day, perhaps, women at high risk for this disease could select foods that have been enriched with indoles.

Folk Cures Come of Age. All of us, even those who reject orthodox medicine in favor of a natural approach to healing, owe a debt of gratitude to French chemist Louis Pasteur (1822–1895). It was Pasteur who established that germs are the cause of many diseases—a fact which marked a decline in the use of traditional remedies. As physicians geared up to combat microorganisms, other approaches to healing were dismissed as too old-fashioned or dangerously unscientific.

Ironically, in light of his role in changing medicine's

view of disease, it was Pasteur who demonstrated the effectiveness of one folk medicine staple: garlic. In 1858, he put raw garlic into a bacteria culture and observed the bacteria die, thus validating a remedy that had been used the world over for centuries. From Egypt to Japan, garlic was used for ailments ranging from gastrointestinal and respiratory problems to skin afflictions and wounds.

And garlic's medicinal use continued into the 20th century. In fact, during the early part of the century, this herb was used against tuberculosis. Then, during World War I, garlic was chosen to fight dysentery and typhus; in World War II British medics treated wounds with garlic to ward off infection and gangrene.

While it would be irresponsible for any practitioner to recommend garlic instead of modern antibiotics for the treatment of strep throat, staph, or other serious bacterial infections, the herb still may have legitimate uses for combatting or preventing some common illnesses. For example, experiments have shown that the ancients were right in offering garlic to those with digestive problems. Garlic has also been shown to have anticoagulant properties as effective as those of aspirin, and so may be useful for those at risk for heart attacks.

But garlic is not the only "food cure" whose usage has been validated by recent research. Remember the old adage "an apple a day keeps the doctor away"? While this bit of folk wisdom may not be literally true, the fiber in apples may well benefit people with high blood cholesterol, as

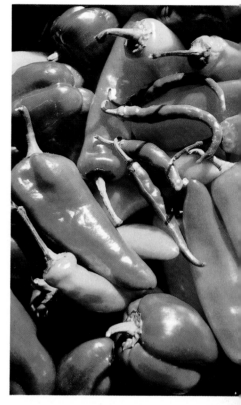

Foods deep in color may also be rich in vitamins, so spice up your diet with peppers for high amounts of A and C.

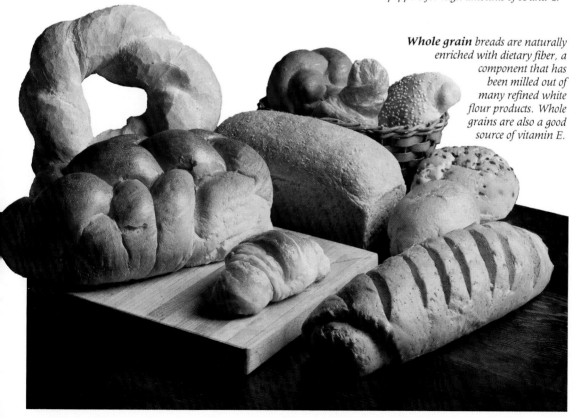

Whole grain breads are naturally enriched with dietary fiber, a component that has been milled out of many refined white flour products. Whole grains are also a good source of vitamin E.

well as those at risk for colon cancer.

And remember when cod-liver oil was a staple in every medicine chest? Cod-liver oil is a rich source of vitamin A, but more promising for preventive health care are omega-3 fatty acids, which are found in fish oil. They appear to reduce blood cholesterol levels, and so may benefit those at risk for cardiovascular disease. For instance, although they subsist on high-fat diets, Eskimos show astonishingly low incidences of heart disease, perhaps because the mainstay of their diet is cold water fish, which contain high amounts of omega-3 fatty acids.

Antioxidants and Free Radicals. Vitamins C and E, and beta-carotene, which the body converts to vitamin A, are under investigation for their potential role in preventing cancer and heart disease. Collectively, they are known as antioxidants.

Antioxidants serve as scavengers of free radicals—unstable molecules that may trigger cancer by altering a cell's genetic code. Free radicals may also contribute to cardiovascular disease, either by damaging artery walls, or by oxidizing LDL (bad) cholesterol, which makes it easier for the cholesterol to adhere to artery walls. In either case, clogged arteries and impeded blood flow are among the possible results.

The high levels of beta-carotene in dark yellow and dark green vegetables like carrots, sweet potatoes, pumpkins, spinach, broccoli, and kale may prove useful in preventing certain types of cancer and heart disease. A long-term study of some 2,000 men found that those who ate relatively few foods containing carotene were more likely to die of lung cancer than those whose diets included more of such foods. But beta-carotene is only one of 500 known carotenoids, and investigation into the disease-inhibiting potential of this group is in its infancy.

Vitamin E, a powerful antioxidant found in margarine and vegetable oils, wheat germ, and whole-grain breads and cereals, may help slow damage to cells done by free radicals, thereby retarding some of the effects of aging. Recently, vitamin C has been associated with a lower risk of cancer of the stomach, esophagus, and cervix. While studies are encouraging, it is too soon to conclude that a diet rich in citrus fruits, or other foods containing vitamin C, will lower your risk for cancer.

The Vitamin Revolution. Aside from the antioxidants, other vitamins are being studied for possible therapeutic use, and for use in the prevention of disease. The role of vitamins in preventing deficiency diseases, such as scurvy and beriberi, is well-established. More controversial are other claims made for these essential nutrients. Because interactions in the body are so complex, it may take scientists years to establish whether it's a vitamin or some other substance that is responsible for certain experimental results.

In the past few decades, the use of vitamin and mineral supplements has aroused considerable passion and contro-

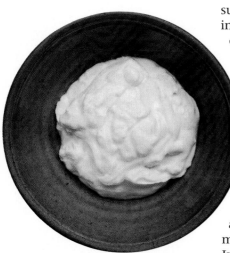

Yogurt, made when special bacterial cultures are added to milk, has long been used as a natural remedy for everything from diarrhea to yeast infections. While yogurt is a good source of protein, B vitamins, calcium, and potassium, there is little evidence that it is a cure-all. However, yogurt made with active bacteria cultures may help settle intestinal problems by encouraging the growth of beneficial bacteria.

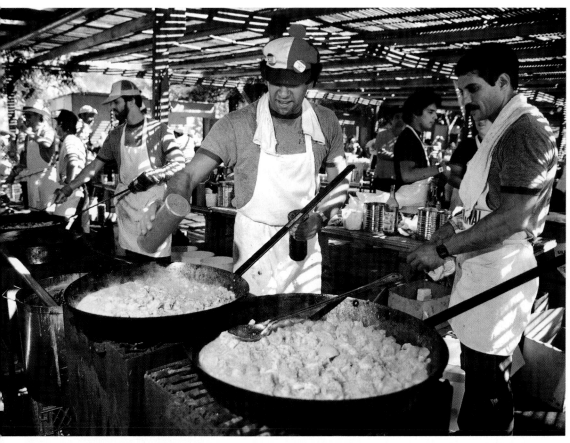

The Garlic Festival *of Gilroy, California, attracts thousands annually in celebration of this aromatic herb. Garlic, an anticoagulant, may be useful for lowering cholesterol and treating hypertension.*

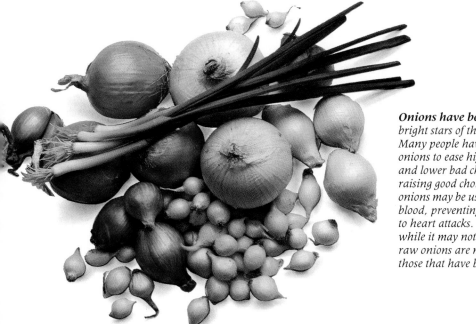

Onions have become *one of the bright stars of the food pharmacy. Many people have successfully used onions to ease high blood pressure and lower bad cholesterol (while raising good cholesterol). Like garlic, onions may be useful for thinning the blood, preventing clots that may lead to heart attacks. But remember, while it may not help your social life, raw onions are more beneficial than those that have been cooked.*

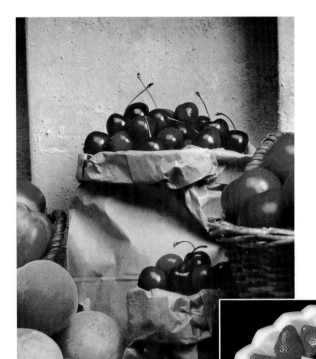

A medley of fruits is an attractive and easy way of putting variety into your family's diet. While almost any mixture will do, be sure to include at least one citrus fruit, such as orange or grapefruit, as these fruits are especially high in vitamin C. An antioxidant, this nutrient has been linked to lower incidences of certain cancers. Citrus fruits also have phytochemicals that may prove useful in preventing diseases.

Cherries, peaches, and plums, in fact all fruits, are rich sources of vitamins. But they also offer a delicious way of getting adequate dietary fiber. A number of fruits are now being studied for their potential in preventing everything from cavities to stomach cancer. But regardless of the outcome of this research, fruit should be a mainstay of any well-balanced, varied diet—in part for the vitamin content, but also because some fruits are good sources of complex carbohydrates.

versy. Indeed, the subject is quite complex, and for this reason vitamins and minerals are treated separately in a later section of the book.

Common Ground. While there is certainly no harm in loading up on fiber, fish, and vitamin-rich fruits and vegetables, it is too early to think of these substances as adding up to some sort of magical formula for a lifetime of good health. What much of this research into foods does indicate is that sound nutrition is the first step toward disease prevention. In fact, studies on particular foods validate the recommendation that we eat a wide variety of foods, as each contains substances that may have unique properties for lowering the risk for certain illnesses.

There is little doubt that a well-balanced, low-fat diet can provide protection against many chronic diseases—and in this way diet is the best "natural" remedy available. And the sooner we establish such eating habits the better. However, keep in mind that while changing unhealthy eating habits should certainly be a priority, it is not an instant prescription for reversing chronic conditions. It may take a little time to reap the rewards of sensible eating. ❏

New Studies, Old Wisdom

Nutrition writer Jean Carper suggests that before we turn to drugs and antibiotics for every minor illness, we should consider the vast health resources found in our local supermarkets.

For thousands of years, food has been regarded as potent medicine. But in the last century, pharmaceutical drugs have taken over as magic bullets, making us forget much of our rich heritage in the medical uses of foods. The idea that foods have pharmacological properties that can be used to promote health often seems like folklore, decidedly deficient in the scientific proof required in the twentieth century. That is, until you start looking.

Never before have scientists united in such an exciting investigation into the chemical basis for food's remarkable impact on human health. What was once regarded as quackery, folklore, and medical heresy is being explored with intense seriousness: the theory that food is indeed our largest, most complex pharmacy—a monumental drugstore stocked with an elaborate display of nonprescription drugs of nature's mysterious design.

We are talking about a food pharmacy of unimaginable versatility and complexity, made up of natural laxatives, tranquilizers, beta blockers, antibiotics, anticoagulants, antidepressants, painkillers, cholesterol reducers, anti-inflammatory agents, hypotensives, analgesics, decongestants, digestives, expectorants, anti-motion sickness agents, cancer inhibitors, antioxidants, contraceptives, vasodilators and vasoconstrictors, anticavity agents, antiulcerative agents, insulin regulators, to name a few.

The research shows that foods and their individual constituents perform in similar fashion to modern drugs —and sometimes better—without the dreaded side effects. For example: when antibiotics fail to heal a wound, sugar almost always works. Yogurt boosts immune functioning better than a drug designed for that purpose, cures diarrhea more quickly than a standard

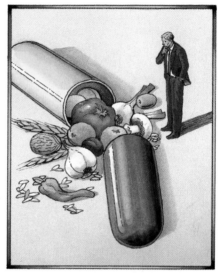

It's time to recall food's healing power.

antidiarrheal drug, and contains agents that are stronger antibiotics than penicillin. Onions raise beneficial HDL-cholesterol levels in the blood more effectively than most prescription heart medicine. Garlic compounds match aspirin in preventing blood clots that may lead to heart attacks and strokes. Fish (notably mackerel) equals most diuretics in depressing mild high blood pressure. Ginger surpasses Dramamine in suppressing motion sickness. A couple of tablespoons of sugar at bedtime are as effective as a sleeping pill. Red wine knocks off bacteria about as well as penicillin.

This global inquiry into the therapeutic powers of food is not a trivial pursuit. It is heady and heavy scientific stuff, commanding the attention and energy of some of the world's leading scientists and physicians. It is already producing a remarkable new understanding of the power of foods to cure and prevent numerous diseases.

Excerpted from The Food Pharmacy *by Jean Carper.*

What Else Is in Food?

*In addition to nutrients, foods contain substances that are essential
for good health. But many also have things that most of us neither want
nor need: added sugar, salt, preservatives, and artificial colors.*

WATER, FIBER, FLAVORS, COLORS, natural carcinogens and anticarcinogens, and pesticide residues are among the tens of thousands of non-nutritive components of our food supply. With one exception, anything we eat or drink that doesn't contribute energy, or calories, can be considered a non-nutritive component. The exception is alcohol, which contributes calories but no nutrients.

Many non-nutrient food components are easily identified, while others are just beginning to be found. In the latter group are hundreds or perhaps thousands of phytochemicals. These are naturally occurring substances in plants that can both help and harm us. Some phytochemicals may contribute to aberrations in cells that become cancerous, while others may serve to block cancer initiators or promoters in the body.

Water, the Life-Sustaining Drink. Anyone who has worked outside on a hot day or exercised rigorously during the summer knows the discomfort of dehydration: dry mouth, hot flushes, headache. Like oxygen, water is essential to our survival. In fact, between 55 and 65 percent of our body weight is water. Water provides the medium for blood, lymph, perspiration, digestive juices, and other bodily fluids, and it allows the nutrients from the food we eat to enter cells, and the waste products to be removed. Natural health practitioners commonly recommend that we consume six to eight glasses of water daily. Drinking plenty of water and avoiding such beverages as coffee and alcohol are routinely recommended to those following a natural medicine regimen.

The Role of Fiber. An important but indigestible food component, fiber is the part of edible plants that the human digestive system cannot process. After fat, carbohydrate, and protein have been digested, dietary fiber remains in the colon where it helps to guard against constipation by increasing the volume and fluid content of stool. Some types of fiber, like oat wheat bran, the pectin in apples and grapes, and the guar gum in beans, may lower elevated blood cholesterol. Fiber may also work with certain bacteria to manufacture chemicals that inhibit the formation of cancer cells in the colon.

The National Cancer Institute recommends 20 to 35 grams a day. The average American consumes about 12 grams of dietary fiber daily.

Because it's difficult to calculate exactly how much dietary fiber a particular food supplies, the best approach is to eat recommended quantities of fruit and vegetables, including both raw and cooked, preferably with their high-fiber skins. Unprocessed or minimally processed grains and

---

The Whole Food Difference

"Many of us have only vague notions about what our food was like in its fresh and natural state. Between the fresh, natural, whole food and its refined, fractioned commercial product there is an abyss of lost nourishment, even when the refined food has been enriched. In whole foods there is a balance between calories and other nutrients, a certain density of nourishment that is lacking in many refined foods. The basic requirements of human nutrition are water, carbohydrate, protein, a broad range of vitamins and minerals and a little fat or oil. Whole foods contribute to many of these needs at once; refined foods often contribute to only one or two."
— From "Laurel's Kitchen" by Laurel Robertson, Carol Flinders, and Bronwen Godfrey

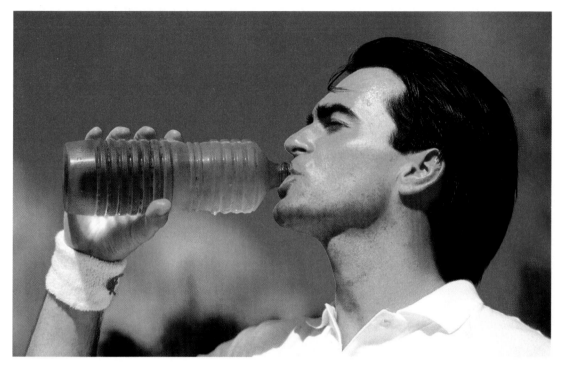

cereals, and dried peas and beans are among the best low-fat sources of both protein and fiber. Nuts and edible seeds like sunflower, sesame, and pumpkin seeds are high in fiber but also relatively high in fat.

For years, food producers and manufacturers have been adding natural and synthetic fibers to food to improve its texture. More recently, oat bran and other types of fiber have been added to foods to boost their appeal to those concerned with cholesterol.

Direct and Indirect Additives. Food companies in the United States rely on some 3,000 additives as preservatives, colors, flavorings, texturizers, moisture protectors, bleaching agents, foaming agents, firming agents, and more. Our present-day diet contains many more additives than it did 30 years ago. But in terms of quantity, if we subtract sugar and salt, the two items that account for most of all additives in food, the other intentional additives (such as caffeine and BHT, a common preservative) comprise about one percent of our total food intake.

The unintentional or indirect additives encompass potentially about 12,000 chemicals used in packaging, some of which "migrate" to the foods under certain conditions; thousands of chemicals that farmers use on crops to keep pests away, to make fruit trees mature sooner, or to otherwise improve the harvests; 20 growth hormones used in animal feed, an array of plant and animal growth regulators, and environmental contaminants.

Who's Regulating What. Some non-nutritive additives come under the jurisdiction of the U.S. Food and Drug Administration, whose mandate since 1938 has been to en-

Many people consider drinking 6 to 8 glasses of water daily an essential part of their health regimen. Water flushes the system, and this, some believe, rids it of accumulated toxins. If you have doubts about the purity of your local supply, consider bottled water or install a water filtering system at home.

Intercropping and high-tech insect vacuums are two alternatives to using potentially toxic pesticides. For instance, here a field of wheat is intercropped with red clover, a forage plant that provides the double bonus of repelling aphids and adding nitrogen to the soil. The strange-looking contraption (below) was designed to vacuum beetles from vegetable and bean crops.

sure the safety of our food supply. Amendments to the law broadened its jurisdiction so that no additive can be used that has been shown to produce cancer in laboratory animals or other suitable tests (saccharin is the exception to this rule). The law requires that additives pass safety tests performed by manufacturers before they can gain entree to our supermarket shelves. The F.D.A. also sets limits on the allowable amount of pesticide residues in raw agricultural products.

The U.S. Environmental Protection Agency regulates the pesticides, herbicides, fungicides, and other chemicals that farmers use to grow food crops. The F.D.A. and the U.S. Department of Agriculture regulate about 60 percent of the food produced in the United States, with the states responsible for the other 40 percent.

Many naturopaths, herbalists, and other practitioners of natural medicine advise us to eat only unprocessed, whole foods. They fear that we know less than we should about both the short-term and long-range impact of food additives. And what we do know about the impact of pesticides and other environmental contaminants is not altogether reassuring.

Continuing Doubts. Although the U.S. government has banned several food colors derived from coal tar that proved to be carcinogenic, consumer advocates are not convinced that all the remaining food colors have been adequately evaluated for safety. There are questions whether we know enough about the interaction among preservatives, pesticides, and other additives. There is some evi-

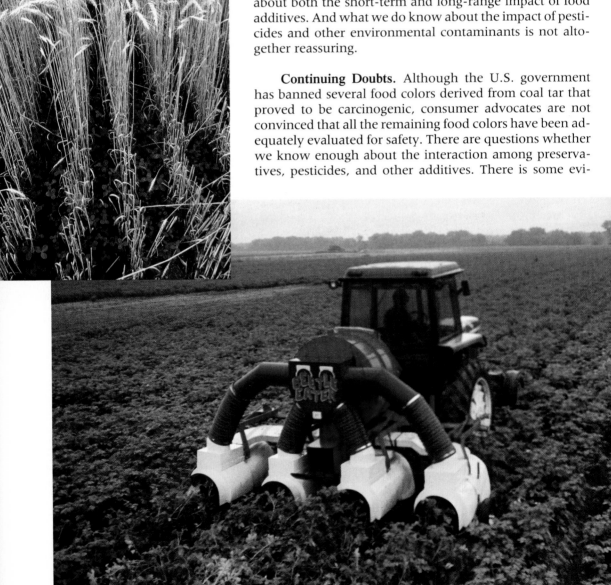

dence, for example, that sorbic acid and its salts, which are common preservatives, can combine with nitrites, popular food additives, to produce a chemical compound that may cause genetic mutations.

Still, additives do offer certain benefits for the health-conscious consumer, too. They allow us to eat a wider variety of food than we could eat if we had to depend exclusively on those grown or produced in season and in our own community. Additives extend the shelf life of certain foods by preventing the growth of bacteria. They allow food to be shipped considerable distances without spoiling or turning rancid, or with only minimal harm. The year-round availability of citrus fruit and many vegetables has been cited as one of the dietary factors contributing to the decline in the incidence of stomach cancer in the United States.

Choose Fresh Foods. The potential toxicity of various additives can be reduced by eating the widest possible variety of foods with an eye on those that are minimally processed. Eating a low-fat, high-fiber diet makes it easy to avoid foods that are overloaded with certain additives.

Fruit and vegetables sold at a farmer's market are generally harvested within a day of being put on sale, so it's more likely that they will not be sprayed with pesticides and then coated with wax to extend their shelf life, as they might be if they were being shipped to a produce distribution warehouse. Lightly steamed fresh vegetables contain minimal amounts of naturally occurring sodium, but canned vegetables tend to be processed with salt and other additives. High-fiber whole-grain breads from a local bakery are bound to have far fewer preservatives, bleaches, and other additives than mass-produced white bread.

A Convergence of Botany and Food Technology. Within a few years, scientists may be able to tell us a lot about how foods, components of foods, and man-made additives can contribute to initiating cancer or to halting its development. And that's only the beginning. Dr. Herbert Pierson, a toxicologist who has worked at the National Cancer Institute, looks forward to the day when "we could produce orange juice with the phytochemical content of 20 oranges or fat-free beef stroganoff with high concentrations of allium," the powerful phytochemical in garlic and onions. ❑

Food Safety

For the most part, our food supply is considered safe, but many people are still concerned with the long-term effects of some additives and preservatives. One alternative is to buy organically grown foods. Another is to avoid foods containing potentially harmful additives. Michael F. Jacobson, Ph.D., an expert on food safety and the author of SAFE FOOD, feels that consumers should know about the preservatives and additives that are commonly used. Consider the following:

- Waxed produce. Waxes can seal pesticides in food, which can be very difficult to wash off. In addition, fungicides, used to retard spoilage, are sometimes combined with the wax. At least two fungicides in use are listed as probable human carcinogens.

- Growth hormones and antibiotic feed additives. The hormones have been implicated in the development of breast cancer and other cancers in humans. Feeding livestock antibiotic-laced feed can promote strains of bacteria that are resistant to our present arsenal of antibiotic drugs, putting humans at risk of dangerous infections.

- Artificial Colors. Red No. 3 (erythrosine) was banned from cosmetics and some food because it produced thyroid tumors in rats. But it is still used in pistachio nuts, maraschino cherries, and other foods. Used in processed foods and some medicines, Yellow No. 5 (tartrazine) can cause hives, runny nose, headaches, itching, or breathing problems in sensitive individuals.

- Nitrites. Sodium nitrite is added to bacon and other processed meats, such as ham and bologna, as a preservative and flavor enhancer. Upon heating, and even when in the stomach, nitrite may combine with other compounds (secondary amines) to form powerful cancer-causing chemicals (nitrosamines).

Understanding Food Sensitivities

Foods can trigger a wide range of unpleasant effects. However, not all adverse food reactions are caused by allergies. Omitting suspect foods then reintroducing them one at a time may help you identify the culprit.

THE OLD ADAGE that "one man's meat is another's poison" pretty well describes how some people react to certain foods. Adverse reactions to foods run the gamut from itchiness and lightheadedness to migraines and bloating—reactions commonly referred to as allergies. But the fact is that among adults food allergies are rather rare, and are only slightly more common among children. So what are these myriad reactions some people have to certain foods?

Food Allergies. What distinguishes one kind of food reaction from another is the specific way in which the body rejects the substance. In an allergic response, the immune system mistakes a particular food for a harmful substance (like a virus or bacteria) and launches an attack, releasing into the bloodstream antibodies known as immunoglobulin E (IgE). Histamines and other chemicals also cascade into the system, producing a host of allergic symptoms, ranging from swelling, hives, and cramping, to a potentially deadly reaction known as anaphylactic shock.

But foods don't have to aggravate the immune system in order to trigger ill effects. Many people have what are known as sensitivity reactions to certain foods, and experience symptoms such as stuffed sinuses, irritability, headaches, or fogginess.

If an allergy or sensitivity is suspected, many physicians recommend an elimination diet. The regime begins by excluding all suspected foods from the diet. If symptoms disappear, the foods are reintroduced one at a time, to see when and if the problem recurs. If it does, then the culprit has been identified and that food is banned from the diet. A more controversial solution involves desensitizing patients to problem foods by conditioning the body to accept increasingly larger amounts of the food.

Intolerances. Chronic migraines, diarrhea, gas, bloating, and other unpleasant symptoms are sometimes the result of an inability to digest milk. Known as lactose intolerance, this condition is due to the lack of an enzyme in the digestive tract which is normally in charge of breaking down milk sugar. While some with this enzyme deficiency can tolerate milk in

Lobster, milk, eggs, and peanuts are among the foods that often produce symptoms in sensitive individuals. Some people experience very severe, life-threatening allergic reactions, and for them total abstinence from the offending food is a must. This is fairly easy in the case of lobster, but milk, eggs, and even peanuts are common ingredients in a great many processed foods and baked goods.

small amounts, others have trouble with all foods containing lactose, including ice cream, many baked goods, and cream sauces. Avoidance is the main "cure" for a food intolerance, although a lactose additive, which contains a dose of the missing enzyme, is available, and may be helpful for some sufferers. In addition, yogurt, aged cheese, buttermilk, and other dairy products whose sugars have been broken down by fermentation are often well tolerated by sensitive individuals. ❑

SEARCHING OUT FOOD SENSITIVITIES

People can eat certain foods for years without apparent harm and then suddenly have a bad reaction to them. Finding the culprit, writes Dr. John Postley, is a painstaking task.

The complexities of food allergies were brought home to Dr. John Postley when, one day, his wife Elaine, who was never ill, unexpectedly complained of dizziness and feelings of general ill health. At that time, she was treated successfully with antihistamines. A few years later, however, her mysterious illness reappeared, this time taking the form of frequent headaches and a stuffy nose.

"I attributed her problems to the pressures of a heavy academic schedule," Postley writes, "and the physical stresses of pregnancy. It did not occur to me to connect her symptoms with our frequent outings to the ice-cream parlor where Elaine indulged her passion for vanilla ice cream with chocolate sauce."

Elaine's headaches and sinus infections increased and worsened. She felt seriously ill almost all the time. According to Postley, "She spent whole weekends in bed with a heating pad on her head, trying to recuperate enough to return to work on Monday morning."

Postley's own field of medical specialty was adult asthma, an illness in which allergies often play a role. Now he set about trying to find the various possible reasons for his wife's health problem. "I studied and experimented," he relates in his book *The Allergy Discovery Diet*, "and I began to track the

relationships between foods and such symptoms as migraine headaches and joint stiffness. Very soon I realized that the only way to empirically discover the precise foods troubling Elaine was to make a list of suspect ingredients and test them one by one."

The Postleys scrutinized Elaine's diet. They paid special attention to "hidden" food additives, examining every food label with great care. Then, using a trial-and-error system, each food — or food additive — was first dropped from her diet and later reinstated.

It turned out that dairy products and chocolate were the causes of Elaine's illness. "This amazed us; Elaine had been eating these foods all her life, without suffering adverse reactions. Elaine's experience is a vivid example of acquired sensitivity to one or more familiar foods resulting from prolonged and repeated exposure to those foods. For Elaine," Dr. Postley writes, "this meant no more bowls of vanilla ice cream with chocolate sauce, but as intervals of health began outlasting those of illness (and three inches vanished from her hips and waistline) she considered the trade-off well worthwhile."

Excerpted from The Allergy Discovery Diet *by Dr. John E. Postley, M.D. with Janet Barton.*

Shopping, Storing, Cooking

After making a commitment to more healthful eating, follow through by reading labels, choosing the most nutritious varieties of food, and cooking so as to preserve both flavor and nutrients.

FRESH VEGETABLES MAY lose only half as many nutrients when they are microwaved as when they are boiled. Dark salad greens supply more nutrients than lighter lettuces. The life of milk products is cut in half if their temperature rises to 50 degrees F. A sweet potato, baked whole, retains about 90 percent of its vitamin C, but keeps only about 30 percent if it's halved before baking. As these examples show, selecting the most nutritious foods and knowing how best to cook and store them can make a big difference.

Whole-grain and enriched breads and cereals are not only an excellent source of fiber, but provide high concentrations of B vitamins and several minerals as well. Texture is a better guide than color when it comes to judging the nutritional value of bread. Whole-grain bread tends to be dark, firm, and chewy. Bread that is dark-hued but soft to the touch may be colored with caramel or other additives and lacking in significant amounts of whole-wheat flour or other whole grains. Minimally processed or un-

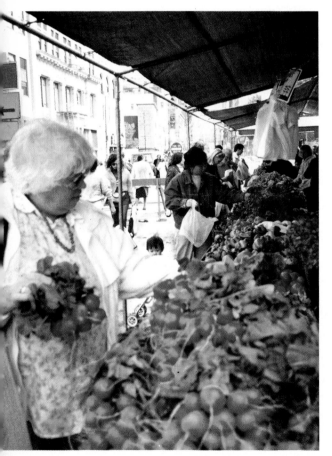

Farmers' markets *have become a fixture in many cities. This one, on the edge of New York's Greenwich Village, offers an array of freshly picked fruits and vegetables. Removing the leafy tops before storing radishes in a refrigerator will help keep them from drying out.*

Cabbage, *a rich source of vitamin C, has many other virtues as well. Versatile, inexpensive, and available year round, it can be used in a variety of dishes, from cole slaw to rich, savory stews.*

processed grains such as barley, bulgur, and brown rice are more nutritious than white rice.

Avoid meat that is marbled with fat, which is typical of the Prime grade. Choice beef is leaner than Prime. A trimmed cut of Good, or Select, beef has an average of 20 percent less fat than a comparable cut of Choice. When buying fish, check for red gills, firm flesh, and protruding eyes. If you don't intend to use meat, poultry, or fish right away, freeze it. Steaks, chops, and roasts will remain unspoiled in a refrigerator for three to five days; ground meat and fresh poultry, one or two days; and fresh fish for a day.

Savvy Shopping. When it comes to fruits and vegetables, deep color is often a good indicator of high nutritional content, especially in vegetables. For example, the best sources of beta-carotene, which the body converts into vitamin A, can be found in orange and yellow plants like carrots and sweet potatoes, and dark-leafed greens. Romaine contains about eight times as much beta-carotene as iceberg lettuce, while kale has about 27 times as much.

Freshly harvested produce generally packs the most nutrients. Store most greens and broccoli in plastic bags or in a vegetable crisper at temperatures just slightly above freezing. Canned foods should be stored at about 65 degrees to minimize vitamin loss.

If you don't live where fresh-caught fish and seafood is

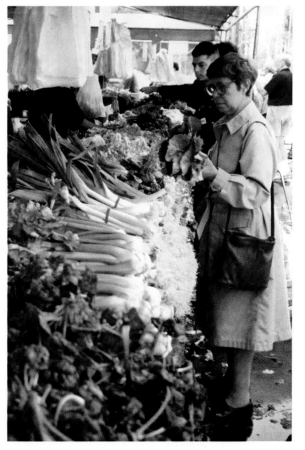

Buying produce directly from a farmer is the best way to ensure freshness. Not only that, but the attractive, colorful displays at many farmer's markets may tempt you to try new, more interesting varieties.

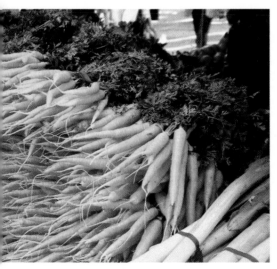

When selecting fresh carrots, look for straight, bright orange ones with feathery green tops. Avoid those with cracks or rootlets, for these are signs of age. Before eating, pull off the tops and scrub the carrots, but don't remove the vitamin-rich peels.

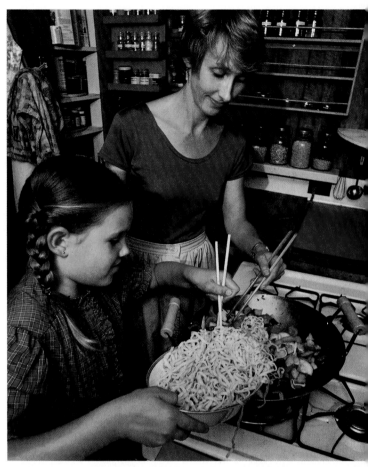

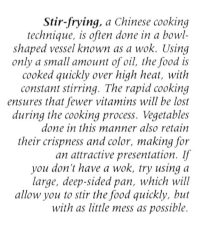

Stir-frying, a Chinese cooking technique, is often done in a bowl-shaped vessel known as a wok. Using only a small amount of oil, the food is cooked quickly over high heat, with constant stirring. The rapid cooking ensures that fewer vitamins will be lost during the cooking process. Vegetables done in this manner also retain their crispness and color, making for an attractive presentation. If you don't have a wok, try using a large, deep-sided pan, which will allow you to stir the food quickly, but with as little mess as possible.

sold or if your local market doesn't stock fresh-looking produce, check out a grocer's freezer case. The vitamin contents of well-wrapped frozen meats, fish, and poultry are almost the same as that of the fresh varieties. Keep your own freezer set at a temperature of 0 degrees or below. Some foods are even better frozen than fresh. For example, a package of frozen broccoli, which contains mostly nutrient-rich florets, or buds, can have more beta-carotene than the same weight of fresh broccoli that has been in the refrigerator for a few days. Frozen foods should be used within several months of purchase. It's a good idea to keep a grease pencil handy to mark on the package the date of purchase.

A Clean Bill of Health. If you are concerned about such additives as pesticides and herbicides in fruits and vegetables, you might look for certified organic produce. The "organically grown" label refers to produce grown virtually without synthetic chemical fertilizers and pesticides. Organically grown foods are often sold in natural-food stores, farmers' markets, and increasingly in grocery stores. Look also for meat and poultry with labels stating that the animal was raised without antibiotics or feed additives.

Anticipated changes in food labeling laws will make it easier to judge how nutritious fresh and processed foods are, and the types of fat they contain. Ingredients appear on labels in the order of their volume. In addition, the U.S. government is preparing a plan for the national certification of food as organic, which would eliminate the patchwork of regulations that exist in more than 20 states.

Preserving Nutrients, Avoiding Fat. Exposure to air and water increases vitamin and mineral losses from foods, especially vitamin C, which is water-soluble. To keep nutrient loss to a minimum, postpone slicing vegetables until it's time to prepare them; better still, cook them unpeeled and whole. Cooking vegetables as close to serving time as possible will also help preserve their nutrients. Fruits and vegetables shouldn't be soaked before cooking, nor boiled in a lot of water. But rinsing off produce may clean the surface of pesticide residues.

Eating vegetables raw or lightly steamed preserves the most nutrients. Steaming is also recommended for fish. Pressure cooking, microwaving, and stir-frying with minimal oil are other techniques that minimize the loss of vitamins and minerals. For cooking meats, broiling or roasting is preferred to braising and stewing, in which high heat and long cooking times promote nutrient losses.

Trim fat from meats and poultry before cooking. Remove the skin from poultry whenever possible. Discarding the skin from a half breast of roasted chicken may trim the fat content from 8 grams to only 3. Using non-stick pans when sauteeing or braising can also help keep fat intake down. To minimize fat consumption, avoid frying foods.

Food-Poisoning Prevention. Although many people prefer rare meat, and, indeed, some delicate nutrients are more likely to survive in lightly cooked than in well-cooked meat, high temperature is likely to destroy any harmful bacteria in undercooked eggs, meat, and poultry. For maximum safety, cooked red meat should reach an internal temperature of at least 160 degrees, poultry should reach 180 degrees, and fish, 140 degrees.

Salmonella bacteria, the most common cause of bacterial food-borne illness, is often transmitted to people through raw foods of animal origin. Diarrhea, cramps, and headaches are symptoms of food-borne illnesses. Botulism, which is caused by bacteria growing in canned foods, can be fatal. Never use cans with bulges or other defects.

When a meal is finished, divide the leftovers into small portions to speed the cooling process and refrigerate them immediately. Do not allow meat, poultry, fish, and dairy products to remain at room temperature for more than two hours: moist, warm food can provide a fertile breeding ground for bacteria. For the same reason, defrost frozen food in the refrigerator, not on the kitchen counter. ❑

How to Calculate Fat Content

The fat content of any food is easy to calculate if you know the total calories and fat content in grams. In scientific terms, a calorie is a measurement of the amount of heat it takes to raise the temperature of a gram of water by 1 degree Celsius.

- Each gram of fat contains about 9 calories. Each gram of protein and carbohydrate contains about 4 calories. On a hot dog package, the label may say that each frank has 170 calories, from 7 grams of protein, 1 gram of carbohydrate, and 15 grams of fat.

- Multiply 15 grams of fat by 9 (calories per gram of fat). The result shows that 135 calories come from fat.

- Then divide total calories, which is 170, into fat calories, which is 135. The result is 0.79.

- Multiply by 100. The answer reveals that 79 percent of the calories in the frank come from fat.

Putting Diets in Perspective

Surprisingly, athletes have nearly the same nutritional needs as dieters. To achieve their goals, they both need to follow the fundamental rules of healthful eating.

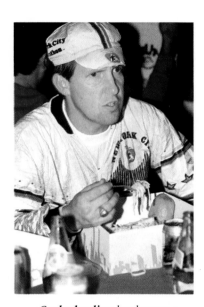

***Carbo loading** has become a tradition of the New York City Marathon. The night before the race, runners from around the world gather to eat heaping plates of pasta. This pre-race feast is designed to give athletes the energy they need to complete the distance.*

AMATEUR AND PROFESSIONAL ATHLETES ALIKE often seek foods they believe will enhance performance, strength, and overall conditioning. Dieters, both those who want to shed a few pounds and those who are obese, also look to eating plans for help. What does the athlete in peak condition have in common with the unfit, overweight dieter? Both need foods that are low in fat and high in fiber and complex carbohydrates. The major distinction between these different groups is in total caloric intake. A runner who is training for a marathon may need to eat a pound of pasta for lunch or dinner to compensate for the energy expended, while someone on a weight-loss diet may be limited to a cup of pasta per meal.

Of course, no single diet can provide the same health benefits for everyone. Factors such as age, sex, build, and activity level make one person's needs different from another's. Adolescents and premenopausal women need more calcium-rich foods than other people. Women who consume too little calcium for many years may be at greater risk for osteoporosis, a bone-thinning and -weakening disease that afflicts mainly postmenopausal women. Children undergoing growth spurts and pregnant women have a higher-than-average need for iron to prevent anemia.

First and foremost, we all need the more than 40 nutrients that food supplies. The U.S. government has set guidelines for levels of essential vitamins and minerals that will ensure well-being for nearly all healthy individuals. These are known as the Recommended Dietary Allowances, or RDA's. A diet that provides variety, balance, and moderation will supply these allowances.

Phantom Fuel for Sports. For years, America's favorite "muscle food" was protein. Athletes, notably bodybuilders, bought protein powders in the belief that protein goes directly into muscles after being eaten. Such efforts to stoke up on protein were misguided. The body uses protein for growth, tissue replacement, and repair. It stores any excess as fat, rather than converting it to muscle.

Carbohydrates are far and away the best fuel for athletes and those exercising for fitness. For a workout or competition, athletes should make carbohydrates the focus of their diets, amounting to between 60 and 70 percent of their total calories. According to sports nutritionist Nancy Clark, their fat intake should not exceed 25 percent of calories. Protein intake should be modest. Like armchair athletes, the active runner, cyclist, swimmer, and all others performing sports should make sure that they consume carbohydrates of the high-fiber, complex type and that their protein sources are low in fat.

Compare these percentages and eating guidelines to

the new nutrition. The variations are surprisingly small: 60-70 percent carbohydrates for athletes, 55 percent or more carbohydrates for the rest of us; fat intake not to exceed 25 percent for the very active, versus 30 percent for the rest of a healthy population. For those of us at special risk for coronary artery disease, fat consumption should probably not exceed 20-25 percent. Everyone should eat only modest amounts of protein, choosing mostly from low-fat foods.

Taking It Off Sensibly. Most diet experts and successful dieters have discovered that a varied low-fat, high-carbohydrate diet, combined with exercise, is more effective than gimmicks and expensive prepackaged meals. A balanced diet rich in carbohydrates raises the ratio of lean body weight to fat. And exercise improves this ratio even further. A person can lose more fatty tissue with exercise than by dieting alone.

There is no mystery to losing weight. When the body expends more energy (calories) than it takes in, it uses calories stored in the tissues. A pound of body fat equals about 3500 calories; to lose one pound a week, it's necessary to cut 500 calories a day from a maintenance-level diet or increase activity by 500 calories.

Drastic calorie reductions are ill-advised. A diet that dips below 1200 calories for women and about 1400 for men may cut out essential nutrients. Also, rapid weight loss on super low-calorie and low-carbohydrate diets comes largely from lean tissue and water because the body burns protein to perform functions usually fueled by carbohydrates.

On a high-carbohydrate diet with adequate protein and nutrients, however, the body breaks down fat instead of muscle. Complex carbohydrates also take up more space in the stomach than fats and proteins, so people feel full on fewer calories. In one study, college students lost weight when they were allowed to eat anything they wanted plus 12 slices of low-calorie, high-fiber bread a day. Evidently the bread satisfied them so that they didn't eat as many high-calorie foods as usual.

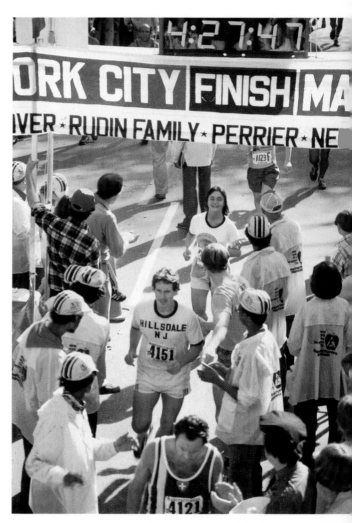

Marathon runners need foods that will keep their muscles supplied with energy even in the late stages of the race. These foods turn out to be complex carbohydrates—the very staples that form the heart of today's high-fiber, low-fat diet.

The Extra Burden of Obesity. Overweight people often don't eat much more than their lean, muscular friends, but because they have a higher ratio of fat to lean body weight, their bodies metabolize food differently. The flabby executive weighing 220 pounds doesn't need as many calories as a muscular wrestler also weighing 220 pounds who carries little fat, because fat can be maintained with fewer calories.

An added problem for significantly overweight people is the enzyme responsible for depositing fat into fat cells, lipoprotein lipase (LPL). When more than 15 percent of body weight is lost, this enzyme goes into overdrive. Months or even years after the diet is over, this enzyme can still be abnormally active, making it more difficult to return to eating normal quantities without gaining weight.

CASE HISTORY

RUNNING ON EMPTY

Sports nutritionist Nancy Clark reports that when a weight-loss diet turned into a cycle of starving and binging for one athlete, he decided it was time to look for professional help.

"Weight-conscious athletes who constantly diet to be unnaturally thin are prime candidates for disordered eating patterns. Food, for these athletes, is not fuel. It's 'The Fattening Enemy' that thwarts their desire to be thin. Their goal is thinness at any price — often a price of anguish and impaired athletic performance.

"Pete, a 42-year-old runner, never was concerned about his weight until he began running 2 years ago. He felt fat compared to other runners and decided to diet. He'd grind through a 10-mile run, eat very little during the day, then devour any food in sight. Pete said, 'I feel so guilty about the boxes of cereal, crackers, and cookies I devour. After a binge, I won't eat dinner with my wife and children. Instead I'll go for another run to burn off the excess calories. My kids get mad at me for eating all the cookies. My wife complains that I'm neglecting the family. I'm disappointed in myself for being such a failure. I'm embarrassed that I'm unable to do something as simple as lose a few pounds. I can't even eat normally now. I either diet or binge.'

"To help Pete better balance his food and exercise goals and normalize his disordered eating patterns, I measured his percent body fat (an excellent 8 percent), determined how many calories his body required each day, and devised a meal plan to stabilize his eating. Like many of my clients, he dieted too hard for someone with little excess fat to lose. His weight goal was well below the set point weight he could comfortably maintain.

"Pete unrealistically restricted his calories. He would run 10 miles in the morning, which expended about 1000 calories, but he would eat nothing until lunch, when he limited himself to 450 calories. No wonder he longed for food before dinner — he was starving! I advised him to stop dieting and start eating breakfast and lunch, and to then eat reasonably at night. He changed his habits and stopped his evening binges.

"Pete followed my recommendations to eat 2600 calories divided more evenly throughout the day. 'I no longer act like a maniac in front of the refrigerator, eating whatever I can get my hands on,' Pete said. 'I've decided against losing any more weight; my body just doesn't want to be thinner. I do feel great. I have energy at work. I'm less irritable. My running is improving. And most importantly, I feel in control of my food.'"

Excerpted from Nancy Clark's Sports Nutrition Guidebook *by Nancy Clark.*

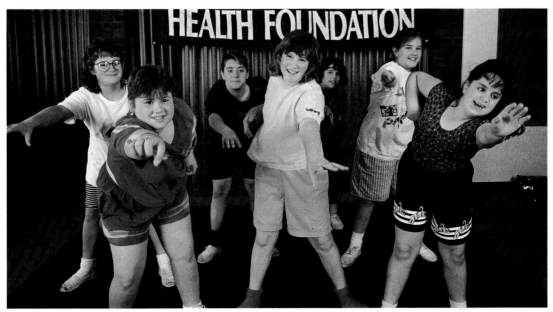

The Diet Treadmill. A government survey says that half of all women and a quarter of all adult men are on a diet at any given time. The scales tell a woeful tale of weight gain. A survey by the National Center for Health Statistics showed that the average American weighed four to six pounds more in 1980 than in 1960.

With so many people concerned about their expanding waistlines, it's no wonder that many reach for the latest quick-fix diet plan, usually one that promises immediate and effortless results. Almost anyone who follows a reducing diet will take off weight initially; however, the first pounds lost are mostly water, which the body releases as it taps into its stores of protein and fat to create energy.

The Hazards of On-Off Dieting. Keeping weight off is as important as—though often more difficult than—taking it off. Constant dieting divides life into periods of deprivation and periods of self-indulgence. In fact, the more often people diet, the more likely they are to regain the weight they lose, a phenomenon that nutritionists call the yo-yo syndrome. The body converts the calories in food into energy to fuel activities, such as making the heart beat or playing tennis. When caloric intake drops sharply, the body's basal metabolic rate (the rate that energy is expended at rest) slows so that available energy is conserved—the "starvation response." With frequent dieting, the body becomes ever more efficient at turning down the metabolic thermostat, so that with each diet it becomes tougher to stay slim.

Unlike dieting, exercise should be a lifelong routine. Exercising three or more times a week not only burns calories and builds muscle, but the feeling of well-being may encourage people to continue their weight-loss efforts after their initial enthusiasm wanes. In addition, exercise speeds up the rate at which the body uses calories during a workout and sometimes for up to three hours afterward. ❑

Moderate exercise can help dieters of all ages take weight off, and keep it off. Exercise works, in part, by speeding up the metabolic rate, so calories are burned more quickly and more efficiently. It is never too early to tackle weight problems. But overweight children should be encouraged to lose weight slowly and sensibly, just like their adult counterparts.

The New Vegetarian

What many considered to be somewhat offbeat is now considered a healthy choice. A vegetarian diet is actually a further modification of the new nutrition's low-fat, high-fiber prescription for health.

MANY OF US were raised to believe that a diet lacking in meat was tantamount to slow suicide. We'd either fade away from want of protein, or if that didn't get us, we'd succumb to gustatory despair after being forced to live on nothing but rabbit food. However, many people around the world live on meatless, or nearly meatless, diets for economic, religious, or cultural reasons—and have throughout history. In fact, our own culture's reliance on meat has more to do with our prosperity than it does with any real need for flesh foods in our diets.

Some argue that humans are meant to be vegetarians. For example, unlike lions, say, we lack flesh-tearing fangs. Like herbivores, our canine teeth are short. In addition, our molars are flattened for crushing food and our jaws are mobile for grinding fibrous plants into bits. Our digestive tracts, too, are designed more for digesting plant foods than animal foods. Our intestines are very long, giving fibrous plant foods the opportunity to be broken down and their nutrients absorbed. Carnivores, on the other hand, have shorter intestinal tracts. This allows them to digest meat quickly and eliminate wastes, possibly before toxins have a chance to accumulate.

A Question of Health. A more compelling reason to think about vegetarianism involves health. Some studies show that vegetarians have lower levels of blood cholesterol and lower blood pressure than meat eaters—meaning that their risk for heart disease is also lower. Many vegetarians eat large quantities of broccoli, carrots, citrus fruits, and other foods thought by some to contain chemicals effective in inhibiting or preventing the growth of cancer cells. A diet lower in fat and high in these protective chemicals may be linked to lower incidences of certain cancers.

Some also feel that because our bodies are designed to digest food slowly, meat, which can be high in saturated fat, stays in the intestinal tract too long; the toxins produced there may be related to our high rates of colon and rectal cancer. These cancers tend to be much rarer among the Japanese and others who stick to essentially meat-free diets.

Guidelines for a Healthy Diet. A strict vegetarian diet is one wholly lacking in animal products of any kind, including fish, poultry, dairy products, and eggs. However, ovo-lacto vegetarians eat eggs and dairy products, and lacto vegetarians will eat dairy products, while avoiding eggs. In addition, many people are part-time vegetarians, or eat fish while still maintaining an essentially meat-free diet.

Most people considering a meat-free diet are concerned about getting adequate protein. Recent nutritional research suggests that protein needs can be easily satisfied

---

Complementary Proteins

"Virtually all traditional societies used grain and legume combinations as their main source of protein and energy. In Latin America it was corn tortillas with beans, or rice with beans. In the Middle East it was bulgur wheat with chickpeas or pita bread falafel with hummus sauce (whole wheat, chickpeas, and sesame seeds). In India it was rice or chapaties with dal (lentils, often served with yogurt). In Asia it was soy foods with rice.

"In each case, the balance was typically 70 to 80 percent whole grains and 20 to 30 percent legumes, the very balance that nutritionists have found maximizes protein usability."

— Excerpted from "Diet for a Small Planet" by Frances Moore Lappé

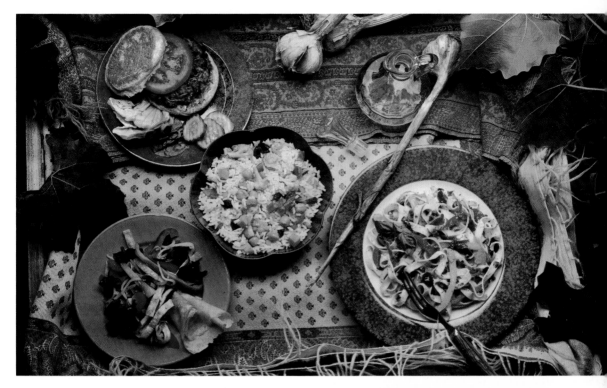

as long as your diet includes a wide variety of vegetables, legumes (like chickpeas and lentils), grains, and fruits.

Many vegetarians advise combining foods in order to be sure of getting complete protein. A typical combination would be rice and beans. These foods complement each other, with each providing amino acids (which comprise protein) that the other lacks. But nutritionists stress that while such combinations will ensure adequate protein intake, eating almost any mixture of nutritious foods will provide enough protein to meet daily adult requirements.

The only real nutritional caveat applies to strict vegetarians (vegans). Because their diets are based exclusively around plants, vegans run a slight risk of developing a vitamin B_{12} deficiency. Derived almost exclusively from animal products, this vitamin is essential for the functioning of most cells in the body, and a prolonged lack can cause serious damage to the central nervous system. Our bodies tend to conserve B_{12}, so a deficiency can take three or more years to show up. Nutritionists may urge those embarking on a vegan regime to take B_{12} supplements.

Making the Switch. If you decide to switch to a vegetarian diet, the first thing to remember is that cutting meat is not a license to overindulge in dairy products, or other foods equally rich in saturated fats. That said, there is no danger in dropping meat from your diet "cold turkey." However, if you're trying to switch your family over to vegetarianism, you may wish to do it in stages to give them some time to adjust to the change. Most people start by eliminating red meat, then gradually phase out poultry, and finally fish. ❏

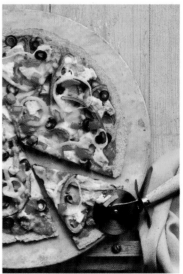

Many vegetarian cooks look to other cultures for inspiration. Noodles, rice, and tofu (top) provide the basis of many meatless meals, with vegetables, beans, and a wealth of other ingredients contributing to an endless variety of dishes. Pizza (below), one of our nation's favorite fast foods, can be quite nutritious. Boost the fiber and vitamin content by using whole wheat flour in the crust and adding a topping of fresh vegetables; cut down on the fat by choosing a low-fat cheese.

Macrobiotics: A Matter of Balance

This approach to healthy living fosters an awareness of the constant fluctuations within body and mind. By choosing foods carefully, adherents strive to strike a balance in order to maintain optimum health.

MORE THAN SIMPLY A DIETARY REGIMEN, macrobiotics is a basic approach to healthful living that stresses the notion of balance. As a philosophy, macrobiotics—from the Greek roots *makros* (big or long) and *bios* (life)—is loosely derived from the ancient Chinese concept of yin and yang, the law of complementary opposites in nature.

According to this system, the universe consists of a balance of yin qualities—death, cold, darkness, female—and yang qualities—life, heat, light, male. There would be no darkness without light, cold without heat, life without death, males without females. So, too, foods are either yin or yang (to a greater or lesser degree) and are classified according to several criteria, including climate (tropical regions producing very yin foods, cold regions very yang), pH (acid or alkaline), and taste (sweet or salty).

The Aim of the Diet. In order to achieve balance in life, one must strike a balance between the two extremes. Some foods, like sugar or honey, are considered very yin; others, like meat and eggs, are considered very yang. Grains, particularly brown rice and other whole grains, are closest to the middle and are the foods around which the daily diet is planned. An overindulgence in yin foods is said to bring on worry and resentment, while an excess of yang foods produces hostility and aggressiveness. So proponents of macrobiotics say that if you're feeling a little yin, eat yang foods (or vice versa) and your equilibrium will be restored.

In addition to focusing

The preferred utensils *in macrobiotic cooking are cast iron, stainless steel, and enamel pots, and ceramic and tempered glass ovenware. Macrobiotic cooks do not use copper or aluminum, as these give off traces of metal which may affect the vitamin content of food. Wooden or bamboo spoons, ladles, spatulas, and natural-bristle vegetable brushes are also used.*

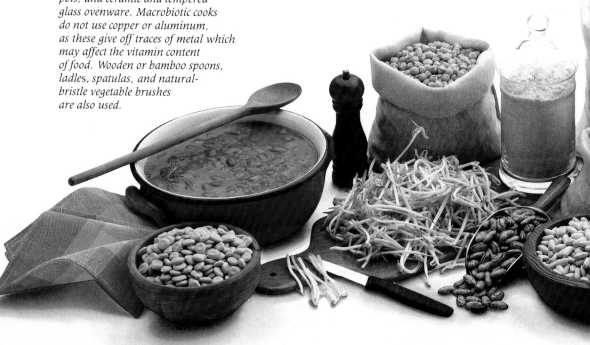

on diet, many macrobiotic enthusiasts carry the notion of balance into other areas of their lives. For many, it is a way of summoning emotional as well as physical well-being by striking a better balance among such things as work, exercise, relaxation, meditation, and relationships.

A False Start. In the 1960's a few food faddists took macrobiotics to extremes, cutting out all foods but brown rice. Needless to say, such food regimens are at best boring and at worst lethal. But unfortunately it was the extremists who first brought macrobiotics to the attention of the public. While advocates of macrobiotics do suggest avoiding foods that are either excessively yin or yang, the guidelines for such a diet do not differ greatly from those of many vegan diets.

The ideal macrobiotic diet is based on a few fundamental principles rather than on particular foods. Michio Kushi, one of the strongest advocates of macrobiotics, describes the diet as "flexible according to season, climate, and personal need." This means eating foods native to your region, preferably in season, and avoiding those that have been processed or treated. In general, whole grains make up about 50 percent of the daily diet, and vegetables constitute another 25 percent. Beans and soy-derived products, such as tofu, make up another 10 percent, as do seeds, nuts, fruits, and fish; and the final 5 percent comes from a soy-based broth known as miso. Among the foods that are generally to be avoided are red meat, sugar, dairy products, eggs, and coffee.

The Benefits of Macrobiotics. Like recent dietary guidelines established by the U.S. Surgeon General, macrobiotic diets are low in fat, cholesterol, and calories, and high in fiber and fresh vegetables. Indeed, medical studies have shown that a person on a macrobiotic diet tends to have far lower blood pressure and cholesterol than the average American. One thing to keep in mind when considering the macrobiotic approach is variety, without which it may be difficult to get adequate amounts of iron, calcium, and vitamins D and B_{12}. Therefore children and pregnant women in particular may be better off on a less restricted diet. In recent years, some enthusiasts have touted their diet as a cancer cure, a claim disputed by most medical experts. While the macrobiotic regimen is similar to the cancer-preventive program of the American Cancer Society, there is no evidence that diet alone can cure cancer. ❑

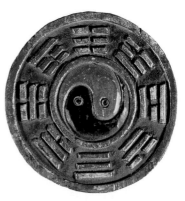

Considering the Yin and Yang of Foods

Feeling too yin? Eat yang foods, and vice versa.

Moderately yin foods include leafy green vegetables, tofu, nuts and seeds, citrus fruit, and sugar-free jams.

Some moderately yang foods are root vegetables; fish and shellfish; cottage cheese; beans and peas.

Brown rice and whole grains are the most balanced foods, and these form the basis of the macrobiotic diet.

Avoid excess. Among foods with extreme yin are sugar and sweets, strong spices, alcohol, tea, and coffee. Meat, poultry, hard cheeses, and eggs are extremely yang foods.

Healthy Eating Around the World

Mealtime provides the perfect forum for introducing children to the pleasures of fresh, wholesome foods. From what we now know, youngsters are not immune to the effects of excess dietary fat. In fact, fat may start accumulating in the arteries at a very early age. The key is to start children off right by serving low-fat, minimally processed meals and snacks.

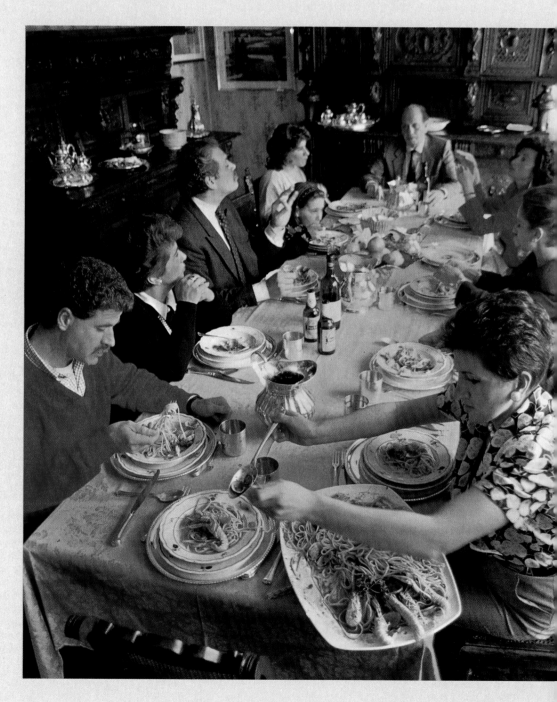

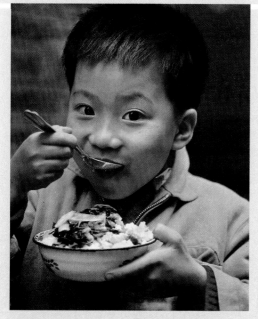

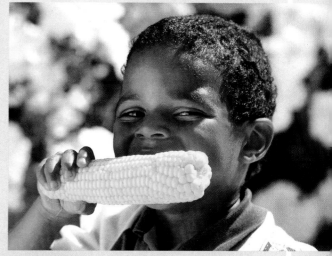

Many children turn their noses up at vegetables, a bad habit that may put them at greater risk for diseases later in life. But even the pickiest eaters love corn on the cob.

In China, where the incidence of heart disease is among the lowest in the world, even young children relish fresh green vegetables. Along with rice, these healthy foods provide the bulk of their daily diets.

Watermelon rind is so thick that there is very little risk of contamination from pesticides. When serving watermelon to small children, do not leave them alone, as the numerous seeds present a choking danger. Better yet, select a seedless variety.

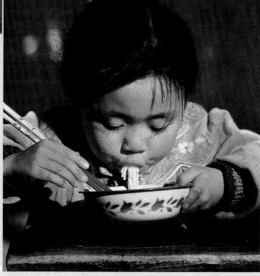

Noodles pose a challenge to young eaters, one they seem to enjoy. Serve noodles with broth, vegetables, or a light sauce.

Southern Italian lunches are festive family affairs, featuring plates of healthful dishes, such as pasta with fresh fish.

The Role of Vitamins and Minerals

These important nutrients are essential to good health since they help the body use the energy stored in food. If you eat a balanced, varied diet, vitamin and mineral supplements are probably unnecessary.

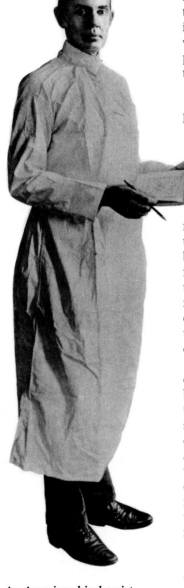

An American biochemist, *Elmer McCollum, discovered the first vitamin, vitamin A, in 1913. Once scientists were able to isolate these substances in food, they could further explore the links between diet and health.*

A SURPRISING NUMBER OF PEOPLE take vitamin or mineral supplements each day as a kind of nutritional insurance— usually without understanding how they work and what they do. Nutrients such as riboflavin, vitamin C, zinc, and many others are essential to good health, but they are no substitute for food. In fact, vitamins and minerals are facilitators that enable the body to make use of the energy stored in food. These nutrients in and of themselves are of little value to the body. Simply taking vitamin and mineral supplements without eating food is like sending in bricklayers to build a wall, but neglecting to supply the bricks.

What They Do. Crucial to the normal maintenance of healthy cells, vitamins perform an extraordinary range of functions in the human body. They not only help convert food into usable energy, but they also assist in the manufacture of blood cells, hormones, and the chemicals of the nervous system.

Vitamins are divided into two categories: water-soluble and fat-soluble. The four fat-soluble vitamins, A, D, E, and K, are absorbed into body fat and may be stored for later use. If taken in excess, however, some fat-soluble vitamins can accumulate in toxic amounts. Vitamin C and the eight B vitamins are all water-soluble, meaning that they dissolve in body fluid, and most of the excess is eliminated through sweat or urine. As a result, there is little concern about toxic overdoses (although excessive doses of B_6 can be toxic).

Minerals play a part in the maintenance of immune cells, in blood coagulation, in the synthesis of oxygen in the blood, in bone formation, and in numerous other functions. Some, such as calcium, phosphorus, and magnesium, are necessary in fairly large amounts. The need for others, known as trace minerals, is much smaller. In fact, although they are present in human tissue, a few of these trace elements play such dubious roles that they are considered nonessential. The essential trace minerals include iron, zinc, fluoride, and copper. Any of these minerals, whether essential or nonessential, is toxic if ingested in sufficient amounts for long enough periods.

How Necessary Are Supplements? For years, controversy has raged between those who believe supplements are necessary and those who say that they are at best a waste of money and, at worst, a hazard to health. With few exceptions (notably vitamins D and K), the human body cannot make its own vitamins or minerals, so they must be obtained from foods. The traditional view holds that a balanced diet will supply all the vitamins and minerals

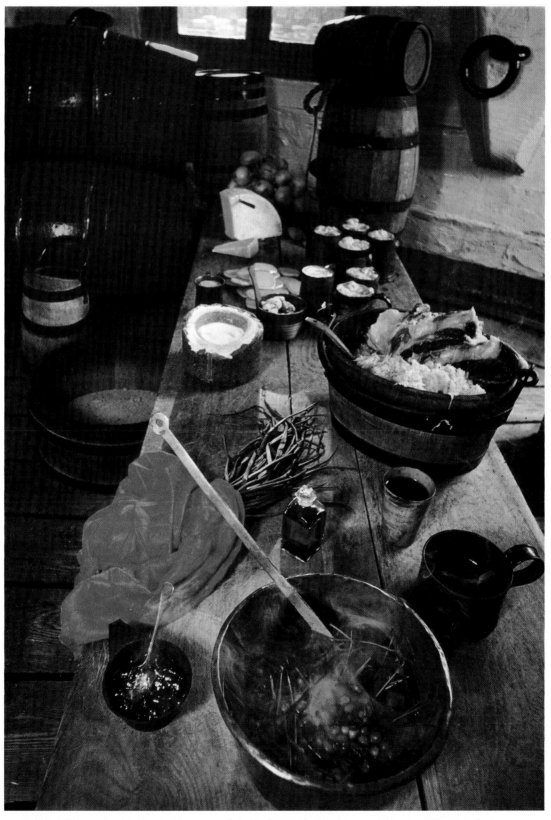

Famed British navigator *Captain James Cook in the late 18th century served his Australia-bound crew a version of this stew of cabbage, leafy greens, and other vegetables. Cook thus became the first ship commander to prevent scurvy, a disease that commonly afflicted sailors whose diets lacked vitamin C.*

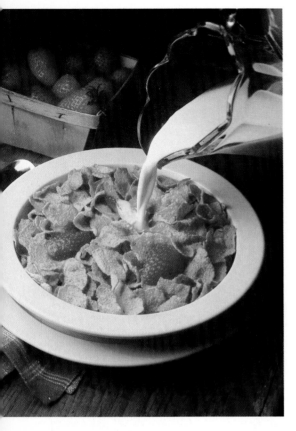

Nutrient Partners

Although all vitamins and minerals influence one another, some have special biochemical partnerships that affect how well they are absorbed by the body. Vitamin C enhances the absorption of iron, which is why topping a bowl of iron-enriched cereal with strawberries — excellent sources of Vitamin C — is a tasty as well as healthy choice. Other nutrient partners include vitamin D and calcium, vitamin E and selenium, vitamin B_{12} and folic acid, and calcium and magnesium.

that are necessary to maintain good health.

The opposing argument for supplements is that many modern diets lack balance. In fact, they are so loaded with processed and refined foods that they cannot provide adequate amounts of essential vitamins and minerals. Furthermore, because many people skip regular meals and instead rely on fast foods, and nutritionally vacuous snacks, supplements may be a necessity. Other proponents of supplements claim that the chronic stress brought on by fast-paced lives can increase our need for these important nutrients.

Orthodox medicine agrees that certain people who are susceptible to deficiencies can benefit from supplements of vitamins and minerals. Among these are the elderly, people taking certain medications, patients recovering from burns or major illnesses, and pregnant and nursing women. In addition, cigarette smoking and heavy drinking can rob the body of nutrients, as can crash or fad diets.

In recent years, scientists have started to investigate possible therapeutic uses for vitamins and minerals. For example, vitamins A, B_6, C, and E, and the mineral zinc have all been suggested as possible immune system boosters. A growing number of researchers think that beta-carotene and C and the trace mineral selenium may reduce the risk of certain types of cancer. But while such research holds considerable promise, results have been inconclusive.

What the Numbers Mean. Supplement bottles often contain a confusing array of chemical names and numbers. Most list daily requirements as a percentage of the U.S. RDA. These are the allowances set by the U.S. Food and Drug Administration, but are based on the National Academy of Science's Recommended Daily Allowances (RDA). The numbers expressed are not the *minimum* required to maintain health, but they reflect the *highest* recommended amount. Some physicians and nutritionists believe the numbers are too low because they are based on the needs of healthy people who maintain good diets. Others feel that the U.S. RDAs are too high, and that as little as two-thirds the amount may satisfy most people's dietary needs. In any case, both sides agree that people with chronic health problems, those recovering from illness, and those with conditions that prevent these vital nutrients from being absorbed from food may have greater requirements for nutrient supplements.

Choosing a Supplement. The shelves of many drug and health food stores are lined with vitamin and mineral supplements, many geared toward a specific problem or lifestyle. Some promise to provide athletes with extra energy, others to ease stress, and still others promise to boost the immune system. For most consumers, the most important factors to keep in mind are the balance of vitamins and minerals in a formula, the expiration date, and the solubility. Some supplements take so long to dissolve that they pass through the body without releasing any nutrients. You can test a supplement's solubility by dropping it into a glass of water; it should dissolve in less than an hour.

The balance of nutrients is important because certain vitamins and minerals can enhance or inhibit the body's ability to absorb and utilize others. For instance, vitamin C enhances the absorption of iron, particularly inorganic iron derived mainly from plants. But too much vitamin C may interfere with the absorption of copper. In general, when choosing supplements keep in mind that vitamins and minerals interact in the body in complex ways.

Despite abundant rhetoric to the contrary, there is no real distinction between natural and synthetic supplements, as far as how well the body utilizes the nutrients. Synthetic vitamins are usually fermented from food sources using microorganisms similar to those used to make yogurt, cheese, or beer. Natural vitamins are extracted from plant sources, but some chemical process is required to extract the vitamins.

If you decide to take a daily multi-vitamin, read labels carefully. But be aware that, unlike drugs, supplements do not have to meet government standards for safety and effectiveness. Nor do supplement manufacturers have to

In remote regions of Siberia, where daylight is virtually non-existent during the winter months, children receive treatment with ultraviolet light to prevent rickets, a bone disease caused by lack of vitamin D. The so-called sunshine vitamin, vitamin D is manufactured in the skin when it is exposed to the ultraviolet rays of the sun. This treatment has recently come into question due to the danger of skin cancer from ultraviolet radiation.

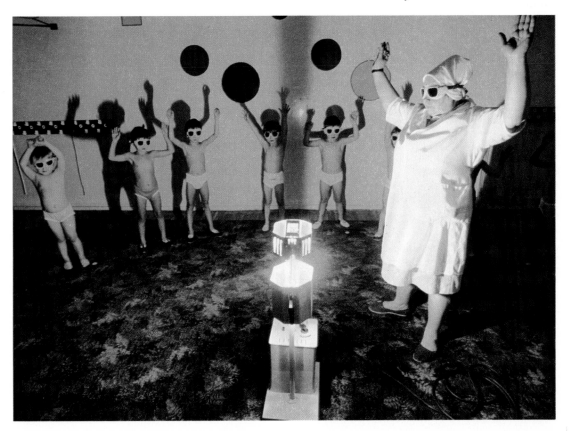

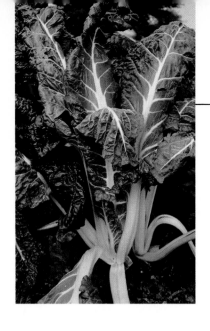

The Role of Vitamins and Minerals

comply with guidelines on potency, purity, or quality, although according to the Council for Responsible Nutrition, an industry trade group, many do meet these standards.

Vitamin and Mineral Chart. Consult the chart below for a quick refresher on the primary role of each nutrient, and the best food sources for insuring that you meet your daily requirements. Fat-soluble vitamins are stored in the liver and fatty tissue, so they need not be consumed each day, while water-soluble vitamins are stored only briefly, so should be part of your daily diet. ❏

	Vitamin	Main Role	Good Food Sources
Fat Soluble	**A** *(retinol)*	Needed for maintenance of skin, mucous membranes, bones, teeth, and hair; vision; and reproduction.	Retinol sources: fish liver oils, egg yolks, butter, cream. Beta-carotene sources: leafy green and yellow vegetables.
	D *(calciferol)*	Helps body absorb calcium and phosphorous; needed for bone growth and maintenance.	Vitamin-D fortified milk and milk products, margarine, egg yolks, fish liver oils, liver.
	E *(tocopherol)*	Helps form red blood cells; prevents oxidation damage.	Vegetable oils, nuts, seeds, green leafy vegetables, whole grains.
	K	Needed for blood clotting.	Green leafy vegetables, vegetable oils, egg yolks, liver.
Water Soluble	**B₁** *(thiamin)*	Needed for nervous system function; helps release energy from carbohydrates.	Whole grains, enriched breads and cereals, seeds, nuts, legumes, dried yeast, potatoes, pork, kidney, liver.
	B₂ *(riboflavin)*	Helps release energy from foods.	Green leafy vegetables, enriched breads and cereals, fish, poultry, milk and milk products, liver, meat.
	Niacin	Needed for nervous and digestive system functions; helps release energy from foods.	Enriched bread and cereals, poultry, fish, legumes, liver, meat.

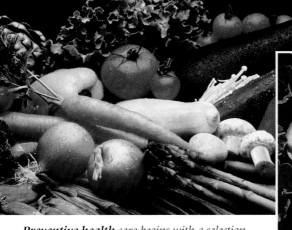

Preventive health *care begins with a selection of fresh fruits and vegetables, especially those that are rich in beta-carotene and vitamin C. These nutrients are antioxidants and may offer protection from certain cancers and heart disease.*

Main Role	Good Food Sources	Water Soluble
Needed for metabolism; helps form red blood cells.	Dried yeast, whole grains, fish, legumes, bananas, nuts, potatoes.	B_6 *(pyridoxine)*
Helps form red blood cells; contributes to neural function.	Liver, meats, seafood, eggs, milk and milk products.	B_{12} *(cobalamin)*
Helps form red blood cells and genetic material.	Leafy green vegetables, fruit, whole grains, legumes.	Folic acid
Helps metabolize nutrients.	Whole grains, legumes, green leafy vegetables, milk, egg yolks, liver, kidney.	Pantothenic acid
Involved in metabolism of fatty acids; helps release energy from carbohydrates and amino acids.	Cauliflower, liver, egg yolk, legumes, nuts.	Biotin
Promotes formation, growth, and maintenance of bones and teeth; repair of tissues; resistance to infection.	Citrus fruits, tomatoes, potatoes, cabbage, green peppers.	C *(ascorbic acid)*

	Mineral	Main Role	Good Food Sources
Macro-minerals	**Calcium**	Needed for bone and tooth formation; heart function and blood coagulation; muscle contraction.	Milk and milk products; canned sardines and salmon with bones; green leafy vegetables.
	Phosphorus	Plays a role in bone and tooth formation; helps release energy from nutrients.	Milk, cheese, poultry, fish, whole grains, nuts, meat, legumes.
	Magnesium	Bone and tooth formation; nerve conduction and muscle contraction; aids in release of energy.	Green leafy vegetables, nuts, whole grains, legumes, milk.
	Sodium	Regulates fluid and acid-base balance; nerve transmission; muscle contractibility.	Table salt, processed foods.
	Potassium	Nerve transmission; muscle contraction; helps maintain blood pressure.	Bananas, prunes, raisins, potatoes, cereals, legumes.
	Chloride	Regulates fluid and electrolyte balance; forms part of gastric juice.	Table salt, processed foods.
	Sulfur	Needed to make hair, nails, and cartilage; tissue formation.	Fish, egg yolks, clams, wheat germ, legumes, meat.
Trace Elements	**Iron**	Formation of hemoglobin; involved in enzyme activities related to energy storage and availability.	Soybean flour, liver, beans, clams, peaches, prune juice, green leafy vegetables, blackstrap molasses, raisins.
	Zinc	Component of enzymes and insulin; aids in wound healing, growth, tissue repair, and sexual development.	Seafood, eggs, fish, whole grains, meats, legumes.
	Iodine	Needed to form thyroid hormones.	Iodized salt, seafood, milk and milk products.
	Copper	Involved in iron absorption and metabolism; helps form red blood cells and nerve fibers.	Organ meats, oysters, nuts, legumes, nuts, seeds,

Main Role	Good Food Sources	Trace Elements
Needed for bone formation; involved in several enzyme reactions.	Tea, coffee, legumes, nuts.	**Manganese**
Bone and tooth formation.	Fluoridated tap water, tea, coffee, sardines with bones.	**Fluoride**
Helps insulin work efficiently in glucose metabolism.	Dried yeast, whole grains, peanuts, wheat germ.	**Chromium**
Has close metabolic interrelationship with vitamin E; involved in certain enzyme systems.	Whole grains, liver, seafood.	**Selenium**
Forms part of an enzyme.	Whole grains, legumes, liver.	**Molybdenum**

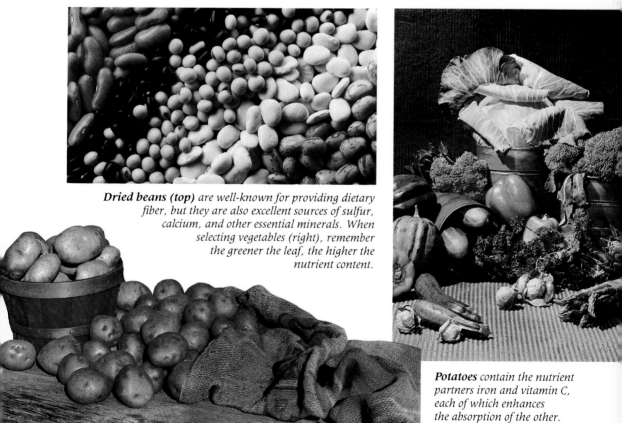

Dried beans (top) are well-known for providing dietary fiber, but they are also excellent sources of sulfur, calcium, and other essential minerals. When selecting vegetables (right), remember the greener the leaf, the higher the nutrient content.

Potatoes contain the nutrient partners iron and vitamin C, each of which enhances the absorption of the other.

Vitamins and Minerals as Therapy

Some health practitioners use vitamins and minerals to treat ailments, despite a lack of widespread approval. While some applications are standard medical treatment, many others are controversial.

IT IS NOT UNCOMMON FOR PRACTITIONERS of natural medicine to use nutrient supplements for problems as diverse as depression, diabetes, blood clots, and menstrual cramps—conditions for which orthodox physicians would be more likely to prescribe drugs. Not surprisingly, controversy surrounds much of this therapy.

The majority of orthodox practitioners maintain that there just are not enough conclusive studies to support the use of vitamins and minerals in the treatment of illness. But based on published data and on their own clinical observations, many nutrition-oriented physicians and practitioners feel that the use of supplements is justified, and that they would be wasting valuable time awaiting the outcome of lengthy research.

Megadoses. In recent years taking megadoses (amounts that considerably exceed the U.S. RDAs) of certain vitamins and minerals has become popular, both to enhance general health and to treat specific illnesses. Nobel laureate Linus Pauling, perhaps best known for his theories on vitamin C and the common cold, is among the advocates of megavitamin therapy. Pauling contends that the U.S. RDAs are completely inadequate for maintaining optimal health—a contention disputed by most orthodox physicians and the bulk of published research.

Many of Pauling's ideas have focused on vitamin C, and its use in combating not just colds, but a number of common diseases. He explains that while most mammals manufacture their own vitamin C, humans cannot and are therefore dependent upon food sources. According to Pauling, our dietary sources do not supply nearly enough to ensure optimal health, which, he contends, is not simply the absence of disease, but a state of mental and physical well-being.

Despite Pauling's claims for the use of megavitamins, most scientists take the position that the practice is wasteful and potentially dangerous. They point out that excessively high doses of vitamins A, D, and B_6, and some minerals, including selenium, can produce dangerous or unpleasant effects. Furthermore, there is little data on the long-term effects of megadoses. Pregnant women are advised against taking excessive amounts of any vitamin or mineral, particularly vitamin A, which can cause fetal abnormalities.

Vitamins as Therapy. Natural practitioners and nutritionally oriented physicians are not the only ones using vitamins and minerals to treat specific ailments. Among orthodox physicians, it is standard medical practice to prescribe zinc for patients undergoing dialysis, for alcoholics suffering from cirrhosis who have vision problems, and

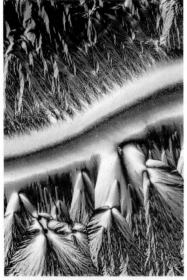

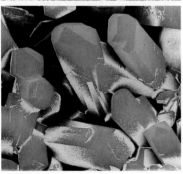

Rainbow-hued micrographs *present a colorful picture of crystalline vitamin C. Scientists study these types of images to get a clearer idea of the vitamin's molecular structure. This information may in turn yield data on how vitamin C works in our bodies.*

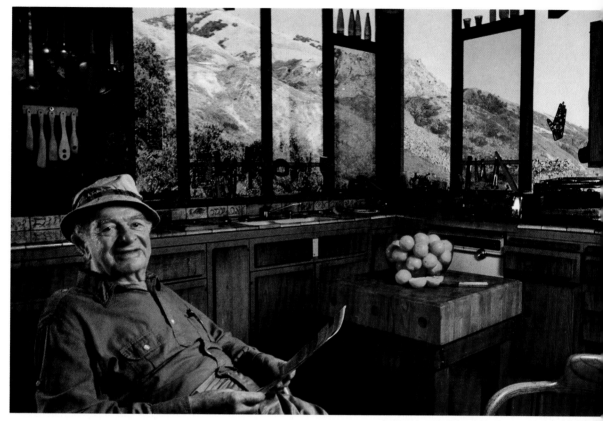

for others suffering deficiencies. In addition, almost all of us drink fluoridated tap water, which helps to prevent tooth decay. Other established uses include iron for the treatment of iron-deficiency anemia, B_{12} for pernicious anemia, vitamin A (Accutane) for severe acne, and niacin to lower triglyceride and cholesterol levels in patients suffering from coronary artery disease. This last usage is said to be safer (and probably cheaper) than any of the widely used prescription drugs.

The Latest News. But what of the myriad other claims for the therapeutic uses of vitamins and minerals? Studies reported in the popular press often give the impression that preliminary results are conclusive, giving rise to distorted notions about what we can expect from certain supplements. Take calcium, for example. While most physicians would recommend calcium supplements for those patients at risk for osteoporosis, there is still little conclusive evidence that the mineral alone will have much effect on adults, particularly after the onset of the disease. Yet reports in magazines and newspapers touting the benefits of the mineral sent many women racing to the pharmacy. Similarly, the studies on vitamin C and the common cold were hardly conclusive, a fact that didn't prevent countless numbers of people from taking preventive doses each day.

For consumers, it is far too complex and time consuming a task to try to sort out the facts from the fallacies. While taking a daily multivitamin supplement doesn't demand

A staunch advocate of using megadoses of vitamin C to enhance health and prevent and treat a variety of illnesses, Dr. Linus Pauling consumes 18,000 mg daily, which is 300 times the recommended daily allowance for adults. Pauling, who has won Nobel prizes for chemistry and peace, would like to see a greater reliance on vitamins and minerals, and less on drugs.

Candidates for Supplements

Even if your diet is balanced and varied, certain conditions or events can put you at risk for a deficiency. Orthodox and natural medicine practitioners do not routinely agree on the benefits of supplements. However, there is a general consensus that the following have nutrient needs that are less apt to be met through diet alone.

- Pregnant women and nursing mothers, who need larger amounts of many nutrients.
- The chronically ill, who take medications. Dozens of drugs inhibit nutrient absorption or deplete nutrients.
- Heavy drinkers, who may need folic acid, thiamin, and other vitamins.
- Cigarette smokers, whose vitamin C levels are often low.
- Dieters, whose calorie intakes may not be sufficient to supply all required nutrients.
- The elderly, who tend to absorb nutrients less efficiently from foods.
- Those recovering from infection or surgery. Supplements may help the body overcome the stress of illness.
- Strict vegetarians (vegans), who may need vitamin B_{12}.
- Women of child-bearing age, who may need iron.

any particular expertise, you should not attempt to treat specific ailments or injuries with vitamins and minerals without expert advice. Alan R. Gaby, M.D., a physician and proponent of the use of supplements for treating certain conditions, has spent considerable time analyzing and interpreting the data from current research. Based on his findings, Dr. Gaby offers the following opinions on possible therapeutic uses for vitamins and minerals.

Thiamin (B_1). Sometimes called the morale vitamin, thiamin plays an important role in maintaining mental health. The need for thiamin increases during periods of physical and emotional stress, and natural practitioners frequently recommend the vitamin to patients suffering from depression. In addition, thiamin is sometimes used for air and sea sickness, hangovers, shingles, and various types of neuralgia.

Riboflavin (B_2). Some natural medicine practitioners use riboflavin to treat certain drug-induced psychoses, as well as eye fatigue. Other health practitioners use riboflavin supplements for alcoholics, who often suffer from a deficiency of the vitamin. It is occasionally suggested as a cure for dandruff.

Niacin (B_3). An established treatment for elevated cholesterol and triglycerides, niacin is also used to treat alcoholics, who are often vitamin deficient. Niacin has been suggested as a treatment for migraine headaches as well. More controversial is the use of niacin by natural medicine practitioners for treatment of schizophrenia, autism, anxiety, depression, hypoglycemia, diabetes, and arthritis.

Pantothenic Acid (B_5). Supplements of pantothenic acid are used to support weak adrenal glands and to treat various symptoms of allergy. Pantothenic acid may help relieve constipation, promote healing of peptic ulcers, and overcome the intestinal paralysis that follows abdominal surgery. The vitamin has been used as a component of vitamin B complex in comprehensive treatment programs for fatigue, anxiety, depression, and hypoglycemia. Creams containing pantothenic acid have been reported to help a wide range of skin conditions, including eczema.

Vitamin B_6. Also known as pyridoxine, this vitamin is frequently recommended for various premenstrual symptoms, including premenstrual tension, acne, fluid retention, and migraines. Vitamin B_6 may also counteract the depression that birth control pills sometimes produce. In addition, it has been used to treat diabetes, heart disease, carpal tunnel syndrome (a nerve disorder of the hands), arthritis, hyperactivity, asthma, certain types of skin problems, and mental illnesses. B_6 may also help prevent toxemia of pregnancy, some forms of bladder cancer, and calcium oxalate kidney stones. Among orthodox physicians, vitamin B_6 is the established treatment for one rare type of anemia, and it is also used to prevent the side effects from certain anti-tuberculosis drugs.

Vitamin B_{12}. Natural medicine practitioners often give vitamin B_{12} injections to patients suffering from fatigue, anxiety, depression, poor memory, insomnia, and other complaints. The vitamin is also used to treat various types of neuritis and neuralgia, and seems to relieve asthma in some cases. Reports suggest that vitamin B_{12} may be of value in treating seborrheic dermatitis, hepatitis, and some eye problems. Vitamin B_{12} injections are the established mode of treatment for pernicious anemia, a rare blood disorder.

Biotin. This vitamin is often prescribed to infants with eczema, and other skin conditions. Some research suggests a role for biotin in treating diabetes. In addition, patients on kidney dialysis may benefit from biotin, since it seems useful in managing some of the side effects associated with dialysis.

Folic acid. This B complex vitamin may be useful for treating canker sores and cervical dysplasia, a condition that

The elderly are often at a greater risk for vitamin and mineral deficiencies, the result of age, medication, or poor diet. For one thing, after the age of 55, metabolism slows and nutrients are absorbed less efficiently. Furthermore, certain drugs can impair the body's ability to absorb calcium, increasing the likelihood of bone ailments.

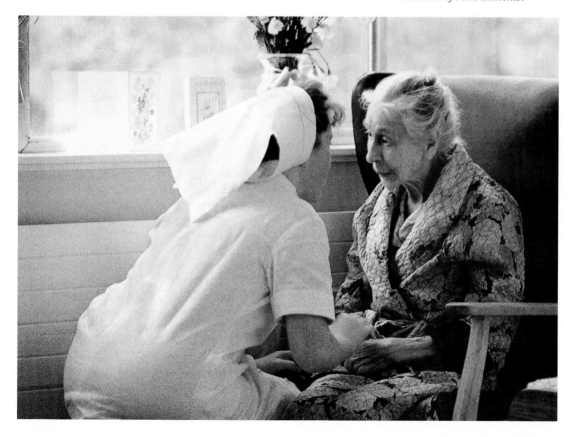

is sometimes a precursor to cervical cancer. Large doses have been used to prevent and treat heart disease, psoriasis, and gout. Folic acid may help prevent some birth defects.

Vitamin C. An antioxidant, vitamin C may prove useful in preventing certain cancers, as well as in protecting the body against the harmful effects of pollution, smoking, and radiation therapy. The vitamin is also being studied for its possible role in improving immune function. Some research indicates a possible role for vitamin C in the treatment or prevention of cardiovascular disease, diabetes, gallstones, eye diseases, viral and bacterial infections, mental disorders, asthma, allergies, and spinal-disc degeneration. Natural practitioners often give vitamin C supplements to aid in wound healing and increase resistance to stress.

Vitamin A. Natural practitioners use vitamin A to treat acute infections, acne and other skin conditions, to stem excess menstrual bleeding, to prevent and treat peptic ulcers, and to promote the healing of cuts and wounds. Beta-carotene, the water-soluble precursor to vitamin A that is found in certain fruits and vegetables, is an antioxidant that may be useful for preventing some cancers, cardiovascular disease, and mitigating the effects of aging.

Vitamin D. Women going through menopause may benefit from supplements of vitamin D, which increases absorption of dietary calcium. In combination with calcium, vitamin D is said to alleviate hot flashes, night sweats, leg cramps, and other symptoms of menopause.

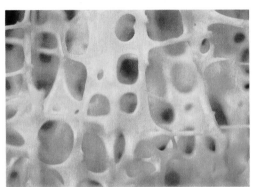
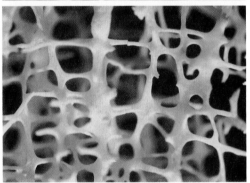

These magnified photographs of a spinal vertebra show the dramatic difference between healthy bone (top) and bone that has been thinned and weakened by osteoporosis (bottom). Although there is considerable scientific debate about how to treat this disease, there is less doubt as to how to prevent it. Eating calcium-rich foods and performing weight-bearing exercise beginning in adolescence are two of the recommended strategies.

Vitamin E. As an antioxidant, vitamin E may help prevent some cancers and cardiovascular disease. Because the vitamin keeps cholesterol and polyunsaturated fats from breaking down into harmful substances in the body, nutrition-oriented physicians use vitamin E for a number of cardiovascular conditions.

In addition, vitamin E may improve circulation and help prevent blood clots. These same antioxidant properties may help protect against the adverse effects of air pollution and other toxins, and may slow the aging process.

Among women, vitamin E has also been reported to alleviate fibrocystic breast disease, prevent miscarriages and other complications of pregnancy, and to relieve premenstrual tension. Some research suggests that vitamin E may help prevent cataracts.

Vitamin K. In combination with vitamin C, vitamin K may relieve nausea and vomiting during pregnancy. It may help those with recurrent nosebleeds or heavy menstrual bleeding, probably due to its role in blood clotting.

Calcium. Best known for its possible role in preventing osteoporosis, calcium has also been used to treat high blood pressure and elevated cholesterol and triglyceride levels. Calcium-deficient diets are often blamed for osteoporosis, a bone-thinning disease most commonly seen in post-menopausal women. However, some nutrition-oriented physicians are convinced that other nutrients besides calcium are important for maintaining bone mass. They suggest taking vitamin D along with calcium supplements to ensure proper absorption.

Calcium may help relieve menstrual cramps, muscle cramps, anxiety, and insomnia. Recent studies suggest a possible link between calcium and the prevention of colon cancer.

Iron. This mineral is routinely used to treat iron-deficiency anemia, a condition that most commonly afflicts women of child-bearing age. While supplements can cure iron-deficiency anemia, taking them unnecessarily may produce iron overload, which may lead to a variety of other health problems. Some practitioners recommend iron to control excessive menstrual bleeding, and to treat a condition called restless leg syndrome.

Magnesium. Magnesium therapy may be helpful for a wide range of conditions, including high blood pressure, heart disease, premenstrual syndrome, migraines, asthma, and fatigue. The mineral has been shown to prevent recurrences of calcium oxalate kidney stones and to relieve some of the symptoms associated with mitral valve prolapse. Some practitioners believe that magnesium may also help alleviate anxiety, depression, and hyperactivity.

Selenium. An antioxidant, selenium has been studied for its possible role in preventing cancer. While the results of these studies are contradictory, there is a possible association between insufficient selenium and increased cancer risk. Its antioxidant properties may help slow the aging process.

Natural medicine practitioners use selenium to treat arthritis and connective tissue disorders, and to prevent cataracts and age-related vision loss. Selenium-sulfide shampoos are commonly used to control dandruff.

Chromium. Deficiencies are fairly common in the United States, perhaps due to low levels of chromium in soil and a reliance on processed foods. Natural medicine practitioners, as well as some orthodox physicians, believe that chromium deficiencies may contribute to diabetes and hypoglycemia, and recommend supplements for those at risk. The mineral may also be useful in lowering cholesterol, and for treating hypertension and cardiovascular disease.

Zinc. This mineral has found wide use among natural practitioners. Zinc has been reported to benefit individuals suffering from some forms of arthritis, acne, boils, skin ulcers, peptic ulcers, infertility, loss of taste and smell, and enlarged prostate glands. ❏

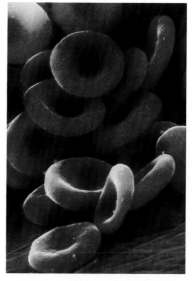

Red blood cells, seen here enlarged hundreds of times, require iron to transport oxygen throughout the body. But they also need adequate amounts of folic acid and vitamin B_{12} for proper maturation. Without these nutrients, the cells fail to develop, leading to a condition known as megaloblastic anemia. In some cases, the deficiency is due not to a dietary lack, but to an inability to absorb the nutrients from food.

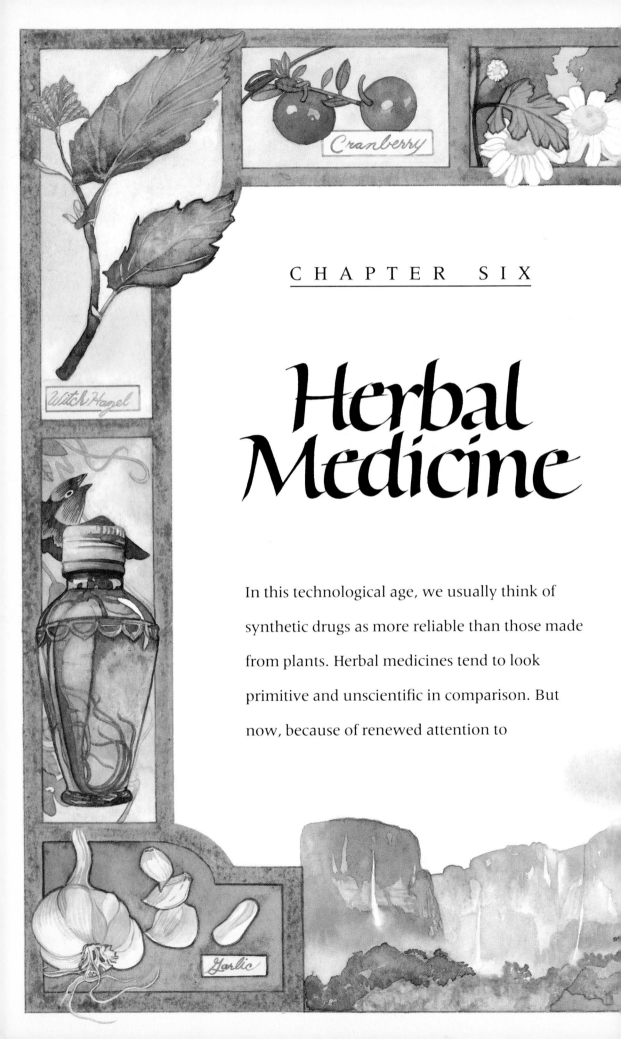

Herbal Medicine

In this technological age, we usually think of synthetic drugs as more reliable than those made from plants. Herbal medicines tend to look primitive and unscientific in comparison. But now, because of renewed attention to

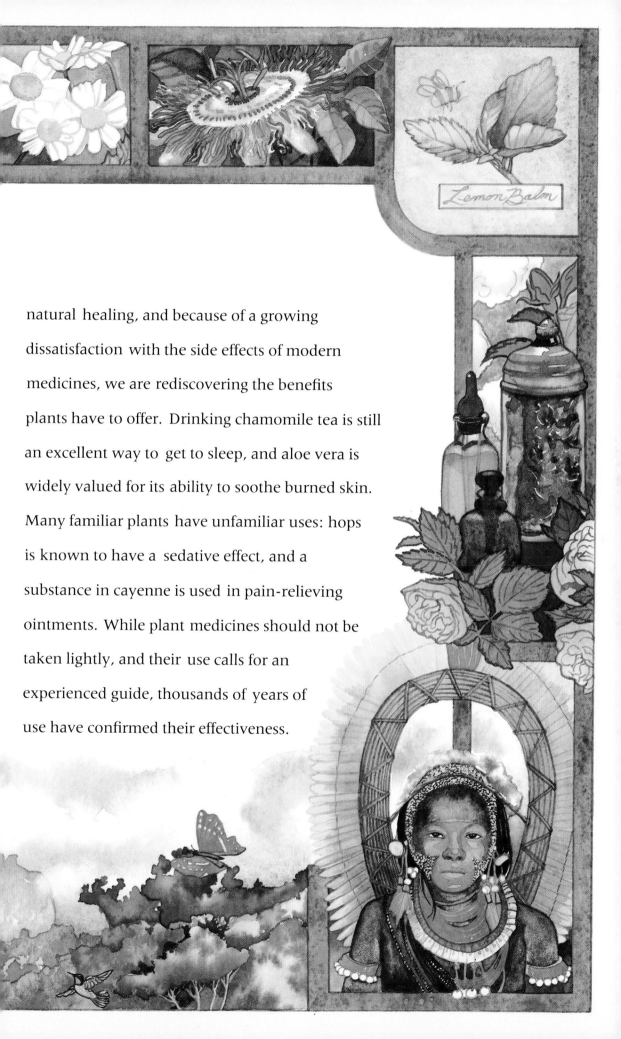

natural healing, and because of a growing dissatisfaction with the side effects of modern medicines, we are rediscovering the benefits plants have to offer. Drinking chamomile tea is still an excellent way to get to sleep, and aloe vera is widely valued for its ability to soothe burned skin. Many familiar plants have unfamiliar uses: hops is known to have a sedative effect, and a substance in cayenne is used in pain-relieving ointments. While plant medicines should not be taken lightly, and their use calls for an experienced guide, thousands of years of use have confirmed their effectiveness.

Lemon Balm

Healing with Herbs

Although herbs have been used for centuries to treat a range of ailments, reliable information on herbal medicine has been hard to come by. But recent studies have validated many of the claims made for healing plants.

THE USE OF PLANTS to heal or combat illness is probably as old as humankind—a fact that has not been ignored by medical science. The pharmaceutical industry grew out of the use of herbs for treating specific complaints, and many of today's prescription drugs are extracts from plants administered in controlled doses. And the search continues for new drugs among the many wild plants as yet untapped for their medicinal riches.

But among herbalists, who nowadays often combine a knowledge of chemistry with an appreciation of folk wisdom, the use of potent plant extracts runs counter to the very essence of herbal medicine. The reason is that the active ingredients that give plants their medicinal properties are tempered by other compounds in the plant, and often act more gently to produce the desired effects. These same compounds, according to some, also reduce side effects.

Years of use and misuse have taught us that plants are not always benign. To understand fully the legitimate uses of healing herbs, folklore and anecdote must give way to science. While mint and chamomile are far less potent than foxglove, for example, any self-treatment should begin with a full appreciation of what a given plant can or cannot do.

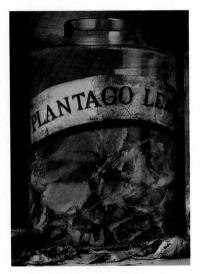

***Tools of the trade** for the nineteenth-century pharmacist included these glass jars with tin lids for airtight storage of herbs. Mortar and pestle were used to grind herbs and drugs, while presses extracted the juice of plants. Often the juices were mixed with alcohol to prevent spoilage.*

Herbal History. Every culture in the world has relied on local herbs and plants to treat illness. For instance, clay tablets dating from about 4000 B.C. reveal that the Sumerians had apothecaries for dispensing medicinal herbs, including licorice and thyme. The *Pen Tsao*, a Chinese text written around 3000 B.C., contained some 1,000 herbal formulas, which were probably a compilation of remedies that had been in use for thousands of years.

But the use of herbal remedies did not end with the ancients. When the Pilgrims landed in Plymouth in 1630, the community quickly set about establishing herb gardens, which contained the medicinal varieties that they had transported from the Old World. As the settlers were soon to discover, Native Americans had their own healing plants, including cascara sagrada and goldenseal.

The history of medicinal plants reveals that trial and error played leading roles in establishing the herbal arsenal. But unfortunately for herbal medicine as a whole, so did magic and a number of illogical systems, including prescribing herbs on the basis of shape or color. For instance, liver-shaped leaves were often recommended for diseases of the liver, red herbs for blood problems, and so forth. As medicine became an increasingly academic discipline, plant medicine took on the doubtful air of a pseudoscience.

But the effectiveness of many herbal remedies has not been overlooked. In fact, even now, with the heavy emphasis on synthetic drugs, some 25 percent of all prescription drugs

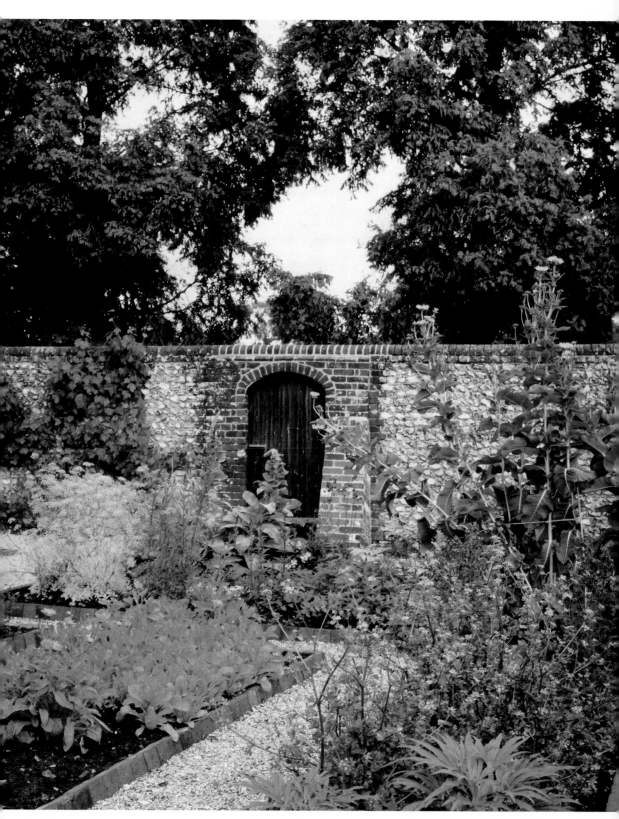

*A **physician prescribing** medicine in the seventeenth century in Great Britain might have relied on the plants grown here in the Petersfield Physic Garden in Hampshire. The use of plants as medicine dates back several millennia. Civilizations in India, China, and Greece that flourished before the Christian era also used medicinal plants. Today botanical gardens in major cities worldwide continue cultivating and preserving such plants.*

in the United States are derived from plants. However, these plant-derived drugs are no less potent, and produce no fewer side effects, than synthetic medicines. And it is the potency and toxicity of drugs, both plant-derived and synthetic, that has led many people back to herbal remedies.

Herbal Medicine Today. While the use of herbs is moving increasingly to the mainstream, it still falls to the consumer to find the most reliable information from the many books and periodicals available on the subject. Now that the United States is experiencing a "green wave" of interest in plant medicines, the Food and Drug Administration may finally be pressured to create a new form of over-the-counter regulation. Currently, the FDA classifies traditional plant drugs as foods or food additives. Therefore, their labels cannot list any medicinal uses or dosage information.

To reach the status of an over-the-counter medicine, plants must go through a rigorous, and costly, testing pro-

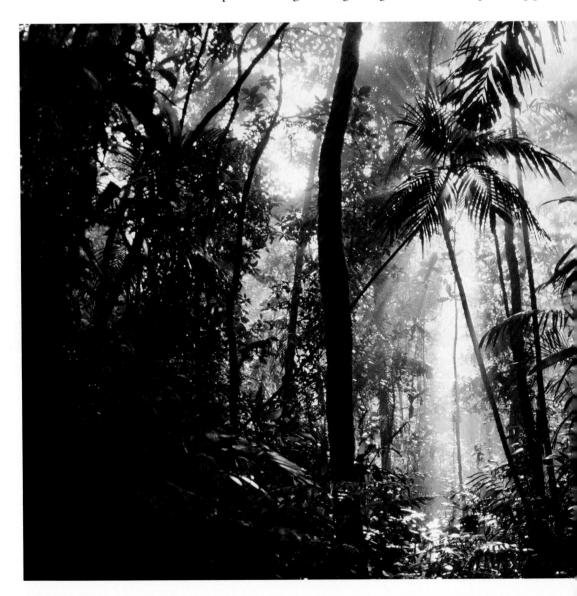

cess. Presently there is little incentive for either the government or pharmaceutical companies to foot the bill. One solution may be for the FDA to create a "traditional medicine" category, modeled on an approach used in European countries. Such a system would provide consumers with traditional usage information, as well as recommended dosage. It would also provide information about scientific tests and results.

Common Healing Herbs. The 60 plants discussed on the following pages represent a selection of healing plants commonly used in the West. Included also are a number of household spices, such as basil, thyme, and rosemary, which have long been used in traditional medicine.

The activity of the herbs mentioned on these pages refers to their observed pharmacological effects. These observations have been drawn from empirical data based on historical use, from clinical studies, and from pharmacological

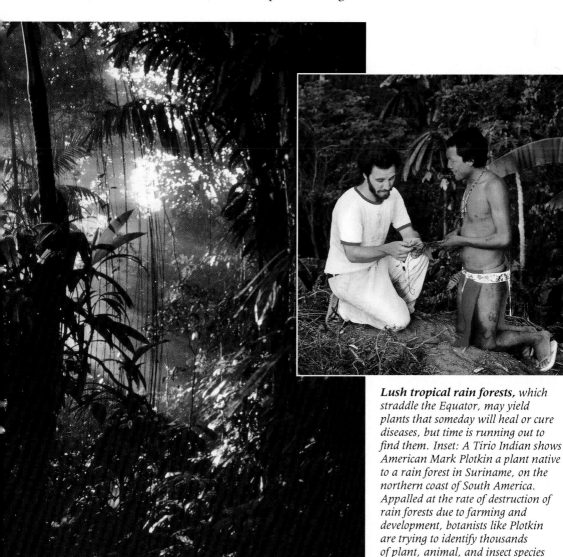

Lush tropical rain forests, *which straddle the Equator, may yield plants that someday will heal or cure diseases, but time is running out to find them. Inset: A Tirio Indian shows American Mark Plotkin a plant native to a rain forest in Suriname, on the northern coast of South America. Appalled at the rate of destruction of rain forests due to farming and development, botanists like Plotkin are trying to identify thousands of plant, animal, and insect species before they disappear forever.*

tests conducted on humans and animals. While all the herbs are safe when used in reasonable amounts, they still must be approached responsibly.

One of the biggest myths attending the use of herbs today is the idea that because something is "natural," it is therefore completely safe. This is a dangerous notion. Some of the most virulent poisons come from the plant kingdom. Underscoring this point is the fact that some of the strongest prescription drugs available are derived from plants that are toxic in their natural state.

Common plant names are unreliable, for they may vary from region to region. For this reason, we have also provided scientific names, which are standardized throughout the world. A plant's scientific name, written in Latin, consists of two parts. The first is the plant's genus (similar to a person's family name), and the second is the species (like a person's first name).

In addition to discussing folklore or historical uses of the plant, each entry describes any testing that has been done, the parts of the plants used, and the compounds that are responsible for its medicinal benefits—a complex problem, for a plant's effects may actually result from an interaction of its many compounds.

The U.S. term for government-approved drugs is Generally Recognized as Safe. Each entry also lists the plant's status in other countries. In the United Kingdom, the Ministry of Health produces a General Sales List (GSL), which lists herbs that can be used medicinally without restrictions. In Canada, traditional medicinal plants qualify for a Drug Identification Number; France has a similar policy, and the words "Traditionally used for" must appear on the label. In Germany, a commission, known as Commission E, reviews the safety of herbs, and issues monographs on those approved for over-the-counter sales.

In the spirit of a unified Europe, the European Economic Community has established the European Scientific Cooperative for Phytotherapy (ESCOP). This group formulates policy and issues monographs on plants intended to be included in the *European Pharmacopoeia*. In Japan, where many people use traditional medicine, healing herbs may be listed in the *Japanese Pharmacopoeia*.

Traditional Chinese medicine uses its own collection of herbs, according to a complex methodology, and their use is discussed in another part of the book. Ayurvedic medicine of India also uses herbs that may be unfamiliar in the West. The system as a whole is discussed elsewhere in the book. ❑

An Herb-User's Guide

Herbal remedies should be taken only when you need them. If you lack experience in the use of herbal medicines, here are a few points to keep in mind.

■ **Be careful of your sources.** Herbs are not subject to the same government scrutiny as pharmaceutical drugs; there's no independent guarantee of purity or potency. Therefore, it's up to you to select reputable brands.

■ **Choose the most reliable forms.** Tinctures and freeze-dried herbs are prepared using techniques for preventing spoilage and loss of potency. Dried herbs, which are sold in bulk, powdered, or encapsulated, may lose potency rapidly because of their exposure to air.

■ **More is not better.** When taking an herbal remedy, take the recommended dosages at the suggested intervals. As with pharmaceuticals, overdosing with herbs can have ill effects.

■ **Monitor your reactions.** At the first sign of an allergic reaction, stop the medication. Or, if the herb doesn't seem to be working, discontinue it; not all remedies work for everyone.

■ **Take no risks.** Never attempt self-medication for serious ailments or injuries; see a doctor or go to a hospital emergency room. Pregnant or lactating women, the very young or old, and people who are taking medication should not use herbal remedies without their physician's approval.

The Value of Using Whole Plants

Medical science has overlooked the healing properties of whole plants, writes Dr. Andrew Weil. Isolating only one element from a plant may well reduce the plant's effectiveness.

A single event in 1803 signaled one of the early milestones in the development of scientific medicine. In that year a young German pharmacist isolated morphine from opium, obtaining for the first time a pure active principle from a crude vegetable drug. This work was valuable and important, both theoretically and practically. It revolutionized medical therapeutics and did indeed put an end to the superstition and uncertainty of herbal treatments. It also created new problems of its own.

In their enthusiasm at isolating the active principles of drug plants, researchers of the last century made a serious mistake. They came to believe that all of a plant's desirable properties could be accounted for by a single compound, that it would always be better to conduct research and treat disease with the purified compound than with the whole plant. In this belief, they forgot the plants once they had the active principles out of them, called all the other principles "inactive," and advanced the notion that prescribing refined white powders was more scientific and up-to-date than using crude green plants.

The erroneous idea that plants and isolated active principles are equivalent has become fixed dogma in pharmacology and medicine. As a physician with a background in botany who has studied the effects of medicinal plants, I find it difficult to explain to my colleagues that purified drugs are not the same as the plants they come from.

In general, isolated and refined drugs are much more toxic than their botanical sources. They also tend to produce effects of more rapid onset, greater intensity, and shorter duration. Sometimes they fail to reproduce desirable actions of plants they come from, and sometimes they lack natural safeguards present in those plants. They also lend themselves to methods of administration favoring abuse and toxicity.

The possibility that secondary compounds of medicinal plants may be valuable in their own right or may

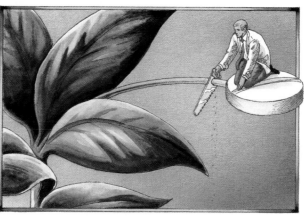

There's more to plants than extracts alone.

modify the effects of dominant compounds in good ways seems unremarkable to me. Nevertheless, I find I have to explain it to physicians and pharmacologists with great patience. Many of them seem to resent the suggestion that natural substances may be better than man-made ones.

All I can say is that I find such a difference, at least in the case of medicinal plants versus isolated drugs. Whenever I have had a chance to experience treatment with a plant and treatment with a refined derivative of the plant, I have found the latter [the refined derivative] to be more dangerous and sometimes less useful.

Excerpted from *Health and Healing* by Andrew Weil, M.D.

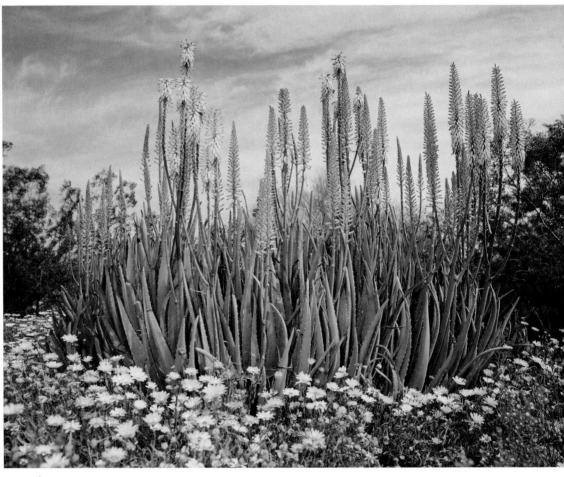

Aloe Vera

ALOE VERA *Aloe barbadensis*

□ **History and Uses.** Nowadays a surprising number of people take advantage of the skin-softening properties of aloe vera in some way. It has long been used in folk medicine, and modern research indicates that when applied externally, aloe vera restores skin tissues and may aid the healing of burns and sores. It can also be used on blemishes and dandruff, and it works cosmetically to keep skin soft.

While aloe seems to be most potent when taken fresh from the leaf, it is an ingredient in several skin creams and shampoos. However, these products contain only small amounts of aloe.

Aloe gel has also been taken internally for stomach disorders, while dried aloe latex—a different substance derived from the leaf—is a strong laxative.

□ **Plant Parts and Active Compounds.** Leaf gel and sap. Aloin.

□ **Regulatory Status.** US: The leaf gel is Generally Recognized as Safe (GRAS) as a food. UK: *British Pharmacopoeia.* Canada: Approved as an over-the-counter laxative. France: Traditional Medicine. Germany: Commission E approved as an over-the-counter drug. Japan: *Japanese Pharmacopoeia.*

ANISE Pimpinella anisum

☐ **History and Uses.** Anise, with its nippy licorice flavor, has been used for centuries in both foods and medicines. The ancient Greeks, including Hippocrates, recommended it for coughs. Ancient Romans used anise in a special cake that concluded their enormous feasts. They included it not only for its flavor, but to aid digestion and ease flatulence. The ancients also used anise as an aphrodisiac, for colic, and to combat nausea.

Today anise is still used for coughs, in both syrups and lozenges. Drinking a tea made from the crushed and steeped seeds is said to aid digestion and ease gas pains. Some herbalists also recommend the tea to nursing mothers to increase milk flow. Anise is considered safe when taken in reasonable amounts.

☐ **Plant Part and Active Compounds.** Seed. Anethole and other aromatic compounds.

☐ **Regulatory Status.** US: Generally Recognized as Safe. UK: General Sales List. Canada: Approved as an over-the-counter drug. France: Traditional Medicine. Germany: Commission E approved as an over-the-counter drug.

ASTRAGALUS Astragalus membranaceus

☐ **History and Uses.** Primarily used in traditional Chinese Medicine, astragalus has only recently become popular among Western herbalists because of its purported effects on the immune system. Although there is some evidence, based on experiments done in test tubes, that it stimulates the immune function, there is no scientific evidence that this same effect can be produced in humans. There is evidence, however, that astragalus may have value in protecting the liver, and it is used by some herbalists to lessen the severity and duration of colds.

☐ **Plant Part and Active Compounds.** Root. Polysaccharides.

☐ **Regulatory Status.** US: None. UK: None. Canada: None. France: None. Germany: None. Japan: *Japanese Pharmacopoeia.*

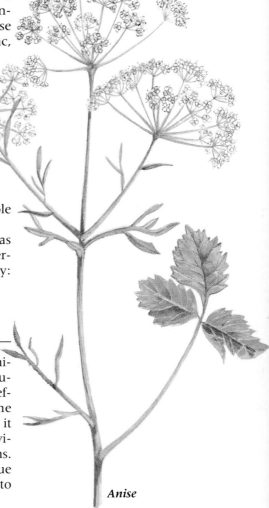

Anise

BASIL Ocimum basilicum

☐ **History and Uses.** *Herbe royale* to the French, a sign of love to Italians, and a sacred herb in India, basil has a rich and fanciful history, and a reputation for both good and evil. Some ancient herbalists believed that basil damaged the internal organs and caused the spontaneous generation of scorpions inside the body.

Various cultures of the world have found their own uses for basil. In the Far East it has been used as a cough medicine, and in Africa it has been used to expel worms. American colonists considered basil the essential ingredient in a snuff used to ease headaches. One folk remedy says that tea made with basil and peppercorns will reduce fever.

While most herbalists prefer other, more effective herbs, basil is still recommended for a variety of home remedies. The herb is a carminative, meaning that it relieves gas, and when brewed in tea is said to aid digestion. Basil tea may also be useful for relieving stomach cramps, vomiting, and constipation.

□ **Plant Part and Active Compounds.** Leaf. Volatile oils (up to 28 percent methyl cinnamate).

□ **Regulatory Status.** US: Generally Recognized as Safe. UK: General Sales List. Canada: Approved as an over-the-counter drug. France: Traditional Medicine. Germany: Not yet Commission E approved.

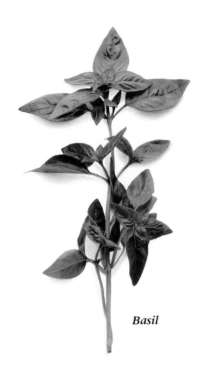

Basil

BLACK COHOSH *Cimicifuga racemosa*

□ **History and Uses.** Long known to Native Americans, black cohosh has been used to treat a variety of ailments, including rheumatoid arthritis, edema, and sore throats. Its primary reputation, however, rested on its ability to relieve menstrual cramps and the pains of childbirth. For this reason it was often known as "squawroot."

Modern herbalists still recommend black cohosh for menstrual problems. This may be explained by the fact that extracts from the roots have effects similar to the hormone estrogen. Herbalists also recommend a tea from the roots as a sedative. Current experiments suggest that extracts from the plant's rhizome may have anti-inflammatory effects, and so may be useful in treating neuralgia and arthritis. Black Cohosh is generally considered safe, although large doses should be avoided because of possible toxicity. Consult an experienced herbal practitioner before using black cohosh during pregnancy.

□ **Plant Part and Active Compounds.** Root. Black cohosh contains a number of potent alkaloids and glycosides.

□ **Regulatory Status.** US: None. UK: None. Canada: Approved as an over-the-counter drug; with the exception that it is not to be used during pregnancy. France: None. Germany: Commission E approved as an over-the-counter drug.

BONESET *Eupatorium perfoliatum*

□ **History and Uses.** Don't be misled by the name: boneset doesn't mend broken bones. A favorite of Native Americans and American colonists, boneset was believed to relieve break-bone fever, caused by a strain of influenza virus, hence the name. It was also thought that a strong infusion of boneset would relieve indigestion, malaria, and snakebite.

Herbalists are showing renewed interest in boneset

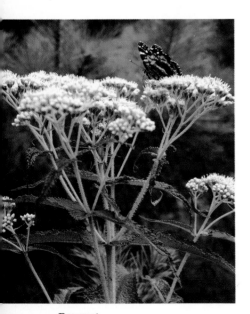

Boneset

to treat fevers due to colds and flu. It is also used as an expectorant to break up mucus. Boneset is considered safe when consumed in reasonable amounts.

□ **Plant Parts and Active Compounds.** Leaves and flowering tops. Flavonoids and terpenoids.

□ **Regulatory Status.** US: None. UK: General Sales List. Canada: Approved as an over-the-counter drug. France: None. Germany: Approved only for use in homeopathic medicine.

BUCKTHORN *Rhamnus frangula*

□ **History and Uses.** Alder Buckthorn was known as early as the second century A.D., when the Greek physician Galen wrote about it. Once credited with the power to protect against demons and witches, it is now known mainly as a laxative. Herbalists often recommend buckthorn tea, made from the bark, to ease constipation. Buckthorn compresses are used to relieve minor skin irritations.

□ **Plant Part and Active Compounds.** Bark. Anthraquinones.

□ **Regulatory Status.** US: Approved as an over-the-counter laxative. UK: General Sales List. Canada: Approved as an over-the-counter drug. France: None. Germany: Commission E approved as an over-the-counter drug. Proposed ESCOP (European Scientific Cooperative for Phytotherapy) monograph for *European Pharmacopoeia*.

BURDOCK *Arctium lappa*

□ **History and Uses.** Just as the burrs of the burdock plant will attach themselves to any passerby, so has burdock attached itself everywhere in the world of folk medicine. It has been used to treat rheumatoid arthritis, indigestion, kidney trouble, dropsy, high fevers, gout, leprosy, and dandruff. And in Shakespeare's play *As You Like It*, burdock was a symbol of lingering annoyance.

Most commonly, burdock root was brewed as a tonic, which was used as a "blood purifier," a diuretic, a mild laxative, and in the treatment of acne and other skin conditions. A poultice made with crushed burdock root is said to be an effective remedy when applied to sores and bug bites. While burdock's widespread application has not stood the test of time, scientific studies have focused on possible value as an external antiseptic.

□ **Plant Part and Active Compounds.** Root. Inulin, a starch (up to 50%).

□ **Regulatory Status.** US: None. UK: General Sales List. Canada: Approved as an over-the-counter drug. France: Traditional Medicine. Germany: Not yet Commission E approved as an over-the-counter drug.

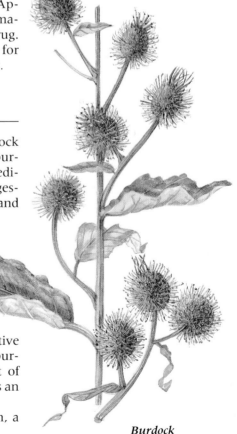

Burdock

CASCARA SAGRADA *Rhamnus purshiana*

☐ **History and Uses.** Used primarily as a laxative, cascara sagrada was first used by Native Americans, and is still in use today. The name means "sacred bark," a reference to the medicinal part of the plant. Cascara sagrada is popular for the relief of constipation, and it is reported to restore the bowel to a healthy tone, making repeated use of the remedy unnecessary. Small doses of tonic prepared from the bark are sometimes taken to ease digestion. Cascara sagrada extracts are found in many over-the-counter preparations in the United States. The bark is considered safe when aged for at least a year, however, it should never be used by pregnant women.

☐ **Plant Part and Active Compounds.** Bark. Anthraquinone glycosides.

☐ **Regulatory Status.** US: Generally Recognized as Safe; approved as an over-the-counter drug. UK: General Sales List. Canada: Approved as an over-the-counter drug. France: None. Germany: None.

CATNIP *Nepeta cataria*

☐ **History and Uses.** Catnip is a popular ingredient in a variety of traditional remedies. Catnip tea is best known as a sleep aid, but it is also recommended to ease menstrual pain, to help soothe the nerves, and as an insect repellent. Compresses applied to the forehead are said to relieve headaches.

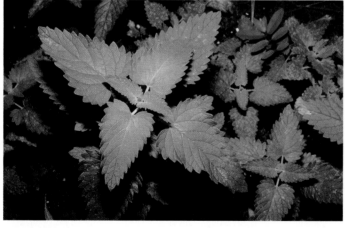

Catnip

Felines of the world, of course, also appreciate the effects of catnip. But rather than eating the plant, they inhale a volatile oil given off by the plant's leaves.

☐ **Plant Parts and Active Compounds.** Leaves and other above-ground parts. Nepetalactones.

☐ **Regulatory Status.** US: Generally Recognized as Safe. UK: General Sales List. Canada: Approved as an over-the-counter drug. France: None. Germany: None.

CAYENNE *Capsicum annuum and C. frutescens*

☐ **History and Uses.** Cayenne pepper has been known to the natives of the tropical Americas for thousands of years, but it was Christopher Columbus who first introduced it to the Old World. Since then, it's had a variety of uses, both culinary and medicinal. Perhaps best known today as an ingredient in hot sauces, cayenne has been recommended as a digestive aid, as a treatment for toothache, and as a way to ward off chills at the onset of a cold.

Capsaicin, the active ingredient in cayenne, is so effective in relieving pain that it has literally become a hot topic for research. Ointments made from capsaicin stop joint and muscle pain by "confusing" pain transmitters; it temporarily upsets the chemical balance in the sensory nerve cells that relay pain messages from the skin. Several over-the-counter products containing capsaicin as the active ingredient can be used externally to ease arthritic pain.

☐ **Plant Part and Active Compounds.** Fruit. Capsaicin.

☐ **Regulatory Status.** US: Generally Recognized as Safe; approved as an over-the-counter drug. UK: General Sales List. Canada: Approved as an over-the-counter drug. France: None. Germany: Commission E approved as an over-the-counter drug. Japan: *Japanese Pharmacopoeia*.

CHAMOMILE *Matricaria chamomilla*

☐ **History and Uses.** A soothing cup of chamomile tea has long been a popular way to take the edge off a long, hard day. Indeed, some studies have shown the herb to be an effective mild sedative, and so it has been used to combat insomnia. To get the strongest possible effects, the tea should be steeped in a closed vessel for at least ten minutes.

Chamomile has a number of other uses as well. The oil of chamomile is sometimes prepared as an extract, which, when applied to the skin, may help reduce inflammations, and thereby alleviate the pain of arthritis. The extract may also be used to heal wounds.

When taken internally, chamomile is said to aid digestion and relieve menstrual cramps, as well as settle acute stomach upset.

This variety of chamomile, *Matricaria chamomilla,* is known as German chamomile. A related plant, Roman chamomile (*Anthemis nobilis*), is less common but has similar effects. Both plants have feathery green leaves and delicate daisy-like flowers that, when crushed, give off a faint scent reminiscent of apples. And both grow along roadsides, in meadows, and other abandoned places.

☐ **Plant Parts and Active Compounds.** Flowers. Chamazulene and alpha bisabolol, both found in the flower's volatile oil.

☐ **Regulatory Status.** US: Generally Recognized as Safe. UK: General Sales List. Canada: Approved as an over-the-counter drug. France: Traditional Medicine. Germany: Commission E approved as an over-the-counter drug.

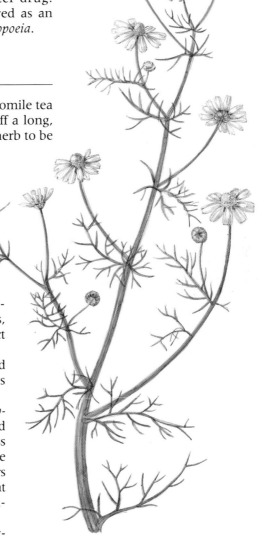

Chamomile

CINNAMON Cinnamomum zeylanicum

☐ **History and Uses.** Cinnamon is a common ingredient in folk remedies for colds, flatulence, nausea, and vomiting. It has been shown to be a carminative (releasing gas in the stomach and intestines), and so is useful for settling an upset stomach and for alleviating diarrhea. Cinnamon has also been used as a treatment to stimulate the appetites of anorexics.

Consumers should note that the variety of cinnamon available for home use is actually derived from cassia bark. It is a related species and is said to produce similar effects.

☐ **Plant Parts and Active Compounds.** Tree bark. Cinnamic aldehyde, eugenol, and tannins.

☐ **Regulatory Status.** US: Generally Recognized as Safe. UK: General Sales List. Canada: Approved as an over-the-counter drug. France: Traditional Medicine. Germany: Commission E approved as an over-the-counter drug.

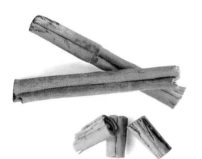

Cinnamon

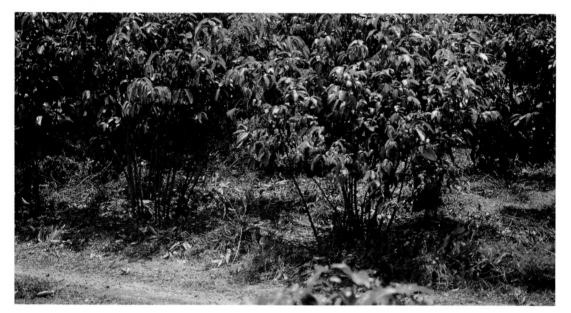

CRANBERRY Vaccinium macrocarpon

☐ **History and Uses.** More than a mere garnish on the Thanksgiving table, cranberries are proving to be a very useful natural remedy. While folk practitioners have often recommended the berries for bleeding gums, some recent research suggests what many people have thought all along: cranberry juice may help fight urinary infections caused by certain bacteria. However, the treatment is only useful as a preventive measure, not as a cure for an existing ailment.

☐ **Plant Part and Active Compounds.** Fruit. Flavonoids.

☐ **Regulatory Status.** No regulatory status applies; cranberries are sold as a food, although concentrated cranberry extracts in capsules have recently been introduced as food supplements.

DANDELION *Taraxacum officinale*

□ **History and Uses.** Medical panacea or ubiquitous weed? While there's little doubt about the tastiness of a dandelion leaf salad or a glass of dandelion wine, this common plant has medicinal uses as well. Once recommended for liver, kidney, and gallbladder problems, it is best known as a mild laxative, an appetite stimulant, and a diuretic. The leaves also contain high levels of potassium.

The bane of lawn tenders across the country, dandelions were transported to the New World by early European settlers, then brought to the Midwest as food for bees.

□ **Plant Parts and Active Compounds.** Leaf and root. The starch inulin (about 25%), bitter principles, sesquiterpenes.

□ **Regulatory Status.** US: Generally Recognized as Safe. UK: General Sales List. Canada: Approved as an over-the-counter drug. France: Traditional Medicine. Germany: Commission E approved as an over-the-counter drug.

ECHINACEA *Echinacea angustifolium and E. purpurea*

□ **History and Uses.** Commonly found growing wild in the central plains, echinacea has long been known to the Native Americans of that region, who used it to treat toothaches, snakebites, and insect bites.

Today echinacea is still used, and research has shown that it may have value in fighting infections and healing wounds. It is also used to stimulate the immune system, and may help ease colds and sore throats.

□ **Plant Parts and Active Compounds.** Leaves and roots. Echinacoside, polysaccharides, isobutyl amides.

□ **Regulatory Status.** US: None. UK: General Sales List. Canada: Approved as an over-the-counter drug. France: None. Germany: Commission E approved as a drug.

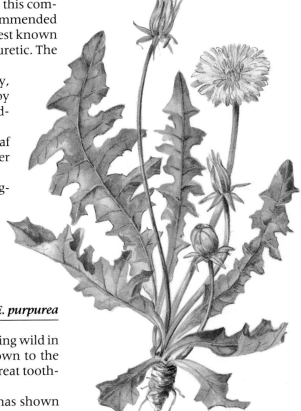

Dandelion

ELDER *Sambucus nigra*

□ **History and Uses.** Elder has a long and varied history. Archaeologists have traced its cultivation to Stone Age sites in Europe. Legends have associated this flowering shrub with witches and spirits, while folk practitioners have used it as an insect repellent, a purgative, and a blood purifier. Many people have at one time tasted elderberries in such foods as preserves and pies. Some may even have sampled a glass of homemade elderberry wine.

Today, elder flowers are brewed in tea, which is mainly prescribed as a mild stimulant and to induce perspiration. The tea is thought to be most effective when the elder flowers are mixed with peppermint leaves and yarrow flowers. In addition, elder extracts are included in a number of commercially available cold remedies. While elder flowers are safe, avoid the roots, stems, and leaves, and use only ripe berries.

☐ **Plant Parts and Active Compounds.** Flowers. Triterpenes, flavonoids.

☐ **Regulatory Status.** US: Generally Recognized as Safe. UK: General Sales List. Canada: Approved as an over-the-counter drug. France: Traditional Medicine. Germany: Commission E approved as an over-the-counter drug.

ELECAMPANE *Inula helenium*

☐ **History and Uses.** Known to the ancient Greeks and Romans, elecampane was among the many herbal preparations prescribed by Hippocrates. Its Latin name may be a reference to Helen of Troy, who in one version of the story is said to have been holding a bunch of elecampane when abducted by Paris.

Elecampane may help soothe itchy skin and minor cuts, and it has been used to induce perspiration in the case of cold or flu. However, the herb's real value is as an expectorant. Prescribed for chronic coughs and bronchitis, elecampane has also been recommended for the treatment of asthma. Researchers are taking a close look to see if the herb has a chemical compound that may be an antibiotic.

☐ **Plant Parts and Active Compounds.** Root. Inulin, a starch (up to 44%), volatile oil, and sesquiterpenes.

☐ **Regulatory Status.** US: Generally Recognized as Safe. UK: General Sales List. Canada: Approved as an over-the-counter drug. France: Traditional Medicine. Germany: None.

EUCALYPTUS *Eucalyptus globulus*

☐ **History and Uses.** The eucalyptus tree came to the Americas and other continents by way of Australia, where it's the mainstay of the koala's diet. You may already have experienced its healing properties. The leaves from the eucalyptus tree contain a pungent oil that helps clear sinuses and soothe mucus membranes. For this reason, it is a popular ingredient in throat lozenges, toothpastes, mouthwashes, and balms.

Bronchial congestion may be relieved by mixing a few drops of the oil with boiling water, and then inhaling the rising steam. When applied directly to the skin and scalp, eucalyptus oil is said to help ease sore muscles, chapped skin, and dandruff.

Warning: take care to avoid getting eucalyptus oil in the eyes, as it can be extremely irritating. If it happens, immediately rinse eyes with water.

☐ **Plant Parts and Active Compounds.** Leaf. Essential oil, primarily composed of eucalyptol.

☐ **Regulatory Status.** US: Generally Recognized as Safe. UK: General Sales List. Canada: Approved as an over-the-counter drug. France: Traditional Medicine. Germany: Commission E approved as an over-the-counter drug.

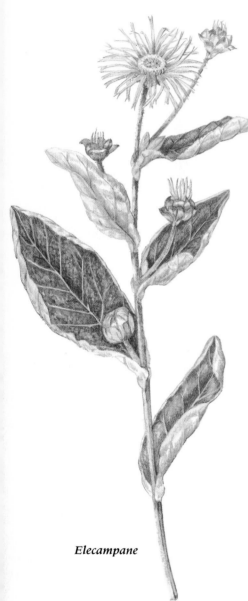

Elecampane

EVENING PRIMROSE *Oenothera biennis*

☐ **History and Uses.** This fragrant plant, which waits until early evening to open its flowers, has something of a reputation as a cure-all. Fans of evening primrose swear that it promotes weight loss, lowers blood cholesterol and blood pressure, and is effective in treating numerous other common ailments.

Evening primrose is native to North America and grows wild in fields, roadsides, and waste areas. Native Americans from the Great Lakes region used the entire evening primrose plant as a sedative and a painkiller. It has also been used to treat a variety of ills, from asthmatic coughs to stomach problems. Today oil from the seed is taken orally for atopic asthma (asthma due to allergy), atopic eczema, and migraines. Most recently, it has been claimed that the oil is effective in the treatment of premenstrual syndrome. Other research suggests that evening primrose oil may have anti-clotting factors, and so may be useful in the prevention of heart attacks that are caused by a blood clot blocking a blood vessel.

☐ **Plant Parts and Active Compounds.** Seed. Fatty oil containing the essential fatty acid GLA (gamma linolenic acid).

☐ **Regulatory Status.** US: None. UK: General Sales List. Canada: Approved as an over-the-counter drug. France: None. Germany: Approved for use as a food.

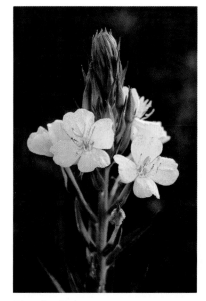

Evening Primrose

Eucalyptus

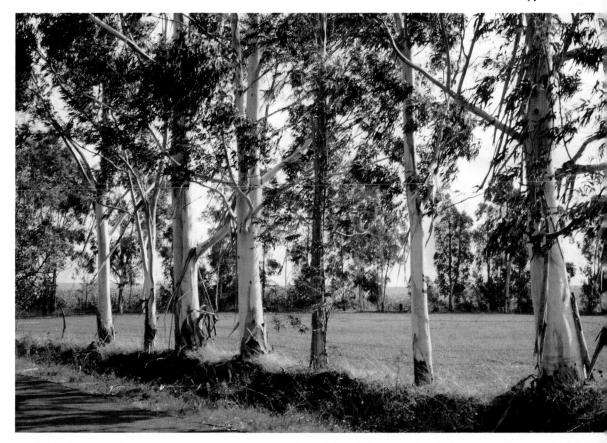

FENNEL *Foeniculum vulgare, or F. officinale*

□ **History and Uses.** Most people are only aware of fennel's use in salads, soups, and stews. Its licorice-like flavor was much in demand as early as the Middle Ages, but even before that, early practitioners, including Hippocrates, were prescribing parts of the plant to increase milk supply in lactating women. And others thought that fennel could provide protection against witches and all manner of spiritual intruders.

Today, fennel is primarily known for its soothing properties. A carminative, it is recommended to ease stomachaches and to aid digestion. Taken in a tea or in extracts, fennel has also been used as an aid to stimulate the appetites of anorexics.

□ **Plant Parts and Active Compounds.** Seed (actually the dried ripe fruit). Volatile oil (about 8% of the seed), consisting mainly of anethole.

□ **Regulatory Status.** US: Generally Recognized as Safe. UK: General Sales List. Canada: Approved as an over-the-counter drug. France: Traditional Medicine. Germany: Commission E approved as an over-the-counter drug. Japan: *Japanese Pharmacopoeia.*

Fennel

FENUGREEK *Trigonella foenum-graecum*

□ **History and Uses.** A prized healing herb in ancient Egypt, India, Greece, and Rome, fenugreek has at times been prescribed for tuberculosis, bronchitis, sore throats, diabetes, anemia, rickets, and waning sexual desire. It has also been used as an expectorant, a laxative, and a fever fighter.

While it is no longer considered a cure-all, fenugreek is known today for having some effective medicinal properties. The secret lies in the seeds, which contain mucilage, a slimy substance that soothes and protects sore or inflamed tissues. Poultices, ointments, and lotions containing fenugreek are recommended for treating skin irritations and wounds, while a tonic brewed from the seeds is said to ease stomach ailments.

□ **Plant Parts and Active Compounds.** Seed. Mucilage (up to 40%), oil.

□ **Regulatory Status.** US: Generally Recognized as Safe. UK: General Sales List. Canada: Approved as an over-the-counter drug. France: Traditional Medicine. Germany: Not yet Commission E approved.

FEVERFEW *Tanacetum parthenium*

□ **History and Uses.** One of the earliest references to feverfew was in the writings of the Greek herbalist Dioscorides. In the first century A.D., he recommended the herb for "all hot inflammations and hot swellings," which may have been a reference to arthritis. Feverfew was also used to treat menstrual cramps and headache pain, as well as to aid digestion, repel insects, and soothe insect bites. But the herb's popularity waned, even among dedicated herbalists.

Recent research is now restoring feverfew's reputation as a pain reliever. Studies of migraine sufferers indicate that feverfew is effective in reducing the number and severity of headaches, as well as alleviating the nausea and vomiting that often accompany them. In addition, some claims have been made about feverfew's effectiveness against rheumatoid arthritis, but these claims are as yet unproven.

The best way to get feverfew's benefits is by eating two or three of the fresh leaves daily. The leaves must be taken for a prolonged period, as it may take some time for the herb's medicinal properties to become effective. Eating feverfew leaves, either fresh or freeze-dried, has been shown to be safe, although no long-term studies have been conducted. The only adverse reactions appear to be temporary mouth ulcers in a small percentage of users.

□ **Plant Parts and Active Compounds.** Leaf. Parthenolide.

□ **Regulatory Status.** US: None. UK: General Sales List. Canada: Approved as an over-the-counter drug. France: None. Germany: Not yet Commission E approved.

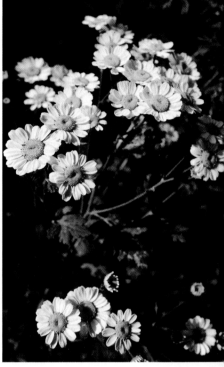

Feverfew

GARLIC *Allium sativum*

□ **History and Uses.** For centuries an amazing array of magical and medicinal powers has been attributed to garlic. It has been used for protection against vampires as well as to enhance sexual prowess. The Egyptians prescribed garlic to build up physical strength, while the Greeks used it as a laxative. Garlic is given some credit for providing immunity to those who ate it during the plague years in Europe. The Chinese have traditionally used it to lower elevated blood pressure.

Early in this century, garlic was used to treat tuberculosis, and as an antibiotic for battle wounds during World War II. Although today most people think of it as a culinary ingredient rather than a potent medicine, scientists have not totally ignored garlic's potential as a healing agent.

Louis Pasteur, the great 19th-century French chemist, was the first to prove garlic's antiseptic properties, and since then hundreds of studies have established the value of garlic as an effective destroyer of bacteria, fungi, viruses, and parasites. Modern-day antibiotics such as penicillin may have overshadowed garlic as a remedy; yet it is still regarded by many herbalists as an effective preventive for colds, flu, and other infectious diseases. Garlic is also used to treat some lower tract problems, such as gas pains and intestinal worms.

Recent research has also shown that garlic has great potential for treating cardiovascular conditions. Various controlled studies have shown that it can reduce cholesterol and triglyceride levels in blood. Experiments also indicate that garlic affects the blood in another important way—by reducing the blood's ability to clot. The herb's capacity to lower high blood pressure has also been proven in tests involving both laboratory animals and humans.

Scientific attention has also turned to garlic's potential as an anti-cancer agent. Experiments with animals suggest that garlic may inhibit or even reverse the growth of certain tumor cells. In another area of research, some studies involving the immune system indicate that garlic may stimulate immune functions by making "killer cells" more active against invading microbes, and perhaps cancer cells as well. But these results are preliminary, and much more work needs to be done before garlic can be recommended to prevent cancer.

Garlic is considered a safe herbal remedy. However, some people are allergic to garlic, and others may experience stomach or intestinal upset. No one is immune to garlic's distinctive odor, which lingers on the breath and the skin. In large amounts, garlic may have toxic effects, such as stomach ulcers and anemia.

□ **Plant Parts and Active Compounds.** Bulbs. Before a bulb of garlic is crushed or chopped it contains few medically active compounds. But once it is cut, chemical reactions occur that create dozens of new compounds. Two of the many newly formed sulfur-containing compounds are allicin, which gives garlic its antibiotic properties, and ajoene, which is an anticoagulant. Allicin is responsible for garlic's strong odor.

Many of garlic's medicinal compounds are destroyed through processing, some studies suggest, and so it may be best to use fresh garlic, and not dried or powdered forms. However, this point is controversial.

□ **Regulatory Status.** US: Generally Recognized as Safe. UK: General Sales List. Canada: Approved as an over-the-counter drug. France: Traditional Medicine. Germany: Commission E approved as an over-the-counter drug.

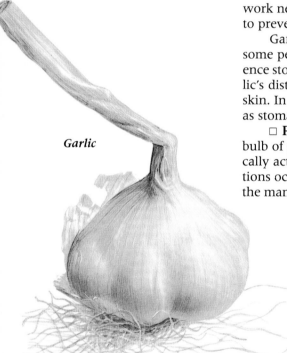

Garlic

GINGER Zingiber officinale

□ **History and Uses.** Known to most people as a food and a spice, ginger has been used medicinally for centuries. Practitioners of Chinese medicine discovered its healing properties at least 2500 years ago, and in China it remains popular for treating colds, nausea, seafood poisoning, and other ailments. But ginger was valued in Greece, India, and many other countries as well. For example, Tibetans used it to help those recuperating from illness and in Japan a ginger-oil massage was given to help alleviate spinal and joint problems.

Today, ginger tea is still prescribed for stomachaches and to aid digestion. A mild stimulant, it is also used to help promote circulation, especially on cold winter days. But current research has come up with some novel ways of using ginger. For instance, powdered ginger has been shown to be more effective for treating motion sickness than some well-known commercial remedies. One added benefit is that ginger does not cause drowsiness, as do many over-the-counter remedies.

A common folk remedy recommends ginger for the treatment of burns. Fresh gingerroot is mashed to release its juices, which are then applied to the burned area. Some who have tried the remedy report that relief is instantaneous, and that a single application will suffice for easing the pain of minor burns.

□ **Plant Parts and Active Compounds.** Rhizome (underground lateral root). Essential oils, gingerols, shogaols, zingerones (phenylalkylketones).

□ **Regulatory Status.** US: Generally Recognized as Safe. UK: General Sales List. Canada: Approved as an over-the-counter drug. France: None. Germany: Commission E approved as an over-the-counter drug. Japan: *Japanese Pharmacopoeia.*

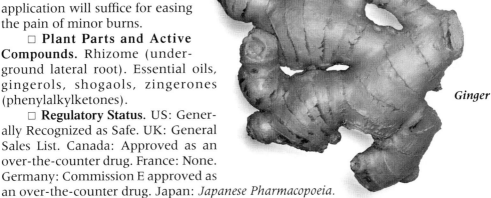

Ginger

GINKGO *Ginkgo biloba*

□ **History and Uses.** The oldest species of tree in the world, dating back some 200 million years, the ginkgo is native to the Far East. So it is not surprising that the Chinese have made the best use of the tree's healing properties. Practitioners of Chinese medicine have traditionally used the gingko's fan-shaped leaves to treat bronchial, asthmatic, and pulmonary conditions.

Today ginkgo is the subject of considerable study in Europe, but increasingly in the United States, too. It has been shown to dilate arteries, veins, and capillaries, thereby increasing peripheral circulation, as well as blood flow to the brain. For this reason, gingko may have potential for treating senility, short-term memory loss, tinnitus (ringing in the ears), and a range of vascular diseases. Ginkgo extracts are regularly prescribed in Asia and Europe to improve mental functions.

□ **Plant Parts and Active Compounds.** Leaf. Flavonoid glycosides and diterpenes (including some unique terpene structures called ginkgolides).

□ **Regulatory Status.** US: None. UK: None. Canada: None. France: Approved as an over-the-counter drug. Germany: Commission E approved as an over-the-counter drug.

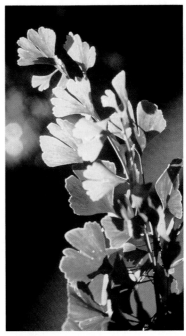

Ginkgo

GINSENG *Panax ginseng*

□ **History and Uses.** A Chinese text dating from the first century A.D. describes ginseng as "enlightening to the mind, and increasing the wisdom. Continuous use leads to longevity." This description of ginseng's powers is strikingly similar to claims made today. For instance, ginseng tea is often taken by people who believe it will promote long life and soften the effects of aging.

A subject of considerable scientific study around the world, ginseng has captured the interest of doctors, researchers, and herbalists alike. Ginseng is most commonly used as a tonic to enhance general health and stimulate the central nervous system. In tests to lower blood cholesterol, ginseng has shown positive results. It has not been proven to promote long life or cure old age, but it may have a slight positive effect on the cardiovascular system—and without the side effects of many drugs.

Other studies report that ginseng prevents heart disease, inhibits blood coagulation, and protects cells from radiation damage. The Chinese have long used ginseng as an aphrodisiac, but there are no studies lending support to this claim. With the herb receiving more and more clinical attention worldwide, ginseng may well be the source of important discoveries in future years.

Ginseng's reputation was tarnished by an uncontrolled study published in 1979 in the *Journal of the American Medical Association*. The article contained erroneous reports of ginseng producing high blood pressure, and irritability. This study has been discredited by reputable scientists. In general, thousands of years of ginseng usage attest to its safety when used in reasonable amounts.

□ **Plant Parts and Active Compounds.** Root. Saponins called ginsenosides.

□ **Regulatory Status.** US: Generally Recognized as Safe. UK: General Sales List. Canada: None. France: Traditional Medicine. Germany: Commission E approved as an over-the-counter drug. Japan: *Japanese Pharmacopoeia.*

GOLDENSEAL *Hydrastis canadensis*

□ **History and Uses.** Goldenseal root has a long history of use among Native Americans. The Cherokees, for example, used it for sore eyes, mouth ulcers, tuberculosis, and edema. They also mixed it with bear grease for use as an insect repellent. Settlers, too, learned of its antiseptic and wound-healing properties, and it was later included in a commercial tonic for gastric ailments.

Today, the herb is relatively rare and expensive, the result of both overzealous harvesting and drought. While goldenseal doesn't have the following that it once had, it is still recommended for some disorders. For instance, goldenseal root is reported to cleanse the liver and blood, as well as to restore digestive functions, and so is sometimes prescribed for alcoholics. In addition, in some circles it is a

Ginseng

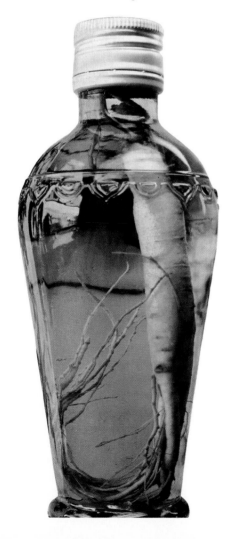

popular remedy for colds and flu. The tea, which is extremely bitter, is commonly recommended for mouth sores, including cracked, bleeding lips and cankers. When used as an eyewash, the tea may soothe the itchiness of certain allergies. In fact, a popular commercial eyedrop intended to reduce eye irritation contains berberine, a major alkaloid of goldenseal. It works by constricting blood vessels in the eyes.

The responsible use of goldenseal is considered safe in reasonable amounts. Though there is little real evidence of any adverse reactions, some herbalists caution against the use of the herb during pregnancy, as it may cause uterine contractions.

□ **Plant Parts and Uses.** Root and rhizome. Alkaloids hydrastine, berberine, canadine, and hydrastinine.

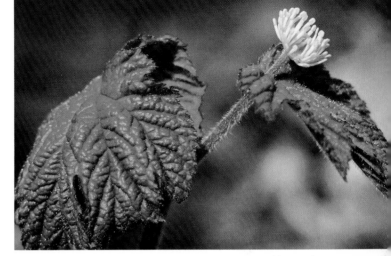

Goldenseal

□ **Regulatory Status.** US: Goldenseal was formerly listed as official in the pharmacopoeia of the United States from 1830-1840, and again from 1865 to 1936. It currently has no regulatory status. UK: General Sales List. Canada: Approved as an over-the-counter drug. France: *French Pharmacopoeia.* Germany: Not yet Commission E approved.

HAWTHORN *Crataegus oxyacantha*

□ **History and Uses.** A common tree in the English countryside, hawthorn has long been used in folk and clinical medicine to treat heart ailments. Experimental studies have determined that hawthorn works in two ways: it dilates blood vessels, which eases blood flow and lowers blood pressure, and it strengthens the heart itself. In Germany, physicians commonly prescribe preparations with hawthorn for minor heart conditions, especially those due to the effects of aging.

Hawthorn also acts as a mild sedative, so it may be useful when heart problems are brought on by stress or nervousness. However, hawthorn extracts are cumulative, so it must be taken over an extended period for the full effect. Hawthorn is considered a safe and effective medicine, but if you suspect that you have heart problems, see a physician before embarking on self-treatment.

□ **Plant Parts and Active Compounds.** Leaf, flowers, and fruit. Flavonoids.

□ **Regulatory Status.** US: No regulatory status. UK: Prescription drug. Canada: None. France: Traditional Medicine. Germany: Commission E approved as an over-the-counter drug.

HOPS *Humulus lupulus*

☐ **History and Uses.** A well-known soporific and flavoring, hops has been used for centuries by herbalists and brewmasters alike. Some Native Americans took the blossoms for their sedative effects, and also dried the flowers for use in a toothache remedy.

Today, hops is prescribed in cases of nervousness, mild anxiety, and sleeplessness. In addition, as an anti-spasmodic, it may ease diarrhea and intestinal cramps. Hops may be taken as a tea (often in combination with valerian and other sedative herbs), in extracts, or capsules, and its safety has been confirmed by centuries of use in brewing and as a food flavoring.

☐ **Plant Parts and Active Compounds.** Lupulin, a chemical complex found in the glandular hairs of the strobiles (flower cones). Volatile oil, flavonoids, resins including bitter acids.

☐ **Regulatory Status.** US: Generally Recognized as Safe. UK: General Sales List. Canada: Approved as an over-the-counter drug. France: Traditional Medicine. Germany: Commission E approved as an over-the-counter drug.

HORSE CHESTNUT *Aesculus hippocastanum*

☐ **History and Uses.** Native to Asia and southeastern Europe, horse chestnuts were long used by the Turks, not for their own ailments, but for their horses' respiratory problems. By the 18th century, horse chestnuts had been introduced to North America, and Native Americans began exploiting the fruits of these stately trees for human use. They discovered that when crushed, the fruits eased the pain and inflammation of hemorrhoids.

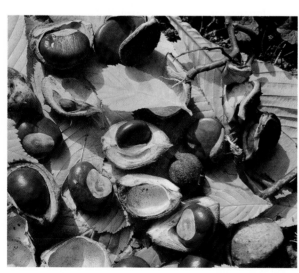

Horse Chestnut

Today, horse chestnuts are used in the treatment of a number of circulatory problems, including varicose veins, blood clots, and hemorrhoids. An extract sold commercially is popular in Europe for arthritis and other complaints—and there is some scientific evidence that horse chestnuts may indeed have anti-inflammatory properties. Horse chestnut extract is also available as a salve, which may be applied to ease sore muscles and leg cramps. These remedies are widely available in Germany and are just beginning to be marketed in the United States.

☐ **Plant Parts and Active Compounds.** Fruits. A mixture of saponins collectively called aescin.

☐ **Regulatory Status.** US: None. UK: General Sales List. Canada: None. France: Traditional Medicine. Germany: Commission E approved as an over-the-counter drug.

HYSSOP *Hyssopus officinalis*

□ **History and Uses.** A traditional herb used since biblical times, hyssop has long been popular for treating mild respiratory problems. In folk medicine, hyssop tea or gargle is taken as an expectorant, and also to relieve colds, coughs, hoarseness, and sore throats.

A member of the mint family, hyssop is a carminative, meaning that it aids digestion and helps to relieve gas. Some claim that it speeds the digestion of fat, and recommend drinking hyssop tea with fatty meats or fish. In addition, extracts of hyssop are used in liqueurs and candies.

Used externally, hyssop may be useful for treating sores. One caveat about this herb: it has been erroneously reported that hyssop leaves contain penicillin. They do not.

□ **Plant Parts and Active Compounds.** Herb. Volatile oil, hyssopin, tannin, flavone glycosides, a terpenoid called marrubin (also found in horehound).

□ **Regulatory Status.** US: Generally Recognized as Safe. UK: General Sales List. Canada: Approved as an over-the-counter drug. France: Traditional Medicine. Germany: None.

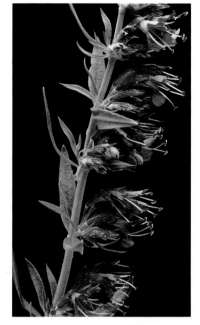

Hyssop

JUNIPER *Juniperus communis*

□ **History and Uses.** The juniper berry has many fans, though few are actually seeking its medicinal benefits. Best known as the flavoring in gin, sauerkraut, and other foods and spirits, the fragrant berries are also an active ingredient in many herbal formulas.

Native Americans drank juniper berry tea to relieve arthritis, stomachaches, and colds. While they are still taken for these ailments, juniper berries are primarily used for their diuretic action.

Experts caution against the use of juniper berries during pregnancy as they may stimulate uterine contractions. Because of their diuretic action, extended use (more than six weeks) may cause problems for people with weak or damaged kidneys.

□ **Plant Parts and Active Compounds.** Berry. Volatile oil, sugars, ascorbic acid, tannins, juniperin.

□ **Regulatory Status.** US: Generally Recognized as Safe. UK: General Sales List. Canada: Approved as an over-the-counter drug. France: Traditional Medicine. Germany: Commission E approved as an over-the-counter drug.

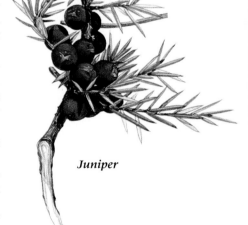

Juniper

LAVENDER *Lavandula officinalis*

□ **History and Uses.** Known as an herb of love in the Middle Ages, lavender's fragrant flowers continue to inspire devotion. The blossoms are a familiar ingredient in many herbal sachets, and lavender-filled pillows have long been used for their purported calming effects.

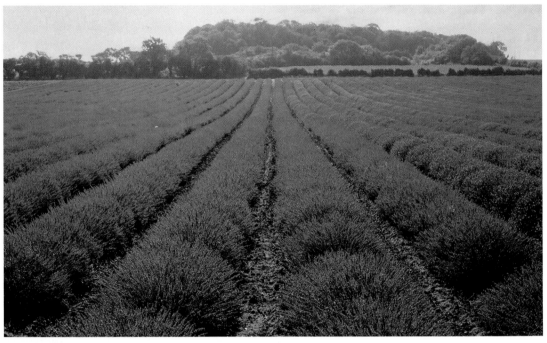

Lavender

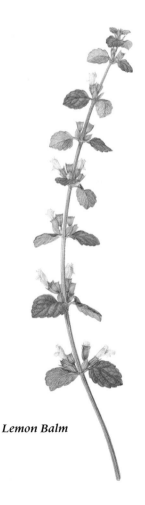

Lemon Balm

Lavender flowers may also be brewed in tea. The aroma is soothing, and the mild carminative action of the blossoms may be useful for settling an upset stomach that often accompanies nervousness and irritability. The flowers are also reported to stimulate bile flow, and so are sometimes included in herbal formulas recommended for liver and gall bladder problems.

□ **Plant Parts and Active Compounds.** Flowers. Volatile oil, tannins, coumarins, flavonoids.

□ **Regulatory Status.** US: Generally Recognized as Safe. UK: General Sales List. Canada: Approved as an over-the-counter drug. France: Traditional Medicine. Germany: Commission E approved as an over-the-counter drug.

LEMON BALM *Melissa officinalis*

□ **History and Uses.** Lemon balm has a long history of use, not only for its mild medicinal benefits, but also because of its pleasant lemony aroma. For instance, the Arabs relied on it to treat depression and anxiety, while the English included it in furniture polish.

Lemon balm is now widely used in herbal teas, both for its flavor and its mild carminative and sedative properties. The tea is recommended to induce perspiration and relieve fever due to colds and flu, and to ease menstrual cramps, insomnia, headaches, and nervousness.

□ **Plant Parts and Active Compounds.** Herb. Volatile oil and polyphenols.

□ **Regulatory Status.** US: Generally Recognized as Safe. UK: General Sales List. Canada: Approved as an over-the-counter drug. France: Traditional Medicine. Germany: Commission E approved as an over-the-counter drug.

LICORICE *Glycyrrhiza glabra* and *G. uralensis*

☐ **History and Uses.** Licorice is one of the world's most widely used medicinal plants. Many people think of it as a flavoring for candy, but in fact most "licorice" sticks sold in this country are flavored with anise oil. Licorice itself was used by the Egyptians, Romans, Greeks, and Chinese to treat coughs and chills, and research has shown that it does have expectorant, anti-allergic, and anti-inflammatory properties. In addition, licorice contains mucilage, a substance that coats and soothes inflamed membranes, and so may be useful for treating ulcers and constipation.

Today, licorice is the subject of much study, primarily for its active compound glycyrrhizin. This substance produces the herb's anti-inflammatory and anti-allergic effects. But there is also some evidence that licorice may be useful for preventing and healing gastric ulcers, and it may offer an effective treatment for chronic hepatitis. In addition, licorice extracts stimulate the adrenal glands, and so have been used for patients suffering from Addison's disease (adrenal insufficiency), a particular boon for those who are allergic to the conventional medication. Further studies, albeit on mice, have shown licorice to counter the effects of two tumor-producing agents. It may also suppress the enzyme that leads to tooth decay from sugar.

In general, licorice and its extracts are safe for normal use. However, long-term or excessive ingestion can produce serious side effects. Symptoms include headache, lethargy, sodium and water retention, loss of potassium, high blood pressure, and possible heart failure. Such reactions, however, are rare, a fact demonstrated by licorice's widespread use in herbal teas, and as a flavoring in foods and tobacco.

☐ **Plant Parts and Active Compounds.** Root and rhizome. Glycyrrhizin (an extremely sweet triterpene glycoside), flavonoids and isoflavonoids, coumarins, polysaccharides.

☐ **Regulatory Status.** US: Generally Recognized as Safe. UK: General Sales List. Canada: Approved as an over-the-counter drug. France: Traditional Medicine. Germany: Commission E approved as an over-the-counter drug. Japan: *Japanese Pharmacopoeia.*

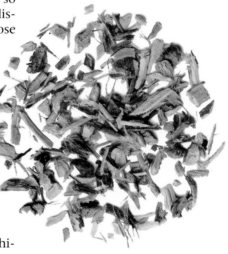

Licorice

MA HUANG *Ephedra sinica*

☐ **History and Uses.** For thousands of years, practitioners of Chinese medicine have relied on ma huang tea to treat asthma, flu, and even arthritis. In the early part of this century, Chinese scientists isolated two important alkaloids from the herb: ephedrine and pseudoephedrine. These alkaloids clear up mucus, open clogged breathing passages, and stimulate the central nervous system, and are now commonly used in many over-the-counter and prescription allergy and asthma medications.

Ma huang is considered safe in reasonable doses. However, because it can raise blood pressure, it is best avoided by those with high blood pressure.

An American cousin, mormon tea (*Ephera nevadensis)*, is similar to ma huang, but contains no ephedrine. The herb is found in the Southwest, and is used to treat arthritis pain.

□ **Plant Part and Active Compounds.** Herb. Ephedrine and pseudoephedrine.

□ **Regulatory Status.** US: Approved as an over-the-counter drug. UK: Pharmacy use only. Canada: Approved as an over-the-counter drug. Germany: Commission E approved as an over-the-counter drug. Japan: *Japanese Pharmacopoeia.*

MARSHMALLOW *Althaea officinalis*

□ **History and Uses.** No longer used in the puffy white candy that bears its name, marshmallow is known primarily for alleviating sore throats and other ailments. The roots of the marshmallow contain mucilage, a gelatinous substance found in plants. When mixed with water, marshmallow root helps soothe irritation and inflammation due to dry coughs, bronchitis, urinary tract infections, colitis, and other problems. When used as a gargle, marshmallow may provide instant relief to inflamed throat tissues. Marshmallow root may also be taken to ease constipation, and when applied topically, to soothe skin abrasions.

□ **Plant Parts and Active Compounds.** Root. Mucilage.

□ **Regulatory Status.** US: Generally Recognized as Safe. UK: General Sales List. Canada: Approved as an over-the-counter drug. France: Traditional Medicine. Germany: Commission E approved as an over-the-counter drug.

Marshmallow

MILK THISTLE *Silybum marianum*

□ **History and Uses.** Milk thistle has a long history of use in European folk medicine, and was frequently prescribed as a liver tonic and digestive aid. In addition, lactating women were sometimes given the herb to stimulate production of their milk. While this last use has been disproven, medical science has confirmed milk thistle's effectiveness in treating certain types of liver disease. Some studies have shown that extracts of the herb are beneficial for treating cirrhosis, hepatitis, and some other chronic liver problems.

Milk thistle's active ingredients are a complex of compounds known collectively as silymarin. These substances protect the liver against certain chemical toxins, and increase the function and regeneration of the organ. In addition, silybin, one of the compounds contained in the herb, is an antidote to the deadly deathcap mushroom, whose poison acts to destroy liver cells. But to be effective, the antidote should be administered intravenously.

□ **Plant Parts and Active Compounds.** Seed. The extract of the seed contains a complex of three flavolignans collectively referred to as silymarin.

□ **Regulatory Status.** US: None. UK: None. Canada: None. France: Traditional Medicine. Germany: Commission E approved as an over-the-counter drug.

MULLEIN *Verbascum thapsus*

□ **History and Uses.** People have long made use of the long-stemmed mullein to heal, to soothe, and even to protect. For instance, according to Homer, the Greek hero Ulysses used the herb to protect himself from the temptress Circe, and in other times it was used to counter the charms of witchcraft.

Less romanticized today, mullein, which contains mucilage, is used as an expectorant, as well as to soothe inflamed mucous membranes. Mullein is an old European remedy for chest conditions, and is still considered useful for treating sore throats, chest colds, and hoarseness. When applied topically, it may offer relief for burns, chilblains, and arthritic joints. Mullein also has astringent properties, and so is useful in healing open wounds. In earlier times, traditional herbalists soaked yellow mullein flowers in oil, which was then used to treat earaches.

□ **Plant Parts and Active Compounds.** Leaves. Mucilage.

□ **Regulatory Status.** US: Generally Recognized as Safe. UK: General Sales List. Canada: Approved as an over-the-counter drug. France: Traditional Medicine. Germany: None.

MYRRH *Commiphora molmol*

□ **History and Uses.** Prized since ancient times for its fragrance and healing properties, myrrh is perhaps best known for its frequent mention in the Bible. The most famous reference is Matthew 2:11, where myrrh is one of the gifts brought to the infant Jesus by the wise men. Later, Mark reported that before Jesus was crucified, he was offered a sedative consisting of a cup of wine laced with myrrh, which he refused. Finally, after his death, Jesus' body was prepared with large amounts of myrrh and aloe.

Today myrrh is still popular for its resinous scent, but herbalists have many other uses for it as well. The herb has astringent and antiseptic properties, meaning it is useful for cleansing and healing wounds, including bedsores. Myrrh is also a common ingredient in mouthwashes and gargles, and is prescribed for sore throats, gingivitis, and sore gums.

As in Bible times, myrrh is a popular incense, and it can also double as a mosquito repellent since the smell of burning myrrh drives these pests away.

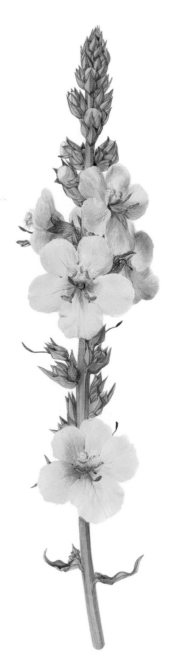

Mullein

□ **Plant Part and Active Compounds.** Gum resin. Volatile oil, resins, gums. Myrrh is used as a food flavoring.

□ **Regulatory Status.** US: Generally Recognized as Safe. UK: General Sales List. Canada: Approved as an over-the-counter drug. France: Traditional Medicine. Germany: Not yet Commission E approved.

NETTLE *Urtica dioica*

□ **History and Uses.** Brush against the leaves of the "stinging nettle," and you'll quickly discover the key to this herb's nickname. The bristly hairs covering the leaves are actually hollow tubes filled with an irritating liquid. When a person or animal brushes against the leaves, the hairs inject their fluid, producing an itchy, burning rash that may last for hours.

Nettle

But, while harvesting the plant may pose some problems, dried nettles have long been used by herbalists, mainly as a diuretic. In addition, nettles have astringent properties, and when applied to the skin they may relieve eczema and numerous other skin problems.

More controversial is their use for treating arthritic conditions. According to some users, when nettle leaves are allowed to sting the skin over sore joints, arthritic pain is eased instantly. Apparently, nettles act as counter irritants, relieving pain in the afflicted area. Although this usage has not been scientifically validated, it is still popular with some physicians in Germany. A recent study on freeze-dried nettles (in capsule form) indicated potential benefits for hay fever sufferers, but evidence was not overwhelmingly convincing.

Dried nettles are considered safe for internal consumption, but the skin rash produced by the fresh leaves may be very irritating to some people.

□ **Plant Part and Active Compounds.** Herb. Chlorophyll (large amounts), histamine, acetylcholine.

□ **Regulatory Status.** US: None. UK: General Sales List. Canada: Approved as an over-the-counter drug. France: Traditional Medicine. Germany: Commission E approved as an over-the-counter drug.

PASSION FLOWER *Passiflora incarnata*

□ **History and Uses.** Native Americans made poultices from the leaves of the passion flower, which they applied to bruises and other injuries. Today, the whole plant—leaves, stems, and intricate blossoms—is used medicinally.

Although the name suggests otherwise, passion flowers have been found to have mild sedative effects. For reasons not yet fully understood, the plant depresses the central nervous system. For this reason, when taken in tea, capsules, or extracts, passion flowers may be useful for treating insomnia and nervousness, and for lowering high blood pressure.

Passion flowers are usually combined with other sedative herbs in mixtures prescribed for a variety of nervous conditions. In addition, the plant has anti-inflammatory properties, which may make it useful in the treatment of arthritis.

□ **Plant Parts and Active Compounds.** Entire herb (flower, stem, leaf). Flavonoids and an alkaloid.

□ **Regulatory Status.** US: Generally Recognized as Safe. UK: General Sales List. Canada: Approved as an over-the-counter drug. France: None. Germany: Commission E approved as an over-the-counter drug.

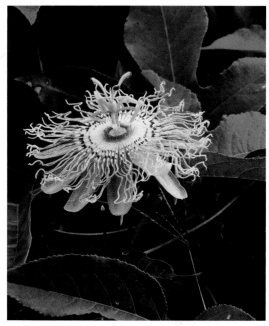

Passion Flower

PEPPERMINT *Mentha piperita*

□ **History and Uses.** The Greeks may have crowned their heroes with wreathes of laurel, but they relied on peppermint for curing their ailments. One of the oldest of all medicinal herbs, peppermint was used for everything from hiccups to "sea serpent" stings. The Greeks were not alone in recognizing this aromatic plant's many virtues. In medieval times, many people depended on its aroma to rid their houses of vermin and noxious odors, and some suggested mixing peppermint leaves with salt as a treatment for dog bites and rabies.

Today, peppermint is better known for its soothing effects on the stomach. An anti-spasmodic and a carminative, the herb is useful for relieving indigestion, nausea, and intestinal gas. In addition, peppermint tea is recommended for headaches, as a mild sedative, and even to treat some upper respiratory conditions. Applied externally, oil of peppermint may help relieve muscle and nerve pain. To ease bronchial symptoms, some herbalists recommend putting a few drops of the oil into boiling water, and inhaling the menthol fragrance.

Peppermint tea is considered to be quite safe when consumed in normal quantities. The concentrated oil should be used sparingly, with internal use being limited to just a few drops.

□ **Plant Parts and Active Compounds.** Leaf and distilled oil. Menthol.

□ **Regulatory Status.** US: Generally Recognized as Safe. UK: General Sales List. Canada: Approved as an over-the-counter drug. France: Traditional Medicine. Germany: Commission E approved as an over-the-counter drug. Japan: *Japanese Pharmacopoeia.*

PSYLLIUM *Plantago ovata* **and** *P. major*

□ **History and Uses.** Called the "mother of herbs" in an old Anglo-Saxon poem, the leaves of this hardy roadside plant have long been used to soothe minor bites and stings. They were also applied to blisters, and their astringent properties were said to stop bleeding. In the New World, Native Americans used psyllium leaves to treat abrasions, sprains, gout, and as a wash for sore eyes.

Today, psyllium is practically a household word. However, it is prized not for its leaves, but for its tiny seeds. The seeds are coated with mucilage, a gelatinous material that swells upon contact with moisture. For this reason, psyllium seeds and their husks are a popular bulk laxative, one that is especially useful for cases of chronic constipation.

Psyllium is but one member of the large plantain family, and the leaves of several related species are still used for minor insect stings and bites.

□ **Plant Parts and Active Compounds.** Seed, seed husks, and leaves. Mucilage (10 to 30 percent), primarily in the seed husk.

□ **Regulatory Status.** US: Approved as an over-the-counter drug. UK: General Sales List. Canada: Approved as an over-the-counter drug. France: Traditional Medicine. Germany: Commission E approved as an over-the-counter drug. Japan: *Japanese Pharmacopoeia.*

ROSEMARY *Rosmarinus officinalis*

□ **History and Uses.** A well-known culinary herb, rosemary also has a long history of medicinal use. European herbal practitioners used it as a tonic and stimulant, as well as to treat stomach upset, digestive disorders, and headaches. The richly scented camphor oil in its leaves is said to invigorate the circulatory and nervous systems, and so rosemary is frequently given to older people and those recovering from illness. Rosemary hair tonic is sometimes recommended for preventing baldness, but there is little hard evidence in support of this usage. As with most culinary herbs and spices, rosemary is considered safe when used in reasonable amounts.

□ **Plant Part and Active Compounds.** Leaves. Volatile oil containing camphor and other compounds, flavonoids, phenolic acids.

□ **Regulatory Status.** US: Generally Recognized as Safe. UK: General Sales List. Canada: Approved as an over-the-counter drug. France: Traditional Medicine. Germany: Commission E approved as an over-the-counter drug.

SAGE *Salvia officinalis*

□ **History and Uses.** The powdery-green leaves of the sage plant have, at one time or another, been offered as a cure for just about everything. In the Middle Ages, the herb

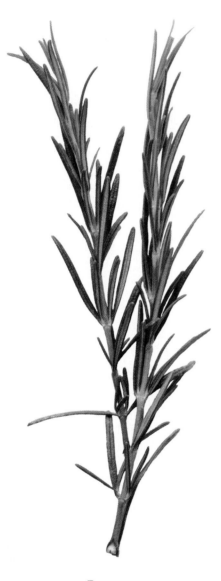

Rosemary

was popular for colds, fevers, epilepsy, and constipation, while Native Americans used it to heal sores and to clean their teeth.

Today, sage is best known for its astringent and drying properties, and is especially useful for easing cold symptoms. When used as a mouth rinse or gargle, sage may help to alleviate the irritation of cankers and sore throats.

As with most herbs, sage should not be taken during pregnancy (except as flavoring in foods). Professionals caution that prolonged use of sage oil or extract may result in convulsions. Herbalists contend that excessive use of sage tea can reduce milk output in lactating women, but this has not been confirmed by scientific studies.

☐ **Plant Part and Active Compounds.** Leaves. The oil contains thujone, cineol, and camphor.

☐ **Regulatory Status.** US: Generally Recognized as Safe. UK: General Sales List. Canada: Approved as an over-the-counter drug. Germany: Commission E approved as an over-the-counter drug.

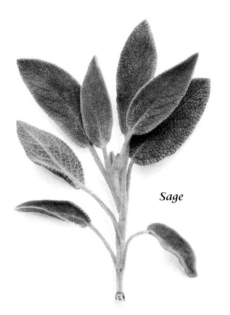

Sage

SAW PALMETTO *Sabal serrulata/Serenoa repens*

☐ **History and Uses.** Saw palmetto is a popular remedy for urinary tract disorders, particularly in males. It is often said that any man who lives long enough will suffer from prostate problems. This nagging disorder makes one of the most basic of human functions, urination, difficult. Some studies suggest that saw palmetto berries and extracts may ease prostate symptoms. In Germany, saw palmetto extracts are also used to treat obstructions of the bladder. The berries and extract are considered safe, and produce no adverse side effects.

☐ **Plant Part and Active Compounds**. Fruit. Essential and fixed oils, a liposterolic compound, and high molecular weight polysaccharides.

☐ **Regulatory Status.** US: None. UK: General Sales List. Canada: Approved as an over-the-counter drug. Germany: Commission E approved as an over-the-counter drug.

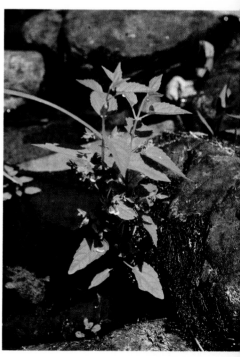

SCULLCAP *Scutellaria lateriflora*

☐ **History and Uses.** Scullcap, a sedative herb, has traditionally been used to treat hysteria, nervousness, and as an anti-spasmodic for muscle spasms and tension. In the 19th century it gained a reputation as a rabies cure, and was dubbed "Mad Dog" scullcap. Indeed, it was effective in easing the muscle spasms associated with the disease, but it did not produce a cure.

Today, scullcap is widely used in herbal formulas (often in combination with other calming herbs such as hops and valerian) prescribed to treat a range of problems, including mild anxiety and epilepsy. It is considered safe in reasonable amounts.

Scullcap

☐ **Plant Part and Active Compounds**. Entire plant. Mainly scutellarin, a flavonoid, iridoids, tannins, and volatile oil.

☐ **Regulatory Status**. US: None. UK: General Sales List. Canada: Approved as an over-the-counter drug. France: None. Germany: None. Japan: *Japanese Pharmacopoeia*.

SENNA *Cassia angustifolia and C. senna*

☐ **History and Uses**. Common along the banks of the Nile in Egypt and Sudan, senna leaves and pods found early use in Arab medicine as safe and effective laxatives. Today, the plant is still widely recognized for these same properties, although the pods are considered to have milder action than the leaves.

The use of senna is generally considered safe. However, as with any stimulant laxative, long-term usage may produce dependency. Consumers should exercise moderation when using senna, as too much may cause nausea and severe stomach upset. Also, as with most stimulant laxatives, senna is best avoided during pregnancy.

☐ **Plant Parts and Active Compounds**. Leaf and fruit. Anthraquinone glycosides known as sennosides A and B, and aloe emodin.

☐ **Regulatory Status**. US: Generally Recognized as Safe; an over-the-counter drug. UK: General Sales List. Canada: Approved as an over-the-counter drug. Germany: Commission E approved as over-the-counter drug. Japan: *Japanese Pharmacopoeia*.

SHEPHERD'S PURSE *Capsella bursa-pastoris*

☐ **History and Uses**. Named for its pouch-shaped seed pods, herbalists have traditionally recommended shepherd's purse to stem internal and external bleeding. However, some researchers believe it may be a white fungus often found growing on the plant that has the remarkable anti-hemorrhagic properties.

Shepherd's purse has also been used for urinary tract infections and to lower fevers.

☐ **Plant Part and Active Compounds**. Herb. Flavonoids, polypeptides.

☐ **Regulatory Status**. US: None. UK: General Sales List. Canada: Approved as an over-the-counter drug. France: Traditional Medicine. Germany: Commission E approved as an over-the-counter drug.

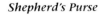

Shepherd's Purse

SLIPPERY ELM *Ulmus fulva*

☐ **History and Uses**. Native Americans used slippery elm as a salve for skin injuries, such as burns and chapped lips. And, in fact, their remedy has been shown to have validity. The bark of the elm contains mucilage, a gelatinous substance that swells in water. When applied to wounds, or when taken internally, the mucilage coats the injured area, bringing soothing relief.

Today, slippery elm is often used in lozenges to ease sore throat pain and smoker's cough. In addition, a powdered form of the bark is useful for treating burns, boils, and minor wounds. Slippery elm is considered non-toxic and safe for external and internal usage.

☐ **Plant Part and Active Compounds.** Bark. Mucilage.

☐ **Regulatory Status.** US: None. UK: General Sales List. Canada: Approved as an over-the-counter drug. France: None. Germany: None.

ST. JOHN'S WORT *Hypericum perforatum*

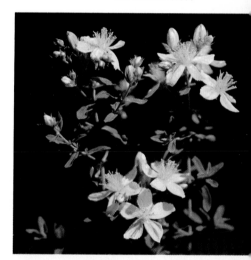

St. John's Wort

☐ **History and Uses.** Traditionally used to drive off demons and evil spirits, St. John's wort has recently shown promise against a more tangible enemy: viruses. In fact, the plant is being tested as a possible treatment for HIV infection, the deadly virus that attacks the immune system. Hypericin, a pigment in the plant, has been shown in experiments to have anti-HIV activity.

Beyond these novel uses, St. John's wort has anti-anxiety, anti-inflammatory, and sedative properties, and has been useful for treating a range of ailments, from depression and bed-wetting, to colds and arthritis. Used topically in a salve, the herb may be applied to open wounds, and it does seem to promote healing.

St. John's wort is relatively safe for human use. However, hypericin, the plant's red pigment, causes photosensitivity (supersensitivity to the sun's rays) in livestock that graze large quantities of the herb. For this reason, in the 1970s it was deemed unsafe by the FDA, although it still enjoyed widespread use in Europe. While the FDA has not totally rescinded its classification of St. John's wort, the consensus of opinion holds that the herb is safe for human use, as long as quantities ingested do not approach those of cows and sheep grazing on the open range.

☐ **Plant Parts and Active Compounds.** All above-ground parts of the herb. Hypericin and essential oil.

☐ **Regulatory Status.** US: Generally Recognized as Safe as a flavoring. UK: General Sales List. Canada: Approved as an over-the-counter drug. France: Traditional Medicine. Germany: Commission E approved as an over-the-counter drug.

THYME *Thymus vulgaris*

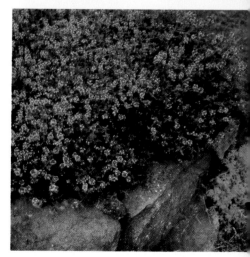

Thyme

☐ **History and Uses.** Thyme is considered by herbalists as one of nature's most powerful antiseptics. Its active ingredient, thymol, is germicidal, and has found wide use in toothpastes and mouthwashes, as well as some topical ointments. Thymol is also an expectorant and cough suppressant, and is a common ingredient in syrups prescribed for coughs and bronchitis.

The herb itself may be brewed in tea, and some herbalists recommend it as an excellent gargle for sore throats and tonsillitis. In addition, thyme's carminative properties make it a good choice for upset stomach, although the taste is a little strong for many people.

☐ **Plant Part and Active Compounds.** Leaves. Thymol.

☐ **Regulatory Status.** US: Generally Recognized as Safe. UK: General Sales List. Canada: Approved as an over-the-counter drug. France: Traditional Medicine. Germany: Commission E approved as an over-the-counter drug.

TURMERIC *Curcuma longa*

☐ **History and Uses.** Primarily used as a spice, turmeric lends its fragrance and flavor to many Indian curries. But it has also enjoyed long use for its purported health benefits. In India, an extract of turmeric is sold as an eyewash for conjunctivitis. In addition, traditional Chinese and Ayurvedic practitioners combine turmeric with other herbs to relieve gas, liver problems, toothaches, sores, and a number of other conditions.

Some research seems to confirm turmeric's use for protecting the liver. There is also evidence that the ingestion of the active compound curcumin may protect the liver by increasing bile secretion, which aids in the digestion of fats.

☐ **Plant Part and Active Compounds.** Rhizome (underground stem). Volatile oil, curcumin.

☐ **Regulatory Status.** US: Generally Recognized as Safe. UK: General Sales List. Canada: Approved as an over-the-counter drug. France: Traditional Medicine. Germany: Commission E approved as an over-the-counter drug.

UVA URSI *Arctostaphylos uva-ursi*

☐ **History and Uses.** Also known as bearberry, the leaves of this evergreen shrub have been used for centuries to treat a range of ailments. Native Americans mixed it with tobacco leaves and smoked it, and made a poultice of the leaves for use on sprains and sore muscles. But mainly uva ursi has been regarded as a diuretic.

Its real value lies in its antiseptic activity in the urinary tract, but only under alkaline conditions. Uva ursi teas, capsules, and extracts are useful for treating inflammations of the tract, as well as cystitis. The leaves also contain a fair amount of tannin, and taken over time may irritate the stomach. Some people tolerate uva ursi more easily by adding an equal amount of peppermint leaves to the mixture. Uva ursi is safe for short-term use, but should be avoided during pregnancy.

☐ **Plant Part and Active Compound.** Leaves. Arbutin.

☐ **Regulatory Status.** US: None. UK: General Sales

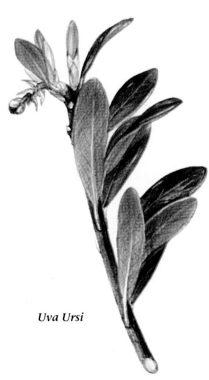

Uva Ursi

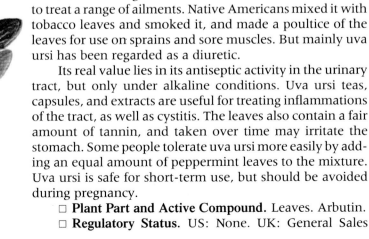

List. Canada: None. France: Traditional Medicine. Germany: Commission E approved as an over-the-counter drug. Japan: *Japanese Pharmacopoeia.*

VALERIAN *Valeriana officinals*

□ **History and Uses.** A popular and reliable sleep aid, valerian has not always been used for its sedative properties. In ancient Greece it was prescribed for digestive problems, nausea, and urinary tract disorders, while Native Americans relied on another species of valerian for treating cuts and wounds.

However, recent research has lent support to valerian's use as a sedative. Studies have indicated that active ingredients in the plant's pungent root both depress the central nervous system and relax smooth muscle tissue (involuntary muscles, such as those that control the intestines and the blood vessels).

In controlled tests, the herb has been shown to lessen the time needed to fall asleep, and it also produces a deep, satisfying rest, similar to that of many commercial sleep aids. In addition, valerian doesn't cause "sleep hangovers" the next morning, nor does it produce dependency as some prescription sleeping pills can.

But valerian is not just useful for inducing sleep. It has also been found effective for calming nervous stomachs, and may be taken during the day to relieve symptoms of stress.

Tinctures and capsules are widely available, and are especially popular in Europe. But valerian is also effective in other forms, including teas and liquid extracts—although many people are put off by valerian's strong smell.

Cats, on the other hand, are wildly attracted to the pungent roots of valerian, which contain a chemical similar to one that may be found in catnip.

Valerian is generally considered safe, but, like most other medicinal herbs, should not be used to treat infants. In addition, pregnant women should consult their obstetricians before using valerian or any other herbals.

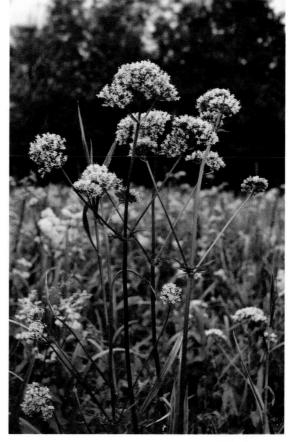

Valerian

□ **Plant Part and Active Compounds.** Root. Essential oil, valerenic acid, and chemically unstable compounds called valepotriates.

□ **Regulatory Status.** US: Generally Recognized as Safe. UK: General Sales List. Canada: Approved as an over-the-counter drug. Germany: Commission E approved as an over-the-counter drug. Japan: *Japanese Pharmacopoeia.*

WINTERGREEN *Gaultheria procumbens*

☐ **History and Uses.** Once a popular flavoring in candies and gum, wintergreen has also enjoyed long use as an herbal remedy. Native Americans, including the Sioux, Penobscot, and Nez Percé nations, among others, used wintergreen tea to treat arthritis pain and sore muscles. Later, the settlers used the leaves of the herb for similiar purposes, as well as to alleviate headaches and colds.

In the 1800s pharmacologists discovered that the plant's essential oil is composed of approximately 90 percent methyl salicylate, a chemical closely related to aspirin. It's the oil that gives wintergreen its anti-inflammatory, mildly analgesic properties. Today, wintergreen is widely used in over-the-counter balms and ointments for the temporary relief of arthritis pain, sciatica, and muscle pain. In addition, when brewed in tea, wintergreen is sometimes used as a diuretic.

Wintergreen tea is considered safe in reasonable amounts. When applied to the skin, oil of wintergreen preparations are also considered safe, although they may cause skin irritation. Taken internally, oil of wintergreen is poisonous, except in very small amounts. Artificial flavorings have now replaced the natural oil in most "wintergreen" sweets.

☐ **Plant Parts and Active Compounds.** Leaves. Essential oil (approximately 90% methyl salicylate).

☐ **Regulatory Status.** US: Generally Recognized as Safe; an over-the-counter drug. UK: General Sales List. Canada: Approved as an over-the-counter drug. Germany: Commission E approved as an over-the-counter drug.

WITCH HAZEL *Hamamelis virginiana*

☐ **History and Uses.** The leaves and bark of this flowering shrub have long been used in traditional medicine, and the plant's forked branches are often the material of choice for divining rods. While witch hazel's effectiveness for dowsing is dubious, the astringency of the leaves and bark (due to the high tannin content) does make the plant a reasonable choice for treating various skin conditions.

Today, witch hazel is a common ingredient in a soothing lotion bearing its name, as well as in commercially available eye drops, aftershave lotions, and cosmetics. In addition, witch hazel preparations have been found to be effective for treating hemorrhoids. When used externally, witch hazel has no adverse side effects.

☐ **Plant Part and Active Compounds.** Leaves. Tannins.

☐ **Regulatory Status.** US: Approved as an over-the-counter drug. UK: General Sales List. Canada: Approved as an over-the-counter drug. France: Traditional Medicine. Germany: Commission E approved as an over-the-counter drug.

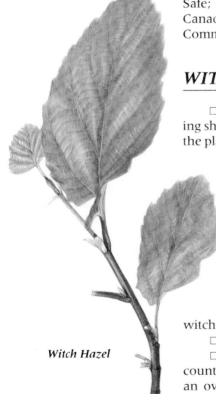

Witch Hazel

YARROW *Achillea millefolium*

□ **History and Uses.** A fragrant, flowering plant that is popular in potpourris and herbal preparations, yarrow is said to have been used by the Greek hero Achilles (hence its genus name) to stop the bleeding of his warriors' wounds. Native Americans and colonists also used yarrow for its healing properties, both as a tea to treat digestive disorders and fevers, and as a poultice to treat cuts and burns. They also chewed the leaves to relieve toothache pain.

Modern medicine has not confirmed yarrow's use as a blood coagulant, but recent research seems to demonstrate its value as an anti-spasmodic. Yarrow's astringent action is also useful in cases of diarrhea and dysentery. In addition, the herb has been used as an anti-inflammatory (to treat arthritis), a diuretic, and as an antiseptic.

Some herbalists recommend steeping an infusion of yarrow leaves and flower tops, which is drunk to reduce fever or to stimulate appetite. A poultice made from the flowers or the whole plant may be applied to swollen joints, as well as to cuts and wounds.

While yarrow use is considered safe, it should not be taken by pregnant women.

□ **Plant Part and Active Compounds.** Flowers. Volatile oil, sesquiterpene lactones, flavonoids.

□ **Regulatory Status.** US: None. UK: General Sales List. Canada: Approved as an over-the-counter drug. France: Traditional Medicine. Germany: Commission E approved as an over-the-counter drug. ❑

Yarrow

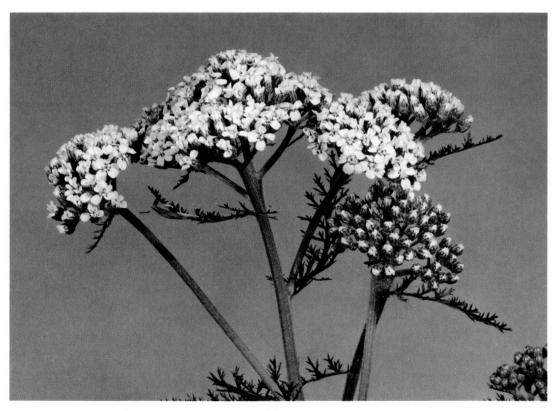

Aromatherapy: Soothing Scents

Concentrated oils from flowers, fruits, and other parts of plants form the basis of aromatherapy. These fragrant extracts are used to relax, stimulate, and relieve pain.

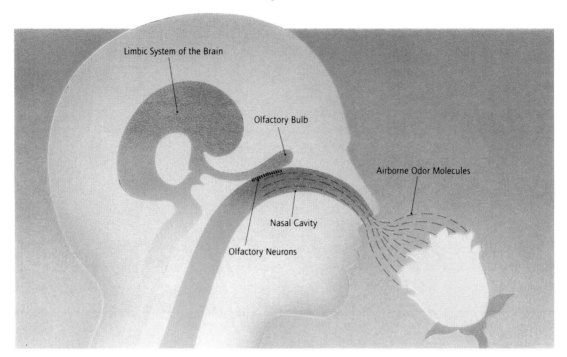

Limbic System of the Brain

Olfactory Bulb

Airborne Odor Molecules

Nasal Cavity

Olfactory Neurons

*As **airborne odor** molecules are drawn into the nasal passage, they strike nerve cells, or olfactory neurons. Nerve impulses are transmitted to a pair of olfactory bulbs that connect with the limbic system, which is the seat of memory and emotion. Thus, we very rapidly become aware of scents. Often certain ones, such as cooking smells or a familiar perfume, stir the emotions.*

IN MOST PEOPLE, THE SENSE OF SMELL is the most acute of the five senses—by one estimate, it is 10,000 times more sensitive than any of the other senses. As we breathe in, odor-bearing molecules activate receptors in the nasal cavity; these translate into nerve impulses, which rapidly reach the olfactory bulbs in the brain. These bulbs are directly connected to the limbic system, which is the seat of memory, emotions, and sexual arousal. Scientists have established that scent does, indeed, provide a potent link to memory and emotion. Just one whiff of a substance laden with childhood associations—such as the cooking smells of your mother's kitchen or the aroma of your grandfather's pipe tobacco—can vividly recreate an entire world.

Soothing Scents. Long before science came to examine the sense of smell, people tried to harness the elusive properties of fragrances in incense and other burnt offerings, as well as perfumes. But can scents actually heal? Scientific explanations are scanty, but proponents of aromatherapy claim that certain scents can ease physical maladies like headaches, as well as emotional conditions like nervousness and irritability.

Aromatherapists use some 40 highly concentrated aromatic oils, each of which is designed to treat specific ailments. These so-called essential oils are derived from the roots, flowers, leaves, bark, wood, and resin of plants, trees, and herbs, as well as the rinds of lemons and oranges. They are often combined with carrier oils like soy, almond, and evening primrose oils, or diluted in alcoholic solutions.

Most often the oils are inhaled, applied during a massage, or added to a bath. Inhaling a bowl of steaming water that contains a few drops of cinnamon and other oils may help clear up congested nasal passages. A combination of eucalyptus, thyme, pine, and lavender oils is said to ease sinusitis and bronchitis when inhaled several times a day.

The skin absorbs oils relatively quickly, so arthritis sufferers may be advised to suffuse their baths with juniper oil to ease their aching joints. Another common prescription is a rosemary and olive oil rub to ease muscle pain.

When using essential oils in self-care, it is important not to exceed the recommended amount. The oils are very potent—some may be up to 100 times more concentrated than dried versions of the same substances—and can be poisonous in anything above minuscule amounts. Some people take essential oils in capsules, in honey-flavored water, or in other forms, but this practice is not recommended due to questions of safety. Essential oils should be taken internally with caution and only as directed by a knowledgeable practitioner.

A Fragrant Export. Aromatherapy may be fairly new in the United States, but its use has been long established in Europe. In France, pharmacies sell aromatic oils, and health insurance plans cover prescriptions for them. A French chemist, René Gattefossé, is considered the father of modern aromatherapy. Nearly a century ago, when Gattefossé burned his hand while working in his laboratory, he plunged the hand into a container of lavender oil. According to Gattefossé, his wound healed quickly, without scarring or infection. During World War I, a French army physician used essential oils to treat burns and other combat injuries suffered by soldiers.

Today, researchers at a New York hospital are investigating whether fragrances can help relax patients who feel claustrophobic when they are undergoing certain diagnostic procedures. One psychologist reports that he has reduced anxiety in such patients by pumping the smell of vanilla into the procedure room.

In another arena, a professor of medical psychology has been studying whether pumping pleasant aromas into subway tunnels can lower the incidence of violent crimes. And in Japan, researchers are studying how various fragrances affect worker productivity.

While it is not clear how scents work to ease anxiety or increase productivity, some offer non-Western rationales for the treatment. For instance, proponents say that the oils carry a plant's vital energy, which raises the user's vital energy. ❏

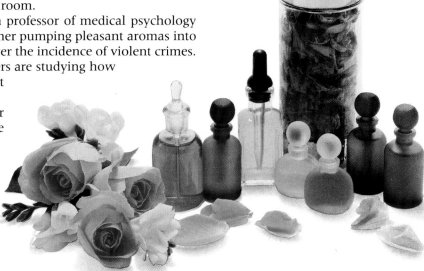

Petals, leaves, roots, and other plant parts contribute their oils to scents that relax or invigorate. Some aromatic oils may ease such ailments as headaches and bronchitis.

Bach Flower Remedies

Concocted from a variety of plants, Dr. Edward Bach's remedies aim to ease the inner conflicts that, in his view, produce illness. While his methods were intuitive, some of his ideas have proven quite sound.

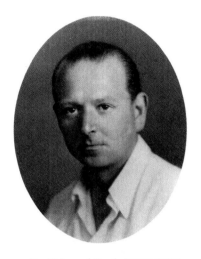

Dr. Edward Bach (1886-1936) used heat and sunlight to prepare his famous flower remedies. With some of the plants, he placed their flowers in glass bowls filled with pure spring water and left them sitting in the sun for three hours. At the end of this process, the flowers were discarded and the water was preserved in brandy, known as the Mother Tincture. Another method involved boiling the twigs, catkins, or flowers of the healing plant in pure spring water for half an hour before preserving the water in brandy. Today, the remedies are still prepared using these precise methods.

"TREAT THE PATIENT and not his disease," observed Dr. Edward Bach, a British physician who invented an unconventional system of therapy using flower-based remedies. Although trained in bacteriology and pathology, Bach found himself rejecting orthodox medicine's use of drugs for treating the symptoms of illness. Instead, he embraced homeopathy, an alternative healing method whose practitioners take into account a patient's personality and lifestyle when choosing a course of treatment.

A Sixth Sense. After serving for several years as a physician in a homeopathic hospital in London, Bach decided to abandon homeopathy and pursue his interest in plant-based remedies. Bach was convinced that negative emotions predispose people to illness and create roadblocks to healing. He suspected that certain flowers could encourage a sunnier outlook, and so dissipate the negative feelings that are preventing the body from healing itself. In the early 1930s he left the city for rural Wales, where he began studying the local wildflowers.

Forsaking his scientific training, Bach wandered through the countryside of England and Wales, using his intuition as a guide. If he was worried, fearful, or suffering from other negative feelings, he would hold his hand over various plants, and try to sense which species of flower was most effective in alleviating his concerns.

Over time, Bach identified 38 healing plants, which corresponded, one to one, with his classification of negative human emotions. He further refined the categories, arranging the 38 into seven groups, each representing a mental state that could, according to his theory, contribute to sickness and interfere with healing: apathy, fear, uncertainty, loneliness, oversensitivity, despair, and overconcern for the welfare of others.

Just how common plants can vanquish such emotions as envy, fear, anger, and anxiety is unknown. Bach conducted extensive research into these matters, but he failed to convince many of his medical peers. Yet for more than a half-century, enthusiastic patients have used these remedies, confident that they will be effective.

Choosing a Remedy. Perhaps the most appealing aspect of the Bach flower remedies is that they are based on a heart-felt concern for the emotional issues that are a part of all of our lives. For example, white chestnut is intended to calm those who can't let go of a problem, turning it over obsessively in their minds. These people might be prone to insomnia or headaches. Gentian can aid those who are depressed for a particular reason, Bach asserted, but mustard is the appropriate remedy for those whose black moods or feelings of despair come on with no apparent cause.

Today, Bach remedies are precisely prepared according to his original recipes, using the same species of flowers, trees, and grasses. Parts of plants are either boiled or immersed in spring water and exposed to sunlight for several hours. Afterward, the plants are discarded and the water is preserved in brandy.

The user chooses an appropriate remedy based on Bach's classification of negative emotions. To take a dose, the user puts a few drops of the remedy in a beverage, or places it directly under the tongue, four times a day until the symptoms disappear (usually one to 12 weeks, according to proponents, although minor ailments may respond much more quickly).

Bach remedies, taken singly or in combination, are available without a prescription. Many people rely on them because they are non-toxic and virtually free of side effects. The remedies are sold at some health-food stores and pharmacies, and by mail order from distributors who import the floral essences from England (many of the plant species are found only in Great Britain). Probably the best known is the Rescue Remedy, which is composed of five of the 38 remedies. Sometimes referred to as an emergency remedy, it is used mainly for treating the emotional effects of sudden trauma (brought on by bad news, for example), as well as episodes of panic, anxiety, or dread.

Recognizing how well a remedy has worked is as simple as it is subjective. When you experience a resurgence of such positive emotions as joy, self-confidence, and courage, you know that you have achieved the desired result.

Current Trends. Although Bach rejected science, it is science that is now lending credence to some of his ideas about the nature of disease. In the past few years, scientists in the fledgling field of psychoneuroimmunology have begun to trace the complex hormonal, neurological, and immunological functions that link emotions and health.

Among the preliminary findings is that emotions may indeed influence physical well-being—perhaps by strengthening our immune response when we're feeling good, or making us more vulnerable to illness when we're feeling depressed, stressed, or anxious. In some ways these new ideas echo the words of Edward Bach when he wrote, "Thus, behind all disease lie our fears, our anxieties, our greed, our likes and dislikes. Let us seek these out and heal them, and with the healing of them will go the disease from which we suffer." ❑

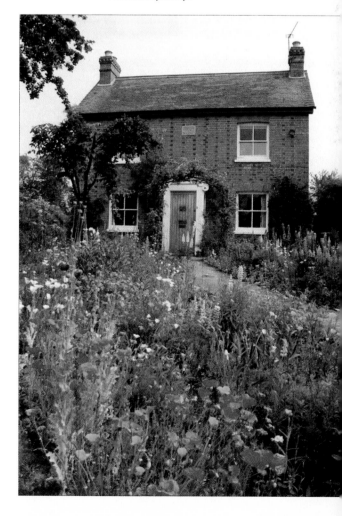

Wildflowers grow in profusion *around the home of Dr. Bach in the Oxfordshire village of Sotwell. Since his death, his residence has been converted into a research and education facility.*

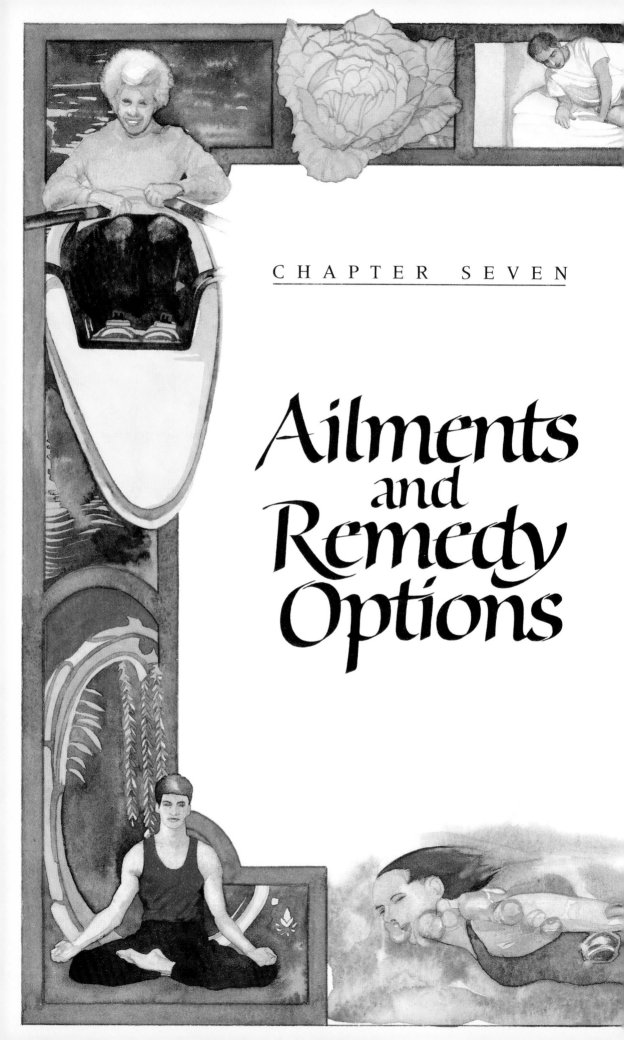

CHAPTER SEVEN

Ailments
and
Remedy
Options

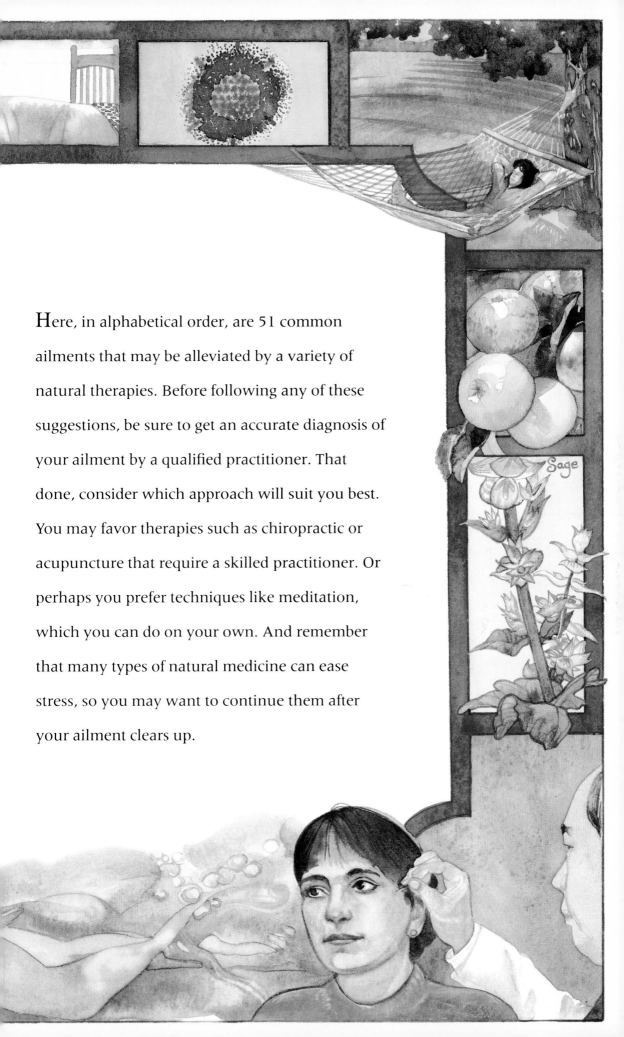

Here, in alphabetical order, are 51 common ailments that may be alleviated by a variety of natural therapies. Before following any of these suggestions, be sure to get an accurate diagnosis of your ailment by a qualified practitioner. That done, consider which approach will suit you best. You may favor therapies such as chiropractic or acupuncture that require a skilled practitioner. Or perhaps you prefer techniques like meditation, which you can do on your own. And remember that many types of natural medicine can ease stress, so you may want to continue them after your ailment clears up.

Complementary Therapies

Practitioners of both orthodox and natural medicine agree that you should see a doctor when you need a diagnosis. If you want to know what options you have in treatment and self-care, consult this guide.

When You Should Seek Medical Help

Most people know enough to call an ambulance in an emergency such as a serious automobile accident. The need for immediate medical care is also obvious in cases of severe burns, broken bones, heatstroke, and poisoning, either from an animal bite or from a toxic substance. Here are some other conditions that should receive immediate medical treatment:

- Difficulty breathing or severe wheezing or shortness of breath.
- Severe or persistent vomiting or diarrhea.
- Significant bleeding from any source — mouth, rectum, or urinary tract — or coughing up blood.
- Sudden, severe pain in the chest or in the abdomen.
- Sudden dizziness or change in vision.
- Slurred speech or loss of speech.
- Persistent numbness in the extremities.

DRAWING ON WISDOM as old as ancient China and as new as today's computer printout, natural medicine relies on both physical and mental healing techniques. Practitioners of natural medicine sometimes use their hands to apply therapy, as in chiropractic, osteopathy, shiatsu, reflexology, and massage. Others, notably homeopaths, base a diagnosis and treatment plan not just on symptoms, but also on the patient's personality traits and emotions. Hypnotherapists may rely on harnessing mental powers to change a physical condition like pain or asthmatic reactions.

By and large, the alternatives to orthodox medical care in this chapter emphasize relieving symptoms, alleviating stress, and preventing recurrences. The ailments included are among the most common disorders. With illnesses that often respond well to drug therapy like insulin for diabetes, these alternatives may be considered an adjunct to orthodox care. When remedies are discussed for chronic illnesses such as emphysema, the approach will likely include ways to manage symptoms of these diseases.

Handling Emergencies. Acute medical and surgical emergencies are not among the ailments listed here. When these situations arise, there is no substitute for immediate, aggressive treatment. Life-saving surgery is essential for such conditions as appendicitis, obstructed bile ducts, and brain hemorrhages. Illnesses like bacterial pneumonia and heart attacks, and emergencies involving head trauma and severe burns are among the situations that call for drug therapy, sophisticated monitoring devices, and other medical interventions.

A proper diagnosis is essential for all but the most minor illnesses like the common cold. Once you have a diagnosis and decide to try a form of natural medicine, consider what types you find most appealing. Be flexible and realistic: understand that what has worked for a friend with similar problems may not work as well for you. If you choose a type of natural medicine as an alternative to orthodox medicine or as an adjunct to it, there are several other things to keep in mind.

The First Step. Begin by finding a reputable practitioner. Referrals from friends and families can help. Inform the physician who diagnosed your problem that you want to try a form of natural medicine. Possibly he or she can make a referral.

States vary in their licensing requirements for practitioners. For example, to practice homeopathy in the United States, a practitioner must be licensed as a physician or doctor of osteopathy. A chiropractor must have graduated from an accredited chiropractic college and pass a yearly re-

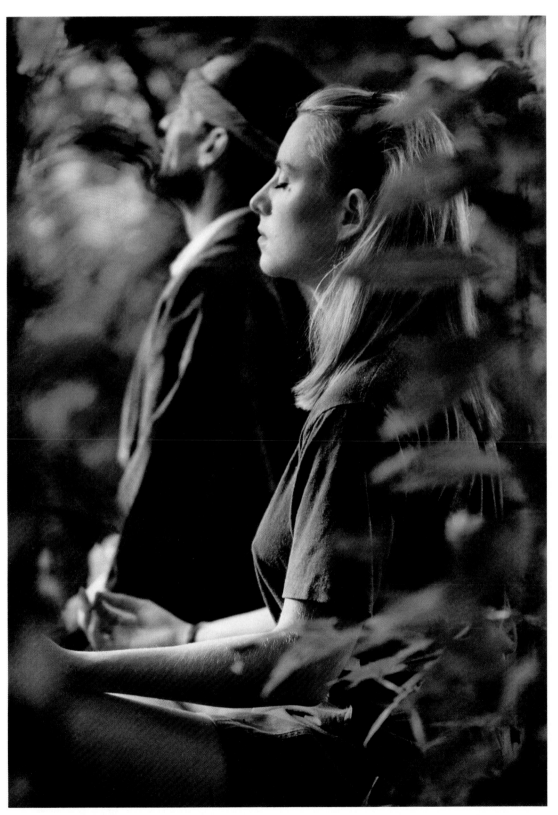

More and more *people are incorporating meditation into their daily routine—a habit that may offer protective health benefits. Regular practice can help relieve symptoms of stress, including hypertension, and so reduce the risk of certain diseases. Because it requires no special equipment, meditation can be done anytime and almost anywhere. In fact, these people are enjoying an early morning session in New York City's Central Park.*

licensing examination administered by a state licensing board. A local clinic or a medical society may be able to guide you to qualified practitioners.

If you know that you have an existing medical condition or suspect that you have one, be sure to notify the practitioner. For example, massage may not be recommended for infection, inflammation, severe back problems, joint diseases like arthritis, and circulatory problems like varicose veins and thrombosis. Likewise, certain yoga postures

---

CASE HISTORY

THE DANGERS OF SELF-DIAGNOSIS

When writer Joan Tedeschi suffered from a pain in her foot,
she tried a number of natural remedies, but still found no relief.
So what went wrong?

"The problem started with an annoying pain in my left foot when I walked. For several weeks I ignored it, attributing the pain to the shoes and boots I wore, or the impact of the hard city sidewalks. I was taking care of a sick relative at that time and didn't listen to my own body's complaints.

"I reported the discomfort to my chiropractor, whom I visit regularly. She adjusted me as usual and suggested that I might be straining my foot as a result of my general misalignment. She didn't look at my foot or recommend a foot doctor. I asked two massage therapists for help. One suggested self-massage a few times a day to relax the muscles, and the other advised alternating hot and cold packs. I tried it all, but to no avail.

"Someone suggested my pain was emotional and signified ambivalence about moving forward in my life. I tried being more positive about myself, and soaked my foot in epsom salts. I did my usual yoga routine and concentrated on strengthening and stretching my foot. The pain continued.

"After several weeks of advice and treatments, the only thing I was sure about was that the pain was worse. I finally started calling podiatrists. Although it was Saturday, I found one who agreed to see me. He examined my foot and diagnosed the trouble as sesamoiditis, an inflammation of the area surrounding the sesamoid bone. He gave me a whirlpool treatment, which felt good, and ultrasound, which was so unpleasant, I fainted. I hobbled home to rest. My foot still hurt, but at least I now knew what was wrong, or so I thought.

"That night my foot began to throb, and the pain increased so much that I almost fainted again. Sunday morning, I phoned the podiatrist to report what had happened. He said that the bone was probably broken, and told me to come in for an x-ray. This time he was right, and he sent me to a foot surgeon to determine the best course of treatment. It turned out I had a stress fracture of the sesamoid bone. The doctor covered me from toe to knee with a plaster cast and sent me off on crutches.

"While I waited for three weeks to see if the foot would heal without surgery, I had time to think about the lessons I had learned. They include: Stay in touch with your body's signals and don't ignore pain. It's often necessary to consult a doctor before trying home remedies. Once the condition is diagnosed, decide which treatments are appropriate. If I had consulted the right person immediately, I might have been walking comfortably a lot sooner."

must be avoided by those with circulatory or cardiovascular ailments, or some types of back pain.

This guide lists natural medicine remedies alphabetically by ailment and by remedy option from acupuncture to yoga. Its aim is to give a representative sampling of the wide variety of therapies for treatment; however, it is not possible to include all therapies for each ailment. Some of the therapies are discussed in much greater detail elsewhere in the book, for example, massage on pages 156-163, and yoga on pages 214-221. For information on the therapeutic use of herbs, see pages 288-327. Additional therapeutic uses of vitamin and mineral supplements advocated by some practitioners are described on pages 282-287. A directory of resources can be found on pages 411-413.

Generational Distinctions. What constitutes good preventive care and sensible self-treatment for an adult does not apply equally well to young children or the elderly. It is not always safe to ignore certain medical conditions in a child that could be considered insignificant in an adult. A sore throat in an adult, for example, may be merely a cold symptom, but in a child it may signal tonsillitis or strep throat, a bacterial infection. If strep throat is left untreated, there's a risk that serious complications like rheumatic fever and kidney inflammation may develop. Similarly, a short bout of diarrhea is no cause for alarm among healthy adults, but in young children and the elderly, it can lead to serious problems.

Among the elderly, various conditions may require special approaches to treatment. Manipulative therapy like chiropractic and osteopathy has to take into account that bones become brittle with age. In addition, when choosing nutrient supplements as a remedy option, the elderly must consider the fact that they may absorb certain vitamins and minerals less easily than younger people.

In a Class by Themselves. Pregnant women must be especially cautious both for themselves and for the developing child. Taking megadoses of vitamin A, for example, can cause birth defects. Performing certain yoga postures or other exercises can place too much stress on the abdominals and back muscles, which may already be strained by the demands of pregnancy. Certain ailments, such as high blood pressure, can pose special problems for expectant mothers. Women who are pregnant should get medical attention at regular intervals and should consult their physician about any therapies in this chapter that are of interest to them.

Acquired Immunodeficiency Disease Syndrome, or AIDS, is not covered here. The extraordinary complexity of this disease and the rapidly changing approaches to its treatment put it beyond the scope of this book. ❏

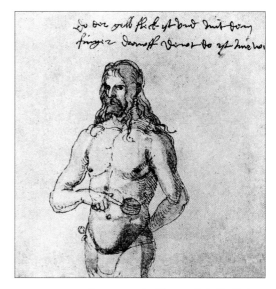

An accurate diagnosis is the first step in any treatment plan. Unable to see his doctor, Albrecht Dürer (1471–1528), the German painter and engraver, sent his physician a sketch with a note scribbled at the top that read "and where my finger points, there is the pain." Modern scholars now think that Dürer was suffering from a disease of the spleen.

Acne *The most common type of skin disorder, acne is a skin eruption seen most prominently on the face but sometimes on the neck, chest, back, and shoulders as well. It generally begins during puberty and often ends by the time the teenage years are over. Occasionally the condition lasts longer, even into the 30s and 40s, or it first develops in adulthood. Although men may have acne, those adults most likely to be affected are women who use oil-based cosmetics or women who are menstruating.*

Teenage boys are more likely to have acne than girls because adolescent males secrete more androgen, a male sex hormone that contributes to acne. The sebaceous glands, located just beneath the skin's surface, produce an oily substance called sebum, which keeps the skin healthy by lubricating the tissue. These glands, located at the root of each hair follicle, start overproducing sebum when male hormones become especially assertive in adolescence. Whiteheads, blackheads, pimples, and cysts may form when sebum and debris on the skin clog pores on the surface of the skin. Sebum and bacteria on the skin can also work in concert to produce acne.

ORTHODOX MEDICINE

Fortunately for most acne sufferers, the condition may subside on its own or with a minimum of treatment. Over-the-counter medications with benzoyl peroxide sometimes alleviate the problem. Superficial acne may also respond to creams, gels, or liquids that contain antibiotics or topical tretinoin, a combination of vitamin A acid and retinoic acid.

For deep acne, an oral antibiotic like tetracycline may be prescribed. The drug Accutane has been hailed as a revolutionary improvement in acne treatment, but it can have very serious side effects. It can cause fetal abnormalities, so physicians are advised not to prescribe it for pregnant women. In addition, women who take Accutane are urged to use contraceptive techniques and to avoid pregnancy for one to three months after the Accutane therapy has ended. If recurring acne outbreaks leave unsightly scars, removing the top layer of skin with a high-speed sanding device may be considered. This process is known as dermabrasion.

COMMON-SENSE CARE

Keeping your face and hair clean is the first order of business to avoid acne or minimize its impact. The face should be cleaned gently, but not scrubbed excessively, with a mild soap, which is better than a specially formulated antibacterial soap. Use water-based cosmetics, not oil-based. Do not squeeze pimples. Do not wear elasticized headbands, turtlenecks, or other tight-fitting apparel that may trap sebum near the scalp, neck, and shoulders.

Experts differ on whether to recommend sunlight, which dries out the skin and may slightly speed the healing of small pustules and papules. There is also debate whether ultraviolet sunlamps provide the same benefit as sun.

NATURAL MEDICINE THERAPIES

■ **HOMEOPATHY**: Remedies recommended for severe acne include Kali bichromicum for chronic acne, and sulphur for inflamed or infected pustules that are worse when washed.

■ **HYDROTHERAPY**: Gently rubbing the skin of the arms, legs, and trunk with a loofah sponge and cold water can stimulate healing.

■ **NATUROPATHY**: Treatment aims at helping the body cleanse itself and eliminate waste products that overburden the system. A practitioner may recommend a diet to help guard against infection and aid in regulating hormone levels. Such a diet will include foods like whole-grain cereals, and fresh fruit and vegetables, including vegetable juices, such as carrot, beetroot, and cabbage. The suggested diet may exclude refined products and foods high in fat, such as cheese, fatty meat, cakes, white bread, and sweets. Fasting briefly to cleanse the system may also be recommended. Sore or bleeding spots can be treated with warm water and sea salt or calendula ointment.

■ **SHIATSU**: Stimulating points on the forearm, hand, face, base of the skull, and upper chest may bring some relief. Such therapy may increase circulation, relieve muscle tension, adjust hormonal imbalances, and boost the immune system. Treatment will concentrate on points on either side of the spinal cord and in the legs.

■ **VITAMIN AND MINERAL THERAPY**: Supplements of vitamins A and E and the mineral zinc may be recommended. The B complex vitamins and C may also help. Acne that erupts before and during menstruation may be improved with added vitamin B_6.

Allergies *Exaggerated immune reactions to common substances that are swallowed, injected, or inhaled, or that touch the skin or the eyes, allergies can make an otherwise healthy person feel miserable. Symptoms include wheezing, coughing, choking, runny nose, sneezing, tearing, and itching. The skin, respiratory system, stomach, intestines, and the eyes are typically affected. Allergic reactions occur when the body starts producing antibodies to fend off allergens, the substances that provoke such discomfort and irritation.*

The most common environmental allergens are grass and tree pollens, mold spores, dust mites, and animal dander. Eating certain foods and food additives, and being stung by insects can trigger allergic reactions in sensitive people. Children can inherit a tendency to develop allergies. Such common disorders as eczema, hives, hay fever, and asthma are often attributed to allergic reactions.

See also Asthma, Eczema, Hay Fever.

ORTHODOX MEDICINE

Treatment varies according to the different causes and symptoms. Antihistamines are usually the first choice to relieve such symptoms as sneezing, itchy eyes and nose, and post-nasal drip. A nasal spray containing cromolyn sodium may be prescribed and, as a last resort, oral steroids to control severe symptoms. For allergens related to disorders like eczema, corticosteroid creams and ointments are

typically prescribed. As prevention, cromolyn sodium and corticosteroids may be given before symptoms develop. For patients whose allergy does not improve with any other technique, a program of immunotherapy that can last several months or as long as three years may be tried. This involves injections of the offending substance in gradually increasing doses to build up a tolerance to the allergen.

COMMON-SENSE CARE

Perhaps the best advice is the simplest: avoid the food, plants, animals, drugs, dust, or other substances that trigger an allergic reaction. If the allergen is airborne, clean living and working spaces frequently. Wear a face mask when doing chores. Get rid of dust, molds, and mildew. Discard old rugs, pillows, furniture, and stuffed animals,

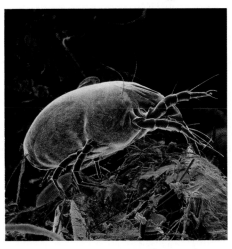

Dust mites *can cause misery for allergy sufferers. They thrive in furniture, pillows, and carpets.*

which provide breeding grounds for molds and dust mites. Air-conditioners can decrease your exposure to pollen. A dehumidifier and an air purifier, cleaned frequently, may help.

Certain common foods can trigger allergies—items like eggs, corn, wheat, yeast, dairy products, citrus fruits, and food additives. Forgoing these foods for three weeks, then reintroducing them one by one, may help identify the source of the problem. However, often food allergies are masked or hidden, so consult a physician trained in nutrition before starting an elimination diet.

Smoking exacerbates allergic reactions. Give up cigarettes, if you haven't already.

NATURAL MEDICINE THERAPIES

■ **ACUPUNCTURE:** Initial treatments will seek to alleviate such common symptoms as skin eruptions, nasal congestion, itching, wheezing, and watery eyes. When the symptoms have subsided, a therapist may focus on the underlying weaknesses that cause hypersensitivity to various substances.

■ **BACH FLOWER REMEDIES:** Clematis is recommended for general oversensitivity; mimulus for fear of getting an allergic reaction; impatiens if there is irritation of the skin or mucous membranes. Rescue Remedy may soothe allergic rashes.

■ **HOMEOPATHY:** Practitioners may approach allergies as a manifestation of hypersensitivity in the entire body, or they may prescribe treatment for specific symptoms. For allergic conjunctivitis, belladonna, euphrasia, and apis may be given. For allergies with upper-respiratory tract symptoms like wheezing and sneezing, remedies include arsenicum, euphrasia, nux vomica, sabadilla, and wyethia.

■ **HYPNOTHERAPY:** Allergy sufferers may find that hypnotic techniques help them relax and alleviate the stress that often accompanies an allergic reaction.

■ **NATUROPATHY:** To control symptoms and possibly eliminate food allergies, the first step may be a fast or a raw-food diet aimed at cleansing the digestive system and colon. Symptoms and conditions that food allergies may cause or can aggravate include migraine and tension headaches, fatigue, depression, nasal congestion, asthma, eczema, irritable bowel syndrome, and rheumatoid and osteoarthritis. A diet that is low in dairy products, which can contribute to mucus production, may be recommended for the long term.

■ **OSTEOPATHY:** Treatment will seek to balance the involuntary nervous system with spinal and cranial adjustments.

■ **SHIATSU:** Points on the forearm, elbow, abdomen, collarbone, and elsewhere can be stimulated to relieve symptoms. Therapy aims not only to enhance the immune system, but also to provide relaxation, which can be important to allergy sufferers.

■ **VITAMIN AND MINERAL THERAPY:** Generally recommended are vitamins A, B_6, and C, the mineral calcium, and a compound mineral supplement.

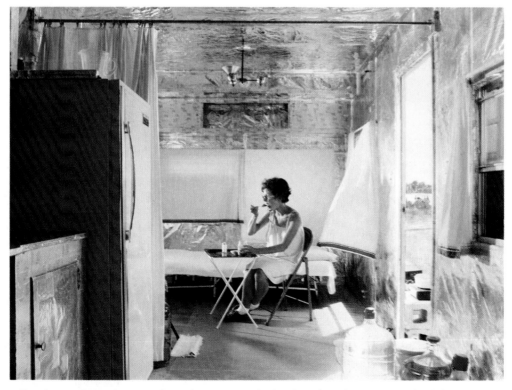

Allergies can be an inconvenience for many people, but for a few, they require radical changes. Sensitive to air pollution, household dirt, and chemicals in various products, this woman scrubs the ceiling and walls of her trailer, then lines them with aluminum foil to guard against contamination.

Anemia *Anemia has been identified as a reduction of red cells or hemoglobin in the blood, which carries oxygen throughout the body. Anemia occurs when there is bleeding, when bone marrow cannot produce enough red blood cells, when those produced have a defect, or when something interferes with the survival of red blood cells.*

Iron-deficiency anemia, caused by heavy or recurring bleeding, is the most prevalent form of the disorder. Persistent bleeding is associated with diseases of the digestive tract, including gastritis, inflammatory bowel disease, and colon and stomach cancer. Other diseases, including leukemia and kidney disease, can produce anemia. Some types of anemia can be traced to genetic disorders.

In children and adolescents, anemia can often be traced to insufficient dietary intake of iron. Loss of blood in menstruation is typically the cause of anemia among girls and women. In men, chronic occult bleeding in the gastrointestinal tract often leads to iron-deficiency anemia. Signs and symptoms of anemia include fatigue, pallor, irritability, loss of appetite, headaches, soreness in the mouth, chest pain, and breathlessness.

See also Cancer, Headaches, Menstrual Problems.

ORTHODOX MEDICINE

Physicians may recommend that you change your eating habits to increase your iron intake, and they may prescribe iron or folic acid supplements. Pregnant women, menstruating women, and the elderly are the most likely to need such supplements. For anemia caused by massive blood loss, which can occur during surgery or as a result of serious injuries sustained in accidents, blood transfusions are often required.

COMMON-SENSE CARE

Eating foods that contain adequate, easily absorbed sources of iron may be the best insurance policy for anemia prevention. A balanced diet that provides the Recommended Daily Allowance of iron is generally sufficient to guard against anemia. Certain chemicals interfere with iron absorption, for example, tannin in tea, polyphenols in coffee, and cadmium in cigarettes. Other important nutrients are folic acid, used by bone marrow to produce blood, and vitamin B_{12}.

NATURAL MEDICINE THERAPIES

■ **NATUROPATHY:** A practitioner may recommend such iron-rich foods as egg yolks, red meat, fish, and poultry; green leafy vegetables; whole grains and enriched breads and cereals; such legumes as lentils, and lima beans; dried prunes and apricots, raisins, wheat bran, blackstrap molasses, and sunflower seeds. Liver, kidney, and other organ meat are also high in iron but are among the foods highest in cholesterol.

Dietary sources of folic acid and vitamin B_{12} may be suggested. Foods rich in folic acid include wheat germ, brewer's yeast, leafy green vegetables, and mushrooms. Vitamin B_{12} is found in all animal food, yeast extracts, and some breakfast cereals. Iron is absorbed best when foods rich in vitamin C are eaten at the same meal as iron-rich foods, for example, eating an orange with an egg sandwich. At mealtime, avoid coffee, strong caffeinated teas, and colas, which all contain substances that hinder iron absorption.

■ **VITAMIN AND MINERAL THERAPY:** In addition to iron supplements, recommendations may include iron salts, copper, and vitamins B_6, B_{12}, and C. Iron overload can cause diabetes and other medical problems, so therapy should be monitored carefully.

Arteriosclerosis *A general term for diseases of the cardiovascular system, arteriosclerosis is one of the changes that aging produces. Arterial walls become thick and lose their elasticity. When they cannot dilate and constrict fully, blood clots are more likely to occur. Also known as hardening of the arteries, arteriosclerosis increases the risk of aneurysms, blood clots, and strokes.*

Atherosclerosis, a related condition, may contribute to heart disease and other serious problems. Atherosclerosis develops when deposits of cholesterol and other fatty substances accumulate on the walls of arteries, creating blockages. Platelets may begin to adhere to the substances, known as plaque, further hindering the flow of blood. Health risks are greatest when plaque clogs the coronary arteries and the carotid artery, which supplies blood to the brain. Blockages that prevent the aorta, which is the body's main artery, and its branches from processing blood adequately also pose serious dangers. Sometimes an artery will be 90 percent blocked before symptoms appear.

Obesity, smoking, high blood pressure, diabetes, certain genetic traits, and being male increase the risks of atherosclerosis. Another risk factor is a diet high in total fat, saturated fat, and cholesterol. This is the diet that people in developed countries usually eat.

See also Diabetes, Heart Disease, High Blood Pressure.

ORTHODOX MEDICINE

There is no drug therapy for either arteriosclerosis or atherosclerosis. Drugs can be prescribed for risk factors, including medication to lower high blood pressure and blood cholesterol. Anticoagulant drugs may help minimize clotting and decrease the risk of an embolism (arterial blockage).

Vascular surgery can be performed to repair arteries that are narrowed, blocked, or weakened. Coronary artery bypass is the most common vascular procedure. The surgeon replaces a diseased coronary artery or several arteries with a vein removed from the patient's leg. Balloon angioplasty can be performed to widen the narrowed or blocked sections of an artery. A physician inserts a catheter with a balloon attached, inflates the balloon to distend the artery, then removes the catheter and balloon.

COMMON-SENSE CARE

Losing excess weight, eating fewer foods high in saturated fat and cholesterol, controlling elevated blood pressure and diabetes, giving up smoking, and exercising regularly are among the best measures for preventing complications of atherosclerosis

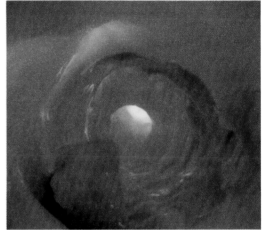

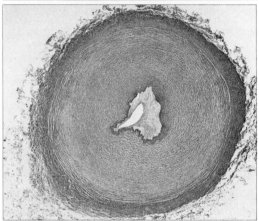

The build-up *of arterial plaque that is beginning to clog the artery seen above can progress over time to produce an almost total blockage (bottom photo), which hampers the flow of blood.*

like coronary heart disease. Foods high in water-soluble fiber like oat bran and pectin may reduce the absorption of cholesterol in tissues and may elevate blood levels of high-density lipoproteins, the so-called good cholesterol.

NATURAL MEDICINE THERAPIES

■ ACUPUNCTURE: Acupuncture can be used to break the habit of smoking, a risk factor for cardiovascular problems.

■ NATUROPATHY: Through diet, exercise, and lifestyle changes, it is possible to limit and perhaps reverse the damage of atherosclerosis. A practitioner may suggest eliminating dietary fats and oils, meat, and dairy products, except for non-fat milk and yogurt, and increasing your consumption of complex carbohydrates, such as grains, fruits, vegetables, and legumes. Onions, garlic, and ginger are said to reduce blood cholesterol levels. Such aerobic exercises as brisk walking, running, and swimming are often recommended; however, if you have a heart condition, are obese, or are generally sedentary, consult a physician before starting an exercise regimen.

■ VITAMIN THERAPY: Supplemental vitamin E may help prevent atherosclerosis by raising levels of high-density lipoproteins, the "good" type of cholesterol. The antioxidants beta-carotene and vitamins C and E may be recommended as preventive measures.

■ YOGA: Stress is considered by some a risk factor in cardiovascular diseases, and yogic deep-breathing exercises can be relaxing. The cobra pose, fish pose, and salutation to the sun can also relax you. Meditation can be an important part of a yoga program aimed at reducing stress.

Arthritis *An umbrella term for more than 100 joint disorders, arthritis is generally an inflammation of one or more joints. It can affect virtually any joint, and symptoms range from mild aches and stiffness to severe pain and crippling deformity. Osteoarthritis, also known as degenerative joint disease, is the most common arthritic disorder. It is a result of the wear and tear on the joints that aging produces. Inheriting a tendency for defective cartilage and engaging in injury-producing activities like football and ballet can increase your likelihood of developing osteoarthritis. Shock-absorbing cartilage between the bones of the joints becomes rough and worn, allowing the bones to rub together when the joints are flexed.*

Rheumatoid arthritis is one of the most debilitating forms of the disease. It is a systemic disorder that affects not only joints, but also surrounding tissues, mostly in the hands, feet, and arms. Rheumatoid arthritis has been described as an autoimmune disease, in which one part of the body attacks another.

Other forms of related joint diseases are ankylosing spondylitis, which is arthritis of the spine, and infective arthritis, which can develop when bacteria from a wound or an infection in the bloodstream invade a joint. Gout, a metabolic disorder that may cause pain in hand, knee, and toe joints, often produces arthritis as its primary symptom.

See also Pain, Chronic, and Gout.

ORTHODOX MEDICINE

Although the past half-century has seen rapid advances in surgery and drug therapy for various forms of arthritis, there is no cure; however, most patients notice some improvement without drugs. Exercise often gets the highest priority. Other approaches include heat, weight loss for the obese, and such forms of joint protection as canes, walkers, and splints on weakened joints.

Aspirin or another member of the family of nonsteroidal anti-inflammatory drugs like ibuprofen may be suggested. If these do not relieve pain, corticosteroids may be injected into joints. The next course of treatment for rheumatoid arthritis may involve gold compounds, D-penicillamine, or hydroxychloroquine. For severe rheumatoid arthritis, immunosuppressive drugs may be prescribed; as a last resort, surgery may be performed. Procedures include fusing or replacing diseased joints with prosthetic devices. Hip replacement is typically the most successful joint-replacement surgery.

COMMON-SENSE CARE

A regular exercise program can contribute substantially to joint mobility and pain reduction. The combination of exercise and physical therapy can help slow the rate of joint deterioration. For severe attacks, curtailing some daily activities or remaining in bed for a day or two may diminish the pain. Soaking in a warm bath may provide relief. Applying cold compresses or hot packs to the affected area can also help.

An arthritic person who is overweight should shed excess pounds to reduce joint strain. Rather than taking sleeping pills, tranquilizers, and narcotic painkillers, which can be addictive, consider over-the-counter pain relievers like acetaminophen, aspirin, and ibuprofen. Folk remedies include wearing copper bracelets and anklets, and rubbing a clove of garlic on painful areas.

NATURAL MEDICINE THERAPIES

■ ACUPUNCTURE: The acupuncturist will stimulate various meridians, depending on where arthritis symptoms appear. When therapy is most successful, it can reduce pain and restore mobility to affected joints.

■ ALEXANDER TECHNIQUE: For arthritis sufferers, it is important to learn how to sit down and stand up, and how to lift and carry objects in ways that will protect the joints. Sessions with an experienced practitioner can help relieve pain.

■ HOMEOPATHY: A homeopath will recommend remedies appropriate to the symptoms, including ruta, rhus tox, bryonia, and pulsatilla.

■ HYDROTHERAPY: Swimming can take the weight off joints and help increase flexibility and reduce pain. Ocean swimming is especially good for most arthritics, although swimming in salt water can occasionally pose problems, so it helps to consult a physician. Taking a shower or

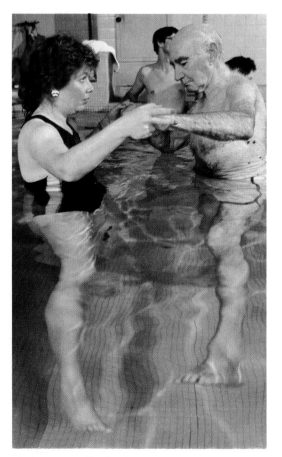

Many types of hydrotherapy *can relieve the pain and stiffness common to arthritis patients. Here, a patient is guided by a therapist.*

soaking in a warm bath may alleviate pain by relaxing muscles and joints that have become stiff.

■ HYPNOTHERAPY: Some arthritis patients find hypnosis helpful when anxiety and depression accompany the condition.

■ MASSAGE: Regular massage can relieve pain and increase mobility. Massage should never be used on a joint that is inflamed, swollen, or extremely painful; instead, knead or rub the area around the affected joint, not the joint itself. An oil used in massage combines rosemary, lavender, and marigold in an almond oil base.

■ NATUROPATHY: A largely vegetarian low-fat diet with plenty of salads and lightly cooked vegetables is frequently recommended. Raw fruit and vegetable juices may be suggested. Practitioners may urge arthritics to avoid dairy products and other foods that may cause allergies. Goat's milk and the cheese and yogurt made from it may be substituted. Other foods to avoid may include red meat, products made with white flour, citrus fruits, salt, sugar, caffeinated drinks, alcohol, and food additives. Fasting may be recommended to rid the body of toxins that accumulate in the joints; however, fasting should only be done under medical supervision.

■ REFLEXOLOGY: Massage may relieve pain and inflammation when directed to the reflex areas relating to the affected joints and to the areas for pituitary, adrenals, and parathyroid glands, kidneys, and solar plexus.

■ SHIATSU: Therapy can be effective in relieving pain and stiffness. For the hands, press a point at the end of the crease between the forefinger and thumb; for the hips, press a point at the hollow at the sides of the hips at the joint between the pelvis and leg; for the knees, a point in and under the kneecap in the outer depression and a point located three thumbs' widths down from the kneecap in the hollow on the outer edge of the shin.

■ VITAMIN AND MINERAL THERAPY: For osteoarthritis, a practitioner may recommend vitamins C and E and niacinamide. For rheumatoid arthritis, the minerals zinc and copper can help, as well as vitamin B_6 and calcium pantothenate. Other supplements used for arthritis include alfalfa tablets and fish oil.

■ YOGA: Yogic exercises can help

increase mobility and relieve stress by promoting relaxation. A qualified teacher can suggest postures to help ease specific arthritic conditions. Yoga may also build a positive self-image, which can be important in dealing with arthritis.

Asthma *Wheezing, being short of breath, coughing, and feeling tightness in the chest may be symptoms of asthma, a disorder of the respiratory system. The airways that permit the lungs to process air go into spasm and become narrowed, and breathing is hampered. Inflammation often accompanies these spasms. Asthma attacks, which vary from mild to life-threatening, can be triggered by exertion, such as exercise, by getting a cold, and by inhaling cigarettes or breathing cigarette smoke. Other agents that can trigger asthma include food and the food additive sulfite, drugs, molds, dust, feathers, and animal dander. Sudden changes in weather can also set off an attack.*

The illness often begins in childhood. Attacks tend to become less frequent or even disappear in adulthood. Psychological stress can prompt an attack or can worsen one. More often than not, there is a family history of allergy or asthma.

See also Allergies.

ORTHODOX MEDICINE

When an attack begins, a bronchodilator drug may be used. Medication can provide relief by relaxing the muscles surrounding the constricted and congested airways, or bronchioles, leading to the lungs so that the airways will open up. Drugs can be inhaled or taken in tablet form. Anti-inflammatory medications like corticosteroids may be prescribed when spasms are triggered by inflammation.

Another way to get medication into the bronchioles is through a nebulizer, a kind of inhaler that propels medication into the lungs with air- or oxygen-pressure. Oxygen may be administered at home or in a physician's office, where injections may be given if needed. An attack so severe that there is a risk of not getting enough oxygen requires hospitalization. An asthmatic patient in extreme respiratory distress may be hooked up to a ventilator, a machine that forces oxygen or air into the lungs.

COMMON-SENSE CARE

Prevention is the key to managing asthma. Some of the same rules apply as with managing allergies. Living quarters and workspaces should be kept as dust-free as possible. If vacuuming and dusting do not improve the situation, you might have to remove carpeting and draperies, where dirt and dust accumulate.

If you are asthmatic, avoid close proximity to trees, flowering shrubs, and plants during the pollen season. Avoid other potential irritants like fur and feathers. Do not smoke and stay out of smoke-filled rooms. If you go outside in very cold weather, covering your nose and mouth with a scarf or mask can help prevent problems by warming and moisturizing the air you breathe.

Deep breathing exercises are helpful. Asthmatics, particularly those who are affected by exertion, should choose their exercise carefully. Avoiding sports that are performed outdoors in cold weather is advised. Team sports that allow for periods of rest are generally better than aerobic exercise, which demands continued effort.

NATURAL MEDICINE THERAPIES

■ ACUPUNCTURE: Therapy may be applied to several points on the lung meridian, and on the back, chest, and hands to relieve coughing and other symptoms.

■ ALEXANDER TECHNIQUE: To correct bad posture that may aggravate an asthmatic condition, the Alexander technique may be recommended. The technique may also enable asthmatics to relax during attacks and prevent a panicked response that can worsen the problem.

■ BACH FLOWER REMEDIES: Larch, mimulus, mustard, and holly are the commonly recommended remedies.

■ CHIROPRACTIC: Treatment aims to correct any partial dislocations or skeletal misalignments that could block nerves serving the respiratory system.

■ HOMEOPATHY: Homeopathy can offer

remedies for long-term improvement as well as for acute attacks. Aconite, arsenicum album, cuprum metalicum, and phosphorus are common treatments.

■ HYDROTHERAPY: Swimming, especially the breast stroke, can help strengthen the lungs and improve breathing.

■ HYPNOTHERAPY: Asthmatics use hypnosis and self-hypnosis to achieve relaxation. Some can even control the narrowing of the bronchial passages.

■ MASSAGE: Massaging the neck, shoulders, and back can relieve muscle tension and release phlegm in the lungs.

■ NATUROPATHY: Asthmatic children are frequently allergic to many foods; a naturopath may be able to determine which allergens to avoid. For adults and children, minimizing the frequency and severity of attacks may require such changes in diet as reducing or eliminating dairy products and sugar, which may increase mucus production; and eating more fresh fruits, vegetables (especially garlic and onions), and less highly processed foods.

■ OSTEOPATHY: Like chiropractic, osteopathy seeks to correct skeletal misalignments, primarily in the spine, that may interfere with the normal functioning of the body's systems. Osteopathy and naturopathy are often used together.

■ REFLEXOLOGY: Pressure on such points as the tips of the fingers and the middle of the palm can relax you and improve breathing. Also, massage the whole foot frequently.

■ SHIATSU: To get relief during an attack, press points in the center of the chest and at the "V" of the collarbone. If the attack continues or worsens, consult a doctor immediately.

■ T'AI CHI: Regular t'ai chi sessions can aid relaxation and improve breathing.

■ VITAMIN AND MINERAL THERAPY: Asthmatics may benefit from supplements of vitamins A (in beta-carotene form), C, B_6, B_{12}, E, and pantothenic acid, and the minerals calcium, manganese, and magnesium.

■ YOGA: The cobra, the cat (pelvic lift), and back rolls (spinal massage) are among the best postures for asthmatics. Abdominal lifts and breathing exercises help the lungs. Daily relaxation sessions may contribute to reducing tension, which in turn may lessen the number and severity of attacks.

Athlete's foot *A minor but uncomfortable skin condition, athlete's foot is usually caused by a fungal infection. Cracked, peeling skin between the toes and over the sole, especially the instep, is common. The skin itches and feels sore. Blisters may develop.*

ORTHODOX MEDICINE

Non-prescription powders, lotions, and creams that contain antifungal agents may clear up the problem. Benzoic acid and aluminum chloride solutions are also used. Whitfield's tincture or ointment may be used. If prescription creams are ineffective, a prescription may be given for the antifungal drug griseofulvin, which comes in pill, capsule, and liquid form.

COMMON-SENSE CARE

To prevent athlete's foot, dry the feet thoroughly, including the area between the toes, after bathing or showering. If you shower regularly in locker rooms, wear rubber clogs in the shower and locker area so that your feet do not touch the floor. After drying feet, dust them with talcum powder. Wear sandals or other open-toed shoes that allow air to circulate freely but avoid vinyl footwear. Alternate shoes from day to day so that each pair dries out between wearings. Wear cotton socks, instead of those made of wool or synthetics, which absorb moisture poorly. If you are especially vulnerable to the fungus, go barefoot in hot weather to allow perspiration to evaporate. A folk medicine treatment calls for bathing your feet in hot tea to alleviate symptoms.

NATURAL MEDICINE THERAPIES

■ HOMEOPATHY: Calendula ointment can be useful.

■ HYDROTHERAPY: Soaking your foot in warm salt water for five to 10 minutes at a time can help kill the fungus. In addition, soaking softens the skin so that antifungal medication can penetrate better.

■ NATUROPATHY: An application of buffered vitamin C powder to the affected areas may be recommended. Calcium ascorbate and sodium ascorbate are less likely to irritate the skin than vitamin C powder.

■ SHIATSU: A point to press is located at the base of the little toe where the little toe and fourth toe meet.

Pillows Provide Support While You Sleep

- If you suffer from back pain, a task as simple as getting out of bed in the morning can become very hard. Here's how to minimize the effort. If you are on your stomach or back, roll over on your side, then bring your knees up to about your hip level. Keep your legs bent and your body relaxed.
  - Gently lower your feet to the floor and use your arms to push yourself up into a sitting position. You can reverse this procedure to get back into bed. Be sure that you sleep on a firm mattress.

Using this method minimizes pressure on your back.

Back pain

Nearly everyone suffers from back pain at one time or another. Fortunately, most such episodes are brief. Among the causes of back pain are incorrect posture; poor muscle tone, especially in the abdomen; sitting in awkward positions; and a sedentary lifestyle, such as spending most of your day at a desk or driving a car for hours.

Straining to do manual labor or other work that involves lifting and carrying heavy loads can trigger back pain. Other mechanical causes include stress and compression fractures, torn muscles, and strained ligaments. Among the diseases and disorders that can cause back pain are tumors, kidney diseases, arthritis, cystitis, gallstones, cancer, and emotional stress.

Back pain often develops as the result of an accident in which discs or vertebrae sustain damage. The term "slipped disc" is frequently used to describe a disc prolapse, which is a structural disorder that may involve one or more discs pressing on a nerve root or on the spinal cord.

See also Arthritis, Cancer, Cystitis, Gallstones, Sciatica.

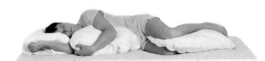

On your side: three pillows offer support.

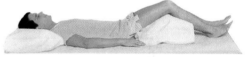

On your back: pillows for the head, knees.

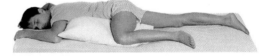

On your stomach: try to keep one leg bent.

ORTHODOX MEDICINE

Resting briefly, usually for only two days, is commonly recommended for acute low back pain. The next step may be a series of exercises focused on stretching and strengthening. Referral to a physical therapist depends on the severity of the pain. A corset or a brace to support the back may be suggested. For acute pain, anti-inflammatory drugs, painkillers, and muscle relaxants may be prescribed. Physicians may recommend surgery for chronic pain when there is weakness or numbness, which are symptoms of nerve compression.

COMMON-SENSE CARE

Strategies for avoiding or minimizing back pain include practicing good posture and learning how to lift, push, and carry heavy objects without straining. When sitting, choose chairs with a firm seat and adequate lower back support. Perform gentle exercises daily to tone back and abdominal muscles and prevent stiffness.

Such activities as walking, swimming, cycling, and rowing are good for the back. If you have recurring back pain, avoid sports like football, tennis, and squash, which involve sudden and often back-wrenching movement. Women should not wear high heels exclusively. When seated, avoid crossing your legs. When standing, do not remain stationary. Periodically shift your weight from leg to leg, or prop one foot on a chair rung. To prevent back problems, sleep on a firm mattress on your back or your side, with a pillow under your head.

NATURAL MEDICINE THERAPIES

■ **ACUPUNCTURE**: Treatment will concentrate on points on either side of the spinal cord and in the legs.

■ **ALEXANDER TECHNIQUE**: A practitioner can teach you how to sit, stand, and move properly to prevent back problems and to relieve pain.

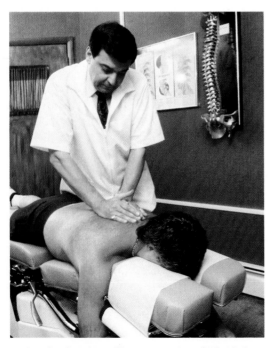

Lower back pain sufferers sometimes find relief when chiropractors manipulate their spines.

■ **CHIROPRACTIC**: A practitioner will treat the problem with spinal adjustments. Ice packs and ultrasound therapy may be used to augment manipulation.

■ **HOMEOPATHY**: Remedies appropriate for soreness and pain include arnica, rhus toxicodendron, and bryonia.

■ **HYDROTHERAPY**: Swimming and other water exercises are recommended for many back problems. Also potential pain relievers are sitz baths with Epsom salts. Ice packs may be recommended for the first several days of pain. Once inflammation has subsided, a hot water pack can be helpful.

■ **MASSAGE**: A qualified practitioner may massage the entire body but will concentrate special attention on the affected area. For a backache, gliding strokes are relaxing, and kneading will help reduce stiffness. For acute back pain, consult a physician before you try massage therapy.

■ **OSTEOPATHY**: If the problem is a slipped disc, a practitioner may first relax the contracted spinal muscles, then gently stretch the spine to relieve pressure on the injured disc. Treatment for a disc problem may require six or more sessions. Lesser injuries, such as a pulled muscle, may improve after only one session.

■ **REFLEXOLOGY**: Treating areas on the foot that relate to the lower spine, kidneys, urinary tract, and hips may ease pain.

■ **SHIATSU**: Pressing points on the lower spine and elsewhere can bring relief. Begin therapy on the side of the back that is pain-free, then switch to the other side. Warning: shiatsu should not be used on anyone with a slipped disc, a high fever, a contagious skin disease, or who takes cortisone medication.

■ **VITAMIN AND MINERAL THERAPY**: Vitamin D, in conjunction with calcium, and vitamin C are important for the development and health of bones and nerve functions. Vitamin C may benefit those with deteriorating discs. Other recommendations may include vitamin E and the minerals magnesium, manganese, phosphorus, and zinc.

■ **YOGA**: A good way to strengthen and relax muscles, yoga will improve bad alignment and posture, which often contribute to back pain; however, it is important to discuss your condition with a qualified yoga teacher before beginning classes. Certain postures, such as the cobra and the plow, may be too dangerous.

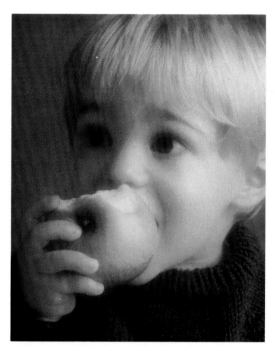

Apples rate highly *as natural breath fresheners, along with cinnamon sticks, parsley, and mint.*

Bad breath *Bad breath, or halitosis, is an unpleasant mouth odor caused mostly by poor dental hygiene and smoking. Drinking alcohol and eating such pungent food as onion and garlic can cause breath odors, as can the normal fermentation of food particles in the mouth and stomach. Infections of the sinuses, nose, lungs, gums, and tonsils can contribute to bad breath.*

See also Periodontal Disease.

ORTHODOX MEDICINE

A physician may offer advice on improving dental hygiene and recommend a mouthwash or breath freshener. If necessary, the underlying infection will be treated.

COMMON-SENSE CARE

Brush and floss after every meal or as often as practicable. Do not overlook brushing your tongue. Avoid cigarettes, alcohol, and spicy foods if you worry about breath odor. Eating apples can contribute to fresher breath. Sucking on cinnamon sticks, or chewing anise or fennel seeds, fresh mint leaves, or parsley may sweeten your breath.

NATURAL MEDICINE THERAPIES

■ **AROMATHERAPY:** Peppermint oil in water makes a good gargle for occasional bad breath.

■ **HOMEOPATHY:** Kali phos may be recommended to remove bitter taste in the mouth on awakening, and mercurius solubilis to eliminate a metallic taste.

■ **VITAMIN AND MINERAL THERAPY:** Vitamin C and the mineral zinc may be recommended if tooth decay or periodontal problems are causing bad breath.

Boils *Boils are inflamed, infected, pus-filled nodules on the face, underarms, back of the neck, and other areas of the body. Typically, a hair follicle under the skin becomes infected by a strain of the staphylococcus bacteria. The area around the boil may become red and tender. Boils may recur for months or years without an underlying disease, but occasionally recurrences indicate diabetes mellitus or another disease that lowers the body's immune capacity.*

See also Diabetes.

ORTHODOX MEDICINE

Applying hot compresses to the affected area can hasten healing by bringing the boil to a head so that it can rupture and the pus can drain. If the boil does not respond to such treatment in three days, if a high fever develops, or if new boils occur, a physician may prescribe an antibiotic or recommend a surgical procedure known as lancing.

COMMON-SENSE CARE

Apply hot compresses to bring the boil to a head. After it bursts, bathe the area with warm water and lemon juice or Epsom salts, and cover with a sterile dressing. Remove the dressing two or three times a day for several days and apply a warm, wet compress. Keep the area around the boil clean but be sure to treat the boil gently. Showers may be better than baths to prevent the spread of infection.

NATURAL MEDICINE THERAPIES

■ **AROMATHERAPY:** Add a few drops of thyme oil to a cup of warm water and use this to bathe the boil to help prevent scarring. Other recommended oils include bergamot and lavender.

■ **HOMEOPATHY:** At the beginning, when the boil is painful, hot, and shiny, belladonna is recommended. If the boil doesn't respond or when the boil starts to point, hepar sulphuricum may help. Silica may be used once the boil breaks; arsenicum for boils when there is burning pain, and lachesis if the skin becomes blue or purple.

■ **NATUROPATHY:** A practitioner may recommend a diet of raw vegetables and fruit during the first two to seven days after the boil appears. Poultices can be made from crushed fenugreek seeds or grated raw cabbage leaves. A hot, soft baked onion can be applied to the boil to bring it to a head.

■ **VITAMIN AND MINERAL THERAPY:** Zinc may be recommended to improve healing, and it can be taken after the boil has disappeared to prevent recurrences. Vitamins A, C, and B complex, and a compound mineral supplement can also be helpful.

Bronchitis *Bronchial congestion, a hacking cough, chest pain, and shortness of breath are symptoms of bronchitis. Acute bronchitis often develops during the late stages of an upper respiratory tract infection, and it is most common in the winter. The airways that connect the windpipe to the lungs become inflamed. If a fever develops and persists longer than a few days, it is important to consult a physician to determine if pneumonia, a serious complication, has set in. Smokers and those with lung disease are most likely to develop bronchitis, although anyone with a bad cold or flu is potentially at risk for acute bronchitis.*

Chronic bronchitis, the more serious form, develops gradually and gets progressively worse. Its symptoms are virtually identical to those of acute bronchitis, except that there is no fever or infection. Chronic bronchitis is often associated with emphysema, another lung disease. Allergies, smoking, and exposure to industrial chemicals can be

contributing factors in chronic bronchitis.

See also Allergies, Colds, Coughs, Emphysema.

ORTHODOX MEDICINE

For acute bronchitis, rest is often recommended, especially for those who run a fever. A cough suppressant and an antibiotic may be prescribed. Drinking lots of fluids and using a humidifier can help.

For chronic bronchitis, a physician will commonly prescribe a bronchodilator drug, which can be inhaled or taken as a tablet. Such a drug helps widen the airways that have been narrowed by the disease, due to either mucus congestion or contraction of the muscle walls in the airways, and thus improves breathing.

COMMON-SENSE CARE

To avoid acute and chronic bronchitis, stop smoking or do not start in the first place. Since acute bronchitis usually develops from a severe upper respiratory tract infection, the elderly, the very young, and those with weakened immune systems should be careful to avoid exposure to anyone with such ailments, especially during the winter. Drinking a lot of fluids helps loosen secretions and promote productive coughing.

Steam can alleviate symptoms. Take a long shower or soak in a steam-filled bathtub. You can also stand over a sink or large pot filled with simmering water and inhale, keeping far enough away from the steam that you don't get burned. You may find relief by applying hot, wet towels to your chest for several minutes. Then dry off, dress warmly, and go to bed in a warm room. Avoid places that are dusty or smoke-filled. Room humidifiers can help. Exercising regularly and practicing breathing techniques can help build up resistance to bronchitis and other lung problems. Relocating from an area with poor air quality to one with less pollution can sometimes aid chronic bronchitis sufferers.

NATURAL MEDICINE THERAPIES

■ **ACUPUNCTURE:** Treatment often involves points on meridians for the lungs, stomach, and urinary bladder, among others.

■ **ALEXANDER TECHNIQUE:** Correcting

poor posture and movement patterns can help improve breathing techniques.

■ **AROMATHERAPY:** The essential oils of pine, cajeput, eucalyptus, and sandalwood can be used as inhalants either in a bowl of hot water, or as drops on a paper towel. They can also be applied during a massage.

■ **HOMEOPATHY:** For sudden attacks, when movement is difficult and the patient craves cool drinks, bryonia is often recommended. A homeopath may suggest aconite for fever, and kali bichromate if the mucus is stringy, thick, and difficult to cough up. Pulsatilla may be recommended if the cough is dry at night but wet during the day.

■ **HYDROTHERAPY:** Cold water packs on the chest and hot water packs between the shoulder blades may relieve coughing.

■ **NATUROPATHY:** Some practitioners believe that bronchitis is closely linked to improper diet, overwork, and other "bad" habits. Such naturopaths may recommend fasts of one to two days to cleanse the system, followed by a period of eating raw food, sometimes exclusively fruits. Consuming plenty of fluids is often advised; however, bronchitis sufferers are urged to eliminate milk and other dairy products to help reduce mucus.

■ **REFLEXOLOGY:** A reflexologist may stimulate the lymphatic system reflexes to help mobilize the body's self-defense mechanisms. The reflexes for the lungs and bronchioles may be used to improve air flow and reduce inflammation.

■ **SHIATSU:** Applying pressure to points on the throat, neck, and upper back may help by relaxing muscles that spasm when bronchitis causes prolonged coughing.

■ **VITAMIN AND MINERAL THERAPY:** Garlic tablets, vitamins A, B complex, and C may be recommended, as well as the mineral iron. To strengthen respiratory-system muscles and improve breathing for those with severe chronic bronchitis, magnesium and carnitine may be recommended.

■ **YOGA:** Postures that are good for draining mucus, strengthening the lungs, increasing resistance, and encouraging healing include the fish, the mountain, pelvic lift, and the upward-facing dog. Yoga breathing techniques are especially beneficial for bronchitis because they can improve circulation, oxygenate the blood, and condition the lungs. These techniques include the basic yoga breathing, alternate nostril breathing, the snake (or hissing) breath, and the charging (or panting) breath.

Exercises to Enhance Breathing

▪ Performing exercises that strengthen the lungs and the diaphragm, which is the muscle between the chest and abdomen, can help minimize recurrences of such respiratory ailments as bronchitis. This disorder may develop from a bad cold or other respiratory tract infections.

▪ Yoga postures such as the upward-facing dog, shown here, are gentle exercises that nearly everyone can do.

▪ The practice of deep, controlled breathing can help relax those with bronchitis, asthma, hay fever, and other such ailments.

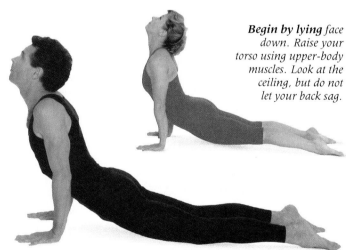

Begin by lying face down. Raise your torso using upper-body muscles. Look at the ceiling, but do not let your back sag.

A modified version *allows those with lower back problems or weak arms to perform this exercise with knees touching the floor and buttocks raised. For more on yoga postures, see pages 214-221.*

Cancer
A group of diseases whose common characteristic is abnormal, unchecked cell growth in bodily organs or tissues, cancer is no longer an automatic death sentence. Many types, including cervical, breast, skin, and colon cancer, respond to therapy and are curable when caught early on.

Overall the incidence of most cancers increases with advancing age; in general, the sooner such cancers are diagnosed, the better the chances of their being cured.

Behavioral and dietary patterns are strongly implicated in the development of certain cancers. For example, smoking is associated with lung, mouth, pharynx, and bladder cancers; alcohol with cancers of the mouth, larynx, and esophagus; a diet high in fat and low in fiber with colon and breast cancers. Sometimes the disease is reversed temporarily or permanently, a condition known as remission. This can happen spontaneously or with the help of various therapies.

See also Constipation, Coughs, Diarrhea, Indigestion, Irritable Bowel Syndrome.

ORTHODOX MEDICINE

Treatments vary according to the type of cancer and the stage of development it has reached when diagnosed. Among the common approaches are surgery to remove a malignant tumor, radiation therapy, hormone therapy, and chemotherapy, which involves anticancer drugs. Often a combination of surgery and other therapies is used.

COMMON-SENSE CARE

To minimize the risk of lung cancer, do not smoke and avoid exposure to passive smoke. To minimize the risk of breast, prostate, and colon cancer, eat a diet low in fat. A high-fiber diet is commonly associated with low colon cancer rates. Abstaining from alcohol or drinking in moderation can minimize the risk of certain types of cancer. The combined effects of heavy drinking and cigarette smoking increase the risk of cancer of the mouth, throat, larynx, and liver.

Overexposure to sunlight can cause you to develop skin cancer, so do not "bake" in the sun and do apply protective lotion when you are outside for any length of time, even on overcast days. Women should periodically have mammography tests to detect early signs of breast cancer and should perform self-examination of the

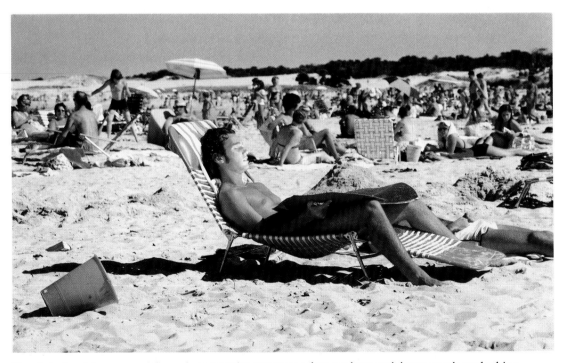

To minimize skin cancer risk, *apply a protective sunscreen when outdoors and do not overdo sunbathing.*

breasts monthly. Women should have regular gynecological checkups that include cervical smear tests to screen for cervical cancer. Anyone with a family history of cancer should be particularly alert to warning signs and should have regular medical checkups.

The seven warning signs of cancer, according to the American Cancer Society, are a change in bowel or bladder habits; a sore that does not heal; unusual bleeding or discharge, especially from the vagina or rectum; a thickening or lump in a breast or elsewhere; indigestion or difficulty in swallowing; an obvious change in a wart or mole; a nagging cough or hoarseness. A sudden, unexplained weight loss also may be a cancer warning sign. Any of these conditions warrants seeing a physician.

NATURAL MEDICINE THERAPIES

■ ACUPUNCTURE: Treatment can be effective in alleviating cancer pain. It may be used as an adjunct to chemotherapy and radiation therapy.

■ HYPNOTHERAPY: Hypnosis may be suggested for pain relief. Hypnosis and self-hypnosis may help some patients boost their disease-fighting immune systems, especially when used in conjunction with meditation, visualization, and other relaxation therapies.

■ NATUROPATHY: To minimize cancer risk, a diet will emphasize whole-grain breads and cereals, which are high in fiber, and raw and cooked fruits and vegetables, which are good sources of vitamin C and beta-carotene. Because certain types of cancer may require special nutritional strategies, it is important for a physician or nutrition specialist to provide dietary guidelines.

■ VITAMIN AND MINERAL THERAPY: Supplements of beta-carotene, which is the precursor to vitamin A, vitamins C and E, and the mineral selenium may be suggested. These are antioxidants, substances that can prevent genetic changes within cells that may contribute to the development of cancer.

■ YOGA: The daily practice of yoga may help alleviate the stress and anxiety that often accompany cancer. Combining yogic exercises with meditation and visualization may assist in pain management and contribute to the body's self-healing capabilities.

Circulatory problems

After varicose veins, one of the most common circulatory problems is a blood clot that attaches itself to a blood vessel. (Clots can also develop to patch up a hole in a blood vessel wall that has been damaged by an injury.) Such clots, or thrombi, occur most commonly in the legs. Symptoms include pain, tenderness, swelling, and skin warmth and discoloration. Clots can become life-threatening when they break off and move to the lungs. Another problem is the development of gangrene, which is the death of skin and underlying tissue due to a cutoff of the blood supply.

If a vein becomes inflamed and a blood clot develops, the disorder is known as thrombophlebitis or, more commonly, phlebitis. Pregnancy, recovery from an operation or an illness that confines a patient to bed for an extended period, a sedentary lifestyle, being overweight, taking birth-control pills, smoking, and the aging process are risk factors for circulatory problems.

See also Hemorrhoids, Migraines, Varicose Veins.

ORTHODOX MEDICINE

For phlebitis in a superficial vein, treatment may involve warm compresses and nonsteroidal anti-inflammatory drugs. For deep-venous thrombosis, treatment varies according to the site and size of the clots. Anticoagulant drugs may prevent other clots from forming. Thrombolytic drugs may be given to break up existing clots. If hospitalization is required, drugs can be administered intravenously. Surgery to remove a blood clot will be performed if there is considerable danger of a clot becoming dislodged from a vein and traveling to the lungs. This life-threatening condition is called a pulmonary embolism.

COMMON-SENSE CARE

The first order of business for anyone with circulatory problems is to quit smoking, because nicotine constricts the veins and

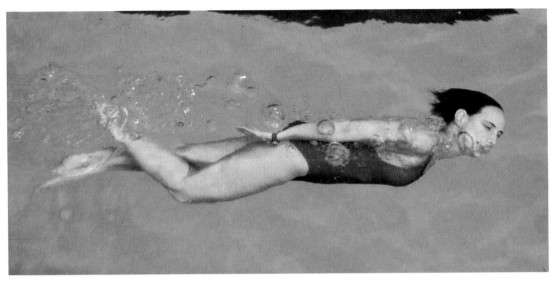

Most people with circulatory problems *are encouraged to exercise regularly; swimming is especially good.*

can permanently damage them. Maintaining a regular exercise program can keep the circulatory system in good working order. Walking and swimming are highly recommended. Taking off excess pounds is essential. Excess weight, particularly in the abdomen, can hamper the return of blood to the heart from the veins, increasing the likelihood of clotting. When you rest, elevate your feet above your head to prevent blood from pooling and minimize the chances of clots developing.

NATURAL MEDICINE THERAPIES

■ **HOMEOPATHY:** For an acute phlebitis attack, hamamelis may be used.

■ **HYDROTHERAPY:** Long soaking baths, or sitz baths, can ease circulation problems. Also recommended are cold compresses and rubbing yourself briskly with a towel that has been soaked in cold water.

■ **NATUROPATHY:** Dietary emphasis may be placed on foods high in fiber, and low in fat, such as fresh vegetables and fruit. Some practitioners suggest avoiding highly refined foods, which tend to be low in fiber and high in fat. Stimulants like coffee, cola, and tea may be banned from your diet.

■ **REFLEXOLOGY:** Stimulating reflexes for the heart and adrenal glands may enhance circulation. Attention will also be given to those reflex areas relating to the site of the circulatory problem, as well as massaging the entire hand or foot.

■ **VITAMIN AND MINERAL THERAPY:** Vitamin C may help prevent blood platelets

from accumulating to form a clot. Some nutritionally oriented practitioners suggest vitamin E supplements to improve circulation in the feet and legs, and niacin to dilate blood vessels. Calcium and magnesium supplements may relieve night cramps in the legs due to poor circulation.

Colds *An infection of the upper respiratory tract caused by one of more than 100 viruses can be termed a cold. The nose, sinuses, throat, larynx, windpipe, and the bronchi, which are airways branching in the lungs, may be affected. Symptoms commonly include sneezing, coughing, congestion, a runny nose, watery eyes, and feeling out of sorts. A low-grade fever, sore throat, chills, muscle aches, and laryngitis may also develop.*

See also Coughs, Sore Throat.

ORTHODOX MEDICINE

Oral decongestants, nasal sprays, and nose drops may provide relief. If over-the-counter brands do not help, a physician may prescribe a spray, drops, or a nasal inhaler. Aspirin or acetaminophen may relieve aches and bring a fever down; acetaminophen is preferred for treating children. An antibiotic will be prescribed only if a secondary bacterial infection develops in the ears, sinuses, lungs, or elsewhere.

COMMON-SENSE CARE

Washing your hands regularly is considered a good preventive measure. If someone in your household or workplace has a cold, be sure that used tissues are disposed of properly. For congestion, try a vaporizer or take a hot shower or bath. Drinking hot liquids like tea and chicken soup may help loosen mucus.

There is no scientific proof that exposure to drafts or sitting in damp rooms makes you liable to catch a cold. Still, it makes sense for the very young, the elderly, and others with weakened immune systems to avoid such situations. They should also avoid exposure to crowds and to confined spaces like buses and airplanes where viruses can be transmitted easily.

Do not smoke when you have a cold. If you get more than one or two colds a year, you may want to examine your diet and lifestyle. As for the old saying, "Feed a cold, starve a fever," you should really feed both because any illness uses up energy, and food replenishes it.

NATURAL MEDICINE THERAPIES

■ ACUPUNCTURE: Stimulating points on the lung, urinary bladder, large intestine, spleen, and stomach meridians may help clear phlegm out of the respiratory system and strengthen the lungs.

■ HOMEOPATHY: Treatment varies according to how the cold developed, what stage it has reached, its symptoms, and other factors. Aconite may be prescribed for a cold in its early stages, for a cold that develops after a sudden chill, or for a cold with fever, headache, and sleeplessness. Gelsemium may be used for a cold that develops during mild but damp weather, and with such symptoms as drowsiness, droopy eyes, and stuffy nose. Other common remedies are allium cepa, belladonna, euphrasia, and natrum muriaticum.

■ HYDROTHERAPY: Cold baths can reduce inflammation; warm baths relax the body and ease muscle aches. Soaking your feet in a warm bath for 10 to 15 minutes before going to bed may boost circulation.

■ MASSAGE: Facial massage can relieve nasal congestion.

■ NATUROPATHY: Practitioners often use such hydrotherapy remedies as Epsom salt baths, hot and cold spraying, and friction rubs to improve circulation, relieve congestion, and ease aches. Dietary recommendations may include avoiding milk products and sugar, which may increase mucus production.

Be sure that your diet includes plenty of fresh fruits and vegetables. Season your food liberally with raw garlic and eat onions regularly; garlic and onions have antiviral effects. Drink increased amounts of juices, soups, and herbal teas.

■ SHIATSU: Efforts may concentrate on points on the face, the back, the base of the neck, the chest, and the arms.

■ VITAMIN AND MINERAL THERAPY: Supplements cannot cure a cold, but some studies show that vitamin C and zinc can ease sore throats and other symptoms. Megadoses of vitamin C may shorten a cold's duration and reduce its severity. A vitamin B complex may be prescribed. Short-term treatment with vitamin A in high doses may help fight colds and other viruses, but a physician must supervise such therapy.

■ YOGA: Performing yoga regularly can help relieve aches, stimulate healing, and relax you. Practice the complete yoga breath frequently.

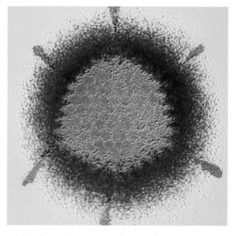

This virus *is just one of more than 100 viruses that can cause the common cold.*

Conjunctivitis *An acute or chronic inflammation of the flexible membrane that seals off the eyeball, conjunctivitis, or pink eye, can be caused by allergies, bacteria, chemicals, or viruses. Wind, smoke, dust, and other environmental factors can contribute to the condition. Its*

symptoms are mild-to-moderate burning sensations, redness, itching, and discharges of mucus or pus. Viral and bacterial conjunctivitis are highly contagious, but they seldom require immediate medical attention.

See also Allergies, Hay Fever.

ORTHODOX MEDICINE

The type of medication depends on what has caused the inflammation. A physician may recommend bathing the eye or using oral antihistamines or decongestant eyedrops for allergies; antibiotic eyedrops or ointments may be used for bacterial infections. When hay fever causes conjunctivitis, steroid eyedrops may be prescribed. Some practitioners treat viral or allergic conjunctivitis with vitamin C eyedrops.

COMMON-SENSE CARE

Conjunctivitis is easily transmitted by hand-to-eye contact, so keep your hands away from your face if you have such viral infections as colds and sore throats, as well as bacterial infections. If the eye problem is an allergic reaction, common causes are chemicals in mascara, contact lens cleaning solutions, animal dander, and airborne pollens. You can switch brands of cosmetics and lens solution, and you can try to avoid exposure to animals and pollen.

Clean the eyes and eyelids with moistened cotton, but do not touch or rub the affected area. A compress (cold if the conjunctivitis is allergy-related, warm otherwise) placed over closed eyes is soothing. Wash towels and facecloths frequently, and do not share them as long as the condition exists. According to folk medicine, poultices for the affected eye can be made from goat-milk yogurt or raw potato, which acts as an astringent.

See a doctor immediately if you have a change in vision, pain in the eyes, or yellow or green discharge. Otherwise, seek medical attention if there has been no improvement in five days.

NATURAL MEDICINE THERAPIES

■ HOMEOPATHY: Belladonna may be used at the beginning, when the eye gets red and teary. If your eyes burn with acrid tears and are sensitive to light, eyebright is

recommended. If there is yellow pus, argentum nitricum or pulsatilla may be prescribed. Apis may be prescribed for severe swelling.

■ VITAMIN AND MINERAL THERAPY: Taking vitamin A may help prevent the recurrences associated with chronic inflammation, but take large doses only under medical supervision. Vitamins A and C and the mineral zinc help the immune system battle viral infections. Vitamin C can help healing and prevent the spread of inflammation.

Constipation *An inability to defecate easily and regularly, constipation is often the result of a diet that is deficient in fiber. It can be a symptom of several ailments, including irritable bowel syndrome, hypothyroidism, and, in rare instances, colon cancer. Most of the time, however, there is no underlying disease. Chronic use of laxatives can cause constipation. It can also be a side effect of antidepressants and other drugs. Occasionally constipation indicates an obstruction or structural abnormality.*

Continued straining and exertion while moving the bowels can lead to the development of hemorrhoids. The condition may become more pronounced during periods of stress, depression, and anxiety.

See also Back Pain, Cancer, Depression, Diverticulitis, Hemorrhoids, Irritable Bowel Syndrome.

ORTHODOX MEDICINE

A change in diet may be advised. Bulk-forming agents like methylcellulose may be prescribed for constipation. Laxatives, enemas, and suppositories may be given as short-term remedies.

COMMON-SENSE CARE

It's easy to get more fiber in your diet by eating such foods as raw fruit and vegetables, especially leafy green vegetables; unprocessed grains like brown rice and whole-grain bread; edible seeds, like sunflower seeds; dried peas and beans, and dried fruit.

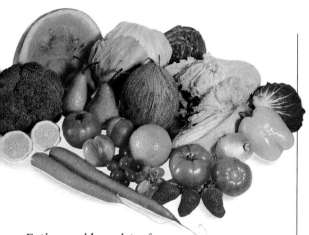

Eating a wide variety of
fruits and vegetables provides dietary fiber, which
can prevent constipation, as well as help treat it.

Eating a tablespoon of raw bran with meals or consuming a vegetable fiber like psyllium may also prove beneficial. It is important to add dietary fiber gradually to minimize gas and bloating, and increase your fluid intake along with the fiber. A program of regular exercise can also promote regularity.

Understanding that regularity can vary from person to person is essential. Not having a daily bowel movement does not in itself signal constipation. However, lack of a movement for a week or a major change in bowel habits that persists calls for consulting a physician.

NATURAL MEDICINE THERAPIES

■ ACUPUNCTURE: The acupuncturist will try to balance the energy in the digestive organs so that they function properly. Choosing specific meridians will depend on the nature of the constipation and accompanying problems like flatulence or tension in the abdomen or back.

■ CHIROPRACTIC: Although it is not generally a chiropractic problem, constipation may be associated with lower back problems. An examination may reveal a weakened or damaged spine, which can respond to chiropractic treatment.

■ HOMEOPATHY: Bryonia is indicated for those with poor stomach-muscle tone. Lycopodium may be prescribed for those who experience gas and bloating. Among other remedies are plumbum, silica, aluminia, platina, sulphur, and nux vomica.

■ HYDROTHERAPY: Hot and cold compresses on the abdomen, and hot and cold sitz baths may be helpful.

■ MASSAGE: To stimulate the colon, massage clockwise, starting at the navel and moving outward over the abdomen, exerting deep, rhythmic pressure.

■ NATUROPATHY: A practitioner may emphasize that chewing food thoroughly ensures the proper breakdown of nutrients before they reach the digestive organs. Eating plenty of fresh fruit, unpeeled when possible, whole grains, legumes, and vegetables supplies dietary fiber, which can promote regularity. Blackstrap molasses is a mild laxative. A teaspoon of molasses can be dissolved in a half cup of warm water.

Exercise may be suggested for toning the muscles involved in elimination and speeding the passage of waste matter through the digestive system.

■ SHIATSU: A common point used to treat constipation is on the back of the hand between the thumb and index finger. Other points are on the abdomen, shin, and elbow crease.

■ VITAMIN AND MINERAL THERAPY: Vitamin C and magnesium aspartate may be given for constipation problems, as well as flaxseed oil or meal. If constipation results from taking antibiotics, acidophilus supplements may be suggested to encourage the growth of intestinal bacteria, which antibiotics can kill.

■ YOGA: Regular practice can contribute to maintaining healthy intestines and bowels. Abdominal contractions, the squat pose, the knee squeeze, and postures that involve bending forward and backward are good for relieving or preventing constipation.

Coughs *A cough is a general term for a sudden, involuntary reflex action that clears pathways of the respiratory system. Coughing can be mild or severe, dry or productive. A productive cough brings up mucus or phlegm. A cough can be symptomatic of a wide range of diseases that includes chronic lung abscess, lung cancer, chronic bronchitis, pneumonia, tuberculosis, hay fever, and asthma, or it may be merely a symptom of the common cold. Smokers may develop a chronic cough.*

See also Asthma, Bronchitis, Cancer, Colds, Hay Fever.

ORTHODOX MEDICINE

Treatment depends on what prompts the coughing. Non-prescription syrups or lozenges containing the ingredient dextromethorphan are often suggested. Medications prescribed for coughs and related disorders may contain codeine and antihistamines. For coughs related to disorders like asthma that constrict the airways to the lungs, a bronchodilator may be recommended.

COMMON-SENSE CARE:

Some people recommend drinking a cup of hot water that contains a tablespoon each of lemon juice and honey. Drinking lots of liquids—soups, teas, fruit juices, and plain water—is good for you. Also inhaling steam, either from a vaporizer or a sink filled with steaming water, will help to loosen the bronchial secretions that cause coughs. Cigarette smoke irritates the bronchial airways, so stop smoking.

If you take a non-prescription cough syrup, you have two basic choices. A suppressant limits the coughing reflex. An expectorant makes a cough less irritating by drawing more liquid into the mouth and airways. Lozenges can be soothing.

NATURAL MEDICINE THERAPIES

■ ACUPUNCTURE: To improve the flow of energy to the lungs, a therapist will use points on the lung meridian in the arms, among others.

■ HOMEOPATHY: Remedies for chronic coughs include aconite, for the initial stage, after you have been exposed to cold, dry winds; belladonna, for a cough that is accompanied by a high fever; bryonia, for a dry and painful cough. Causticum, hepar sulphuris, kali bichromicum, phosphorus, pulsatilla, rumex crispus, and spongia are also prescribed.

■ HYDROTHERAPY: Inhaling steam from a vaporizer or by taking a hot, steamy shower can help relieve nasal congestion and coughs. Cold compresses on the throat and chest may also help.

■ NATUROPATHY: A practitioner may recommend a raw-food diet with uncooked fruit and vegetables, nuts, seeds, herbal teas, and mineral water. It may help to avoid dairy products and other mucus-forming foods. To loosen bronchial secretions, eat raw onions and garlic, prepared horseradish,

and spicy mustard. Hot lemon juice with a teaspoon of honey and glycerine can be soothing.

■ SHIATSU: Applying pressure to points on the chest, throat, neck, and upper back can bring relief and relaxation.

■ VITAMIN AND MINERAL THERAPY: Garlic tablets, which may act as an expectorant, and supplements of vitamins A and C may be suggested.

Cystitis *Among infections of the lower urinary tract, the most common is cystitis, an inflammation of the lining of the bladder caused most often by bacterial infections. Cystitis affects women more frequently than men because women have shorter urethras, the tube from the bladder to the outside of the body, which allows bacteria to enter more easily.*

Symptoms include frequent urination and burning pain during urination, and sometimes pain in the lower abdomen. Symptoms may be mild and disappear quickly; however, in susceptible people, cystitis may recur every few months. In women, bacteria enter the bladder by passing from the vagina through the urethra. Incomplete emptying of the bladder during urination, irritation during intercourse, and improperly fitted diaphragms may increase the risk.

A diagnosis is important both because untreated cystitis can spread infection to the kidneys and other organs and because symptoms of cystitis can mimic those of chlamydia and other sexually transmitted diseases.

ORTHODOX MEDICINE

Although a single megadose of antibiotics will sometimes clear up the infection, more commonly, 3-, 7-, and 10-day courses of antibiotics are prescribed. Surgery may be performed to correct structural abnormalities or remove any obstruction that contributes to recurring persistent cystitis.

COMMON-SENSE CARE

Hot soaking baths, hot water bottles, and heating pads can be relaxing and help alleviate symptoms, especially abdominal pain. Women with cystitis should avoid perfumed soaps, bubble baths, and vaginal deodorants. Wearing cotton underpants and loose clothing that does not bind is recommended. Good hygiene is important: cleanse thoroughly, wiping from front to back to avoid passing fecal bacteria to the urethra. Empty the bladder completely each time you urinate, and both before and after sexual intercourse. Drink a lot of fluids, except for alcoholic beverages.

The use of cranberry juice to prevent or treat cystitis arouses considerable debate among medical practitioners. Some argue that for it to be effective as an antibiotic, a patient would have to drink excessively large quantities. Others point out that cranberry juice contains hippuric acid, an antibiotic, as well as other unidentified substances that make the wall of the bladder slippery, preventing bacteria from adhering.

NATURAL MEDICINE THERAPIES

■ **ACUPUNCTURE:** Treatment may involve points on the kidney, spleen, liver, and urinary bladder meridians.

■ **HOMEOPATHY:** Cantharis is recommended for strong burning pains on urination. Aconite is suggested for the sudden onset of symptoms after exposure to dry cold. Sarsaparilla is given when pain is felt only after urinating.

■ **HYDROTHERAPY:** Spray the pelvic area with warm water, followed with cold water. Also try hot and cold sitz baths in alternation. Hot baths are generally soothing to cystitis sufferers.

■ **NATUROPATHY:** A diet of mild, non-irritating foods may help. A 48-hour fast may be recommended. Avoid citrus fruit and hot, spicy dishes. Replace tea and cola drinks with herb teas and fresh juices. Instead of coffee, try substitutes like chicory and barley extracts.

■ **REFLEXOLOGY:** Massaging the areas related to the urinary tract, kidneys, lower back, and sexual organs can ease symptoms.

■ **VITAMIN THERAPY:** Vitamin C will acidify the urine, which hampers the growth of bacteria. However, do not use vitamin C if you are taking an antibiotic that does not work well in acidic urine.

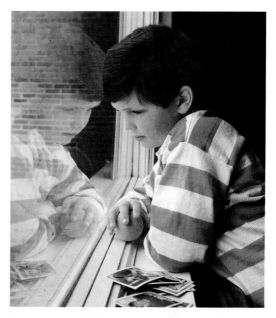

Even young children can experience depression. For children and adults, natural remedies can help.

Depression
Feeling lonely, bored, helpless, alienated, or hopeless are among the emotions associated with depression. When depression interferes with daily living, it can be considered a form of mental illness. Feeling sad now and then is a normal part of life, but losing your self-esteem and interest in other people may signal depression. The risk of depression tends to be highest during adolescence, middle age, and after retirement.

Some forms of depression, like manic-depressive illness, have a genetic component. Others are related to stressful events, such as loss or chronic stress. Often, no precipitating factor can be identified. Among the biological causes of depression are chronic pain; neurological conditions, such as multiple sclerosis, head trauma, and stroke; disorders of the endocrine system, such as hyperthyroidism and hypothyroidism; and infectious diseases such as hepatitis. Drug-related depression sometimes occurs with steroids, antihypertensive agents, sleeping pills, contraceptives, and other medications.

ORTHODOX MEDICINE

The type of the depression, its origins, and its severity determine the treatment. The three approaches are antidepressant drugs, psychotherapy, and shock therapy, also known as electroconvulsive therapy. An estimated one in 15 persons suffers an episode of depression serious enough to require medical attention. Most people who get professional help for depression are treated with drugs or psychotherapy, or a combination of the two. Hospitalization may be required when a person is considering suicide, or is otherwise mentally or physically debilitated by depression.

COMMON-SENSE CARE

Exercise can be a powerful antidote to depression. Vigorous workouts can make you feel better about your appearance and may release chemicals in the body that improve mood. Running, brisk walking, bicycling, and other aerobic exercise, weight lifting, gymnastics, ballet, and other forms of dancing can be effective. Exposure to fresh air and the sun can help a gloomy outlook. As a rule, having a sense of purpose and a fair measure of control over your life makes you less prone to depression. The ideal: create a pleasant environment and surround yourself with positive, understanding people.

NATURAL MEDICINE THERAPIES

■ **ACUPUNCTURE:** The acupuncturist may choose points on the liver, gallbladder, pericardium, heart, stomach, and spleen meridians, aiming to lift depression by stimulating the energy in the liver.

■ **HOMEOPATHY:** Arsenicum, ignatia, and sepia are common prescriptions. Pulsatilla is suggested if depression makes you weep easily, while aurum may be used for a depressed person who becomes suicidal.

■ **MASSAGE:** Having a massage makes a person feel cared for and comforted. It can also stimulate the body's innate healing abilities by improving circulation and cleansing the body of toxins.

■ **NATUROPATHY:** Emphasizing the link between diet and mental health, a practitioner may suggest that you replace fatty and sugary foods with fruits, vegetables, complex carbohydrates, and low-fat protein sources. Advice may include forgoing caffeine and alcohol. A regular program of exercise may be recommended.

■ **VITAMIN THERAPY:** Vitamins C and the B complex and biotin are commonly recommended when nutritional deficiencies seem to contribute to depression. Magnesium supplements and injections of vitamin B_{12} are sometimes recommended.

■ **YOGA:** Regular sessions can improve self-esteem while regulating and toning the body overall. Postures that call for active exertion, such as the salute to the sun, can be beneficial. Rhythmic breathing often eases stress.

Dermatitis *Virtually any skin inflammation not diagnosed as eczema may be considered dermatitis. Some clinicians use the terms interchangeably. Dermatitis can be caused by coming into contact with substances that irritate the skin, by an allergic reaction to drugs, detergents, and other chemicals, and by other causes. Itching and formation of blisters, which sometimes burst open and ooze, are common symptoms. Redness, scaling, and thickening of the skin may occur.*

Dermatitis can affect almost any area on the body. Dandruff in adults and cradle cap in infants are types of seborrheic dermatitis, an inflammation of the glands beneath the skin that open onto hair follicles. Atopic dermatitis,

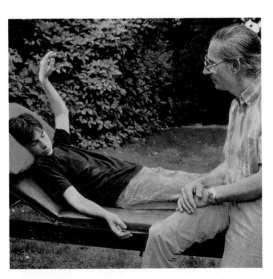

Using hypnotherapy, *some patients with skin disorders such as dermatitis can control itching. For more on hypnotherapy, see pages 120-125.*

which can develop in infancy, is due to a sensitivity to various substances. Statis dermatitis, characterized by scaly red patches on the lower leg, affects mainly middle-aged women who have had multiple births or who have circulatory ailments of the legs.

The most dangerous form is known as generalized exfoliative dermatitis, and hospitalization may be necessary. Symptoms include widespread areas of red, scaly skin, itching, fever, and weight loss.

ORTHODOX MEDICINE

Treatment for severe inflammation may include corticosteroids in ointment, gel, or pill form, and antimicrobial agents if an open sore becomes infected. Antihistamines may be prescribed for itching.

COMMON-SENSE CARE

Try to identify what causes the problem. For dandruff, switch brands of shampoo or hair conditioner. A shampoo that contains selenium sulfide may help. For facial skin problems, switch cosmetic or soap brands. For outbreaks elsewhere, consider changing your laundry detergent and avoiding synthetics and wool clothing, which can irritate the skin. If you have hand dermatitis, or housewife's eczema, wear protective gloves for household chores, preferably vinyl gloves lined with cotton to absorb perspiration. Dry your hands thoroughly after each washing. Apply a mild skin cream or lotion several times daily. Creams and lotions that contain aloe are especially recommended.

NATURAL MEDICINE THERAPIES

■ HYDROTHERAPY: Alternating cold and hot water sprays may relieve symptoms.

■ HYNOTHERAPY: Using hypnosis or self-hypnosis to help you create such sensations as lightness and numbness may alleviate the itchiness and irritation of dermatitis.

■ NATUROPATHY: If a diagnosis indicates that a food allergy causes the condition, dietary changes will be recommended, based on the patient's sensitivities.

■ VITAMIN AND MINERAL THERAPY: Practitioners may recommend vitamins A, C, D, and B complex, which contribute to healthy skin.

Diabetes *A complex disorder, diabetes, or more properly, diabetes mellitus, has been described as a malfunction of metabolism, of the pancreas, and possibly of the immune system. Diabetes can be insulin-dependent or non-insulin-dependent. The pancreas of a diabetic may produce little or no insulin, or else the diabetic is unable to use the insulin produced.*

The hormone insulin regulates the absorption of glucose by the cell. A carbohydrate, glucose is a simple sugar that provides the body's energy needs; excess glucose can be stored in the liver or converted to fat and stored in fat cells. With diabetes mellitus, the level of glucose rises above normal.

Symptoms include increased hunger and thirst, excessive urination, weight loss, and fatigue. The body's ability to metabolize fat is affected, and small blood vessels deteriorate. The disorder hampers the body's ability to fight infections, so diabetics are especially vulnerable to urinary tract, vaginal yeast, and skin infections. If untreated, diabetes mellitus can cause blindness and kidney damage, and increase the likelihood of heart attacks, among other complications.

Diabetes mellitus is more common with advancing age. Those at highest risk of the non-insulin-dependent type are overweight middle-aged or elderly women. Control of diabetes mellitus in pregnant women is an important prenatal consideration. In addition, pregnancy puts a woman at risk for a disease called gestational diabetes.

See also Heart Disease, High Blood Pressure.

ORTHODOX MEDICINE

To maintain the proper insulin level in patients with insulin-dependent diabetes, self-injected insulin is required daily. Proper diet and weight control is also important. This may require coordination among physician, patient, and dietitian. For

Complementary Therapies

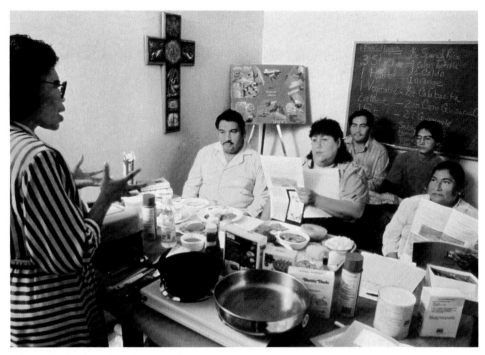

A dietitian advises *Mexican Americans how to lower their risk of diabetes by changing their diet. Eating foods relatively low in fat and sugar are the most common recommendations.*

non-insulin-dependent diabetics, most of whom are obese, dietary control may be sufficient. However, if the proper diet does not adequately regulate the blood glucose level, antidiabetic drugs or insulin may be prescribed.

COMMON-SENSE CARE

The proper diet, which is low in fats and simple sugars and high in fiber and complex carbohydrates, can help balance blood sugar and control weight. Eat meals at approximately the same time every day. Exercise may help the body use insulin. A low-fat diet and aerobic exercise may also help prevent diabetes from developing, an important consideration for those with risk factors.

Frequently diabetics suffer from poor circulation, so do not smoke, and drink only in moderation, if at all. Poor circulation often affects the feet, which are the body part farthest from the heart. To prevent skin ulcers and other problems, choose shoes that fit well.

NATURAL MEDICINE THERAPIES

■ ACUPUNCTURE: Treatment may concentrate on strengthening the stomach, spleen, and kidneys.

■ HOMEOPATHY: A practitioner may choose phosphorus to stabilize blood sugar and energy levels.

■ NATUROPATHY: A diet high in fiber and complex carbohydrates will be recommended. Onions and garlic may be suggested for their possible role in lowering blood sugar. An exercise program that is tailored to the diabetic may be advised. An obese diabetic will be placed on a weight-loss diet.

■ REFLEXOLOGY: Treatment may be applied to reflexes for the pancreas, liver, and the pituitary, thyroid, and adrenal glands. A diabetic who takes insulin should be monitored closely immediately after treatment and again 24 hours later.

■ VITAMIN AND MINERAL THERAPY: Supplements of vitamins A, B_6, C, and E, biotin, niacin, and the minerals chromium, zinc, selenium, and calcium may be suggested. They should be taken only if prescribed by a physician.

■ YOGA: Practiced regularly, yoga helps regulate hormones and other body chemicals, as well as toning the body and contributing to lowered stress levels. Recommended postures include the plow and shoulder stand, which may activate the thyroid gland, and the kneeling pose.

Diarrhea
A common symptom of various disorders, diarrhea is an increase in the frequency and volume of bowel movements, and a change in the consistency to unusually loose movements. Its cause can be as minor as eating something that disagrees with you or as serious as cancer of the colon, ulcerative colitis, and amebic dysentery. Diarrhea is a side effect of some medications. A physician should be consulted when diarrhea lasts more than three or four days or sooner if it is accompanied by vomiting and bloody stools, severe abdominal pain, or lightheadedness and decreased urination, which are symptoms of dehydration.

See also Cancer, Irritable Bowel Syndrome.

ORTHODOX MEDICINE

Treatment varies according to the cause of the complaint. Replacement of lost fluids, minerals, and salts is essential. Antidiarrheal drugs can be taken except when an infection causes the condition; such drugs may prolong the infection. Travelers who suffer from so-called traveler's diarrhea may get relief from liquid medications containing kaolin-pectin or bismuth subsalicylate.

COMMON-SENSE CARE

To prevent dehydration, drink plenty of fluids. Clear liquids like tea, broth, fruit juices, and water are suggested. Avoid milk and fatty foods for several days. If diarrhea is caused by antibiotics, eating yogurt with lactobacilus can restore the proper intestinal balance of bacteria that such drugs may destroy. Consider taking supplements of acidophilus culture in liquid or capsule form. Avoid coffee, tea, and other caffeinated beverages, alcohol, and spicy foods for several days.

If you change your eating habits to increase dietary fiber, do so gradually. The sudden introduction of high-fiber foods is often more than the system can handle, and diarrhea results. To prevent a bout of traveler's diarrhea, avoid salads and other raw food that cannot be peeled, tap water, ice cubes, ice cream, and anything served cold at a buffet table.

NATURAL MEDICINE THERAPIES

■ ACUPUNCTURE: Therapy can be effective in treating chronic and acute diarrhea. Stomach, spleen, and large intestine meridians are among those that may be stimulated.

■ HOMEOPATHY: Aconite is often recommended for diarrhea caused by exposure to dry, cold winds or a sudden surge of fear. If diarrhea is caused by food poisoning, especially meat, arsenicum album is prescribed. For particularly severe attacks with cold sweats, veratrum album is advised.

■ HYDROTHERAPY: Placing ice packs on the lower and middle spine for 10 minutes at a time may help.

■ NATUROPATHY: A naturopath may recommend a 24-hour fast. Meantime, to prevent dehydration and maintain electrolyte balance, drink mineral water, diluted vegetable and fruit juice, or a solution of water with salt and sugar. When you go back to solid foods, begin with such soft foods as boiled rice, bananas, grated apples or applesauce, and dry toast.

■ SHIATSU: Pressure on various points on the navel, the abdomen slightly below the navel, and the feet may help tone abdominal muscles and relieve diarrhea.

■ VITAMIN AND MINERAL THERAPY: Consider taking supplements of vitamin B complex and the minerals potassium and sodium.

Diverticulitis
The presence of small sacs, or diverticuli, on the wall of the colon is diverticulosis, a condition that is usually asymptomatic. Diverticulitis develops when the lining of the sacs becomes inflamed. Serious health problems can occur when the inflammation becomes infected or when there is an obstruction, perforation, or bleeding. Symptoms include fever, chills, constipation, pain, rectal bleeding, tenderness, and rigidity of the area over the intestine. Complications include peritonitis, which is inflammation of the lining of the abdomen, and the development of abscesses and fistulas, or narrow channels, that link different parts of the intestine.

See also Constipation.

ORTHODOX MEDICINE

A high-fiber, high-fluid diet, bed rest, stool softeners, antibiotics, and antispasmodic drugs are the usual recommendations. For severe cases of diverticulitis with infection, hospitalization may be required so that antibiotics can be given intravenously. If there is an obstruction in the colon, the formation of a fistula, an inflammation of the lining of the abdominal cavity, or other complications, surgery may be performed.

COMMON-SENSE CARE

A good way to prevent diverticulosis is to eat a high-fiber diet. Anyone who needs to add more dietary fiber should do so gradually. If necessary, take a psyllium-seed supplement. If you already have diverticulosis, avoid eating seeds, popcorn, and nuts, which can get stuck in diverticula and cause inflammation. Drink plenty of water. Forgo alcoholic beverages. Move the bowels regularly and without straining. Do not rely on laxatives or suppositories to keep you regular because they can become habit-forming. Try to minimize stress and learn stress-reduction techniques. Perform exercises to tone the muscles in the abdomen.

NATURAL MEDICINE THERAPIES

■ ACUPUNCTURE: Therapy can be effective in relieving symptoms. Acupuncture will be applied on several meridians according to what is causing the discomfort.

■ MASSAGE: Various forms of massage are helpful for elimination problems.

■ NATUROPATHY: Practitioners may suggest eliminating red meat, alcohol, drinks that contain caffeine, and refined carbohydrates. Avoiding dairy products can relieve symptoms for some. Dietary suggestions include fresh vegetable and fruit juices, especially carrot, apple, and cabbage juice. Aloe vera juice may help prevent constipation and other colon problems. Fasting may be suggested.

■ VITAMIN AND MINERAL THERAPY: Recommendations may include garlic capsules; vitamin K, which may be destroyed by intestinal tract disorders or antibiotic drugs; vitamin A, which protects colon lining; and vitamin E, which protects mucous membranes.

■ YOGA: Regular yoga practice may help because many postures tone the organs and encourage passage of waste through the system. Yoga can also contribute to controlling stress, which may aggravate problems in the digestive tract.

Eczema *Inflamed skin that itches or develops scales or blisters can be one of several types of eczema. Allergic reactions can trigger eczema. Atopic eczema, which affects young children and those with allergies, is identified by a rash that itches intensely. Other types include hand eczema and aural eczematoid dermatitis, which affects the outer ear and the ear canal.*

See also Dermatitis.

ORTHODOX MEDICINE

To reduce itching, soothing ointment or petroleum jelly may be applied to the affected area. For severe cases, corticosteroids, antibiotics, and antihistamines may be prescribed.

COMMON-SENSE CARE

Most cases respond to over-the-counter lotions and ointments that lubricate the skin and alleviate itching. Keep the affected area clean using mild soap and non-oily shampoo. Try to reduce stress and get adequate rest. Wet compresses can bring relief. Daily friction rubs to boost circulation and hasten renewal of skin tissue can improve the condition. The rubs can be done with a dry towel or a moist cool towel.

NATURAL MEDICINE THERAPIES

■ ACUPUNCTURE: Therapy may be effective in clearing up some cases of eczema. Points to be stimulated include those on meridians for the large intestine, lungs, spleen, and stomach.

■ HOMEOPATHY: Remedies include graphite for outbreaks on the hands and behind the ears; arsenicum for chronic dry eczema; and sulphur and rhus ven for other conditions.

■ HYPNOTHERAPY: Because anxiety and stress are often implicated in skin disorders, hypnosis can help by providing a form of relaxation.

■ **NATUROPATHY:** Food allergy is a common cause of eczema, particularly among children. A naturopath may suggest an elimination diet to identify foods that provoke eczema. Some practitioners advise limiting animal products and foods that contain sugar.

■ **REFLEXOLOGY:** Eczema may respond to therapy using points on both the side and sole of the foot. Reflexes to stimulate include the endocrine glands, solar plexus, and kidneys.

■ **VITAMIN AND MINERAL THERAPY:** Practitioners may recommend vitamins A, C, and B complex to heal eczema and prevent recurrences.

Emphysema *A disease of the very small air sacs in the lungs known as alveoli, emphysema is an incurable respiratory disease. Smoking is virtually always the cause of emphysema, although air pollution may precipitate the condition. In a very few cases, a genetic tendency exists for emphysema.*

See also Bronchitis, Coughs.

ORTHODOX MEDICINE

Treatment generally aims to alleviate such symptoms as shortness of breath, coughing, lung inflammation, and retention of fluids. It may also slow the progression of the disease and minimize disability. A physician will urge the patient to stop smoking, if smoking continues. Bronchodilators and corticosteroids may be prescribed. Oxygen therapy may be used for special breathing problems. If an infection develops, antibiotics will be prescribed.

COMMON-SENSE CARE

Once cigarette smoking has ceased, changes in diet and lifestyle can help maintain general health and minimize respiratory infections and other problems. A low-salt diet is advised to minimize fluid retention. Drinking clear, hot beverages like herbal teas can help clear out passages clogged by mucus.

If your workplace is dusty, dirty, or polluted by toxic chemicals, wear a mask, use a respirator, or consider changing jobs. Emphysema sufferers are vulnerable to acute bronchitis, pneumonia, and other serious respiratory illnesses, so they should stay

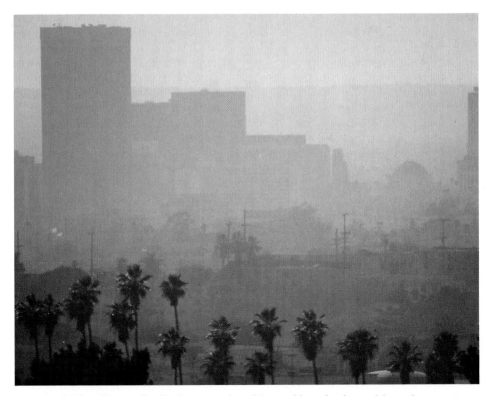

Smog and other forms of pollution *create breathing problems for those with emphysema. In this respiratory disease, distended air sacs make it harder for the lungs to process oxygen.*

away from anyone with a cold or flu and get flu shots annually as a preventive measure.

It is helpful to build up endurance by engaging in regular physical activity; otherwise, the slightest movement will leave you gasping for breath. Perform a mild form of exercise regularly, like walking or playing golf. Breathing exercises can help.

NATURAL MEDICINE THERAPIES

■ ACUPUNCTURE: Points along the lung, urinary bladder, and ren meridians may be stimulated to relieve symptoms.

■ AROMATHERAPY: Eucalyptus extract can be added to steam that is inhaled, and it can be used twice daily in massage oil. Lemon oil is also suggested.

■ HYDROTHERAPY: A cold water pack placed on the chest may relieve congestion.

■ NATUROPATHY: The dietary emphasis is likely to be on foods low in salt and sodium, which can contribute to fluid retention, like raw fruits and vegetables; processed foods tend to be relatively high in sodium. Consuming dishes daily with garlic and onion, preferably raw, is suggested.

■ REFLEXOLOGY: Among the reflexes that can be stimulated for symptom relief are those for the diaphragm, heart, throat, and immunological system.

■ VITAMIN AND MINERAL THERAPY: Garlic capsules can help prevent infection. Vitamins A and C can bolster the immune system and help heal inflamed lung tissue. The mineral magnesium can strengthen the respiratory muscles and reduce the tendency for the bronchi to spasm.

Eyestrain *Eyestrain is a general term to describe minor discomfort, fatigue, or pain in the eyes. Although medical experts vary as to whether the disorder exists, common complaints of eyestrain arise after prolonged periods of reading, watching television, or working on a computer.*

See also Conjunctivitis, Styes.

ORTHODOX MEDICINE

An eye specialist will perform tests to rule out possible eye diseases and to test vision. Corrective glasses or contact lenses will be prescribed if needed, or if you already have them, the prescription may be adjusted.

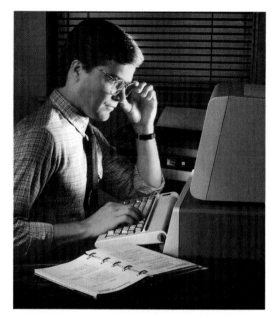

Working at a computer *all day long can strain the eyes. Try taking a break every two hours.*

COMMON-SENSE CARE

When you are reading, position light sources carefully, so that light comes from behind and to the side at shoulder height. Be sure that work spaces are adequately illuminated. Users of video display terminals should spend no more than two hours at a time in front of their screens without taking a break. For relief, bathe the eyes in a weak salt solution, seawater, or a mixture of a teaspoon of honey and a pint of boiled water, used after it is cooled. Blink frequently and perform eye exercises regularly. Try palming your eyes. Place your hands over your eyes so that the little fingers flank the bridge of the nose. Do this several times daily for a few minutes at a time.

NATURAL MEDICINE THERAPIES

■ HOMEOPATHY: Bathe the eyes with four drops of euphrasia mother tincture in 1/4 pint of lukewarm water. Seek the advice of a homeopath or other physician for persistent eyestrain.

■ REFLEXOLOGY: Eyestrain can be a result of tension, and for this reason it may respond to reflexology. Concentrate on the area at the base of the toes.

■ SHIATSU: Massage several key points of the face to get relief. These include the bridge of the nose, the area around the eyes, and below the cheekbones.

■ **VITAMIN AND MINERAL THERAPY:** Taking vitamins A and B 12 daily may be recommended. Eat unprocessed, unsalted sunflower seeds, which are a good source of iron, calcium, and vitamins.

Gallstones *When cholesterol in the liver or gallbladder crystallizes and joins with the bile secreted by the liver to help digest fat, gallstones may form. Many pass through the body unnoticed. Most gallstones produce pain when they get lodged in the cystic duct, which is a fairly small passageway from the liver to the gallbladder. The intensity and duration varies, but at its worst it causes several hours of intense pain. Pain may be felt in the abdominal area, or it may be felt on the right side of the chest, then move to the back or shoulder. Jaundice may develop afterward. Those facing the highest risk are overweight women in their forties or older. A tendency for gallstones is often inherited.*

ORTHODOX MEDICINE

A two-year program of drug therapy with bile acids can dissolve gallstones for some people; however, recurrences are common after therapy has ended. Some drugs are effective in dissolving those gallstones composed of cholesterol; about 75 percent of gallstones are cholesterol, and the other 25 percent are mainly calcium salts. Surgery may be performed to remove the gallbladder. This operation is the most commonly performed abdominal surgery in the United States; however, laparoscopic surgery, which is much less traumatic, has begun to replace it.

COMMON-SENSE CARE

To prevent gallstones, keep your weight under control. If you decide to diet, choose a weight-loss plan carefully. Obese people who rely on rapid-weight-loss diets face increased risk of developing gallstones.

NATURAL MEDICINE THERAPIES

■ **ACUPUNCTURE:** Points on the gallbladder, stomach, liver, kidney, and conception-vessel meridians may be stimulated.

■ **HOMEOPATHY:** Celidonium, berberis, and podophyllum are commonly prescribed.
■ **NATUROPATHY:** To prevent gallstones or to avoid recurrences, follow a low-fat, high-fiber diet that is low in cholesterol. Water-soluble fiber, which is found in fruit, vegetables, pectin, and oat bran, may help lower blood cholesterol levels.
■ **REFLEXOLOGY:** Working reflexes for the liver and gallbladder may bring relief.
■ **SHIATSU:** Applying rhythmic pressure in circles on the lower abdomen around the gallbladder may relieve symptoms. The gallbladder is located under the liver.
■ **VITAMIN AND MINERAL THERAPY:** Recommendations may include vitamins A, C, E, and B complex with choline, which is necessary for cholesterol metabolism, and liver and gallbladder functions. Vitamin D supplements may be suggested for gallbladder ailments, which can hamper the body's ability to absorb the vitamin.

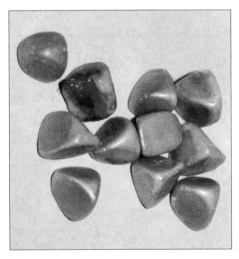

Gallstones, *which contain mostly cholesterol, can reach an inch in diameter.*

Gout *Gout is a metabolic disorder that produces acute attacks of joint pain. Areas affected include the joints at the base of the big toe, foot, ankle, knee, and wrist, and small hand joints. The first attack, which typically affects one joint, usually lasts a few days. If the disorder progresses, more joints may become inflamed, the pain may worsen, and kidney problems may develop. Gout commonly produces a form of arthritis as its primary*

symptom. Being male and obese puts you in a high-risk group.

Gout is caused by a buildup of excess uric acid in the blood that may occur when the kidneys fail to excrete uric acid normally as part of the digestive process or because of overproduction of uric acid. Uric acid is a by-product of the metabolism of protein. The accumulation of uric-acid crystals in joints and surrounding tissues may cause inflammation and pain.

See also Arthritis.

ORTHODOX MEDICINE

Anti-inflammatory drugs can lessen joint pain. The drug colchicine, derived from a crocus plant, may also provide relief for acute attacks of gout. For intense pain, painkillers may be prescribed. Bed rest and adequate fluid intake are recommended. The drug allopurinol is commonly used to inhibit the formation of uric acid. Drugs that promote uric-acid excretion by the kidneys often prove effective.

COMMON-SENSE CARE

Weight reduction and dietary modifications may be the first order of business. Losing weight is advised for those gout patients who are overweight, particularly for the obese. However, fasting should be avoided since it can elevate uric-acid levels in the blood. Limit consumption of foods high in the chemical purine, which forms uric acid. Among these foods are liver and other organ meat; herring, sardines, and other fish; poultry, legumes, spinach, and asparagus. Limit the amount of sweets. Other suggested changes include drinking less alcohol or none at all, exercising regularly, and minimizing stress, which can precipitate a gout attack.

NATURAL MEDICINE THERAPIES

■ ACUPUNCTURE: Therapy aims to decrease pain and swelling, and to enhance wellness overall. The specific meridians treated vary according to which joint or joints are affected. Points on the urinary bladder and stomach meridians may be stimulated for gout in the big-toe joint.

■ HOMEOPATHY: Attention will be paid to specific symptoms as well as constitutional weaknesses that allow for gout to develop. Remedies include belladonna and colchicine.

■ HYDROTHERAPY: Applying hot or cold compresses or ice packs to the affected joint may ease the pain.

■ NATUROPATHY: In addition to avoiding those high-purine foods listed above in Common-Sense Care, you should increase your intake of complex carbohydrates and fluids. The diet should include plenty of fresh fruit and vegetables (except spinach and asparagus). Some practitioners recommend eating cherries, blueberries, and blackberries, which contain a substance that may help prevent attacks by reducing uric-acid levels.

■ REFLEXOLOGY: The spleen and kidney reflexes are most directly involved in uric-acid production. Other reflexes to be stimulated include the pituitary gland and the adrenal gland.

■ VITAMIN AND MINERAL THERAPY: Folic acid, which can inhibit the production of uric acid, may be recommended. Vitamin C, vitamin E, and B complex may also be suggested.

Hay fever *Scientifically known as allergic or seasonal rhinitis, hay fever commonly occurs in the spring, summer, and fall, when tree pollens, grass pollens, and ragweed pollens flourish. The wind carries the substances, or allergens, that produce the characteristic cough, sneeze, watering eyes, drippy nose, and itchy throat.*

See also Allergies, Coughs.

ORTHODOX MEDICINE

If over-the-counter decongestants, antihistamines, and nasal sprays do not relieve symptoms, a physician may prescribe stronger versions of these medications or a corticosteroid spray. Persistent symptoms may require short-term corticosteroid therapy.

Those most severely affected by hay fever sometimes try an intensive program of desensitization. This may involve a weekly, biweekly, or monthly injection with serum that contains pollen extract. Such therapy usually lasts for one to three years.

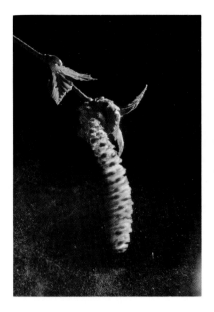

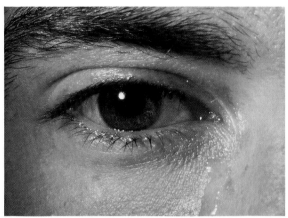

Birch pollen (left) is one of the most irritating of all wind-borne pollens, quickly triggering hay fever symptoms—coughing, tearing, and sneezing. Acupuncture and homeopathy are among the natural medicine therapies that offer relief.

COMMON-SENSE CARE

Staying indoors for weeks at a time or walking around with protective face gear is not very practical, but the need to avoid contact with allergens cannot be overstated. Steer clear of anyone who is smoking; likewise, industrial pollution and household dust can heighten allergic reactions. Air conditioning can help guard against your coming into contact with pollens. Change the filter in your air conditioner and furnace regularly. If you mow a lawn, wear a mask that covers your nose and mouth.

NATURAL MEDICINE THERAPIES

■ ACUPUNCTURE: Stimulating points along the urinary bladder and large intestine meridians may relieve sneezing. If you are affected at the same time each year, weekly acupuncture sessions two or three months prior to hay-fever season might be advisable.

■ HOMEOPATHY: Persistent hay fever may call for remedies that strengthen the immune system, in addition to more specific approaches. For streaming and a sore nose and eyes, euphrasia and arsenicum album are used. Pulsatilla may also be recommended.

■ HYDROTHERAPY: Such treatment as a cold-water plunge, sitz bath, and daily morning friction rubs can ease symptoms.

■ NATUROPATHY: The emphasis is on a diet with a lot of whole grains, raw fruits, vegetables, and garlic. Avoid mucus-forming foods such as dairy products. Some people are persuaded that eating certain foods, including honey, horseradish, mustard, onion, and garlic, can reduce hay fever symptoms. Giving up dairy products may bring relief to those sensitive to casein, the protein in milk, which can increase mucus production. A practitioner may advise against alcoholic drinks, since alcohol can cause mucous membranes to swell.

■ VITAMIN AND MINERAL THERAPY: Beta-carotene and vitamin C can stimulate your immune response. Vitamin C, pantothenic acid, and calcium may alleviate symptoms.

■ YOGA: Performing the basic yoga postures regularly can relieve the stress that may accompany allergic reactions. A nasal wash and a breathing exercise known as kapalabhati may also be recommended.

Headache *A dull ache or piercing pain in the back of the head or at the temples may be a tension headache. This type of pain is typically caused by muscles that contract in the head, neck, or face. Such movements stimulate nerve endings, producing pain that may be felt in only one area of the head or neck, or the entire head.*

Pain from expansion or contraction of the walls of the blood vessels in and near the head causes vascular headaches. Migraine headaches, which sometimes last for days, are generally the most intense form.

Overindulging in alcoholic beverages can produce headaches in the form of hangovers. Sinusitis, toothaches, gum infections, eyestrain, head injuries, and misalignment of the jaw can cause headaches. The onset of a headache may be affected by weather changes, disturbing lights or smells, and emotional stress. Certain foods, like cheese and red wine, and some food additives can trigger a migraine headache in sensitive people.

In rare cases, headaches indicate serious ailments like intracranial infection or tumor, severe high blood pressure, or diseases of the eye, ear, nose, throat, and teeth.

See also Allergies, High Blood Pressure, Menstrual Problems, Migraine, Periodontal Disease.

ORTHODOX MEDICINE

Aspirin, acetaminophen, ibuprofen, or other nonsteroidal anti-inflammatory medications with or without caffeine and phenobarbital are recommended for most headaches. Recurring headaches that do not respond to such medication may be treated with antidepressants, tranquilizers, or sedatives. Often these are given along with psychotherapy. Recurrences accompanied by nausea or vomiting may signal a serious organic problem; likewise, a severe headache accompanied by blurred vision, unsteadiness, or slurred speech requires prompt medical attention.

COMMON-SENSE CARE

Exercising regularly is considered one of the best antidotes to stress and tension, which are regarded by many as the cause of most headaches. When you feel stress, muscles in your neck and shoulders tense up. In addition, stress and anxiety can worsen an existing headache. People who are very driven and competitive may need to find ways to slow themselves down.

Keep track of when headaches occur and try to determine what triggers them. Among the foods and drinks that most commonly cause headaches are chocolate, beverages that have caffeine, and red wine. If you are prone to headaches, avoid the food additives monosodium glutamate, nitrites, and nitrates, and very-low-calorie diets. Get adequate rest.

Drinking coffee is said to alleviate headaches caused by hangovers. Folk medicine remedies include peppermint or menthol oil rubs, and herbal teas.

NATURAL MEDICINE THERAPIES

■ ACUPUNCTURE: The major points for headache relief are on the head, neck,

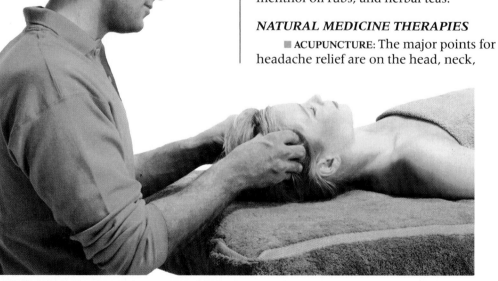

A massage can relieve tense muscles in the scalp, forehead, neck, and shoulders, which often contribute to headache pain. It is also a pleasant way to dissipate emotional stress.

hands, and feet. The location of the pain determines which meridians will receive the most attention. Acupuncture has been effective with both acute head pain and chronic headaches.

■ **ALEXANDER TECHNIQUE:** Correcting posture and movement problems that may contribute to tension headaches can help prevent recurrences in some people.

■ **CHIROPRACTIC:** A headache may be the sign of a skeletal displacement that is suitable for chiropractic therapy.

■ **HOMEOPATHY:** Commonly prescribed remedies include nux vomica for a hangover, sepia for a headache with nausea, and belladonna for violent headaches.

■ **HYDROTHERAPY:** Alternate hot and cold compresses on the forehead and the base of the skull, or hot and cold showers. Ice packs to the head or neck, or cold running water on the head provide relief for some. Others prefer hot showers or baths, or moist hot towels on the back of the neck.

■ **MASSAGE:** Headaches caused by stress, muscular tension, or bad posture may respond to massage and other tension-releasing therapies. Efforts may concentrate on tight muscles in the face and neck, and along the scalp.

■ **NATUROPATHY:** A naturopath may advise changes in diet and lifestyle to prevent recurrences, especially of migraines. Eliminating chocolate, cheese, and alcohol may decrease their frequency. Possible links between headaches and food allergies may be explored. Relaxation and meditation techniques may be recommended.

■ **OSTEOPATHY:** Osteopaths believe that headaches stem from pressure on nerves or blood vessels that can be eased by manipulative therapy.

■ **REFLEXOLOGY:** Massage foot reflexes for the upper spinal column, eyes, ears, throat, and solar plexus.

■ **SHIATSU:** To alleviate pain, the practitioner may stimulate points on the head, neck, hands, feet, and shoulders.

■ **VITAMIN AND MINERAL THERAPY:** The B complex vitamins and vitamin C, as well as calcium, magnesium, and potassium, may be recommended.

■ **YOGA:** The shoulder stand and roll, the cobra, and other postures that release tension in the upper back, shoulders, and neck may be recommended. Yogic breathing exercises can also be helpful.

Heart disease *The leading cause of death in the United States, heart disease, which is known scientifically as coronary heart disease, occurs when the heart sustains damage due to narrowed or blocked arteries within the organ. Such blockages make it impossible for blood to reach the heart*

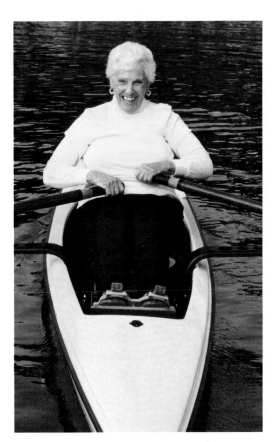

Aerobic exercises *such as rowing, running, and swimming can help lower the risk of heart disease.*

muscle. The most dramatic and potentially life-threatening result of this process is a heart attack, also known as acute myocardial infarction. The severe chest pain known as angina pectoris is a warning that the blood supply to the heart is insufficient, but it is not immediately life-threatening in most cases.

The buildup of deposits of fatty plaque along the arterial walls is a disease known as atherosclerosis. When these fatty deposits multiply and thicken, they become

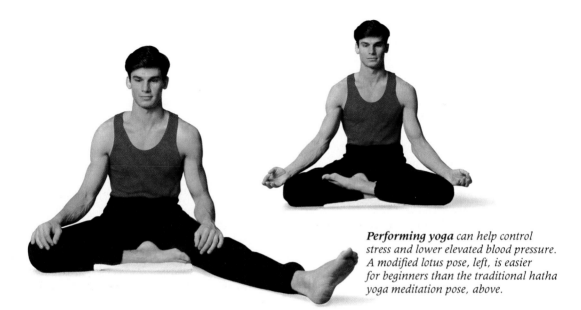

Performing yoga can help control stress and lower elevated blood pressure. A modified lotus pose, left, is easier for beginners than the traditional hatha yoga meditation pose, above.

lesions that can prevent the heart muscle from getting enough blood and, as a result, it becomes oxygen-starved. Chest pain or heart-tissue damage may occur. The seven most significant risk factors for coronary heart disease, in no particular order, are high blood pressure; elevated levels of blood fat, especially certain types of cholesterol; smoking; diabetes mellitus; obesity; being male, and a family history of heart disease occurring before age 60.

See also Arteriosclerosis, Diabetes, High Blood Pressure.

ORTHODOX MEDICINE

A wide range of drugs is available to treat the various forms of heart disease. If a patient with coronary artery disease, characterized by inadequate blood flow through clogged arteries, does not improve with medication, surgery may be performed.

Common surgical techniques are coronary artery bypass, in which one or more veins are grafted to reroute the blood flow, and angioplasty, in which a balloon is inserted to widen a narrowed artery.

Before heart disease progresses so far that it causes a heart attack, or surgery is needed to prevent such an occurrence, a physician will advise a patient on preventive strategies. Three items at the top of the list are to stop smoking, consume fewer high-fat foods, and exercise regularly. Diet and drugs may work in tandem to lower the blood level of the harmful type of cholesterol, LDL cholesterol. A patient who suffers a heart attack may be rushed to a hospital and placed in a cardiac-care unit for treatment.

COMMON-SENSE CARE

People who watch what they eat, control their weight, and exercise regularly tend to have less coronary heart disease and fewer heart attacks than their overweight, sedentary counterparts. Although a genetic tendency toward heart problems may intensify the risk, when you eat sensibly, avoid cigarettes, drink in moderation or not at all, exercise, and learn to control stress, you can provide a form of do-it-yourself health insurance.

A heart-healthy diet emphasizes foods low in fat, and high in complex carbohydrates. This means a minimal amount of red meat and moderate amounts of fish and skinless chicken; several servings daily of fruits and vegetables, and a reduction in foods that are processed and fried. Performing aerobic exercises three to five times a week is recommended to condition the cardiovascular system. Learning how to reduce stress can lower the risk of coronary artery disease.

NATURAL MEDICINE THERAPIES

■ ACUPUNCTURE: Such symptoms of heart disease as muscle spasms may respond to acupuncture. Treatment can help angina patients relax and can ease their pain.

■ **ALEXANDER TECHNIQUE:** This can serve as a preventive approach for those with a tendency for cardiovascular problems.

■ **SHIATSU:** Pressing several places along the inner forearm can be effective in relieving symptoms.

■ **VITAMIN AND MINERAL THERAPY:** To prevent heart disease or help control it if you already have it, you may consider taking vitamins B_6, C, E, vitamin B complex, and beta-carotene, as well as copper, magnesium, and lecithin. Selenium tablets may be suggested, since a deficiency of this mineral has been linked to heart disease. Chromium tablets may help prevent the buildup of cholesterol in arteries.

■ **YOGA:** Relaxation through yoga helps some patients control their blood pressure.

Hemorrhoids *The enlargement of a vein in the rectum creates hemorrhoids, or piles. This disorder, which is a form of varicose veins, can produce itching, pain, bleeding, and, less commonly, mucous discharges. Hemorrhoids can make being seated or moving the bowels difficult.*

See also Circulatory Problems, Constipation, Varicose Veins.

ORTHODOX MEDICINE

Stool softeners, along with a diet high in fiber, are frequently recommended. Topical anesthetic or anti-inflammatory ointments and witch hazel compresses may relieve symptoms. Operations to remove hemorrhoids include cryosurgery, which involves instruments cooled to about -256° F, laser surgery, banding, and formal operative hemorrhoidectomy.

COMMON-SENSE CARE

Many people who have hemorrhoids suffer from constipation and strain to pass stool, so a high-fiber diet is recommended. Among the foods that are high in fiber, a natural laxative, are whole grains, oat bran, and raw fruits and vegetables. If you drink more water and juices, these foods will increase the effectiveness of fiber and soften stool.

Exercise can stimulate muscle tone, which helps overcome constipation. Walking briskly, especially after eating a meal, may also alleviate constipation. Soaking at least twice a day in a warm tub can bring relief.

NATURAL MEDICINE THERAPIES

■ **ACUPUNCTURE:** Points used to heal hemorrhoids and prevent further inflammation, bleeding, and pain are on the meridians for the lung, spleen, stomach, ren, kidney, and urinary bladder.

■ **HOMEOPATHY:** Pulsatilla, nux vomica, witch hazel, and horse chestnut may be used.

■ **HYDROTHERAPY:** Immerse your trunk in a tub filled with six inches of hot water for up to 10 minutes. Some therapists recommend that you follow with a minute of cold water, then get out and rub yourself with a towel that has been soaked in ice water. Dry off, wrap yourself up, and remain warm for at least 20 minutes.

■ **NATUROPATHY:** In addition to suggesting exercises to tone abdominal muscles, a practitioner will recommend a whole-food or raw-food diet that is high in fiber, as well as vitamins and minerals. Such a diet will help prevent recurrences. Avoid very spicy foods, caffeine, and alcohol. Drinking plenty of water daily—at least six to eight glasses—is important.

■ **OSTEOPATHY:** A practitioner may recommend exercises to strengthen weak abdominal muscles. This can help in overcoming constipation.

■ **SHIATSU:** Pressing points on the abdomen, lower back, and back of the leg may bring relief.

■ **VITAMIN AND MINERAL THERAPY:** Vitamin B complex, vitamin E supplements and suppositories, and vitamin C may be recommended.

Hepatitis *An acute or chronic disease of the liver, hepatitis develops most often from an infection that is caused by one of three viruses: type A, B, or C. Other causes include drug reactions, chemicals, and poisons. Symptoms may mimic the flu, with fever, nausea, and malaise, or may be more severe, including jaundice, which turns the skin*

yellow, joint pain, liver failure, and coma.

A form of acute hepatitis known as hepatitis A, or infectious hepatitis, is associated with contaminated food and water. It is spread mainly by fecal-oral contact.

Most of those with the B virus, which is blood-borne, are infected by contaminated blood from a transfusion, during dialysis, through sexual activity, or by intravenous drugs. When hepatitis B develops into chronic hepatitis, cirrhosis of the liver, which impairs liver functioning, and liver cancer may develop. One type of chronic hepatitis may develop from excessive alcohol consumption. The C virus usually appears in someone who has received blood transfusions.

ORTHODOX MEDICINE

There is no cure for acute hepatitis, although symptoms can be treated. Except for those whose immune systems are weak, most cases resolve themselves with no care other than bed rest. Gamma globulin injections are advised for those traveling to areas with a high risk for hepatitis A, to guard against infection. A vaccine is available to prevent hepatitis B. Corticosteroids may be prescribed for chronic active hepatitis.

COMMON-SENSE CARE

If you suspect that you have hepatitis, see a physician immediately for a diagnosis. Get plenty of rest. Avoid drinking alcohol and exposure to toxic chemicals, which can place undue strain on the liver.

Good personal hygiene, practicing safe sex, and getting vaccinations when traveling abroad to certain countries are important precautions. If you visit an area where sanitation standards are inadequate, beware of drinking water that has not been properly decontaminated. Do not eat fish, shellfish, or other food from contaminated water. Avoid unpeeled, uncooked vegetables and fruits—when animal feces are used as fertilizer, they can transmit the virus to the crops.

NATURAL MEDICINE THERAPIES

■ ACUPUNCTURE: Treatment may involve points on the meridians of the liver, gall bladder, and spleen.

■ NATUROPATHY: A diet high in fiber and low in saturated fats and sugary, processed, and fried foods may be recommended. Do not eat raw fish or shellfish, because of the risks of bacterial contamination, or drink alcohol.

■ REFLEXOLOGY: For some types of hepatitis, massaging certain reflex areas can be helpful. Such areas include the liver, gallbladder, intestines, and spleen.

■ SHIATSU: Pressing on the back and the lower edge of the rib cage may ease symptoms.

■ VITAMIN THERAPY: Injections of vitamin C have proved effective in preventing transfusion recipients from getting hepatitis. Vitamin B_{12} and folic acid can help speed recovery from viral hepatitis.

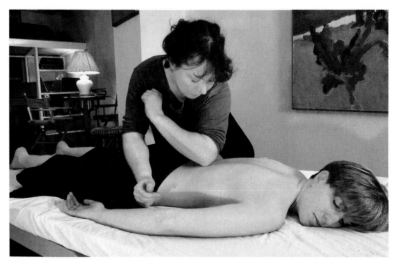

Shiatsu aims to relieve hepatitis symptoms by treating points on the lower back.

High blood pressure *High*

blood pressure refers to levels of the systolic or diastolic blood pressure readings that exceed the norms for a person's age and sex. The systolic pressure measures the pressure exerted by the blood against the artery walls when the heart contracts fully. The diastolic pressure corresponds to the phase of full cardiac relaxation.

What causes high blood pressure, or hypertension, is not fully understood. Primary, or essential, hypertension, is sometimes known as the ''silent killer'' because it is asymptomatic until heart disease, stroke, kidney failure, hemorrhages in the retina, or other problems occur. Being in a family with a history of hypertension is a risk factor, and blacks are twice as likely to become hypertensive as are whites.

Smoking, obesity, excessive alcohol consumption, and having diabetes can worsen the condition. High blood pressure during pregnancy poses special hazards to the mother and the fetus.

See also Diabetes, Heart Disease.

ORTHODOX MEDICINE

Antihypertensive drugs include beta blockers, diuretics, calcium channel agents, and several other types. Medication is usually prescribed for patients with moderate-to-severe hypertension. Opinions vary on whether non-drug treatment alone is adequate for patients with mild hypertension or whether they should also take medication.

COMMON-SENSE CARE

Diet and exercise, which help some people control mild hypertension, may also benefit those with more seriously elevated blood pressure. A sensible weight-control and exercise plan is suggested, especially for the obese. Aerobic exercises like walking, running, and swimming are commonly recommended. Using seasonings other than salt and avoiding those processed foods with high salt or sodium content will aid those

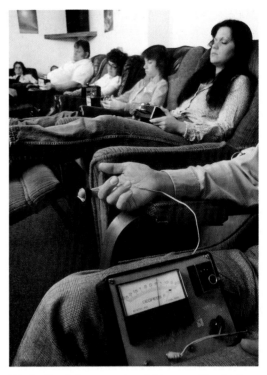

Biofeedback *has proved useful in controlling high blood pressure. See also pages 114-117.*

who are sodium-sensitive. Cut back on alcohol and stimulants like caffeine, or cut them out entirely. If you smoke, stop. Make time each day for stress-reduction and relaxation techniques like biofeedback.

NATURAL MEDICINE THERAPIES

■ ACUPUNCTURE: A practitioner may focus on meridians for the liver and bladder, as well as stimulate several ear points. Blood pressure must be monitored during each session. With severely high blood pressure, acupuncture and shiatsu, or acupressure, can be dangerous.

■ MASSAGE: Having a massage can reduce stress, which may contribute to high blood pressure. Before you get a massage, check with your physician. If he or she approves, tell the person giving the massage that you have high blood pressure.

■ NATUROPATHY: Changes in eating habits and behavior patterns are considered essential. A common recommendation is eating plenty of raw fruit and vegetables, whole grains, and unprocessed foods. Cutting back on the red meat, sugar, and salt in your diet, or even eliminating them entirely, and eating more low-fat, low-cholesterol foods may be suggested.

Some practitioners believe that a potassium deficiency may contribute to hypertension and suggest potassium-rich foods like bananas and potatoes. Garlic and onions have antihypertensive effects. Cucumbers are good diuretics and calming agents. A practitioner will most likely recommend techniques for stress management and relaxation.

■ REFLEXOLOGY: A general foot massage can help you relax. Reflexes to stimulate for hypertension include those for the head, heart, kidneys, and urinary tract.

■ SHIATSU: Regular sessions can reduce tension and promote relaxation. Points to press are on the back of the leg, inner wrist, and elsewhere. As in acupuncture, blood pressure should be monitored.

■ VITAMIN AND MINERAL THERAPY: Recommendations may include vitamins A, C, and E, and the minerals potassium, calcium, and magnesium. Other nutrients that may benefit hypertensives include choline, lecithin, and the trace minerals selenium and zinc.

■ YOGA: Relaxation, breathing techniques, and meditation can help lower blood pressure, but do not assume inverted postures like the shoulder stand.

Indigestion *A catch-all term for such unpleasant sensations as heartburn, abdominal pain, nausea, and flatulence, indigestion usually results from eating or drinking too much or too quickly, or consuming foods that disagree with you. Too little or too much stomach acid can trigger indigestion. Smoking, drinking alcohol, taking certain drugs, and stress can increase stomach acid. Indigestion can be symptomatic of serious disorders like gallstones, peptic ulcer, or inflammation of the esophagus. Immediate medical attention is required if indigestion is accompanied by bouts of vomiting, vomiting blood, or passing very dark stools.*

See also Diarrhea, Gallstones, Ulcers.

ORTHODOX MEDICINE

Over-the-counter and prescription antacids can help, but chronic use can mask serious problems.

COMMON-SENSE CARE

Smoking and drinking can irritate the stomach, so if indigestion troubles you, cut out cigarettes and alcohol. Smokers who experience indigestion frequently should avoid lighting up right before a meal.

Create a pleasant atmosphere for meals. Chew each bite thoroughly. Eating five or six small meals at regular intervals throughout the day may be gentler on digestion than three large meals. Avoid foods that seem to aggravate your stomach. If you are prone to indigestion, don't lie down for two to three hours after eating. As a preventive measure, drink a cup of hot water with a tablespoon of lemon juice before meals. Exercise and relaxation techniques help alleviate stress, which can prompt indigestion or aggravate it.

NATURAL MEDICINE THERAPIES

■ ACUPUNCTURE: Treatment seeks to free the flow of energy in the spleen, which is regarded as the stomach's partner in digestion. Points for other digestive organs are also treated.

■ BACH FLOWER REMEDIES: Agrimony is sometimes recommended for anxiety-related indigestion. Impatiens may relieve emotional irritability and calm the stomach.

■ CHIROPRACTIC: A practitioner can adjust any dislocations that may interfere with digestion.

■ HOMEOPATHY: A practitioner may prescribe nux vomica for gas and heartburn, pulsatilla for bloating, carbo vegetabilis for pain and bloating, ipecacuanha for nausea, and arsenicum album for a burning stomach.

■ HYDROTHERAPY: Placing warm compresses on your abdomen may provide quick relief.

■ NATUROPATHY: For anyone troubled by occasional attacks, eating a light, bland diet or limiting yourself to juices for one or two days afterward may be recommended. Some foods that most often cause heartburn are coffee, tea, caffeinated sodas, alcohol, chocolate, fatty foods, citrus fruits, and gas-producing foods like beans and cabbage. Recurring indigestion may be linked to food allergies or lactose intolerance.

■ REFLEXOLOGY: Among the reflexes that

can be stimulated are those for the pituitary, thyroid, parathyroid, stomach, pancreas, and colon.

■ SHIATSU: Using a clockwise motion (the direction food travels through the system), massage the abdominal area. Pressing shiatsu points on the knee, shin, and abdominal area may relieve indigestion.

■ YOGA: Regular practice of such postures as the posterior stretch and the twist may tone the digestive system.

Insomnia *An inability to fall asleep when you go to bed feeling tired or to sleep through the night without interruption constitutes insomnia, a common sleep disorder. Its causes can be psychological, physiological, or both. Physiological problems include pain, the side effects of medications, various ailments, and withdrawal from such drugs as heroin, barbiturates, sedatives, and antidepressants. People suffering from anxiety, depression, and other psychological disorders may experience insomnia.*

Troubled relationships, a difficult work or school assignment, and other stresses will sometimes keep you up at night. Frequent bouts of insomnia can leave you feeling irritable, depressed, and unable to concentrate; however, such problems usually disappear after a good night's sleep.

See also Depression.

ORTHODOX MEDICINE

Sedative-hypnotic drugs are often prescribed for insomnia sufferers. These medications can be habit-forming, and should be considered short-term measures. It is common to build up a tolerance to sleep-inducing drugs, requiring progressively larger doses. When combined with certain other drugs or with alcohol, sleeping pills can be fatal. If anxiety or depression provokes insomnia that lasts for a prolonged period, counseling may be recommended.

COMMON-SENSE CARE

Among the most important strategies is following a regular schedule for going to bed and getting up. Establish a quiet, soothing routine before bedtime, such as reading, putting on a tape of classical music, or tuning into an easy-listening radio station. Avoid such stimulants as coffee, alcohol, and nicotine. Try drinking warm milk or chamomile tea. Exercise regularly, but not within two hours of going to bed. Sleep in a well-ventilated room.

NATURAL MEDICINE THERAPIES

■ ACUPUNCTURE: Using points on the heart, spleen, and urinary bladder channels, among others, the therapist tries to calm the insomniac's restless spirit.

■ HOMEOPATHY: Some popular remedies include arsenicum album to relieve anxiety, passiflora for uneasy sleep, chamomile, coffea, ignatia, and nux vomica.

■ HYDROTHERAPY: A warm bath before bed can relax both muscles and mind; however, very hot baths can be stimulating, instead of relaxing.

■ HYPNOTHERAPY: A combination of hypnotherapy and psychological counseling can be effective. Self-hypnosis can also be useful.

■ MASSAGE: A full body massage can release tension throughout the body.

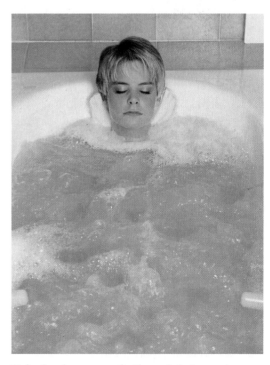

Relaxing in a warm bath can help insomniacs. For more on hydrotherapy, see pages 206-211.

■ NATUROPATHY: A practitioner will urge scrutinizing your diet for hidden sources of caffeine, including cola, tea, chocolate, coffee ice cream, as well as medications that contain caffeine. Some practitioners advise that you eat foods rich in tryptophan, one of the amino acids that comprise protein. Tryptophan, which has been called a natural sedative, stimulates the brain to produce a substance that promotes sleep. Cheddar and cottage cheeses and other dairy products are good sources of tryptophan. Besides dietary changes, recommendations will include exercising daily and practicing relaxation techniques.

■ SHIATSU: Pressing several points on the forehead, ankle, heel, wrist, and base of the skull may help overcome occasional insomnia.

■ YOGA: Stretching, doing relaxation exercises, and practicing such calming postures as the corpse, mountain, locust, and camel can promote sleep.

■ VITAMIN AND MINERAL THERAPY: The minerals calcium and magnesium, and inositol, a vitamin-like nutrient, may help insomniacs.

Irritable bowel syndrome

Waves of abdominal pain accompanied by recurring episodes of diarrhea or constipation are typical indicators of irritable bowel syndrome, or irritable colon, a chronic ailment of the large intestine. Other symptoms include a swollen stomach, mucus in the feces, and gas. Chronic stress, anxiety, and depression are believed to contribute to the disorder, which affects women more often than men. A diagnosis is important since symptoms mimic those of several diseases, including colon cancer, ulcerative colitis, and Crohn's disease, which are inflammatory bowel diseases.

See also Cancer, Constipation, Diarrhea.

ORTHODOX MEDICINE

A combination of dietary changes and antidiarrheal, antispasmodic, or other drugs may be used. Switching to a high-fiber diet and adding fiber in the form of bran or methylcellulose can often help.

COMMON-SENSE CARE

Alcohol, tobacco, and food and drink that contain caffeine can irritate the intestines, so avoid them. Although food sensitivities vary widely, some people find that forgoing sugar, dairy products, or wheat products may alleviate symptoms. A high-fiber diet is generally recommended.

NATURAL MEDICINE THERAPIES

■ ACUPUNCTURE: To clear up intestinal problems, several points on the stomach meridian may be stimulated.

■ BACH FLOWER REMEDIES: Crabapple, which is a general cleansing remedy for the emotions, may be suggested.

■ HOMEOPATHY: Recommended remedies include podophyllum for loose bowel movements, phosphoric acid, aloe, and mercurius (quicksilver).

■ HYPNOTHERAPY: This approach can be useful in controlling pain, diarrhea, and constipation, especially for those who are

Strengthening Exercises

■ Strengthening and toning the abdominal muscles with proper exercise can help minimize problems of the gastrointestinal tract such as irritable bowel syndrome. Pressing the abdominals in toward the spine helps massage the intestines.

■ Begin with as many repetitions as you can do comfortably. Try to work up to 30 repetitions of the pelvic tilt, 40 abdominal curls, and 100 arm pumps.

■ If possible, sit beside a mirror so that you can see yourself in profile to check your posture.

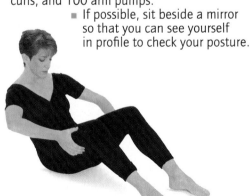

For the pelvic tilt, sit up tall with spine lengthened, knees bent. Tucking your pelvis under you, lower yourself far enough that your lower back is pressed into the floor. Exhale, then inhale as you pull back up to the seated position. Think of scooping the lower abdominals toward the spine as you round your back. Keep your shoulders down and feet flat.

under a lot of stress.

■ NATUROPATHY: A diet rich in complex carbohydrates and fiber may be successful in treating irritable bowel syndrome. If allergies trigger your condition, an elimination diet may identify the offending foods. When lactose intolerance is a factor, avoiding dairy products can help. Drinking peppermint tea or taking peppermint-oil capsules may reduce colonic spasms. Relaxation techniques may be suggested to relieve stress-related symptoms.

■ VITAMIN AND MINERAL THERAPY: Calcium and magnesium are recommended.

■ YOGA: Like any condition that is worsened by stress, irritable bowel syndrome can be improved with regular yoga practice. Abdominal contractions, the solar plexus pose, and other postures that work the abdominal muscles are recommended, along with stretching and relaxing postures. Breathing exercises and meditation can be helpful.

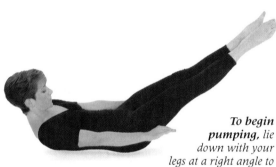

To begin pumping, *lie down with your legs at a right angle to the floor. Lift your head so your chin touches your chest and reach your arms along your sides. Pump the arms up and down in short, quick movements.*

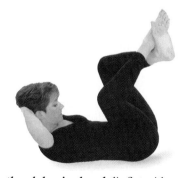

For the abdominal curl, *lie flat with your back against the floor and cross your ankles. With hands behind your head, exhale. Curl up as far as you can. Use your arms to lift your head; keep the abdominals tucked in. Inhale and lower yourself down. If your back begins hurting, stop at once. Your back must be flat when you are supine to avoid straining it.*

Kidney stones *The concentration of calcium, uric acid, and other substances in the urine can lead to the formation of kidney stones. Small stones are often excreted unnoticed, while larger ones can cause problems when they get lodged in the urinary tract. Kidney stones can create extreme pain that radiates from the lower back to the abdomen, pelvic region, genital area, or thighs. Symptoms also include blood in the urine, nausea, chills, and fever. Large stones that have caused no pain or other symptoms for several years can damage kidney tissue. Genetic defects in metabolic processes can increase the chances that a person will develop kidney stones.*

ORTHODOX MEDICINE

If drinking more liquids does not help the stone pass, drugs may be prescribed to reduce stone formation. For years surgery was performed to remove an impacted stone, but a technique that dissolves stones with shock waves, allowing fragments to be excreted, is now preferred. Antibiotics may be prescribed to treat infections associated with kidney stones.

COMMON-SENSE CARE

To dilute the urine and reduce the risk of crystal formation, drink at least three quarts of liquids daily. Reduce your salt consumption if it's more than two or three grams a day. Those with recurrences of calcium oxalate stones should avoid or cut back on asparagus, beets, spinach, Swiss chard, and other vegetables that contain or produce oxalates. Be sure to replace fluids that are lost when exercising, sunbathing, or performing manual labor that causes you to sweat profusely.

NATURAL MEDICINE THERAPIES

■ ACUPUNCTURE: For kidney stones, points along the urinary bladder, kidney, and stomach meridians may be stimulated.

■ HOMEOPATHY: Berberis may be prescribed if sharp pain radiates around the abdomen into the hip and groin. Magnesia phosphorica may be recommended for kidney pain that makes you double over and that is relieved by heat. Aconite, lycopodium, and cantharis are also used.

■ HYDROTHERAPY: To relieve pain, try placing a hot-water bottle or ice pack on the affected area.

■ NATUROPATHY: Maintaining adequate bodily fluids by drinking regularly and avoiding profuse sweating is important if you have a tendency to develop kidney stones. Drinking between three and four quarts of liquids daily will increase urination and ensure that urine is highly diluted, which makes it harder for substances to bind together and form stones. Avoid dairy products, which can increase the body's store of calcium.

■ VITAMIN AND MINERAL THERAPY: Supplements of vitamin B_6 and magnesium are commonly recommended. B_6 may reduce the body's production of oxalate, a mineral salt that combines with calcium and may contribute to the formation of stones. Magnesium increases the solubility of calcium and oxalate, making it more difficult for these compounds to crystallize into stones.

Menopausal problems

When women stop ovulating and having monthly periods, they have reached a stage known as menopause. They undergo various physical changes that are mostly attributed to a drop in the production of estrogen. They may experience hot flashes, night sweats, changes in the skin's elasticity that produces wrinkling, reduced vaginal lubrication, or diminished interest in sex. Fatigue, insomnia, irritability, and nervousness often accompany menopause; however, there is debate over whether menopausal changes or other factors cause these problems, which can last for a few months or several years.

Menopause occurs naturally at about age 50; however, the surgical removal of the ovaries at any age can produce menopause. Post-menopausal women face increased risks of osteoporosis and heart disease.

See also Heart Disease, Insomnia, Menstrual Problems, Osteoporosis.

ORTHODOX MEDICINE

Estrogen replacement therapy is the most common approach to halting hot flashes and other symptoms. If medical factors rule out such therapy, sedative-hypnotic drugs may be an alternative. Estrogen vaginal cream may be prescribed. For recurring episodes of depression, irritability, and nervousness, a physician may prescribe antidepressants and tranquilizers. Psychotherapy may also help.

COMMON-SENSE CARE

A nonprescription lubricating jelly may help alleviate vaginal dryness, which can hinder sexual intercourse. If hot flashes are a problem, avoid very spicy foods, which can make you sweat. Smoking can add to the physical problems of menopause. A lifelong devotion to weight-bearing exercise like walking, running, and cycling can help prevent osteoporosis, the most serious and most common health hazard that menopause poses.

NATURAL MEDICINE THERAPIES

■ ACUPUNCTURE: Therapy aimed at alleviating hot flashes may use points along the urinary bladder, governing vessel, gallbladder, and kidney meridians.

■ HOMEOPATHY: Lachesis, sepia, and sulphuric acid may help suppress hot flashes and control sweating. Bryonia may be prescribed when vaginal walls become dry.

■ NATUROPATHY: Adequate dietary calcium is important for women after menopause, when the rate of loss of bone mass accelerates, heightening the risk of osteoporosis. Calcium-rich foods include chickpeas, lentils, and other dried peas and beans, leafy green vegetables, eggs, sardines with bones, and blackstrap molasses. Dairy products are good calcium sources, but some practitioners urge limiting them to help prevent hot flashes. Forgo coffee and alcohol.

■ VITAMIN AND MINERAL THERAPY: Vitamin E can be effective in alleviating hot flashes. A combination of calcium and vitamin D may be recommended, especially for women receiving estrogen replacement therapy, to reduce hot flashes and backache, and to counteract the loss of bone mass.

■ YOGA: Postures that provide overall conditioning can be helpful when combined with relaxation and meditation.

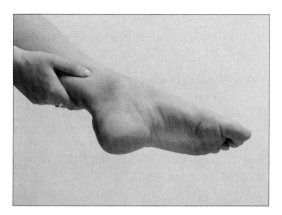

Shiatsu and acupressure may help ease cramps and other problems. For more on such pressure-point therapy, see pages 164-167.

Menstrual problems *The monthly shedding of the lining of the uterus and an unfertilized egg, menstruation begins between ages 11 and 14 for most American girls. Menstrual periods occur once every 21 to 35 days for most women, with a 28-day cycle considered average. Bleeding lasts generally from three to seven days each cycle. Except for interruption by pregnancy, menstruation typically continues until menopause, the cessation of monthly periods. Problems linked to the menstrual cycle include pain in the lower back region, cramps, and tension.*

Some women are affected by what is termed premenstrual syndrome (PMS), a period of physical discomfort and mental distress that precedes the start of the monthly cycle. PMS symptoms include headaches, skin outbreaks, swollen and tender breasts, lethargy, insomnia, depression, and irritability.

Other menstrual problems include the absence of regular periods, or amenorrhea, which can be caused by weight loss, extremely rigorous physical exertion, and stress; abnormally heavy periods, which can signal the development of fibroid tumors, a pelvic infection, or endometriosis, which is the growth of part of the uterine lining in tissue outside the uterus; painful periods; and irregular bleeding.

See also Back Pain, Cancer, Depression, Headache, Insomnia, Menopausal Problems, Migraines.

ORTHODOX MEDICINE

Treatment depends on the particular problem and its underlying cause. Heavy bleeding may decrease with hormone therapy or by switching from an intrauterine device to another contraceptive. A surgical procedure called dilation and curettage (D and C) may be performed to learn the cause of heavy periods. For endometriosis, various drugs including oral contraceptives may be prescribed to suppress ovulation and menstruation. Surgery may be recommended for patients with moderate-to-severe endometriosis.

Among the therapies for PMS are diuretic drugs to relieve fluid retention, progesterone supplements, and oral contraceptives, which regulate the menstrual cycle. Some physicians prescribe vitamin B_6 and magnesium to alleviate PMS symptoms. Psychological counseling may be advised for those who are especially affected by PMS.

COMMON-SENSE CARE

Dietary changes, smoking cessation, and exercise have proved effective in relieving PMS for some women. Avoiding chocolate, coffee, and other food or drink containing caffeine may help those who frequently feel tense and irritable around the time of the menstrual period. Keeping salt intake low will help minimize fluid retention. Cutting back on processed food is one way to avoid excess salt and sodium. For some women, forgoing alcohol and foods high in sugar can ease PMS symptoms. Getting extra sleep and practicing stress-management techniques may offer relief.

NATURAL MEDICINE THERAPIES

■ ACUPUNCTURE: For PMS, points on meridians for the liver and conception vessel may be treated. For other symptoms, points on the kidney, ren, stomach, spleen, urinary bladder, and liver meridians may be used.

■ HOMEOPATHY: Pulsatilla may help defuse tension and alleviate breast pain. Sepia may relieve premenstrual irritability, fatigue, and weepiness. Magnesia phosphorica can be effective for cramps. For more severe pain, caulophyllum or colocynthis may be recommended.

■ **HYDROTHERAPY:** Soaking in a warm bathtub or applying a hot water pack to the lower back can promote circulation and alleviate pain.

■ **MASSAGE:** A therapist may massage the lower back, abdomen, and legs. A self-massage to the abdominal area, using an open hand and moving clockwise, can ease symptoms.

■ **NATUROPATHY:** If premenstrual syndrome (PMS) affects you, eat fewer foods with saturated fat, like meat and dairy products, and more with polyunsaturated fat, such as legumes and whole grains. This diet may improve hormonal balances. Eat plenty of fresh vegetables, especially leafy green vegetables. Avoid salt, which tends to increase water retention. Watermelon, cucumbers, and parsley act as natural diuretics and may help reduce bloating during menstruation. A practitioner may suggest exercises to reduce fluid retention and improve general well-being.

■ **REFLEXOLOGY:** Working the reflex areas for the uterus, Fallopian tubes, ovary, and vagina may bring relief.

■ **VITAMIN AND MINERAL THERAPY:** Women who bleed profusely during their periods may require iron supplements to replace the lost iron. Vitamins A and C and bioflavonoids, which are vitamin-like substances that enhance the absorption of vitamin C, may be suggested to control heavy bleeding or irregular cycles. To relieve PMS, supplements of vitamin B complex, vitamin B_6, and folic acid may ease several PMS problems, including fluid retention. Vitamin E supplements may help relieve breast pain, and calcium combined with magnesium may be recommended for those affected by PMS.

■ **YOGA:** Practicing the corpse pose in the early stages of premenstrual tension may reduce its intensity. Different postures are effective at different times during the menstrual cycle. The cat stretch and half shoulder stand may release tension in the lower abdomen. The pelvic tilt may relieve lower back pain. The cobra, plow, and posterior stretch may also be recommended. Breathing exercises can provide relief from discomfort and promote relaxation.

Migraine *An intense, throbbing headache that lasts for hours or days may be a migraine. Although there is no clear understanding of migraines, researchers often attribute them to overexpansion of one or more branches of the carotid artery, which reaches into the head. Precipitating factors include food allergy or sensitivity, birth control pills and other medications, sleep deprivation, and physical changes of the menstrual cycle. Emotional tension and stress may trigger a migraine or intensify the pain.*

Symptoms include excruciating, throbbing pain on one side of the head or all over the head, sensitivity to sound and light, nausea, and vomiting. If headaches persist, a full physical evaluation may be needed to rule out a serious disease. Migraine sufferers usually experience their first attack between the ages of 10 and 30; for many, attacks cease after they turn 50. Women get more migraines than men, and there is often a family history of such headaches.

See also Allergies, Headache.

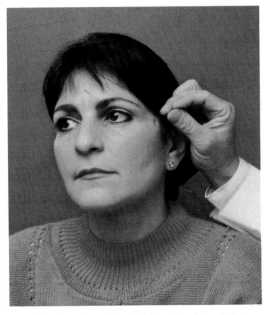

By inserting very thin needles *at points on the patient's face, an acupuncturist can sometimes relieve migraine headaches. For more on acupuncture and other Chinese therapies, see pages 42–51.*

ORTHODOX MEDICINE

Aspirin or acetaminophen will sometimes bring relief. If not, a physician may prescribe a stronger painkiller or a drug such as ergotamine, which constricts the blood vessels surrounding the brain. Drugs used to prevent migraines include beta-blockers and calcium channel agents. For some people, taking an aspirin daily reduces the frequency. Medication may be prescribed to relieve nausea.

Since psychological factors often play a role, some physicians recommend psychotherapy. Stress-reduction techniques like biofeedback may also be suggested.

COMMON-SENSE CARE

Some people are sensitive to food with tyramine, a substance that causes blood vessels to dilate. Among the foods high in tyramine are aged cheese, liver, bananas, eggplant, chocolate, and yeast. Keep a food diary to see if a pattern emerges linking migraine attacks and diet. Avoid situations or substances that seem to trigger migraines. Avoid drinking excess alcohol. For some women, switching from birth-control pills to another form of contraception eases or eliminates migraines.

Managing stress is essential for avoiding recurrent migraines. Exercising regularly, shortening overly long workdays, and practicing a form of relaxation therapy may decrease the frequency of migraines. Stretching neck and shoulder muscles can release tension. Some people find it helpful to go to sleep at the first warning signs or just retreat for several minutes to a quiet, darkened room.

NATURAL MEDICINE THERAPIES

■ **ACUPUNCTURE**: For symptom relief, acupuncture can be effective. Treatment usually concentrates on points for the gallbladder, large and small intestines, liver, and stomach.

■ **CHIROPRACTIC**: A chiropractor may adjust abnormalities in the neck, thoracic joints, and spine that can contribute to head and neck pain.

■ **HOMEOPATHY**: Sanguinaria may be used for a right-sided headache, while spigelia may be advised for a left-sided headache. Other commonly used remedies include iris, natrum muriaticum, and pulsatilla.

■ **HYDROTHERAPY**: Alternating hot and cold compresses can lessen the pain.

■ **NATUROPATHY**: In addition to stressing the need for regular exercise and relaxation, a practitioner may suggest avoiding caffeine and alcohol (especially red wine), red meat, the food preservative monosodium glutamate, and processed meats.

■ **OSTEOPATHY**: To ease pain, an osteopath can make adjustments to enhance circulation and nerve signals to the brain.

■ **REFLEXOLOGY**: Massage may be applied to the areas relating to the head, spine, eyes, sinuses, pituitary gland, and thyroid gland.

■ **SHIATSU**: Points on the feet, lower skull, face, and neck may be stimulated for relief of migraine pain.

■ **VITAMIN AND MINERAL THERAPY**: Niacin, which helps maintain the dilation of blood vessels, and the other B complex vitamins, vitamin C, and the minerals magnesium and calcium may be recommended.

■ **YOGA**: Meditation and relaxation techniques may help prevent attacks as well as relieve symptoms. Postures that release tension in the upper back, shoulders, and neck are particularly recommended, such as the shoulder stand, fish, and cobra. Yoga breathing techniques may also help.

Osteoporosis *A progressive disease in which the bones become thin and brittle as they lose density, or mass, osteoporosis affects postmenopausal women more than any other group. Underweight Caucasian women over 50 who smoke and exercise seldom or not at all face the greatest risk of developing osteoporosis. A family history of the disease is also a risk factor. If your diet has been lacking in calcium for a period of years, your chances of developing this disease increase.*

The onset of menopause hastens the normal bone-thinning process of aging because the ovaries stop producing the female hormone estrogen, which helps to retain bone mass. Bone brittleness and weakness make you especially prone to fractures of the spine, hip, wrist, and other bones.

See also Menopausal Problems.

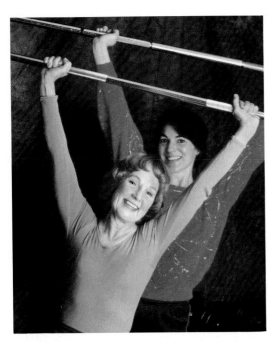

Exercising regularly can help prevent osteoporosis, a bone-thinning disease that mostly affects women.

ORTHODOX MEDICINE

Physicians commonly recommend calcium supplements. Estrogen-replacement therapy is often prescribed for post-menopausal women. Some physicians and nutritionists suggest a high-calcium diet that omits alcohol.

COMMON-SENSE CARE

To prevent osteoporosis or slow its progression, you should pay attention to what you eat and exercise regularly. Make sure that your diet includes plenty of dairy products, green leafy vegetables, shellfish, and other calcium sources. Do not eat excessive amounts of chard and spinach, however. They are high in oxalic acid, a substance that hinders calcium absorption.

Weight-bearing exercise such as running, brisk walking, and rope jumping can help counteract the loss of bone mass if you exercise at least three times weekly. Try to get out in the sun regularly; your skin absorbs the sun's ultraviolet rays, which the body can convert to vitamin D, an important catalyst in the absorption of calcium. Stop smoking, if you haven't already stopped; smoking may reduce estrogen levels. Anyone who develops osteoporosis should take extra care to avoid falls, which can cause already weakened, brittle bones to fracture or break relatively easily. This may mean covering wood floors with carpeting, providing adequate lighting in halls and at staircases, and adding handrails to bathtubs and shower stalls.

NATURAL MEDICINE THERAPIES

■ NATUROPATHY: A low-protein diet, with an emphasis on foods high in calcium, phosphorus, magnesium, and vitamins A and D, may be recommended. Cod-liver oil is a good source of vitamins A and D. A practitioner can suggest a series of weight-bearing exercises.

■ VITAMIN AND MINERAL THERAPY: Calcium and vitamin D tablets are often recommended. Folic acid, vitamin K, and the minerals manganese, silicon, boron, and magnesium may contribute to maintaining bone mass, and supplements may be suggested for post-menopausal women.

■ YOGA: Some practitioners believe that more efficient breathing can provide relief for those with osteoporosis. Diaphragmatic breathing may aid the body as it copes with changing bone structure. Relaxation techniques may also prove useful.

Pain, chronic *Pain that lasts longer than six months is considered chronic pain. Its causes include traumatic injuries, diseases like rheumatoid arthritis and cancer, and conditions for which physicians can find no organic cause, such as lower back pain, chronic headache, and certain types of facial or pelvic pain. On occasion, for no apparent reason, a persistent, severe pain develops months after a wound has healed.*

Psychological factors frequently have a bearing on chronic pain. Often introverted, chronic-pain sufferers tend to become depressed, have sleep disturbances, lack energy, and withdraw from their family and friends.

See also Arthritis, Back Pain, Cancer, Headache.

ORTHODOX MEDICINE

A physician may prescribe painkillers with or without narcotics, antidepressants, anti-inflammatory drugs, and sedatives, among others. Narcotic painkillers may be taken in pill form or by injection. Besides medication, treatment may include various types of psychological counseling; injection of drugs that provide nerve blocks; transcutaneous electrical nerve stimulation (TENS), which sends electrical impulses to nerves just beneath the skin's surface, and surgery on the brain, spinal cord, and nerves. Patients may be referred to a pain clinic.

COMMON-SENSE CARE

Emotional factors can play a role in pain management, so it helps to understand what makes you tense and anxious, and to develop a way of dealing with such situations. Depression, stress, and anxiety can lower your pain threshold, so alleviating the psychic pain may help ease the physical pain. Surrounding yourself with supportive friends and family with whom you can talk easily may help. For stress management and general well-being, eat well-balanced meals in moderation, get enough rest, and exercise regularly. In addition to keeping you fit and aiding in relaxation, exercise may prompt the body to release chemicals known as endorphins, which act as painkillers.

NATURAL MEDICINE THERAPIES

■ ACUPUNCTURE: Therapy can help provide relatively quick relief for some types of chronic pain. A point on the large-intestine meridian is considered the body's most effective pain-relieving point.

■ CHIROPRACTIC: Spinal manipulation may ease pain caused by joint problems or misaligned vertebrae.

■ HYDROTHERAPY: Hot and cold compresses, ice packs, and warm and cold baths are among the forms of hydrotherapy used by chronic-pain sufferers. Cold baths can tone muscles, stimulate circulation, and increase mental alertness, while warm baths can relax you, soothe aching muscles and joints, and possibly help you fall asleep.

■ HYPNOTHERAPY: Considered most effective with chronic pain caused by injury or illness, hypnosis can help you refocus your attention away from the pain and toward some positive aspect of your life.

■ NATUROPATHY: Fatty fish contain substances that may help decrease inflammation, which contributes to pain in such diseases as arthritis, so eating mackerel, herring, salmon, and other fatty fish may be suggested. Biofeedback and other relaxation therapies may be suggested.

■ SHIATSU: Where to apply pressure depends on where pain is felt. For example, a point at the crease in the web of the hand between the finger and thumb may alleviate upper-body pain, arthritis pain, and headaches. A point at the top of the shinbone may ease knee pain.

■ YOGA: Yoga has brought relief to those with rheumatoid arthritis, backache, and other types of chronic pain. Regularly performing yoga postures, breathing and relaxation techniques, meditation, or a combination of these can alleviate pain.

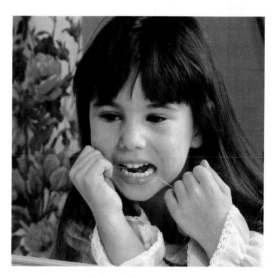

Practicing good dental hygiene, with regular brushing and flossing, is one of the best ways to guard against periodontal diseases.

Periodontal disease *When the gums or any other tissues that support the teeth become inflamed or damaged, periodontal disease is the probable diagnosis. Its most common form is gingivitis, an inflammation of the gums that may cause swelling, bleeding, and bad breath. If left untreated, gingivitis may progress to periodontitis, a disease that occurs when the bones that support the teeth erode and surrounding tissues become inflamed. This is the main cause of tooth loss among adults*

over 35. *The condition may also be the result of uncontrolled diabetes and pregnancy.*

See also Bad Breath, Diabetes.

ORTHODOX MEDICINE

For gingivitis, brushing and flossing teeth several times daily is advised. Those with gum problems need professional dental care two to four times yearly. For periodontitis, such techniques as scaling and scraping can loosen and remove infected matter and diseased tissue. Loose teeth may be splinted. Periodontal surgery and tooth extraction may be recommended.

COMMON-SENSE CARE

Good dental hygiene, including removing dental plaque and food particles by brushing and flossing, is essential as a preventive measure. A diet that lacks adequate vitamin C contributes to gum infections in some people; eating fruits and vegetables that contain this vitamin helps lower the risk.

Keep sugary food and drink to a minimum; sugar promotes the formation of dental plaque. Avoid sticky food, especially as between-meal snacks. Eat plenty of raw, chewy food. Vigorous chewing encourages production of saliva, which helps protect the mouth from decay-causing bacteria. Smoking can aggravate gum problems, so smokers should quit.

NATURAL MEDICINE THERAPIES

■ HOMEOPATHY: For gingivitis, spongy gums, or inflamed tissues, use a tincture of staphysagria (stavescare) three times daily; for gums that are inflamed, bleeding, or retracting, mercurius solubilis may be prescribed. A folic acid solution may be suggested for bleeding and inflamed gums.

■ VITAMIN AND MINERAL THERAPY: A deficiency of vitamins A or C can contribute to periodontal problems. Supplements of vitamin A in the form of beta-carotene may be advised. An imbalance of calcium and phosphorus may be a contributing factor, and supplements can help restore the balance. Applying the oil from a vitamin E capsule can help heal inflammation and relieve sore gums. Lightly brushing calcium ascorbate or sodium ascorbate, which are forms of buffered vitamin C, onto the gums daily may be suggested.

Psoriasis *A skin disorder recognized by its dry, silver, scaly patches, psoriasis involves the rapidly accelerated growth of new skin layers at a rate too fast for old skin to be shed. The scalp, hands, armpits, elbows, knees, lower back, buttocks, and other areas may be affected. A genetic tendency may exist for psoriasis, which often appears initially in early adulthood and tends to recur. In general, it produces little physical discomfort besides itching. The most serious complications are secondary bacterial infections and the development of a form of arthritis.*

See also Arthritis.

ORTHODOX MEDICINE

Topical creams and ointments that contain corticosteroids, coal tar, or anthralin are often prescribed. Exposure to sunlight or to special lamps with ultraviolet light may be advised.

COMMON-SENSE CARE

Properly moisturizing skin with lubricating creams and ointments can help prevent skin disorders. Getting out in the sun can help clear up red patches, but be careful to avoid a sunburn. Taking an oatmeal bath can help loosen scales. A shampoo that contains coal tar is often recommended. When you clean your skin, use a mild soap and avoid intense scrubbing, which can provoke further irritation. Reduce stress, which can precipitate recurrences.

NATURAL MEDICINE THERAPIES

■ BACH FLOWER REMEDIES: Treatments include crabapple if you feel disgust and shame, pine if you are guilt-stricken, and willow for resentment. Rescue Remedy cream or impatiens may relieve itching.

■ HOMEOPATHY: Mercurius may be prescribed when the scalp is affected.

■ HYDROTHERAPY: A practitioner may suggest that you work up a sweat in a sauna. Initial visits should be two minutes daily, gradually increasing to 30 minutes twice daily. Drink two glasses of water before and after using a sauna. Warning: do not use a sauna right after eating a meal, and do not use it if you have a heart problem, or circulatory or tubercular disease.

■ **HYPNOTHERAPY:** Hypnotic suggestion can help control stress, which can trigger a recurrence, as well as alleviate itchiness and skin irritation.

■ **NATUROPATHY:** Liver disorders may be a contributing factor in psoriasis, so common recommendations are to avoid coffee and alcohol, which can impair liver function. A practitioner may emphasize such non-meat protein sources as seeds, whole grains, and legumes. Fish oil can sometimes improve psoriasis, so eat mackerel, salmon, herring, and other fatty fish regularly.

■ **REFLEXOLOGY:** Stimulating points on both the feet and hands may provide symptom relief.

■ **VITAMIN AND MINERAL THERAPY:** Vitamins A and E, folic acid, selenium, zinc, and flaxseed oil may be recommended for treating symptoms.

Sciatica *Throbbing or shooting pain*
that radiates down one leg or both legs is the hallmark of sciatica. The sciatic nerves, which begin at the base of the spinal cord and end in the feet, are the largest nerves in the body. Pressure on a disk in the lower back or a ruptured disk can produce sciatica, which is sometimes accompanied by numbness and weakness. Other causes include osteoarthritis and tumors.

See also Arthritis, Back Pain.

ORTHODOX MEDICINE

Painkillers, muscle relaxants, and anti-inflammatory drugs may be prescribed. Bed rest for two or three days is recommended for acute sciatic pain, which often subsides within six weeks. Physical therapy is often prescribed.

COMMON-SENSE CARE

To reduce pain, ice the affected area several times daily for two or three days. Afterward, a heading pad or hot water bottle may bring relief. Certain exercises can ease sciatic pain; walking and swimming are commonly recommended. Prolonged periods of sitting, especially in chairs that lack adequate back support, can add to your discomfort. Rocking chairs and those with adjustable backs and arm supports are best. Make sure that your posture is correct; slouching can strain the lower back. Practice relaxation techniques if you are under a lot of stress.

NATURAL MEDICINE THERAPIES

■ **ACUPUNCTURE:** Points along the urinary bladder, gallbladder, governing vessel, and large intestine meridians may be stimulated to relieve pain.

■ **CHIROPRACTIC:** A practitioner may ease pain with spinal manipulation and prescribe stretching and strengthening exercises for preventing recurrences.

■ **HOMEOPATHY:** Colocynth is recommended for pain that gets worse in cold, damp weather and when sciatic pain

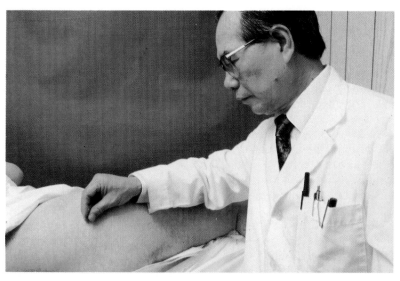

***Sciatic pain**, which is often intense, may disappear after acupuncture therapy.*

extends to the knee or heel. Aconite may be prescribed when the pain is excruciating and the condition prompts fear and anxiety. Magnesia phosphorica may be suggested for intermittent spasms and overall weakness.

■ **HYDROTHERAPY:** A hot water pack on the lower back may relieve pain. Alternating heat treatment with ice packs may help. Swimming and other water exercises in a warm pool are often suggested.

■ **MASSAGE:** A therapist may treat the entire back, then apply a variety of massage techniques to the lower back, buttocks, thighs, and back of the knee. Massage can help relax muscles, thus alleviating pain.

■ **REFLEXOLOGY:** Stimulating points for the hip and sciatic area, lymphatic groin area, and lower back may relieve pain.

■ **SHIATSU:** Pressing on the bladder meridian and at several points on the outside and back of the leg can bring relief.

■ **VITAMIN THERAPY:** Supplements of vitamin B complex may be recommended for nervous system functioning, as well as thiamin (B_1). Inadequate thiamin may erode the sheaths that cover nerve endings, exacerbating sciatic pain.

Shingles *The result of an infection by the same virus that causes chickenpox, shingles most often strikes those older than 50. Nerve roots beneath the skin are affected. An attack of shingles, also known as herpes zoster, is characterized by burning pain and a rash of crusting blisters. The outbreak appears on one side of the face or neck, or in the chest or trunk. After the skin eruptions have healed, neuralgia, or nerve pain, may persist for several months, or occasionally even years.*

See also Pain, Chronic.

ORTHODOX MEDICINE

Painkillers may be prescribed. Anti-viral drugs and corticosteroids may prevent the development of neuralgia. A topical cream that contains capsaicin, the pungent substance in cayenne pepper, can provide relief when neuralgia does occur. If blisters appear near the eye, a patient may be referred to an ophthalmologist.

COMMON-SENSE CARE

When bathing, wash blisters gently. Applying cool, wet compresses, calamine lotion, or cornstarch to blisters several times a day may provide relief and hasten healing. Otherwise, try not to touch or scratch blisters.

NATURAL MEDICINE THERAPIES

■ **ACUPUNCTURE:** Therapy for pain can be effective, especially when neuralgia develops. Points on meridians for the large intestine and the governing vessel may be stimulated.

■ **HOMEOPATHY:** Recommended remedies include arsenicum, for intense burning sensations; mezereum, for pain that is sharp or burning and that lasts after the eruption has subsided; ranunculus bulbosus, for intense pain on the chest or back; and rhus toxicodendron, for itching that becomes intolerable.

■ **HYPNOTHERAPY:** Hypnotic suggestion can help alleviate the burning pain that accompanies shingles, as well as help patients relax, which can aid in managing this disorder.

■ **VITAMIN AND MINERAL THERAPY:** Supplements of the vitamin B complex can help nerve cells regenerate. Also recommended are vitamin C, which can be an effective anti-viral agent, and bioflavonoids, which are vitamin-like nutrients that help the body absorb vitamin C.

Sore throat *Feelings of dryness, scratchiness, irritation, and difficulty in swallowing are typical of sore throats. A red and swollen throat may be the symptom of a cold or other infection; an allergy; childhood diseases like mumps, measles, and chickenpox; and mononucleosis.*

In young children, a sore throat is often the mark of a bacterial streptococcal infection. If not diagnosed and promptly treated, it can lead to such serious complications as tonsillitis, scarlet fever, rheumatic fever, and kidney damage.

See also Allergy, Colds.

ORTHODOX MEDICINE

For a minor sore throat, gargling with salt water may help. Aspirin or acetaminophen is recommended for adults. When there is strep throat, tonsillitis, or another bacterial infection, penicillin or other antibiotics are often prescribed.

COMMON-SENSE CARE

Do not smoke and avoid smoke-filled rooms and polluted environments. Drink lots of liquids and gargle several times a day with a solution of warm water and salt, apple cider vinegar, or lemon juice. Combine the juice of one lemon with a tablespoon of honey, add to a glass of hot or cold water, and drink. Sucking on lozenges, especially those with buffered vitamin C and zinc gluconate, may soothe the throat and help fight infection.

NATURAL MEDICINE THERAPIES

■ ACUPUNCTURE: Treatment may concentrate on conception-vessel, large-intestine, and lung meridians, and on ear points for the lung, pharynx, and larynx.

■ AROMATHERAPY: Inhalations of clary sage, sandalwood, and tea-tree can be soothing. To fight infection, gargle with geranium or lemon oil in hot water.

■ HOMEOPATHY: The most common remedies include aconite, recommended when a sore throat is accompanied by a fever and cold; apis, when swallowing is difficult; baryta muriatica; belladonna, for dryness

and burning sensations; hepar sulphuris; and phytolacca, for severe discomfort.

■ NATUROPATHY: A practitioner may suggest that you limit your consumption of sugary foods and drink large quantities of fluids, especially clear liquids like soup broth, ginger tea, and fruit juices. Eating raw garlic, which has antibiotic properties, may help clear up a strep infection.

■ REFLEXOLOGY: Reflex points for the neck, adrenal glands, and lymphatic area can be stimulated.

■ SHIATSU: Points at the outside of the thumbnail, at the base of the skull, on the chest, and on the upper side of the wrist may be stimulated to relieve discomfort.

■ VITAMIN AND MINERAL THERAPY: Vitamins C and A and beta-carotene may be recommended to boost the body's immune system and enhance healing. The mineral zinc can also help the immune system fight off viruses, bacteria, and other invaders.

■ YOGA: Practice the lion face several times daily to strengthen facial and throat muscles.

Styes
A stye is a pus-filled boil that develops when a follicle of an eyelash becomes infected. Styes, which appear on the eyelid margin at the base of the eyelash, commonly become red and swollen. Although they can be painful, styes are not generally dangerous. They last about five to seven days. They may disappear without coming to a head and draining, or they may come to a head, burst, and heal on their own. Styes that do not heal completely can leave a firm red lump in the eyelid, which may rub the eye and allow new stye growth. Seek medical care if vision is affected, if you have a fever, headache, lethargy, or loss of appetite, or if the swelling is on, or directed to, the inside of the eyelid, rather than the rim.

See also Allergies.

ORTHODOX MEDICINE

Physicians recommend hot compresses or surgical drainage if a stye comes to a head but doesn't drain on its own. Antibiotics may be prescribed if infections recur.

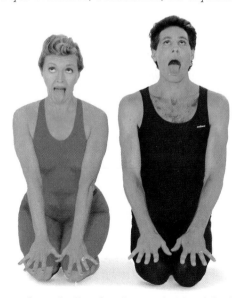

To perform the lion face *for sore throats, sit back on heels, hands on knees, and stick out your tongue.*

COMMON-SENSE CARE

Avoid rubbing the eye or squeezing the stye, especially if it is infected. Warm-to-hot compresses will decrease the pain and bring the stye to a head.

NATURAL MEDICINE THERAPIES

■ HOMEOPATHY: One of the commonest remedies for styes is pulsatilla. When the stye is erupting, aconite may be prescribed to ease the pain, then pulsatilla if the aconite is not effective. Staphysagria may be tried when styes recur every few weeks, especially if you suffer from nervous exhaustion.

■ NATUROPATHY: Eating a raw-food diet of uncooked vegetables or fruit at each meal for one to seven days may help.

■ VITAMIN AND MINERAL THERAPY: Suggestions include taking a multivitamin/multimineral supplement and extra vitamin C and zinc daily. If styes appear frequently, you may have a vitamin A deficiency; however, large doses of vitamin A should be taken only under medical supervision.

Ulcer *A painfully inflamed open sore on the skin's surface or on the mucous membrane of an internal organ may be an ulcer. The most common gastrointestinal ulcers occur in the stomach and the duodenum, which is the tube that connects the stomach and intestines. The term peptic ulcer includes both gastric (stomach) and duodenal ulcers, and it refers to an ulcer caused by acid erosion. Symptoms include bloating, heartburn, and abdominal pain that often strikes within an hour of a meal and lasts for up to three hours. Canker sores are mouth ulcers that may appear on the tongue, inner cheeks, lips, and gums. These sores can be related to food allergies, poor dental hygiene, smoking, stress, and fatigue.*

Smoking, drinking, taking aspirin, corticosteroids, and other drugs, and genetic factors can put you at risk for developing peptic ulcers.

See also Allergies, Indigestion.

ORTHODOX MEDICINE

Antacids in liquid or tablet form may be recommended. Patients should avoid taking aspirin or other nonsteroidal anti-inflammatory drugs or corticosteroids. Drugs known as histamine-2 receptor blocking agents can lower gastric acid levels, relieve symptoms, and aid in healing gastric and duodenal ulcers. The effectiveness of a bland diet is in doubt, although some physicians still favor it for certain patients. Surgery is rarely performed.

COMMON-SENSE CARE

Stop smoking, if you still smoke. Using such stress-control techniques as meditation and biofeedback may alleviate symptoms and minimize recurrences. Avoid coffee, tea, alcohol, and acidic foods like citrus fruit if you have an ulcer of the digestive tract. A food allergy may be a contributing factor. Scrutinize your diet and see if any type of food causes an ulcer flareup. Although milk can neutralize stomach acid, the protein and calcium in milk can also spur the production of more acid, canceling out its benefits.

NATURAL MEDICINE THERAPIES

■ HOMEOPATHY: Peptic ulcers may respond to argentum nitricum, when symptoms include flatulence and cravings for sweets; nux vomica, when symptoms include irritable pain soon after eating; lycopodium, arsenicum album, and anacardium.

■ HYPNOTHERAPY: For both alleviating ulcer pain and managing stress, hypnotherapy may be effective.

■ NATUROPATHY: Although a bland diet may be recommended briefly for peptic ulcers, such a diet can interfere with healing, since it provides insufficient iron and vitamin C. Avoid alcohol and such caffeine sources as colas, chocolate, coffee, and tea. Practitioners may also advise against decaffeinated coffee.

■ SHIATSU: Points on the liver, spleen, stomach, urinary bladder, and conception meridians are commonly treated.

■ VITAMIN AND MINERAL THERAPY: The most common recommendations are vitamins A and E, which some practitioners believe can protect against ulcers caused by stress. For canker sores, vitamin B_{12}, folic acid, and zinc may speed healing, along with vitamin E applied directly to the sore.

Varicose veins *The twisted,*
elongated, unsightly veins that pop out just
beneath the skin's surface are varicose veins.
They are most often found in the legs. Other
sites are the esophagus, scrotum, and anus,
where they take the form of hemorrhoids.

A malfunction in the mechanics of blood
circulation or an inherited weakness of vein
walls causes varicose veins. Normally valves in
the legs keep circulating blood from draining
back down once it has delivered oxygen to the
tissues in the limbs. However, if the valves
fail, blood flows downward, forms pools, and
eventually causes veins near the surface to
become swollen and contorted. Prolonged
periods of standing and lack of exercise can
contribute to the condition; among women,
hormonal changes and pressure on pelvic veins
during pregnancy may lead to varicose veins.

See also Circulatory Problems, Hemorrhoids.

ORTHODOX MEDICINE

When the sight of the distended, bluish veins causes anguish or if the area becomes tender and itches uncomfortably, surgery may be performed to remove the swollen vein. Injecting a chemical into varicose veins in the lower leg may lessen swelling.

COMMON-SENSE CARE

Women with varicose veins in the legs should switch from regular hosiery to elastic support stockings. They should sit with their feet elevated, not with legs crossed, to enhance circulation and rest with their feet propped up with the legs raised above chest level, whenever possible. Preventive measures include not smoking, avoiding obesity, exercising the legs by walking, running, cycling, or swimming, and avoiding standing for long periods.

NATURAL MEDICINE THERAPIES

■ **AROMATHERAPY:** A cool compress with essential oils of cypress, rosemary, and peppermint may soothe affected veins.

■ **HOMEOPATHY:** Pulsatilla and hamamelis may be prescribed for pregnant women with varicose veins.

■ **HYDROTHERAPY:** Sponging your legs with cold water, or spraying water on them, may relieve discomfort.

■ **REFLEXOLOGY:** Massaging reflexes for the colon and the endocrine glands may bring improvement.

■ **VITAMIN AND MINERAL THERAPY:** Vitamins C and E and bioflavonoids, which are substances that enhance the absorption of vitamin C, may improve the condition.

■ **YOGA:** Such positions as the shoulder stand, plow, fish, and inverted corpse can improve drainage of blood and help prevent more varicose veins from forming. ❏

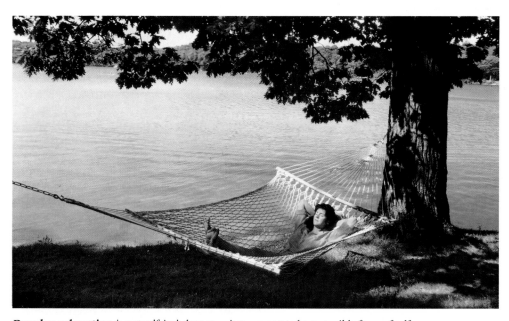

Regular relaxation *is not self-indulgence—it turns out to be a sensible form of self-care.*

Index

Abdominal curl, **202**, 203, 379
Abdominal pain, 334, 376
Aboriginal Australia, 130-131, **130, 131**
Abrasions, 316, 320
Accutane, 283, 338
Acidophilus, 357
Acne, 299, 338-339
Aconite, 346, 351, 355, 358, 359, 363, 380, 388, 389, 390
Acquired Immune Deficiency Syndrome (AIDS), 30, 337
Acupressure, 46, 166-167
  for menstrual problems, **166, 381**
  tips for, **166**
Acupuncture, 9, 27, 44, 46-49, 55, 166, **166**, 170
  for addiction, 47, 144
  for allergies, 340
  as analgesia, 47, 48
  for arteriosclerosis, 342
  for arthritis, 344
  for asthma, 345
  for back pain, 9-10, 348
  for bronchitis, 350
  for cancer, 353
  for chronic pain, 385
  for colds, 355
  for constipation, 357
  for coughs, 358
  for cystitis, 359
  for depression, 360
  for diabetes, 362
  for diarrhea, 363
  for diverticulitis, 364
  for eczema, 364
  for emphysema, 366
  finding practitioner of, 48-49
  for gallstones, 367
  for gout, 368
  for hay fever, 369, **369**
  for headache, 370-371
  for heart disease, 372-373
  for hemorrhoids, 373
  for hepatitis, 374
  for high blood pressure, 375
  for indigestion, 376
  for insomnia, 377
  for irritable bowel syndrome, 378
  for kidney stones, 379
  for menopausal problems, 380
  for menstrual problems, 381
  meridians and. *See* Meridians.
  for migraine, **382**, 383
  for pain, 47, 48, 348, 385

  for sciatica, 387, **387**
  scientific explanations of, 47-48
  for shingles, 388
  for sore throat, 389
  uses of, 46-47
Acupuncture points (tsubos), **45**, 81, 164, **164**, 165
Addiction, 142-144, **142, 145, 147,** 149
  acupuncture for, 47, 144
  causes of, 143-144
  creative therapy for, 138
  dance therapy for, 140
  as disease, 143
  external factors in, 144
  gambling as, **144**
  genetic basis for, 144
  group therapy and, **136**
  insecurity and, 143
  nature of, 142-143
  personality and, 145
  roots of, 145
  self-help groups for. *See* Self-help groups.
  socially acceptable forms of, 145
  as spiritual concern, 145
  treatment options for, 144
  Weil on, 145
Addison's disease, 315
Additives, food, 255-257, 262
Adrenal glands, 91, 315
  reflexology for, **175**
Aerobic exercise, 194-195, **195**, 198, 199, **199**, 200, 203, **209**
  heart disease and, **371**
  See also Exercise.
Aerophobia, **134**
Africa, 170
Agave, **65**
Aging, 8, 250, 310
  exercise and, **197**
  massage and, **157**
  See also Elderly.
Agriculture, U.S. Department of, 243, 256
Agrimony, 376
AIDS (Acquired Immune Deficiency Syndrome), 30, 337
AIDS Memorial Quilt, **141**
Aikido, 223, **227**, 228, 231
Air element, 177
Alaska, **107**
Alcohol, 108, 254
  cancer and, 352
Alcoholics, 146, 310
Alcoholics Anonymous (AA), 143
  Twelve Steps of, **146**
Alcoholism, 142, **142,** 144
  disease concept of, 143, 146
  self-help groups for, 146
  vitamin and mineral supplements and, 284

Aldous Huxley (Bedford), 84
Alexander, F. Matthias, 180, **180, 181,** 183
Alexander Technique, 26, 154, 180-183, 185
  for arthritis, 344
  for asthma, 345
  for back pain, 348
  benefits of, 183
  for bronchitis, 350-351
  carrying bags and, **182**
  for headache, 371
  for heart disease, 373
  lifting and, **182**
  for pain, 182, 348
  posture and, 181-182, **181**
  relaxation promoted by, 182
  replacing habits in, 180-182
  talking on phone and, **181**
Alfalfa, 344
Alienation, 359
Allergic rhinitis. *See* Hay fever.
Allergens, 339, 368
Allergies, 8, 56. 62, 75, 90, 315, 339-340, **340**
  breast feeding and, 14
  bronchitis and, 350
  dust mites and, **339**
  eczema and, 364
  to foods, 258, 339, 340, 346
  hypnotherapy for, 120, 125, 340
Allergy Discovery Diet, The (Postley and Barton), 259
Allium, 257
Allium cepa, 355
Alman, Brian M., 123
Almond oil, 344
Aloe vera, 296, **296**
Alternative medicine:
  definition of, 21
  See also Natural medicine.
Altman, Lawrence K., 25
Aluminia, 357
Aluminum cookware, **270**
Amblyopia, 82
Amebic dysentery, 363
Amenorrhea, 381
American Cancer Society, 247, 271
American Heart Association, 247
American Institute of Homeopathy, 61
American Massage Therapy Association, 161-163
American Medical Association
  chiropractic and, 75
  homeopathy and, 61
  hypnosis and, **22**
  naturopathy and, 79-80
  osteopathy and, 27
Amino acids, 245, 269
Anacardium, 390
Analgesia
  acupuncture as, 47, 48
  See also Pain relievers.

Anaphylactic shock, 258
Anatomy of an Illness (Cousins),
  14-15
Anemia, 62, 264, **287**, 306, 341
Anesthesia, in childbirth, 13
Aneurysms, 341
Anger, 165
  polarity therapy and, 178
  yoga and, 214-216
Angina, 242, 371
Animal bites, 334
Animal magnetism, 120
Animals
  dreaming in, 127
  homeopathy and, 65
  power, 33
Anise, 297, **297**
Ankylosing spondylitis, 343
Anorexia, 302, 306
Antibiotic(s), 28, 62, 253
  garlic as, 13, 307
  in meat and poultry feeds, 257,
    262
Antibodies, 14, 258
Antihistamines, 339
Antihypertensive drugs, 359
Antioxidants, 250, **252, 279**, 343,
  353
Antiseptics, 307, 310, 317, 323,
  324, 327
Anxiety, 97, 312, 321, 323, 344
  creative therapy for, 138
  electrodermal response (EDR)
    for, 115
  hypnotherapy for, 125
  irritable bowel syndrome and,
    378
  meditation for, 102
  shamanistic methods for, 34-
    35
  See also Nervousness; Stress.
Aphrodisiacs, 297, 310
Apis, 340, 356, 389
Appalachia, 30
Appendicitis, 10, 25-26, 334
Appetite stimulants, 303, 306,
  327
Apples, 249-250
Archery, 104
Argentum nitricum, 356, 390
Armoring, 187
Arnica, 348
Aromatherapy, 328-329
  for bad breath, 349
  for boils, 349-350
  for bronchitis, 329, **329**, 351
  for emphysema, 366
  for sore throat, 389
  for varicose veins, 391
Arrythmias, 117
Arsenicum, 340, 350, 360, 364,
  388
Arsenicum album, 346, 363,
  369, 376, 377, 390

Arterial plaque, 342, **342**
Arteries, 246, **246**, 247, 272
Arteriosclerosis, 341-343
Arthritis, 62, 343-345, **344**, 347
  ankylosing spondylitis, 343
  aromatherapy for, 329
  from gout, 367-368
  herbs for, 298, 301, 307, 312,
    313, 315, 316, 317, 318,
    319, 323, 326, 327
  hypnotherapy for, 122, 344
  infective, 343
  massage for, 157
  mud baths for, **212**
  osteoarthritis, 340, 343, 344
  psoriasis and, 386
  quack cures for, 27
  rheumatoid, 298, 299, 307,
    340, 343, 344
  sand baths for, **213**
Artificial food colors, 254, 256,
  257
Art of Seeing, The (Huxley), 84
Art of Survival, The (Gharote and
  Lockhart), 221
Art therapy. *See* Creative
  therapies.
Asanas, 216-218
Aspirin, 37, 249, 253, 326
Asthma, 334, 339, 340, 345-346,
  357
  Alexander Technique for, 180
  chiropractic for, 75
  electromyograph (EMG) for,
    115
  herbs for, 304, 305, 309, 315
  hypnotherapy for, 120, 346
  osteopathy for, 69
  reflexology for, 169
Aston Patterning, 154, 189
Astragalus, 297
Astringents, 317, 318, 320, 321,
  326, 327
AT. *See* Autogenic training.
Atherosclerosis, 341-342, 343,
  371-372
Athletes, **115**, 266
  Alexander Technique used by,
    180
  chiropractic and, 75
  diets and, 264-265
  electrodermal response (EDR)
    used by, 115-116
  massage and, 157
  visualization used by, 118
Athlete's foot, 346-347
Atopic dermatitis, 360-361
Atopic eczema, 364
Aural eczematoid dermatitis, 364
Auras, 99, **99**
Aurum, 360
Australia, 130-131, **130, 131**
Autism, 138, 139
Autogenic training (AT), 123-
  125
  meditation and, 124-125

Autoimmune diseases, 8
Aversion techniques, 134
Awareness Through Movement,
  184, 185
Ayurvedic medicine, **34**, 52-57,
  55, 99, 154, 176, **176**, 177
  assessment in, 56
  cupping in, **56**
  herbs used in, 56-57, 294
  as holistic therapy, 54-55
  institutes of, 57
  practitioners of, 55-56, 57
  prevention in, 54, 56
  sweatboxes used in, **57**
  three life forces in, 52-54
  treatment prescription in,
    56-57
  Western medicine and, 54
  yoga and, 55-56

Babies, 10, 13-14, 62, 65, 325
  colic in, 75, **156**, 297
  cradle cap in, 360
  massage for, **156**
Bach, Edward, 330, **330**, 331,
  331
Bach Flower Remedies, 330-331,
  330
  for allergies, 340
  for asthma, 345
  for indigestion, 376
  for irritable bowel syndrome,
    378
  for psoriasis, 386
Back-lift, **219**
Back massage, **158-163**
Back pain, 9-10, 347-348, **348**
  acupressure for, 167
  Alexander Technique for, 180
  chiropractic for, **73, 75, 75,**
    348, **348**
  electromyograph (EMG) for,
    115
  massage for, 157
  osteopathy for, 9-10, **68**, 69,
    348
  polarity therapy for, 178
  relaxation for, 108
  yoga for, 218-220
Back problems, constipation and,
  357
Back releaser, **202**, 203
Bacteria, bacterial infection, 10,
  248, 249, 253, 257, 334
  immune system and, 88
Bad breath, 349, 385

Balance, 18-21, 23, 154
  acupuncture and, 46
  Ayurvedic medicine and, 52, 54
  Chinese medicine and, **44**, 50
  macrobiotics and, 270-271
  naturopathy and, 76
  osteopathy and, 66
  polarity therapy and, 176, 177, 178. *See also* Polarity therapy.
  reflexology and, 169
  shiatsu and, 164-165
  t'ai chi and, 237
  yoga and, 216, 218
Baldness, 320
Balloon angioplasty, 342
Balls, metal, **26**
Barton, Janet, 259
Baryta muriatica, 389
Basal metabolic rate, 267
Basil, 297-298, **298**
Basketball, 195
Bates, William, 83
Bates eye exercises, 83, 84
Bathhouses, 206, 209
Bathing, 109, 209
Baths of Caracalla, 206
B complex vitamins. *See* Vitamin B complex.
Beads, good-luck, **26**
Beans, 255, **269, 281**
Bearberry (uva ursi), 324-325, **324**
Beatles, 104
Beck, Aaron, 135
Bedford, Sybille, 84
Bedsores, 317
Bedwetting, **125**, 323
Beef, 261
Behavior therapies, 133-134
Belief. *See* Faith and belief.
Belize, 30
Belladonna, 340, 350, 355, 356, 358, 368, 371, 389
Benson, Herbert, 109
Berberis, 367, 379
Bergamot, 350
Bernard, Saint, 104
Besant, Annie, 100
Beta-carotene, 12, 250, 261, 276, **279**, 343, 346, 353, 369, 373, 386, 389
  See also Vitamin A
Better Eyesight Without Glasses (Bates), 83
BHT, 255
Biathalon, **115**
Bicycle, stationary, **195**
Bicycling, 195, **199**
Big toe pose, **217**
Bile ducts, 334
Binocular trick, 135
Bioenergetics, 184, 187
Biofeedback, 91, 114-117, **114, 117**

autogenic training and, 123
  EDR, 115-116
  electroencephalograph, 117
  for high blood pressure, 117, **375**
  home practice of, 117
  limitations and dangers of, 117
  methods of, 114-115
  temperature, 115
  visualization used with, 115
Bioflavonoids, 382, 388, 391
Biotin, 360, 362
  food sources of, 279
  main role of, 279
  therapeutic uses of, 285
Birch pollen, **369**
Birth, 13-14
Bites
  animal, 334
  insect, 299, 303, 307, 320
Black cohosh, 298
Blackheads, 338
Bladder, 321
  cancer of, 352
  infection of (cystitis), 324, 358-359
Blavatsky, Helena Petrovna, 100
Bleeding, 320, 322, 334, 341
Blemishes, skin, 296
Blind children, music therapy for, **140**
Blisters, 320, 360, 364, 388
Bloating, 258
Block, parry, and punch, **234, 236**
Blood
  cleansers for, 299, 310
  clotting of, 308
  coagulation of, 310, 327
  hemoglobin levels of, 97
  white cells of, 88, 90
Blood clots (thrombi), 253, 305, 312, 341, 353
  onions and, **251**
Blood pressure, 246, 305, 307
  garlic and, 13
  high. *See* High blood pressure.
  macrobiotic diet and, 271
  meditation and, 102
  vegetarianism and, 268
Blood vessels, cold treatments and, 208, 209
Bodhidarma, 222-223
Body, healing power of, 8, 11, 15, 18-20
Body-mind balance, 20-21
Bodywork, 154
  acupressure. *See* Acupressure.
  Alexander Technique. *See* Alexander Technique.
  in ancient Egypt, **154**

Aston Patterning, 154, 189
  Bioenergetics, 184, 187
  combinations, 154
  Connective Tissue Polarity, 189
  emotional stresses and, 184
  Feldenkrais Method, 184-185
  goal of, 179
  Hellerwork, 154, 189
  massage. *See* Massage.
  newer methods of, 184-187
  polarity therapy. *See* Polarity therapy.
  reflexology. *See* Reflexology.
  Rolfing, 26, 254, 188-189, **189**
  Rosen Method, 184, 185-187, **187**
  Rubenfeld Synergy, 184, 185, **185**
  shiatsu. *See* Shiatsu.
  Tragerwork, 184, 187
Boils, 323, 349-350
  styes, 389-390
Bones
  broken, 334
  sedentary lifestyle and, 192
  See also Osteoporosis.
Boneset, 298-299, **298**
Boredom, 359
Boron, 384
Boston Lying-In Hospital, 13
Botanical gardens, **291**
Botany, 11
Botulism, 263
Bound-angle pose, **220**
Bowers, Edwin, 170
Brain, 88, 90, 91
  cells of, **89**
  hemorrhages in, 334
  tumor in, 48
  waves, 33, 117
Brain Mind Gym, **110**
Braun, Bennett, 90
Breads, 240, 243, 247, **249**, 257, 260
Breast cancer, 10, 12, 240, 248, 257, 352
Breast disease, fibrocystic, 13
Breast feeding, 13-14
Breath, bad, 349, 385
Breathing, 56, **108**, 315, 345
  Alexander Technique and, 154
  conscious connected, 151
  difficulty in, 221, 334
  exercises for, 44, 51, 109, 351
  as relaxation aid, 109
  in t'ai chi, 237
  in yoga, 214, 216
  See also Respiratory conditions.
Breezestroke, **175**
Brennan, Barbara Ann, 99
Broccoli, 262
Broken leg, 211

Bronchial conditions, 304, 309, 319
Bronchitis, 350-351, 357
  aromatherapy for, 329, **329,** 351
  herbs for, 304, 306, 316, 324, 329, **329,** 351
  osteopathy for, 69
Brown, Barbara, 114, 117
Bruises, 208
Brush knee and press, **234, 236**
Bruxism, 115
Bryonia, 344, 348, 351, 357, 358, 380
Buckthorn, 299
Buddhism, **58,** 100, **103,** 105, 222, **222**
Burdock, 299, **299**
Burns, 296, 309, 317, 322, 323, 327, 329, 334
Butter, 245, 247
B vitamins. *See* Vitamin B complex.

Cabbage, **260**
CAD. *See* Coronary artery disease.
Caffeine, 108, 255
Cajeput oil, 351
Calcium
  addiction and, 144
  drugs and, **285**
  food sources of, 280, **281**
  kidney stones and, 379
  macrobiotics and, 271
  magnesium and, 276
  main role of, 280
  osteoporosis and, 264, 283, **286**
  therapeutic uses of, 287, 340, 346, 348, 354, 362, 369, 371, 376, 378, 379, 380, 382, 383, 384, 386
  vitamin D and, 276
Calcium carbonate, 62
Calcium pantothenate, 344
Calendula ointment, 346
California Nutrition Book, The (Saltman, Gurin, and Mothner), 240
Calming, 313, 330. *See also* Sedatives.
Calories, 247, 254, 263, 265, 271
  exercise and, 267
  frequent dieting and, 267

Cancer, 8, 28, 108, 250, 308, 347, 352-353
  antioxidants and, **279**
  breast, 10, 12, 240, 248, 257, 352
  cervical, 12-13, 250
  of colon, 12, 194, 240, 250, 254, 268, 341, 352, 356, 363
  diet and, 12-13
  of esophagus, 250, 352
  fat intake and, 12, 240
  fiber and, 12, 254
  food additives and, 256
  foods and, 248, 257
  of larynx, 352
  of lungs, 12-13, 250, 352, 357
  macrobiotics and, 271
  of mouth, 352
  nitrites and, 257
  nutrients and, 12, 276
  of pharynx, 352
  phytochemicals and, 254
  of prostate, 12
  quack cures for, 27
  rain forest and, 30
  self-help groups for, 148-149
  seven warning signs of, 353
  skin, **352**
  spontaneous remission of, 92
  of stomach, 250, 257, 341
  stress and, 106
  support groups for, **148**
  of uterus, 12
  vegetarianism and, 268
  visualization exercises for, 10, 118, **118,** 119
  vitamin C and, **252**
Cankers, 321
Cannon, Walter B., 106
Cantharis, 359, 380
Capsaicin, 301
Carbohydrates, 245-247, 254, 264, 265
  complex, 247, **252,** 264, **265**
  simple, 245
Carbo loading, **264**
Carbo vegetabilis, 376
Cardiologists, 24
Cardiovascular disease, 242, 250, 308
  arteriosclerosis, 341-343
  exercise and, 192
  See also Heart disease.
Cardiovascular fitness, 194-195
Cardiovascular system, 310
Carminatives, 298, 302, 306, 313, 314, 319, 324
Carnitine, 351
Carper, Jean, 253
Carrots, 248, **261**
Carrying bags, **182**
Cartilage discs, **73**
Cascara sagrada, 300
Case of Nora, The (Feldenkrais), 186
Castelli, William, 242, **242**
Catholic Church, **95**

Catnip, 300, **300**
Cattail pollen, **38**
Caulophyllum, 382
Causticum, 358
Cayenne, 300-301
Celery, 248
Celidonium, 367
Cells, receptor sites of, 88-90, **88, 89**
Cereal. *See* Grains and cereals.
Cerebral palsy, 69, 139-140, **210**
Certified pastoral counselors, 135
Cervix, cancer of, 12-13, 250
Chado, The Japanese Way of Tea (Sen), 104
Chakras, **34, 53, 54,** 99, 177
Chamomile, 301, **301,** 377
Change, 23
  resistance to, 56
Chanting, 34
Chapped lips, 322-323
Cheese, 243
Cherries, **252**
Chest
  pain in, 334
  reflexology for, **174**
Chest conditions, 56, 317. *See also* Respiratory conditions.
Chilblains, 317
Child abuse, 90, 140, 146
Childbirth, 13-14
Childbirth pains, 298
Children, 62, **91,** 337
  depression in, **359**
  group therapy for, **136**
  healthy eating for, 272-273
  hypnotherapy for, **125**
  overweight, **267**
  stress in, **106**
  See also Babies.
China, 101, 170, 222, 224
  diet in, **273**
Chinese medicine, 21, 42-51, 54, 154, 156, 164, 166-167, 176, 270
  acupuncture in. *See* Acupuncture.
  anatomy as viewed in, 42-44
  assessment in, 44-46
  balance in, **44,** 50
  cupping in, **56**
  food cures in, 50
  herbs used in, **43,** 49-51, **50,** 294
  qi in, 44, 50, 51
  Western validation of, 51
  yin and yang in. *See* Yin and yang.
Chiropractic, 21, **64,** 72-75, **72,** 334, 337
  adjustment techniques in, 73-74, **75**
  for asthma, 345
  for back pain, 73, 75, **75,** 348, **348**

for chronic pain, 385
conditions treated by, 75
for constipation, 357
examination in, 72-73, **74**
for headache, 75, **75**, 371
for indigestion, 376
for migraine, 75, **75**, 383
for sciatica, 387
two kinds of, 74-75
Chiropractors, licensing
    requirements for, 334-336
Chloride, 280
Cholecystectomy with Self-Hypnosis
    (Rausch), 124
Cholesterol, 246, 247, 271
    arteriosclerosis and, 341-342
    fiber and, 255
    gallstones and, 367
Cholesterol, blood levels of, 242,
    242, 246, 247, 249, 250,
    254, 305, 308, 310
    exercise and, 192
    garlic and, **251**
    HDL, 247, 253, 343
    LDL, 247, 250
    macrobiotic diet and, 271
    niacin and, 13
    onions and, **251**, 253
    vegetarianism and, 268
Choline, 367, 376
Christianity, 94, 100, 101
Christian Scientists, 95
Chromium, 362, 373
    food sources of, 281
    main role of, 281
    therapeutic uses of, 287
Cigarette smoking. *See* Smoking.
Cinchona, 60, **62**
Cinnamon, 302, **302**, 329
Circulation, circulatory
problems, **26**, 209, 309, 312,
    320, 353-354, **354**
    biofeedback and, 115
    cupping for, **56**
    dermatitis and, 361
    osteopathy for, 69
    reflexology and, 169
    sand baths for, **213**
Cirrhosis, 316
Citrus fruits, 248, 250, **252**
Clark, Nancy, 264, 266
Clary sage, 389
Claustrophobia, 329
Clematis, 340
Clergy, 135
Cliffhanger, **178**
Clifford, Carolyn, 248
Clinical psychologists, 135
Cocaine addiction, 144
Coconut oil, 247
Cod-liver oil, 250

Coffea, 377
Coffee, 254
Cognitive therapy, 134-135
Colchicine, 368
Cold, bodily effect of, 208-209
Colds, 337, 354-355, **355**, 357
    herbs for, 297, 299, 301, 302,
        304, 308, 311, 313, 314,
        317, 321, 323, 326
    vitamin C for, 282, 283
Colic, 75, **156**, 297
Colitis, 62, 316, 363
Colocynth, 382, 387-388
Colon
    cancer of, 12, 194, 240, 250,
        254, 268, 341, 352, 356,
        363
    diverticulitis and, 363-364
    irritable, 340, 356, 378-379
    spastic, 180
Colostrum, 13-14
Comfrey, 79
Complementary treatments, 9,
    10, 21-22
Compulsive behavior. *See*
    Addiction.
Compulsive eating. *See*
    Overeating, compulsive.
Congestion, 56, 329, 340
Conjunctivitis (pink eye), 324,
    340, 355-356
Connective Tissue Polarity, 189
Conscious connected breathing,
    151
Constipation, 356-357, **357**
    energy blockage and, 167
    fiber and, 254, 356-357, **357**
    herbs for, 298, 299, 300, 315,
        316, 320, 321
    polarity therapy for, 178
    reflexology for, 169
    See also Laxatives.
Consumers' movement, 12, 14
Contraceptive pills, 359
Contusions, 208
Conventional medicine. *See*
    Orthodox medicine.
Cook, James, **275**
Copper, 341, 344, 373
    food sources of, 280
    main role of, 280
    vitamin C and, 277
Copper cookware, **270**
Corn syrup, 245
Coronary artery bypass, 342
Coronary artery disease (CAD),
    21, 221, 240, 265
Coronary heart disease. *See* Heart
    disease.
Corpse pose, 216, **220**
Corticosteroids, 91, 339
Coughing up blood, 334
Coughs, 56, 345, 357-358
    herbs for, 297, 304, 313, 316,
        323, 324
Counselors, 135

Couples therapy, 135, 137
Cousins, Norman, 14-15, 29
Crabapple, 378, 386
Cradle cap, 360
Cramps
    intestinal, 312
    leg, 312
    menstrual. *See* Menstrual
        cramps.
    muscle, 178, 209
Cranberry, 302
Cranial osteopathy, 70-71
Cream, 247
Creative therapies, 138-141, **138,
    139, 140**
    dance, 138, 139-140
    drama, 138, 140-141
    interaction in, 138
    journal writing, 138, 141
    music, 138, 139, **140**
Creativity, 170
Cromolyn sodium, 339
Crossed eyes (strabismus), 82
Crystals, **34**
Cupping, **56**
Cuprum metalicum, 346
Cuts. *See* Wound healing.
Cycling, 195, **199**
Cypress, 391
Cystitis, 324, 347, 358-359
Cysts, acne, 338

Dairy products, 243, 247, 269
    food poisoning and, 263
Dance therapy, 138, 139-140
Dancing, 195
Dandelion, 10, 38, 303, **303**
Dandruff, 296, 299, 304, 360
Dang gui, 49
Deep tissue therapies
    Aston Patterning, 154, 189
    Connective Tissue Polarity,
        189
    Hellerwork, 154, 189
    Rolfing, 26, 154, 188-189, **189**
Deer, **30**
Degenerative joint disease
    (osteoarthritis), 340, 343,
    344
Depression, 56, 135, 323, 330-
    331, 340, 344, 359-360, 377
    in children, **359**
    creative therapy for, 138
    dance therapy for, 140
    exercise for, 194
    hypnotherapy for, 125
    irritable bowel syndrome and,
        378

visualization for, 119
yoga for, 214-216
Dermatitis, 360-361, **360**
Detoxification, for addictions,
144
Diabetes, 56, 194, 306, 334, 341,
342, 361-362, **362**
biofeedback and, 117
Chinese medicine and, 45
dietary fat and, 240
exercise and, 194
multiple personality disorder
and, 90
in Pima Indians, 244, **245**
Diarrhea, 253, 334, 337, 363
herbs for, 302, 312, 327
lactose intolerance and, 258
Dickens, Charles, 61
Diet(s), dieting, 21, 44, 264-267
for athletes, 264-265
balance in, 276
drastic calorie reductions in,
265
exercise and, 267, **267**
high-carbohydrate, 265
macrobiotic, 270-271
naturopathy and, 76, 78, 80
obesity and, 265-266
on-off, hazards of, 267
in polarity therapy, 176, 177-
178
sensible, 265
treadmill, 267
vegetarian, 268-269
vitamin and mineral
supplements and, 284
See also Nutrition.
Diet for a Small Planet (Lappé),
268
Digestive aids, 297, 298, 299,
300, 301, 306, 307, 309,
310, 313, 316, 319, 320,
325, 327
Digitalis, 51
Diphtheria, 11
Disabilities, 138
Disraeli, Benjamin, 61
Diuretics, 299, 303, 313, 318,
324, 326, 327
Diverticulitis, 363-364
Divine healing. *See* Faith healing.
Dizziness, 334
*Dr. Dean Ornish's Program for
Reversing Heart Disease*
(Ornish), 246
Dr. Sheehan on Running
(Sheehan), 192
Doshas, 52-54, 55, 57
Dramamine, 253
Drama therapy, 138, 140-141
Dream-guessing ceremonies, **128**
Dream nets, **128**

Dreams, 126-129, **126**
forgetting of, 127, 128, 129
function of, 127-128
groups for sharing of, 128-129
interpretation of, 133
lucid, **127**, 129
remembering and recording of,
129
REM sleep and, 127, **127,** 128
theories about, 127
unconscious and, 127
working with, 128-129
Dreamtime, 130-131, **130, 131**
Dream Work (Taylor), 129
Dropsy, 299
Drug addiction, 142, **142**, 144
self-help groups for, 146
See also Addiction.
Drugs, medicinal, 8, 253
in childbirth, 13
depression and, 359
herbs vs., 11, 12, 290-292, 295
overuse of, 11, 12, 13, 22, 24,
29
toxicity of, 11-12
Drumming, 33, 34
Drury, Nevill, 35
Duodenal ulcer, 390
Dürer, Albrecht, **337**
Dust mites, **339**
Dysentery, 249, 327, 363

Earaches, 317
Ears
eczema in, 364
infection in, 71
reflexology and, 168
Earth element, 164, 177
Eastern cultures, **103**
energy principle in. *See* Energy,
life.
Japan, 101-102, 164, 170,
209, 222
See also Ayurvedic medicine;
Chinese medicine; Martial
arts; Meditation; Yoga.
Eating, compulsive. *See*
Overeating, compulsive.
Echinacea, 79, 303
Eczema, 305, 318, 339, 340,
364-365
hypnotherapy for, 120, 364
Eddy, Mary Baker, 95
Edema, 298, 310
EDR (Electrodermal Response),
115-116
EEG (Electroencephalograph
Biofeedback), 117
Effleurage, 158-160, **159, 161**
Eggs, 243, 247
allergy to, 258
food poisoning and, 263

Egypt, 170
Eisenberg, David, 48
Elder, 303-304
Elderly, 337
anemia and, 341
exercise for, **197**
massage for, **157**
vitamins and minerals and,
284, **285**
Elecampane, 304, **304**
Electrodermal Response (EDR),
115-116
Electroencephalograph
Biofeedback (EEG), 117
Electromagnetic energy. *See*
Energy, life.
Electromyograph (EMG), 114-
115
Elements. *See* Five Elements.
Elements of Shamanism, The
(Drury), 35
Elimination diet, 258
Emergencies, medical, 10, 11,
12, 21-22, 62, 334
EMG (electromyograph), 114-
115
Emotional health
breast feeding and, 14
yoga and, 220
Emotional problems
childhood pain and, 150
creative therapy for, 138
dance therapy for, 140
drama therapy for, 140-141
Emotions, 14, 21, 68, 91, **133,**
331, 334
Bach Flower Remedies and,
330, 331
bodywork and, 184, 185
faith healing and, 94
polarity therapy and, 178
Rolfing and, 188
See also Stress.
Emphysema, 69, 334, 365-366,
365
Encounter groups, 135
Encounters with Qi (Eisenberg),
48
Endocrine system, 88, 359
biofeedback and, 117
Endocrinologists, 24
Endometriosis, 381
Endorphins, 142, 171
Enemas, 57
Energy, life (qi; prana), 18, 44,
156
acupuncture and, 46
aikido and, 228
chakras and, **34, 53, 54,** 99,
177
Chinese medicine and, 44, 50,
51

faith healing and, 96
Hara and, **165**
homeopathy and, 64-65
polarity therapy and, 154. *See
  also* Polarity therapy.
reflexology and, 169, 170, 171
Reich and, **133**
Reiki and, 99
shiatsu and, 164, 165, **165**, 167
t'ai chi and, 227, **230**, 231,
  235, 237
yoga and, 214
Environmental Protection
  Agency, U.S. (E.P.A.), 256
Ephedrine (ma huang), 51, 315-
  316
Epilepsy, 321
  biofeedback for, 117
  osteopathy for, 69
Episiotomies, 13
Erving, Julius, **184**
Eskimos, 250
Esophagus, cancer of, 250, 352
EST (Erhard Seminar Training),
  135, 151
Estrogen, 248
Ether element, 177
Eucalyptus, 304, **305**, 329, 351,
  366
Euphrasia, 340, 355, 366, 369
European Scientific Cooperative
  for Phytotherapy (ESCOP),
  294
Evening primrose, 305, **305**
Exercise, **20**, **51**, 109, 192-205,
  221, **241**, 265, 267, **267**
  aerobic. *See* Aerobic exercise.
  for arthritis, 343
  basic routine for, 200-205,
    200-205
  benefits of, 192-193, 197
  Chinese medicine and, 51
  cool down, 203
  cycling, 195, **199**
  for flexibility, 194, 197, 199,
    214
  fun of, 297
  heart rate in, 200
  hiking, 195, **198**
  immune function and, 20
  irritable bowel syndrome and,
    378
  for muscular strength and
    endurance, 194, 195-196,
    198-199, 214
  for older people, **197**
  osteoporosis and, **384**
  with other people, 199
  personal trainers for, 199
  planning program of, 194-197
  in polarity therapy, 177-178
  as relaxation, 109
  risks of, 198-199
  road racing, 193

running, **193**, 195, 196, 199
skiing, **198**
on stair machine, **195**
on stationary bicycle, **195**
walking, **194**, 197-198
warm-up, 200-203
water, **208**, **209**, 210-211
See also Martial arts; Yoga.
Exfoliative dermatitis, 361
Expectations, 93. *See also* Faith
  and belief.
Expectorants, 304, 306, 313,
  315, 317, 324
Expressive therapies. *See* Creative
  therapies.
Extended-angle pose, **217**
Eyebright, 356
Eyes
  allergies and, 340
  conjunctivitis in, 324, 340,
    355-356
  crossed, 82
  exercises for, 82, 83, 84
  farsighted, 82
  lazy, 82
  reflexology for, **174**
  sore, 310, 320
  styes and, 389-390
Eyestrain, **82**, **366**, 366-367
Eyewashes, 311, 324

Faith and belief, 21, 39, 93, 94
  in Native American medicine,
    38
  shamanism and, 34
Faith healing, 92, 94-99
  auras and, 99
  belief in, 94
  laying on of hands in, 94, 96,
    97, 98
  Reiki, 27, 99
  therapeutic touch in, 96-97
Families
  addiction and, 144
  genograms and, **137**
  in group therapy, 137
Fanning out, **159**
Farmers' markets, 257, **260**, **261**,
  262
Farsightedness, 82
Fascia, 154, 188, 189, **189**
Fasting, 81
Fatigue, 340

Fats, **241**, 245, 246, 247, 254,
  264, 265
  atherosclerosis and, 342
  avoiding of, 263
  calculating content in foods,
    263
  cancer and, 12, 352
  children and, 272
  as disease risk, 240
  food additives and, 257
  four food groups and, 244
  heart disease and, 242, 246,
    247
  high blood pressure and, 240,
    246
  LPL and, 266
  macrobiotics and, 271
  monitoring of, 247
  monounsaturated, 247
  polyunsaturated, 247
  saturated, 240, 246, 247, 268,
    269, 342
  See also Cholesterol.
Fatty acids, 246, 247
  omega-3, 250
F.D.A. *See* Food and Drug
  Administration, U.S.
Fears, 134
  yoga and, 214-216
  See also Phobias.
Feet
  gout and, 367
  pain in, 75, 336
  reflexology and. *See*
    Reflexology.
Feldenkrais, Moshe, 184-185,
  184, 186
Feldenkrais Method, 184-185
Fencing, Eastern, **224**
Fennel, 306, **306**
Fenugreek, 306
Ferguson, Tom, 24
Fever, 298, 299, 306, 314, 321,
  322, 327
Feverfew, 307, **307**
Fiber, 12, 240, **241**, 245, 252,
  257, 264, 352
  constipation and, 254, 356-
    357, **357**
  macrobiotics and, 271
  recommended amount of, 254
  role of, 254-255
  sources of, **25**, 247, 249, **249**,
    260, **281**
Fibrocystic breast disease, 13
Fibroid tumors, 381
Fight or flight response, 106-108
Finland, 209
Fire element, 164, 177
Fish, 247, 252, 253, 261-262
  cooking of, 263
  food poisoning and, 263
Fish oils, 250, 344
Fitzgerald, William, 170-171
Five Elements, **44**, 164-165, 167,
  177

Flatulence. _See_ Gas.
Flaxseed, 248
Flaxseed oil, 387
Flexibility training, 194, 197,
    199, 214
    martial arts and, 228
    yoga and, 214
Flinders, Carol, 254
Flotation tanks, 110, **111**
Flour, 248, **249**
Flowers
    aromatherapy and, 328-329
    See also Bach Flower Remedies.
Flu, 298, 299, 304, 311, 314, 315
Fluoride
    food sources of, 281
    main role of, 281
    in tap water, 283
Flying, fear of, 134, **134**
_F. Matthias Alexander: The Man
    and His Work_ (Westfeldt),
    183
Folic acid
    addiction and, 144
    food sources of, 279
    main role of, 279
    red blood cells and, **287**
    therapeutic uses of, 284, 285-
        286, 341, 368, 374, 382,
        384, 386, 387, 390
    vitamin B$_{12}$ and, 276
Folk medicine, 9, 13, 30
    definition of, 21
Food and Drug Administration,
    U.S. (F.D.A.), 255-256, 276
    herbs and, 292-293
Food Pharmacy, The (Carper), 253
Food poisoning, 263
Foods
    addiction to, 142
    additives in, 255-257, 262
    allergies to, 258, 339, 340, 346
    antibiotics in, 257
    artificial colors in, 254, 256,
        257
    calculating fat content of, 263
    for children, 272-273
    in Chinese medicine, 50
    cooking of, 260-263
    "designer," 248
    as disease prevention, 248-
        252, 253
    fiber in. _See_ Fiber.
    four groups of, 242-245
    fresh, 257
    frozen, 262
    hormones in, 257
    hospital, 15
    immune function and, 20
    labeling of, 262-263
    macrobiotics and, 270-271
    as medicine, 50
    natural, 12

    nitrites in, 257
    non-nutrient components of,
        254-257
    nutrient loss in, 263
    organically grown, 257, 262,
        263
    regulations on chemicals in,
        255-256
    sensitivities to, 258-259
    shopping for, 260-263
    storing of, 260-263
    variety and, 242, **252**, 257
    water and, 254
    waxed, 257
    whole vs. refined, 254
    yin and yang, 270, 271
    See also Nutrition.
Forceps, 13
Formula feeding of infants, 13,
    14
Four food groups, 242-245
Foxglove, 51
Fragrances, aromatherapy and,
    328-329
Framingham Heart Study, 242,
    242
Francis, Saint, 100
Frank, Jerome, 34
Fraud, health, 27
Free association, 133
Free radicals, 250
Freud, Sigmund, 127, **132**, 133,
    133
Freudian psychoanalysis, 132-
    133, 134, 135
Friction, in massage, 160, **162**
Fruits, 240, 243, 245, **252**, 254,
    257
    additives in, 262
    aromatherapy and, 328-329
    citrus, 248, 250, **252**
    nutrient loss in, 263
    shopping for, 261
Fuller, Betty, 187
Funakoshi, Gichin, 226
Functional Integration, 185
Fungal infections, 248
    athlete's foot, 346-347
Fungicides, 256, 257

Gaby, Alan R., 284
Gallbladder problems, 303, 314
    gallstones, 347, 367, **367**
Galloway, Elliott, 196
Galloway's Book on Running
    (Galloway), 196
Gallstones, 367, **367**
Galvanic skin response (GSR),
    115-116
Gambling, 142, 143, **144**
    self-help groups for, 146
Gangrene, 353

Garden, organic, **19**
Garlic, 13, 248, 249, **251**, 253,
    257, 307-308, **308**, 351,
    358, 364, 366
Garlic Festival, **251**
Gas (flatulence), 258, 297, 298,
    302, 308, 313, 319, 324,
    376.
    See also Carminatives.
Gastritis, 341
Gastrointestinal ulcer, 390
Gattefossé, René, 329
Gellert baths, **77**
Gelsemium, 355
Genetics, 247
    diabetes and, 244
    nutrition and, 240
Genograms, **137**
Gentian, 330
Geranium, 389
Germ theory of disease, 68, 248
Gestalt Therapy, 129, 140, 185,
    188
Gharote, M. L., 221
Ginger, 253, 308-309, **309**
Gingivitis, 317, 385
Ginkgo, 309, **309**
Ginseng, 310, **310**
Glucose, 245
God, 102
Godfrey, Bronwen, 254
Goldenseal, 310-311, **311**
Golden walnuts, **26**
Goleman, Daniel, 108
Golfer's elbow, 75
Gout, 299, 320, 343, 367-368
Graham, Sylvester, 248
Graham cracker, 248
Grains and cereals, 243, 247,
    248, **249**, 254-255, 260,
    261, 270, 271
Grapefruit, **252**
Graphite, 62, 364
Grasping the bird's tail, **232-233,
    235**
Greek medicine, 52, 94
Greeley, Horace, 61
Green, Elmer and Alyce, **117**
Grief, **125**
Group therapy, 136-137, **136**
    self-help groups vs., 148
Growth hormones, 257
GSR (galvanic skin response),
    115-116
Guided imagery, 91, 118. _See also_
    Visualization.
Gums
    bleeding, 302
    periodontal disease and, 385-
        386, **385**
    sore, 317
Gurin, Joel, 240
Gurrumurringu, **130**

H

Habits, breaking of
hypnotherapy for, 120, 122
See also Addiction.
Hahnemann, Samuel, 60, **60, 61, 62,** 63
Hair, 320
Halitosis, 349
Hamamelis, 391
Hamstring stretch, 203, **203,** 205
Hands
eczema of, 364
gout and, 367
pain in, 75
Hand-eye coordination, 82
Handicaps, creative therapies for, 139, **140**
Hand of Fatima, **26**
Hands of Light (Brennan), 99
Hangovers, 370
Hara, **165,** 165
Harmony, 42. *See also* Balance.
Harner, Michael, 35
Harvard Medical School, 11, 12
Hatha yoga, 104, 216
Hawthorn, 311
Hawthorne, Nathaniel, 61
Hay fever, 318, 339, 357, 368-369, **369**
HDLs (high-density lipoproteins), 247, 253, 343
Head
reflexology for, **174**
trauma to, 334, 359
Headache, 62, 330, 340, 369-371
acupressure for, **166,** 167
Alexander Technique for, 180
aromatherapy for, **329**
biofeedback for, 117
chiropractic for, 75, **75,** 371
electromyograph (EMG) for, 115
herbs for, 298, 300, 307, 314, 319, 320, 329, **329**
hypnotherapy for, 120
ice pack for, 208
massage for, **370,** 371
polarity therapy for, 178
reflexology for, 169
tension, 369
vascular, 369
See also Migraine.
Head and shoulder isolation, **201**
Head First, the Biology of Hope (Cousins), 29
Healing, 8, 11
Healing Relationship, The (Solfvin), 96

Health and Healing (Weil), 23, 92, 295
Health education, 29
Health history, keeping record of, 15
Hearing difficulties, 146
music therapy for, 139
Heart ailments, 311
Heart attack (acute myocardial infarction), 10, 242, 253, 305, 334, 371
garlic and, 249
onions and, **251**
relaxation and, 108
Heartburn, 376
Heart disease (coronary heart disease), 93, 108, **242,** 310, 341, 371-373, **371**
antioxidants and, 250, **279**
in China, **273**
dietary fat and, 242, 246, 247
lifestyle and, 28, 221
vegetarian diet and, 221, 246, 268
Heart (pulse) rate
heat treatments and, 208
target, 200
yoga and, 220
Heat, bodily effect of, 208-209
Heatstroke, 334
Heller, Joseph, 189
Hellerwork, 154, 189
Helplessness, 359
Hemoglobin levels, 97
Hemorrhage, 322
brain, 334
Hemorrhoids (piles), 312, 326, 356, 373, 391
Hepar sulphuris, 350, 358, 389
Hepatitis, 315, 316, 359, 373-374, **374**
Herbal remedies, 9, 12, 21, 27, 290-327
for arthritis, 298, 301, 307, 312, 313, 315, 316, 317, 318, 319, 323, 326, 327
for asthma, 304, 305, 309, 315
in Ayurvedic medicine, 56-57, 294
for bronchitis, 304, 306, 316, 324, 329, **329,** 351
in Chinese medicine, **43,** 49-51, **50,** 294
for colds, 297, 299, 301, 302, 304, 308, 311, 313, 314, 317, 321, 323, 326
for constipation, 298, 299, 300, 315, 316, 320, 321
for coughs, 297, 304, 313, 316, 323, 324
for diarrhea, 302, 312, 327
drugs vs., 290-292, 295
guide to using, 294
for headaches, 298, 300, 307, 314, 319, 320, 329, **329**
for high blood pressure, 308, 319

history of use of, 290-292
for insomnia, 300, 301, 312, 314, 319, 325
for migraine, 305, 307
modern-day, 292-293
myths about, 294
in Native American medicine, 37-38, 290
for nausea, 297, 302, 308, 319, 325
safety of, 12, 294
See also Aromatherapy; Bach Flower Remedies.
Herbicides, 256, 262
Herpes zoster, 388
Herrigel, Eugen, 104
High blood pressure (hypertension), 62, 342, 375-376, **375**
biofeedback for, 117, **375**
chiropractic for, 75
cupping for, **56**
dietary fat and, 240, 246
exercise and, 192
fish and, 253
flotation tanks and, 111
garlic and, **251**
herbs for, 308, 319
meditation and, 102, **335**
onions and, **251**
pregnancy and, 337
yoga for, 220
High-density lipoproteins (HDLs), 247, 253, 343
Hiking, 195, **198**
Hinduism, **52**
Hip circle, 205, **205**
Hippocrates, 12, 67, 156, 206
Hirohito, Emperor of Japan, 226
Histamines, 258
Hives, 339
HIV virus, 323
Hoarseness, 313, 317
Hobbies, 109
Hoffman, Ronald, 171
Holding the ball, **232, 235**
Holistic therapies, 9, 10, 94
Ayurvedic medicine as, 54-55
definition of, 21
homeopathy as, **60,** 61
self-care in, 10
Holly, 345
Holmes, Thomas H., 106
Homeopathy, 21, 60-65, **60, 61, 62, 64, 65,** 330, 334
for acne, 338
for allergies, 340
for arthritis, 344
for asthma, 345-346
for athlete's foot, 346

for back pain, 348
for bad breath, 349
for boils, 350
for bronchitis, 351
for circulatory problems, 354
for colds, 355
for conjunctivitis, 356
for constipation, 357
controversy over, 64-65
for coughs, 358
for cystitis, 359
for depression, 360
for diabetes, 362
for diarrhea, 363
for eczema, 364
for eyestrain, 366
for gallstones, 367
for gout, 368
for hay fever, 369, **369**
for headache, 371
for hemorrhoids, 373
for indigestion, 376
for insomnia, 377
for irritable bowel syndrome,
    378
for kidney stones, 379-380
"like cures like" principle in,
    60, **62,** 63, 64
for menopausal problems, 380
for menstrual problems, 381-
    382
for migraine, 383
orthodox medicine vs., 61, 62-
    64
for periodontal disease, 386
practitioners of, 65
for psoriasis, 386
recommendations for, 62-64,
    65
for sciatica, 387-388
for shingles, 388
for sore throat, 389
spread of, in 19th century, 61
for styes, 390
symptoms as seen in, 61, 62,
    64, 65, 334
for ulcers, 390
for varicose veins, 391
visiting a practitioner of, 62
Honey, 28, 245
Honeybee extract, 62
Hopelessness, 359
Hops, 312, 321
Hormone imbalance, 62
Hormone injections, in
    childbirth, 13
Hormones, 88, 90, 91, 246
    exercise and, 194
Horse chestnut, 312, **312,** 373
Hostility, 108-109
Hot tubs, 209
Howe, Elias, 128
Huang-di, Emperor of China, **42**

Humanistic therapies, 135
Humor, **14,** 15
Humors, Greek theory of, 52
Husk Faces, **128**
Huxley, Aldous, 84, 180
Huxley, Laura Archera, 84
Hydromassage, 209-210
Hydrotherapy (water therapy),
    21, **77, 78, 78,** 206-211, **206**
    for acne, 338
    for arthritis, 344, **344**
    for asthma, 346
    for athlete's foot, 346
    for back pain, 348
    bathing, 109, 209
    for bronchitis, 351
    for chronic pain, 385
    for circulatory problems, 354
    for colds, 355
    for constipation, 357
    for coughs, 358
    for cystitis, 359
    for dermatitis, 361
    for diarrhea, 363
    for emphysema, 366
    exercise, **208, 209,** 210-211
    for gout, 368
    for hay fever, 369
    for headache, 371
    heat and cold in, 208-209
    for hemorrhoids, 373
    for indigestion, 376
    for insomnia, 377, **377**
    for kidney stones, 380
    massage, **206,** 209-210
    for menstrual problems, 382
    for migraine, 383
    mineral springs, 206, 210, 212
    for physical rehabilitation,
        210, **210**
    for psoriasis, 386
    relaxation from, 209-210
    for sciatica, 388
    steam treatments, 57, **80**
    thalassotherapy, 206-208
    Turkish baths, **207,** 209
    for varicose veins, 391
Hyperopia, 82
Hypertension. *See* High blood
    pressure.
Hyperthyroidism, 359
Hypnosis, hypnotherapy, 14, **22,**
    27, 120-125, 334
    for allergies, 120, 125, 340
    appeal of, 120
    for arthritis, 122, 344
    for asthma, 120, 346
    autogenic training, 123-125
    best subjects for, 121
    for breaking habits, 120, 122
    for cancer, 353
    for children, **125**
    for chronic ailments, 120, 385
    for depression, 125
    for dermatitis, **360,** 361
    for eczema, 120, 364

eye rolling and, 121
fears about, 121-122
for headache, 120
for insomnia, 377
for irritable bowel syndrome,
    378-379
for migraine, 125
for overeating, 120, 122, 125
for pain, **22,** 120, 122, 385
for phobias, 120
post-hypnotic suggestions and,
    121-122
for psoriasis, 387
recalling suppressed
    experiences with, 121
for relaxation, 122
self-, 91, 122-125, **122**
for shingles, 388
for smoking, 120, 122, 125
for stress, **22,** 120, 122, 123,
    125
for surgery, 124
for ulcers, 390
for warts, 120
what to expect from, 121
Hypothyroidism, 356, 359
Hyssop, 313, **313**
Hysteria, 321

Ice packs, 208
Ignatia, 360, 377
Imagery. *See* Visualization.
Imagined illness, 93
Immune system, immunity, 10,
    340
    balance and, 20
    colostrum and, 14
    diabetes and, 361
    herbs for, 303, 307, 308
    memory of, 91
    mind-body connection and,
        88-91
    mystery of, 88-91
    as network, 88
    nutrients and, 276
    placebo response and, 93
    stress and, 106
    support groups and, 148-149
    visualization and, 118
    yogurt and, 253
Immunization, 10-11
Immunoglobulin E, 258
Immunotherapy, 339
Impatiens, 340, 376, 386

Incest victims, 146
India, 170, 222
Indian (American) medicine. *See* Native American medicine.
Indian (Eastern) medicine. *See* Ayurvedic medicine; Meditation; Yoga.
Indigestion, 69, 178, 376-377
  balance and, 18-20
  See also Digestive aids.
Indoles, 248
Indonesia, healing ceremony in, **33**
Infants. *See* Babies.
Infectious diseases, 10-11, 62, 359
  osteopathy for, 69-70
Inflammation, 209, 312, 315, 319, 323, 327
Inflammatory bowel disease, 341
Influenza. *See* Flu.
Ingham, Eunice, 171
Inner thigh stretch, 205, **205**
Inositol, 378
Insect repellents, 300, 307, 310
Insect stings and bites, 299, 303, 307, 320
Insect vacuums, **256**
Insight program, 135
Insomnia, 22, 330, 377-378, **377**
  biofeedback for, 117
  exercise for, 194
  herbs for, 300, 301, 312, 314, 319, 325
  sugar for, 253
  yoga for, 218-220
  See also Sedatives.
Insulin, 361
Intestinal problems, 70
  cramps, 312
  worms, 298, 308
  yogurt and, **250**
  See also Colon.
Iodine, 280
Ipecacuanha, 376
Iridology, 82, 83-85, **85**
  orthodox medicine vs., 85
Iris (flower), 383
Iris (in eye), 83, 84-85, **85**
Iron, 284
  anemia and, 264, 283, 341
  food sources of, 280
  macrobiotics and, 271
  main role of, 280
  therapeutic uses of, 283, 287, 351, 382
  vitamin C and, 276, 277, **281**
Iron palm training, 225
Iroquois, **128**
Irritability, 314, 377. *See also* Nervousness.

Irritable bowel syndrome (irritable colon), 340, 356, 378-379
Isolation tanks, 110-111
Israelites, 94
Italian foods, **273**
Itching, 167, 304, **360**

Jacobson, Michael F., 257
James, William, 61
Janov, Arthur, 150
Japan, 101-102, 164, 170, 209, 222
Jenner, Edward, **62**
Jensen, Bernard, 84-85
Jesus, 94
Job's Body: A Handbook for Bodywork (Juhan), 179
Jogging and running, **193**, 195, 196, 199
Joint problems, 56, 157, 220, 309
  from gout, 367
  See also Arthritis.
Journal of the American Medical Association, 310
Journal writing, 138, 141
Judaism, 101
Judo, 222, 223, **225**, 227, 228, 229, 230
Juhan, Deane, 179
Juice fasts, 81
Jung, Carl, **103**
Juniper, 313, **313**, 329

Kalachakra mandala, **58, 59**
Kali bichromate, 338, 351, 358
Kali phos, 349
Kapha, 52-54, 55, 56
Karate, 222, 223, **223**, 225-227, 228, 230
  myths about, 226
Katas, 226-227
Kellogg, John, **76**, 78
Kellogg, Will, **76**, 78
Kendo, **224**
Kidney problems, 299, 303, 337, 341, 347
  gout and, 367
  reflexology for, **175**
  stones, 169, 379-380
Kings, divine attributes of, 94
Kirlian photographs, **99**
Kluckhohn, Clyde, 39

Knee problems, 69
  gout, 367
Knee-up pose, **218**
Kneipp, Sebastian, 78
Koans, 100
Korea, 222
Krieger, Dolores, 96, 97, **97**
Kung fu, **222**, 224-225, **226**, 228, 230
Kushi, Michio, 271

Lachesis, 350, 380
Lactic acid, 102
Lactose intolerance, 258-259
Lambrou, Peter T., 123
Lao-tze, 231
Lappé, Frances Moore, 268
Larch, 345
Lard, 245
Larynx, cancer of, 352
Laughter therapists, 15
Laurel's Kitchen (Robertson, Flinders, and Godfrey), 254
Lavender, 313-314, **314**, 329, 344, 350
Lawlis, G. Frank, 34-35
Laxatives, 299, 300, 303, 306, 307, 320, 322
  in Ayurveda, 57
  chronic use of, 356
Laying on of hands, 94, 96, 97, 98. *See also* Faith healing.
Lazy eye, 82
LDLs (low-density lipoproteins), 247, 250
Learning disorders, 138
LeBerge, Stephen, 129
Lecithin, 373, 376
Left heel kick, **237**
Leg, broken, 211
Leg exercises, 203, **203, 204**, 205, **205**
Leg pain, 75, 312
  from sciatica, 387
Leg to Stand On, A (Sacks), 211
Legumes, 247
Leighton, Dorothea, 39
Lemon balm, 314, **314**
Lemon oil, 366, 389
Leprosy, 299
LeShan, Lawrence, 102
Leukemia, 341
Licensing requirements, 334-336
Licorice, 248, 315, **315**
Lie detection tests, 115
Lifestyle, 221
  heart disease and, 28, 221
  naturopathy and, 76, 80
  polarity therapy and, 176
Lifting objects, **182**
Lillard, Harvey, 72

Lilly, John C., 110
Ling, Per Henrik, 156
Lipoprotein lipase (LPL), 266
Lipoproteins
   high-density (HDLs), 247, 253,
      343
   low-density (LDLs), 247, 250
Lips, chapped, 322-323
Liver, 297
   cleansers for, 177-178, 310
   gallstones and, 367
   tonic for, 316
Liver disorders, 70, 303, 314, 324
   hepatitis, 373-374
Ljungdahl, Lars, **14**
Lobster, **258**
Lockhart, Maureen, 221
Loneliness, 359
Longevity, 240, 310
Longfellow, Henry Wadsworth,
   61
Louis IX, King of France, 94
Lourdes, **95**
Love, Medicine, and Miracles
   (Siegel), 18
Low-density lipoproteins (LDLs),
   247, 250
Lowen, Alexander, 187
Lower back releaser, **202**, 203
LPL (lipoprotein lipase), 266
Lungs
   abscess of, 357
   cancer of, 12-13, 250, 352,
      357
   reflexology for, **174**
   See also Respiratory conditions.
Lupus, 148
Lust, Benedict, 78
Lycopodium, 357, 380, 390
Lymph, 69-70
Lymphatic swelling, 79

Macrobiotics, 270-271
Macronutrients, 245
Magnesia phosphorica, 379-380,
   382, 388
Magnesium
   addiction and, 144
   calcium and, 276
   food sources of, 280
   main role of, 280
   therapeutic uses of, 287, 346,
      348, 351, 354, 360, 366,
      371, 373, 376, 378, 379,
      380, 382, 383, 384

Magnesium aspartate, 357
Magnetism theory, 120
Magritte, René, **126**
Maharishi Mahesh Yogi, **101**,
   104
Ma huang (ephedrine), 51, 315-
   316
Malaria, 60, **62**, 298
Mandalas, **58-59**, 103
Manic-depressive illness, 359
Manganese, 346, 348, 384
   food sources of, 281
   main role of, 281
Manley, Elizabeth, 119, **119**
Mantras, 104, 109, **117**
Marathon runners, **265**
Margarine, 247
Marigold, 62, 344
Marital therapy, 137
Marshmallow, 316, **316**
Martial arts, 222-229, **222-229**
   aikido, 223, **227**, 228, 231
   health benefits of, 228
   judo, 222, 223, **225**, 227, 228,
      229
   karate. *See* Karate.
   kendo, **224**
   kung fu, **222**, 224-225, **226**,
      228, 230
   roots of, 222-223
   spiritual dimensions of, 229
   tae kwon do, 226
   t'ai chi chuan. *See* T'ai chi
      chuan.
   variety of styles in, 223
Martin, Gina, 167
Massage, 13, 96, **155**, 156-163,
   334, 336
   acupressure. *See* Acupressure.
   for arthritis, 344, **344**
   for asthma, 346
   in Ayurvedic medicine, **55**, 57
   for babies, **156**
   of back, **158-163**
   for back pain, 348
   choosing a therapist for, 161-
      163
   for colds, 355
   conditions requiring
      physician's approval before
      having, 163
   for constipation, 357
   for depression, 360
   for diverticulitis, 364
   Eastern vs. Western forms of,
      156
   effects of, 157
   effleurage in, 158-160, **159**,
      161
   fanning out in, **159**
   friction in, 160, **162**
   for headache, **370**, 371
   for high blood pressure, 375
   for insomnia, 377

for menstrual problems, 382
   misconceptions about, 157
   for older people, **157**
   petrissage in, 160, **160**
   Polarity therapy. *See* Polarity
      therapy.
   pressure-point, 164-167
   reflexology. *See* Reflexology.
   rolling stroke in, **161**
   for sciatica, 388
   self-, 157, 167
   shiatsu. *See* Shiatsu.
   stretching back muscles in, **163**
   Swedish, 156
   Swedish, basic techniques of,
      158-163
   tapotement in, 160-161, **163**
   thumb circles in, **162**
   vibration in, 161
   water, **206**, 209-210
   what to expect from session of,
      157-158
   yoga and, 218
   See also Bodywork; Deep-tissue
      therapies.
McCollum, Elmer, **274**
Meat-free diet. *See* Vegetarian
   diet.
Meats, 12, 240, 245, 247, 261,
   262
   cooking of, 263
   as food group, 243
   food poisoning and, 263
   nitrites in, 257
   Select grade of, 242, 261
Medical establishment. *See*
   Orthodox medicine.
Medical help, when to seek, 334
Medical school curriculum, 11,
   12
Medical Self-Care, 24
Medicine bundle, 36
Medicine men, 30, 36, **36**, 38,
   39, 94. *See also* Shamans.
Meditation, 56, **58**, 91, 100-104,
   111, **117, 335**
   ancient roots of, 100-102
   autogenics and, 124-125
   benefits of, 102
   forms of, 101
   four paths to, 102-104
   Relaxation Response and, 109
   tips for, 102
   Transcendental, **101**, 104, 109
   yoga and, 214-216, **214**, 221
Memory loss, 309
Menopausal problems, 380, 383
Menstrual cramps, 298, 300,
   301, 307, 314
   acupressure for, **166, 381**
   TENS therapy for, 81

Menstrual problems, 75, 381-382
  PMS, 305, 381, 382
  See also Menstrual cramps.
Menstruation, anemia and, 341
Mental control, 101
Mental disability, 140
Mental illnesses, 8, 359
Mental imagery. *See* Visualization.
Mentastics, 187
Mercurius, 386
Mercurius solubilis, 349, 386
Mercury, **60**
Meridians (zones), **45,** 46, 49, 164, 167
  massage and, 156, 164, 165
  purposes of, 44
  reflexology and, 170
  t'ai chi and, 227
  tongue examination and, 45
  tsubos (acupuncture points) and, **45,** 164, **164,** 165
Mesmer, Franz, 120
Metabolic diseases, 8
Metabolism, 265-266, 267
  diabetes and, 361
  exercise and, **267**
Metal element, 164, 167
Mezereum, 388
Michigan, University of, **134**
Micronutrients, 245
Migraine, 22, 81, 382-383
  acupuncture for, **382,** 383
  chiropractic for, 75, **75,** 383
  herbs for, 305, 307
  hypnotherapy for, 125
  lactose intolerance and, 258
  massage for, 157
  osteopathy for, 69
  reflexology for, 169
  yoga for, 218-220
Milk, 247, 260
  allergy to, **258**
  inability to digest, 258-259
Milk thistle, 316-317
Miller, Don Ethan, 229
Mimulus, 340, 345
Mind, 55, 61
  balance of body and, 20-21
  power of, 14-15
Mind-body connection, 14, 15, 88-93
  and beliefs and expectations, 93
  immune system and, 88-91
  placebo response and, 91-93
  warts and, 92, 93
Minerals, 245, 260, 264, 274-281
  addiction and, 144
  chart of, 280-281
  food preparation and, 263
  macro-, 280
  megadoses of, 282

  supplements of, 250-252, 274-278, 282, 337
  trace elements, 245, 274, 276, 280-281
  See also Mineral therapy; *specific minerals.*
Mineral springs, 206, 210, 212
Mineral therapy, 13, 282-287
  for acne, 339
  for allergies, 340
  for anemia, 341
  for arthritis, 344
  for asthma, 346
  for back pain, 348
  for bad breath, 349
  for boils, 350
  for bronchitis, 351
  for cancer, 353
  for circulatory problems, 354
  for colds, 355
  for conjunctivitis, 356
  for constipation, 357
  for coughs, 358
  for dermatitis, 361
  for diabetes, 362
  for diarrhea, 363
  for diverticulitis, 364
  for eczema, 365
  for emphysema, 366
  for eyestrain, 367
  for gallstones, 367
  for gout, 368
  for hay fever, 369
  for headache, 371
  for heart disease, 373
  for hemorrhoids, 373
  for high blood pressure, 376
  for insomnia, 378
  for irritable bowel syndrome, 379
  for kidney stones, 380
  for menopausal problems, 380
  for menstrual problems, 382
  for migraine, 383
  for osteoporosis, 384
  for periodontal disease, 386
  for psoriasis, 387
  for shingles, 388
  for sore throat, 389
  for styes, 390
  for ulcers, 390
  for varicose veins, 391
Miracles, **95**
Moderation, 42
Modern medicine. *See* Orthodox medicine.
Molasses, 245, 357
Molecular messengers, 88-90, **88, 89**
Molybdenum, 281
Monounsaturated fat, 247
Moran, Victoria, 79

Moreno, J. L., 137
Mormon tea, 316
Mosquito repellent, 317
Mothner, Ira, 240
Motion sickness, 253, 309
Mount Barrille, **107**
Mouth
  cancer of, 352
  sores in, 310, 311
Movement re-education. *See* Alexander Technique.
Moxa cones, **49**
Mucilage, 306, 315, 316, 320, 323
Mucous membranes, 304, 317
Mucus, 54, 299, 315, 340
Mud, 212, **212**
Mullein, 79, 317, **317**
Multiple personality disorder, 90
Multiple sclerosis, 359
Muscle pain, 209, 304, 312, 319, 324, 326, 329
  cupping for, **56**
  polarity therapy for, 178
Muscles, 325
  massage and, 157
  sore. *See* Muscle pain.
  spasms and tension in, 208, 321
Muscular strength and endurance exercises, 194, 195-196, 198-199
  yoga as, 214
Musculoskeletal problems, osteopathy and, 66, 68, 69, 70, 71
Music therapy, 138, 139, **140**
Mustard, 330-331, 345
Myopia, 82
Myrrh, 317-318

Nail-biting, 120
Nancy Clark's Sports Nutrition Guidebook (Clark), 266
Nasal purging, 10, 57
National Cancer Institute, 30, 248, 254, 257
National Center for Health Statistics, 267
Native American medicine, 30, 36-41
  herbs in, 37-38, 290
  medicine men and shamans in, 36
  power animals in, 33
  rituals in, **37,** 38, 39
  sand painting in, **37,** 38
  Sioux ceremony for veterans, 40-41
  sweat lodges in, **41, 57,** 209, **213**
Natrum muriaticum, 355, 383

Natural childbirth, 13, 14
"Natural Doc, The" (Moran), 79
Natural Health, Natural Medicine
(Weil), 145
Natural medicine, 8-15
balance and, 23
body's healing power and, 8,
11, 15, 18-20
choosing of, 26-27
as complement to orthodox
medicine, 9, 10, 15, 21-22
definition of, 21
innovation vs. quack cures in,
27-28
interest in, 8-9, 10, 13
listening to body and, 21
mind-body balance in, 20-21
orthodox medicine contrasted
with, 11, 18-20
and overuse of drugs and
technology, 8, 11, 12, 22-24,
25-26
prevention in, 13, 28
self-care in, 10, 15, 24
See also specific therapies.
Natural products, consumer
interest in, 12
Naturopathy, 21, **64,** 76-81
for acne, 338
for allergies, 340
for anemia, 341
for arteriosclerosis, 342-343
for arthritis, 344
for asthma, 346
for athlete's foot, 346
for boils, 350
for bronchitis, 351
for cancer, 353
for chronic pain, 385
for circulatory problems, 354
for colds, 355
for constipation, 357
for coughs, 358
for cystitis, 359
for depression, 360
for dermatitis, 361
development of, 78
for diabetes, 362
for diarrhea, 363
for diverticulitis, 364
for eczema, 365
for emphysema, 366
for gallstones, 367
for gout, 368
for hay fever, 369
for headache, 371
for hemorrhoids, 373
for hepatitis, 374
for high blood pressure, 375-
376
hydrotherapy in, **77, 78, 80**

for indigestion, 376
for insomnia, 378
iridology and, 83
for irritable bowel syndrome,
379
for kidney stones, 380
for menopausal problems, 380
for menstrual problems, 382
for migraine, 383
orthodox medicine vs., 76
for osteoporosis, 384
for psoriasis, 387
steam treatments in, **80**
for styes, 390
teaching healthy living in, 80
TENS therapy in, 81
toxins and, 80
for ulcers, 390
Nausea, 376
acupressure for, **166**
herbs for, 297, 302, 308, 319,
325
motion sickness, 253, 309
See also Indigestion.
Navaho, The (Kluckhohn and
Leighton), 39
Nearsightedness, 82
Neck, reflexology for, **174**
Neck pain
Alexander Technique for, 180
chiropractic for, **75**
electromyograph (EMG) for,
115
massage for, 157
relaxation and, 108
Neck vertebrae, 75, **75**
Nelson, Randy F., 229
Nerve pain (neuralgia), 298, 319
from sciatica, 387-388
from shingles, 388
Nervousness, 300, 312, 314, 319,
321. *See also* Anxiety; Stress.
Nervous system, 315, 319, 320,
325, 340
chiropractic and, 75
Nesse, Randolph, **134**
Nettle, 318, **318**
Neuralgia. *See* Nerve pain.
Neural pathways, 88
Neurochemicals, 142
Neurological conditions, 359
Neuromusculoskeletal system,
osteopathy and, 66, 68, 69,
70, 71
Neurosis, 150
New Age movement, **34**
New England Journal of Medicine,
15
*New Holistic Health Handbook,
The,* 83
New York City Marathon, **264**
Niacin (vitamin B$_3$)
cholesterol and, 13
food sources of, 278
main role of, 278
therapeutic uses of, 283, 284,
354, 362, 383

Niacinamide, 344
Nicotine, **143**
Nitrites, 257
Noodles, **269, 273**
Norman, Laura, 171
Nose
bleeding from, 208
congestion in, 329, 340
Numbness, 334
Nursing, 13-14
Nursing mothers, 297
Nutrients, 245, 264
balance of, 277
partnerships of, 276
See also Carbohydrates; Fats;
Minerals; Protein; Vitamins.
Nutrition, 240-247
antioxidants and, 250
carbohydrate-based diet and,
245-247
disease prevention and, 12-13,
248-252, 253
folk cures and, 248-250
four food groups and, 242-245
in polarity therapy, 177-178
sports and, 264-265
switching food-consumption
patterns and, 240
U.S. government policy on,
240, 243
variety of foods and, 242, **252,**
257
See also Diet, dieting; Foods;
Nutrients.
Nuts, 255
Nux vomica, 340, 357, 371, 373,
376, 377, 390

Oat bran, 255
Obesity, 28, 62, 194, 244, 264,
342
metabolism and, 265-266
Obstetrical practices, 13-14
Office, relaxation exercises for,
112-113
Oils, 245, 246, 247, 328-329,
329. *See also* Fats.
Ojibway Indians, **128**
Okinawe-te, 226
Older people. *See* Elderly.
Olive oil, 329
Omega-3 fatty acids, 250
Onions, 62, **251,** 253, 257
Ophidiophobia, **134**
Ophthalmologists, 82
Optometrists, 82
Oranges, **252**
Organic produce, 257, 262, 263
Organon of Medicine
(Hahnemann), 63

Orgone, **133**
Orgone box, **133**
Ornish, Dean, 221, 246
Ornstein, Robert, 100
Orr, Leonard, 151
Orthodox medicine
  achievements of, 10-11
  as body-focused, 10, 14, 15
  consumers' movement and,
    12, 14
  cost crisis in, 11, 14, 15
  dangers of, 11-12, 14, 15
  definition of, 21
  as disease-focused, 11
  emergencies and, 10, 11, 12,
    21-22, 62, 334
  eye examination in, 85
  homeopathy vs., 61, 62-64
  interest in alternatives to, 8-9,
    10, 13
  iridology vs., 85
  learning when and when not
    to use, 15
  limitations of, 8
  medical school curriculum
    and, 11, 12
  mind ignored in, 14, 15
  natural medicine as
    complement to, 9, 10, 15,
    21-22
  natural medicine contrasted
    with, 11, 18-20
  natural medicine dismissed by,
    14, 26-27
  naturopathy vs., 76
  osteopathy vs., 27, 67-68
  overuse of drugs and
    technology in, 8, 11-12, 13,
    15, 22-24, 25-26
  specialization in, 22-24
  as "traditional" medicine, 9
Osteoarthritis (degenerative joint
  disease), 340, 343, 344
Osteopathy, 66-71, 334, 337
  for allergies, 340
  for asthma, 346
  for back pain, 9-10, **68**, 69,
    348
  body's healing ability and, 66,
    67
  cranial, 70-71
  founding of, 67
  for headache, 371
  for hemorrhoids, 373
  for migraine, 383
  modern-day, 67-68
  orthodox medicine vs., 27, 67-
    68
  physical exam in, 69, **69**
  practitioner's hands as tools in,
    67
  treatment methods of, 68, **71**
  and wear and tear on body, 71
  what to expect from, 68-69

Osteoporosis, 194, 264, 283, **286,**
  383-384, **384**
Overeaters Anonymous, 149
Overeating, compulsive, 146,
  149
  hypnotherapy for, 120, 122,
    125
Overlook Martial Arts Reader, The
  (Nelson, ed.), 229
Overweight
  in children, **267**
  See also Obesity.

Pain, 334
  abdominal, 334, 376
  acupuncture for, 47, 48, 348,
    385
  Alexander Technique for, 182,
    348
  back. *See* Back pain.
  biofeedback for, 116
  chest, 334
  of childbirth, 298
  chronic, 359, 384-385
  in feet, 336
  headache. *See* Headache;
    Migraine.
  hydrotherapy for, 348, 385
  hypnotherapy for, **22,** 120,
    122, 385
  leg, 312, 387
  menstrual. *See* Menstrual
    cramps.
  as message, 29
  muscle. *See* Muscle pain.
  naturopathy for, 385
  neck. *See* Neck pain.
  nerve, 319
  osteopathy for, 71
  polarity therapy for, 178
  referred, 70
  shamanistic methods for,
    34-35
  shiatsu for, 348, 385
  stomach, 306, 309, 313. *See
    also* Stomach ailments.
  toothache, 301, 303, 312, 324,
    327
  visualization for, 119
  yoga for, 348, 385
Pain relievers, 305, 307
  overuse of, 29
  wintergreen, 326
Painting, 138, **138, 139, 140**
Palm and palm kernel oils, 247
Palmer, Bartlett Joshua, **72**
Palmer, Daniel David, 72, **72,** 74
Palming, 118
Panchakarma, 57
Pancreas, 361
Panos, Maesimund, **64, 65**

Pantothenic acid (vitamin B₅),
  346, 369
  addiction and, 144
  food sources of, 279
  main role of, 279
  therapeutic uses of, 284
Paraplegics, **226**
Parsley, 248
Parting the horse's mane, **232**
Partner stretches, 205, **205**
Passiflora, 377
Passion flower, 318-319, **319**
Pasta, 240, 245, 247
Pasteur, Louis, 248-249, 307
Pastoral counselors, certified, 135
Patanjali, 214
Pauling, Linus, 282, **283**
Peaches, **252**
Peanuts, **258**
Peas, dried, 255
Peczely, Ignatz von, 84
Pelvic infection, 381
Pelvic tilt, 378, **378**
Pelvis, Polarity Squat exercise for,
  178
Penicillin, 253
Peppermint, 319, 324, 349, 391
Peppers, **249**
Peptic ulcer, 62, 390
Periodontal disease, 385-386,
  385
Periodontitis, 385-386
Peripheral vision, 82
Peritonitis, 363
Perls, Fritz, 188
Personality, 334
Perspiration
  excessive, 115, 116
  See also Sweating, therapeutic.
Persuasion and Healing (Frank),
  34
Peruvian bark, 60
Pesticides, **25,** 255, 256, **256,**
  257, 262, 263
Petersfield Physic Garden, **291**
Petrissage, 160, **160**
Pharynx, cancer of, 352
Phlebitis, 353
Phobias, 134, **134,** 135
  electrodermal response (EDR)
    for, 115
  hypnotherapy for, 120
Phosphorus
  food sources of, 280
  main role of, 280
  therapeutic uses of, 346, 348,
    358, 362, 386
Physician's tomb of Ankhmahor,
  154
Phytochemicals, 248, **252,** 254,
  257
Phytolacca, 389
Pierson, Herbert, 257
Piles. *See* Hemorrhoids.

Pima Indians, 244, **245**
Pimples, 338
Pine, 329, 351, 386
Pink eye (conjunctivitis), 324, 340, 355-356
Pitta, 52, 54, 55, 56
Pituitary, **175**
Pizza, **269**
Placebo response, 91-93
  acupuncture and, 48
  homeopathy and, 64
  shamanism and, 34
Plantar warts, 92
Plants, 11, 12, 30, 290
  aromatherapy and, 328-329
  isolating active principles of, 295
  See also Flowers; Herbal medicine.
Platina, 357
Plotkin, Mark, **293**
Plumbum, 357
Plums, **252**
Pneumonia, 10, 334, 357
PNI (psychoneuroimmunology), 88, 90, 91
Poisoning, 334
Poisons
  immune system and, 88
  See also Toxins.
Polarity therapy, 154, **176**, 176-178, **177**
  aim of, 177
  balance of elements in, 177
  cliffhanger exercise in, **178**
  counseling in, 177-178
  diet in, 177-178
  exercise in, 177-178
  squat exercise in, **178**
  typical session of, 177
  yoga in, 178
Polio, 10-11
Pollens, 368
  birch, **369**
Polyunsaturated fat, 247
Pomeranz, Bruce, 47
Positive attitude, 21
  polarity therapy and, 176, 178
Post, C. W., **76**, 78
Postley, John, 259
Posture, 154
  Alexander Technique and, 154, 181-182, **181**
  osteopathy and, 71
Potassium, 303, 363, 371, 376
  food sources of, 280
  main role of, 280
Potatoes, 245, **281**
Poultry, 247, 261, 262
  cooking of, 263
  food poisoning and, 263
Power animals, 33
Prana. *See* Energy, life.
Prayer, 94, 95

Pregnancy, 62, 313, 321, 322, 324, 325, 327, 337, 353
  anemia and, 341
  diabetes and, 361
  heat therapies and, 208
  high blood pressure and, 375
  varicose veins and, 391
  vitamin and mineral supplements and, 282, 284
  water exercise and, **208**, 210
Premenstrual syndrome (PMS), 305, 381, 382
Preservatives, 254, 256, 257
Pressure-point massage, 164-167. *See also* Acupressure; Polarity therapy; Reflexology; Shiatsu.
Prevention, 42
Priests, 94
Primal Prescription (Willoughby), 244
Primal therapy, 150
Procrastination, 56
Prostate cancer, 12
Prostate problems, 321
Protein, 245, 254, 264, 265, 268-269
  complementary, 268, 269
Psoriasis, **28**, 386-387
Psychiatric problems
  dance therapy for, 140
Psychiatrists, 135
Psychoanalysis, Freudian, 132-133, 134, 135
Psychoanalysts, 135
Psychodrama, 137, 140
  for addiction, 144
Psychologists, clinical, 135
Psychoneuroimmunology (PNI), 88, 90, 91, 331
Psychosomatic conditions, 8, 108
Psychotherapy, 101, 132-135, 140
  behavior, 133-134
  in Bioenergetics, 187
  choosing a therapist for, 132, 135
  cognitive, 134-135
  creative, 138-141
  group, 136-137, **136**
  humanistic, 135
  psychodynamic, 132-133, 134, 135
  reasons for choosing, 132
  in Rubenfeld Synergy, 185
Psyllium, 320, 357
Pulmonary conditions, 309
Pulsatilla, 344, 351, 356, 358, 360, 369, 373, 376, 381, 383, 390, 391
Pulse
  diagnosis from, 45, **47**, 54, 56
  See also Heart rate.
Pumpkin seeds, 255
Pure Food and Drugs Act, 27
Pyridoxine. *See* Vitamin B₆.

Qi. *See* Energy, life.
Qi dong, 51
Qinghao, 51
Quackery, 12, 27
Quinine, 60

Racketball, 195
Radiation damage, 310
Rahe, Richard H., 106
Ranunculus bulbosus, 388
Rapid eye movement (REM) sleep, 127
Rattles, 36, **36**, 38
Rausch, Victor, 124
Raynaud's disease, 115
Rebirthing, **150**, 151, **151**
Recommended Dietary Allowances (RDAs), 264, 276, 282
Reconstructive surgery, 10
Rectal cancer, 268
Red blood cells, **287**
Referrals, to natural medicine practitioners, 334-336
Reflexology, 154, **154**, 168-175, **168-175**, 334
  for arthritis, 344
  for asthma, 346
  for back pain, 348
  breeze stroke in, **175**
  for bronchitis, 351
  for circulatory problems, 354
  for cystitis, 359
  for diabetes, 362
  doing it yourself, 173-174
  Eastern origins of, 170
  for eczema, 365
  for emphysema, 366
  for eyestrain, 366
  for gallstones, 367
  for gout, 368
  for headache, 371
  for hepatitis, 374
  for high blood pressure, 376
  for indigestion, 376-377
  for menstrual problems, 382
  for migraine, 383
  for psoriasis, 387
  relaxation sequence in, **168-169**
  for sciatica, 388
  seven basic techniques in, **172**
  for sore throat, 389
  theories on, 171

thumb-walking technique in, **172, 173**
for varicose veins, 391
Western practice of, 170-171
what to expect from session in, 171-173
Reich, Wilhelm, **133**, 187
Reiki, 27, 99
Relaxation, 56, 97, 106-113, 118, 119, **391**
autogenic training for, 123-124
biofeedback and, 114, 115
brain waves and, 117
electromyograph (EMG) and, 115
hypnotherapy for, 122
managing stress with, 108-109
martial arts and, 228
reflexology and, 168, **168-169**
tanks for, 110-111
tips for, 102
water therapy and, 209-210
workplace exercises for, 112-113
See also Meditation; Stress.
Relaxation Response, 109
Religious beliefs, 94, 95, 101. *See also* Faith and belief.
REM (rapid eye movement) sleep, 127, **127**, 128
Rescue Remedy, 331, 340, 386
Resentment, 108-109
Respiratory conditions, 69, 313, 319, 340. *See also* Asthma; Bronchitis; Colds; Emphysema.
Respiratory system, 345
Rest position, **204**
Restricted Environmental Stimulation Therapy (REST), 110
Rheumatic fever, 337
Rheumatism, **212, 213**
Rheumatoid arthritis, 298, 299, 307, 340, 343, 344
Rhinitis, allergic or seasonal (hay fever), 318, 368-369, **369**
Rhus toxicodendron, 344, 348, 388
Rhus ven, 364
Riboflavin. *See* Vitamin B₂.
Rice, **269, 273**
Rickets, 306
Right heel kick, **237**
Rippe, James, 192
Rituals, 39, 94
Road racing, **193**
Robertson, Laurel, 254
Rockefeller, John D., 61
Rodgers, Bill, 157

Role-playing, 140
Rolf, Ida P., 188, **188**
Rolfing (Structural Integration), 26, 154, 188-189, **189**
Rolf Institute, 189
Roll down, **201**
Rolling stroke, **161**
Roman baths, 206
Roosevelt family, genogram of, **137**
Rosemary, 320, **320**, 329, 344, 391
Rosen, Marion, 185, 187, **187**
Rosen Method, 184, 185-187, **187**
Rubenfeld, Ilana, 185, **185**
Rubenfeld Synergy, 184, 185, **185**
Rumex crispus, 358
Running and jogging, **193**, 195, 196, 199
Russian bath, 209
Ruta, 344

Sabadilla, 340
Saccharin, 256
Sacks, Oliver, 211
Sadness, 178. *See also* Depression.
Sage, 320-321, **321**
St. John's wort, 323, **323**
Salicin, 37
Saline, 10
Salmonella bacteria, 263
Salt, 254, 255
Saltman, Paul, 240
Sand, 212, **213**
Sandalwood, 351, 389
Sand mandalas, **58-59**
Sand painting rituals, **37**, 38
Sanguinaria, 383
Sarsaparilla, 359
Saturated fat, 240, 246, 247, 268, 269, 342
Saunas, 209
Saw palmetto, 321
Scams, health-care, 27
Scents, aromatherapy and, 328-329
Schizophrenia, creative therapies for, 138, 139
Schultz, Johannes, 124
Sciatica, 75, 81, 157, 326, 387-388, **387**
Science, 8, 12
Scientific medicine. *See* Orthodox medicine.
Scopolamine, 13
Scullcap, 321-322, **321**
Sculpture, 138, **138**
Scurvy, **275**
Seafood poisoning, 308

Seated forward bend, **219**
Seborrheic dermatitis, 360
Sebum, 338
Sedatives, 298, 301, 305, 311, 312, 314, 318-319, 321, 323, 325. *See also* Insomnia.
Sedentary lifestyle, 192, 347, 353
Seeds, 255
Selenium, 353, 362, 373, 376, 387
food sources of, 281
main role of, 281
therapeutic uses of, 287
vitamin E and, 276
Self-Actualization, 135
Self-awareness, bodily, 21
Self-care, 10, 15, 24
Self-defense arts. *See* Martial arts.
Self-destructive behavior. *See* Addiction.
Self-diagnosis, dangers of, 336
Self-esteem, 135
Self-help (support) groups, 146-149, 221
for cancer victims, 148-149
fellowship and camaraderie in, 148
group therapy vs., 148
as growing movement, 146-148
Twelve Steps in, **146**
when to seek help from, 148
Self-Hypnosis, a Complete Manual for Health and Self-Change (Alman and Lambrou), 123
Self-worth, 96
Selye, Hans, 118
Sen, Soshitsu, 104
Senility, 309
Senna, 322
Sensory deprivation, 110
Sepia, 62, 360, 371, 380, 381
Sesame seeds, 255
Sex
addiction to, 146
waning desire for, 306
Shamanism, 21, 30-35
beliefs and, 34
drumming in, 33
modern, 34-35
workshops in, 35
Shamans, **31, 34**, 36, 94, 100
characteristics of, 32
dangerous job of, 32-33
in healing ceremony, 34
spirit helpers and, 33
trance of, 33
Shaolin monastery, 222-223, **222**, 224, 225
Shaw, George Bernard, 180
Sheehan, G. A., 192
Shepherd's purse, 322, **322**

Shiatsu, 46, 154, 156, 164-166, **165,** 334
  for acne, 338-339
  for allergies, 340
  for arthritis, 344
  for asthma, 346
  for athlete's foot, 346
  for back pain, 348
  for bronchitis, 351
  for chronic pain, 385
  for colds, 355
  for constipation, 357
  for coughs, 358
  for diarrhea, 363
  for eyestrain, **82,** 366
  five elements and, 164-165
  for gallstones, 367
  for headache, 371
  for heart disease, 373
  for hemorrhoids, 373
  for hepatitis, 374, **374**
  for high blood pressure, 376
  for indigestion, 377
  for insomnia, 378
  itchiness relieved by, 167
  life energy and, 164
  for menstrual problems, **381**
  for migraine, 383
  for sciatica, 388
  for sore throat, 389
  Swedish massage vs., 165
  for ulcers, 390
  what to expect from, 165-166
Shingles, 81, 388
Shopping, addiction to, 142, 143, 146
Shortening, 245
Shorter, Frank, 196
Shoulder
  pain in, 75
  reflexology for, **174**
Shoulder stand, **214**
Siberia, **277**
Side stretch, **202,** 205, **205**
Siegel, Bernie S., 18
Silica, 350, 357
Silicon, 384
Simonton, Carl, **118**
Simonton Cancer Center, **118**
Single forward bend, **219**
Single whip, **233, 236**
Sinuses, 56, 304
  reflexology for, 169, **174**
Sinusitis, 10, 69, 329
Sioux ceremony for veterans, 40-41
Sitala, **52**
Sitz bath, 209
Skating, 195
Skepticism, 28
Skiing, 195, **198**
Skin, 56, 167, 296
  biofeedback and, 115
  mud and, **212**

Skin conditions, 120, 299, 318, 326
  abrasions, 316, 320
  acne, 299, 338-339
  allergies and, 340
  athlete's foot, 346-347
  blemishes, 296
  blisters, 320, 360, 364, 388
  boils, 323, 349-350
  burns, 296, 309, 317, 322, 323, 327, 329, 334
  cancer, **352**
  chapped, 304
  dermatitis, 360-361, **360**
  eczema. _See_ Eczema.
  inflammation, 301
  injuries, 322-323
  irritations, 299, 306
  itchiness, 167, 304, **360**
  psoriasis, **28**
  ulcers, 390
Skinner, B. F., 133
Sleep, **107**
  REM, **127,** 128
  See also Dreams.
Sleeping pills, 359
Sleeplessness. _See_ Insomnia.
Slipped disc, 347, 348
Slippery elm, 322-323
Smallpox, **62**
Smith, Robert, 146
Smoking, 142, **143,** 342, 357
  bronchitis and, 350
  cancer and, 352
  emphysema and, 365
  hypnotherapy for, 120, 122, 125
  self-help groups for, 146
  vitamin and mineral supplements and, 284
Snakebite, 298, 303
Snakes, fear of, **134**
Snake venom, **60, 62**
Sneezing, 340
Soccer, 195
Social workers, 135
Sodium, 363
  food sources of, 280
  main role of, 280
Sodium nitrite, 257
Solar plexus, 175
Solfvin, Jerry, 96
Sorbic acid, 257
Sores, 296, 299, 321, 324
Sore throat. _See_ Throat, sore.
Soubiroux, Bernadette, **95**
Sour date kernel, 51
South America, rain forests in, 30
Soybeans, 248
Spas, **28, 77, 78,** 206, **206,** 210, **212**
  seaside, 206-208

Spasms, 312, 327
  muscle, 208, 321
  stomach, 319
Specialization, medical, 22-24
Speech, 334
Speech difficulties, 139
Speigel, Herbert, 121
Spigelia, 383
Spinal manipulation, 72, **73**
Spinal problems, 309
Spinal-twist pose, **220**
Spine, 73
  arthritis of, 343
  Polarity Squat for, **178**
  reflexology for, **175**
Spirits, 30-32, 36
Spiritual healing. _See_ Faith healing.
Spirituality, 14, 30
Spongia, 358
Sprains, 208, 320, 324
Stair-climbing, 195
Stair machines, **195**
Staphylococcus bacteria, 349
Staphysagria (stavescare), 386, 390
Starches, 245. _See also_ Carbohydrates.
Starvation response, 267
Statis dermatitis, 361
Steam treatments, 57, **80**
Steroids, 359
Still, Andrew Taylor, 67, 68, 70
Stimulants, 303, 320
Stings, 320
Stir-frying, **262**
Stomach, 319
Stomachaches, 306, 309, 313
Stomach ailments, 75, 237, 306
  cancer, 250, 257, 341
  cramps, 298
  indigestion. _See_ Digestive aids; Indigestion.
  nervous, 325
  upset, 301, 302, 314, 320, 324
Stone, Randolph, 176
Storytelling, 141
Strabismus (crossed eyes), 82
Strength, muscular
  martial arts and, 228
  yoga and, 214
Strep throat, 337
Stress, 18, 20-21, 23, 68, 91, 100, 106, 118, 134, 325, 334, 340, 343, 345, 347
  asthma and, 345
  Ayurvedic medicine and, **55**
  biofeedback for, **114,** 116, 117
  bodywork and, 184, 185
  in children, **106**
  Chinese medicine and, 51
  exercise and, 194
  fight or flight response and, 106-108
  golden walnuts for, **26**
  hypnotherapy for, **22,** 120, 122, 123, 125
  insomnia and, 377

irritable bowel syndrome and, 378
managing of, with relaxation, 108-109
martial arts and, 228
massage and, 157
meditation and, **335**
polarity therapy and, 177, 178
reflexology and, 169, **173**
shamanistic methods for, 34-35
t'ai chi and, 237
TENS therapy and, 81
vision problems and, 83
yoga and, 214, 218-220
See also Anxiety; Emotions; Nervousness; Relaxation.
Stress test, 198
Strokes, 240, 253, 341, 359
Feldenkrais Method and, 186
relaxation and, 108
Structural Integration. *See* Rolfing.
Stuttering, 115
Styes, 389-390
Subluxations, 72, **73**, 74
Sugar, 28, 109, 245, 253, 254, 255
Sulfur, **281**
food sources of, 280
main role of, 280
Sulphur, 338, 357, 364
Sulphuric acid, 380
Sun, **277**
Sunflower seeds, 255
Sun salutation and warm-up, **215-216**
Support groups. *See* Self-help groups.
Surgeon General's Report on Nutrition and Health, The, 240
Surgery, 334
acupuncture in, 47, 48
hypnosis for, 124
Surigahama sand baths, **213**
Sutherland, W. G., 70-71
Sweating, excessive, 115, 116
Sweating, therapeutic, 212
in Ayurvedic medicine, **57**
herbs for, 303, 304
in Native American medicine, 36-37, **41, 57**, 209, **213**
Swedish massage, 156
Swimming, 195, 210, 346, 348
Swimming (floor exercise), 203-205, **204**
Symptom-oriented view of illness, 18-20
Symptoms, homeopathic view of, 61, 62, **64, 65**, 334
Synergists, 185

Tae kwon do, 226
T'ai chi chuan, 51, **51**, 104, 222, 223, 227, 228, 230-237, **230-237**
for asthma, 346
benefits of, 237
centering in, 235
classes in, 232-235
contradictions and paradoxes in, 231-232
with a partner, 237
postures in, 230, **231-237**, 235-237
roots of, 230-231
Tan tien, 235
Tao, 231
Taoism, 42, 231
Tapotement, 160-161, **163**
Target heart rate, 200
Taylor, Jeremy, 128-129
Tea ceremonies, 104, 105
Tea-tree, 389
Technology, 8, 11, 12, 22, 98
in childbirth, 13
Tedeschi, Joan, 336
Teenagers, addictions and, **142**
Teeth, 321
grinding of, 115
periodontal disease and, 385-386, **385**
Temperature, body, 18
biofeedback and, 115
Tennis elbow, 75
TENS (transcutaneous electrical nerve stimulation) therapy, 81
Tension, 194. *See also* Stress.
Tension headache, 369
Tests, medical, 22
overuse of, 24, 25-26
Tetanus, 11
Thai boxing, 226
Thalassotherapy, 206-208
Theosophical Society, 100
Therapeutic Touch, **97**
Therapy. *See* Psychotherapy.
"Theta" brain patterns, 33
Thiamin (vitamin B$_1$), 284, 388
addiction and, 144
Thigh stretch, 205, **205**
Thinking, 135
This Timeless Moment (Huxley), 84
Thomas, Lewis, 98
Throat, sore, 56, 298, 306, 313, 316, 317, 321, 323, 324, 337, 388-389, **389**
Thrombi. *See* Blood clots.
Thrombophlebitis, 353
Thumb circles, **162**
Thumb-walking, **172, 173**

Thyme, 323-324, **323**, 329, 349-350
Tibet, 101, 222
Time Transfixed (Magritte), **126**
Tinnitus, 309
TM (Transcendental Meditation), **101,** 104, 109
TMJ, 180
Tofu, **269**
Tongue, 45, **46**
Tonics, 320
Tonsillitis, 324, 337
Toothache, 301, 303, 312, 324, 327
Tooth decay, 315
Touch, 96, 98
Therapeutic, 96-97, **97**
Toxins, **255,** 268, 334
fasting and, 81
massage and, 157
mud and, **212**
naturopathy and, 80
polarity therapy and, 177
reflexology and, 169
water and, 255
Trace elements, 245, 274, 276, 280-281
Traditional medicine, 30
definition of, 21
Trager, Milton, 187
Trager Institute, 187
Tragerwork (Trager Psychophysical Integration), 184, 187
Trainers, personal, 199
Transcendental Meditation (TM), **101,** 104, 109
Transcutaneous electrical nerve stimulation (TENS) therapy, 81
Transference, 133
Trauma, 10, 331
Triangle pose, **217**
Triglycerides, 247, 308
Tropical rain forests, 30, **293**
Tsubos. *See* Acupuncture points.
Tuberculosis, 249, 306, 307, 310, 357
Tumors, 315, 347, 381
Turkish baths, **207,** 209
Turmeric, 324
Twelve-step programs, 146-148, 149. *See also* Self-help groups.
Twelve Steps, **146**
Typhus, 249

Ulcerative colitis, 363
Ulcers, 62, 115, 180, 237, 315, 390
Umbanda religious cult, **93**
Universal Life Energy, 99. *See also* Energy, life.

Unmon, 104
Upper abdominal curl, **202,** 203
Upper body stretch, **200**
Uric acid, 171, 368, 379
Urinary tract, 324
Urinary tract disorders, 302, 316,
    321, 322, 325
    cystitis, 358-359
    kidney stones, 169, 379-380
Usui, Mikao, 99
Uterus, cancer of, 12
Uva ursi (bearberry), 324-325,
    324

Valerian, 312, 321, 325, **325**
Vanilla, 329
Varicose veins, 312, 391. *See also*
    Hemorrhoids.
Vascular diseases, 309
Vascular headache, 369. *See also*
    Migraine.
Vata, 52, 55, 56
Vegans, 269, 284
Vegetables, 12, **25,** 240, 243, **246,**
    247, 252, 254, 257, **269,**
    271, **273**
    additives in, 262
    nutrient loss in, 260, 263
    shopping for, 261
    stir-frying of, **262**
Vegetarian diet, 221, 246, 268-
    269
    arthritis and, 344
    heart disease and, 221, 246,
        268
    vitamin and mineral
        supplements and, 284
Veratrum album, 363
Verodoxin, 51
Vertebrae, 72, **73, 75**
    headache and, 75
Veterans, 122
Vibration, in massage, 161
Vichy, **78**
Vietnam veterans, Sioux
    ceremony for, 40-41
Violinists, **71**
Virgin Mary, **95**
Viruses, viral infections, 8, 91,
    323, 354, **355**
    immune system and, 88
    warts and, 92
Vision changes, 334
Vision quests, 36, **41**
Vision therapies, 82-85
    Bates eye exercises, 83, 84
    iridology, 82, 83-85
    prevention in, 82

Visualization, 14, 91, 118-119
    for addiction, 144
    in Alexander Technique, 182
    benefits of, 118-119
    biofeedback combined with,
        116
    for cancer patients, 10, 118,
        118, 119
    guided imagery, 118
    immune system and, 118
    Manley's use of, 119
    in meditation, 216
    in self-hypnosis, 123
    shamanism and, 34, 35
Vital energy. *See* Energy, life.
Vitamin A (retinol), **249,** 250,
    261, 274, **274,** 276, 283,
    339, 340, 346, 350, 351,
    353, 355, 356, 358, 361,
    362, 364, 365, 366, 367,
    376, 382, 386, 387, 389,
    390
    food sources of, 278
    main role of, 278
    megadoses of, 282
    pregnancy and, 282, 337
    therapeutic uses of, 286
    see also Beta-carotene
Vitamin B_1 (thiamin)
    food sources of, 278
    main role of, 278
    therapeutic uses of, 284
Vitamin B_2 (riboflavin)
    food sources of, 278
    main role of, 278
    therapeutic uses of, 284
Vitamin B_3. *See* Niacin.
Vitamin B_5. *See* Pantothenic acid.
Vitamin B_6 (pyridoxine), 274,
    276, 339, 340, 341, 344,
    346, 362, 373, 380, 382
    food sources of, 279
    main role of, 279
    megadoses of, 282
    therapeutic uses of, 284-285
Vitamin B_{12} (cobalamin), 269,
    271, 283, **287,** 341, 346,
    360, 367, 374, 390
    folic acid and, 276
    food sources of, 279
    main role of, 279
    therapeutic uses of, 285
    vegetarian diet and, 284
Vitamin B complex, 144, 260,
    274, 339, 350, 351, 360,
    361, 363, 365, 367, 368,
    371, 373, 382, 383, 388
Vitamin C (ascorbic acid), 15,
    249, 250, **252, 260,** 263,
    274, **275,** 276, **279, 281,**
    282, 283, 339, 340, 341,
    343, 344, 346, 348, 349,
    350, 351, 353, 354, 355,
    356, 357, 358, 359, 360,
    361, 362, 365, 366, 367,
    368, 369, 371, 373, 374,
    376, 382, 383, 386, 388,
    389, 390, 391

addiction and, 144
    cancer and, 276
    colds and, 283
    food sources of, 279
    iron and, 276, 277
    main role of, 279
    Pauling's theories on, 282, **283**
    smoking and, 284
    in sweet potatoes, 260
    therapeutic uses of, 286
Vitamin D (calciferol), 271, 274,
    277, 348, 361, 367, 380, 384
    calcium and, 276
    food sources of, 278
    main role of, 278
    megadoses of, 282
    therapeutic uses of, 286
Vitamin E (tocopherol), **249,**
    250, 274, 276, 339, 343,
    344, 346, 348, 353, 354,
    362, 364, 367, 368, 373,
    376, 380, 382, 386, 387,
    390, 391
    food sources of, 278
    main role of, 278
    selenium and, 276
    therapeutic uses of, 13, 286
Vitamin K, 274, 364, 384
    food sources of, 278
    main role of, 278
    therapeutic uses of, 286
Vitamins, 12, 245, **249,** 250-252,
    252, 263, 264, 274-281, 337
    addiction and, 144
    chart of, 278-279
    fat-soluble, 274, 278
    functions of, 274
    megadoses of, 282
    supplements of, 250-252,
        274-278, 282
    water-soluble, 274, 278-279
    See also Vitamin therapy;
        specific vitamins.
Vitamin therapy, 12-13, 282-287
    for acne, 339
    for allergies, 340
    for anemia, 341
    for arteriosclerosis, 343
    for arthritis, 344
    for asthma, 346
    for back pain, 348
    for bad breath, 349
    for boils, 350
    for bronchitis, 351
    for cancer, 12-13, 10, 353
    for circulatory problems, 354
    for colds, 355
    for conjunctivitis, 356
    for constipation, 357
    for coughs, 358
    for cystitis, 359
    for depression, 360
    for dermatitis, 361

for diabetes, 362
for diarrhea, 363
for diverticulitis, 364
for eczema, 365
for emphysema, 366
for eyestrain, 367
for fibrocystic breast disease,
    13
for gallstones, 367
for gout, 368
for hay fever, 369
for headache, 371
for heart disease, 373
for hemorrhoids, 373
for hepatitis, 374
for high blood pressure, 376
for insomnia, 378
for irritable bowel syndrome,
    379
for kidney stones, 380
for menopausal problems, 380
for menstrual problems, 382
for migraine, 383
for osteoporosis, 384
for periodontal disease, 386
for psoriasis, 387
for sciatica, 388
for shingles, 388
for sore throat, 389
for styes, 390
for ulcers, 390
for varicose veins, 391
Vomiting, 298, 302, 334
Voodoo death, 93

Weil, Andrew, 8-15, **9**, 23, 92,
    145, 295
Weiss, Steven J., 70
Westfeldt, Lulie, 183
Wheezing, 334, 340, 345
Whirlpools, 209-210
White blood cells, 88, 90
White chestnut, 330
Whiteheads, 338
Willoughby, John, 244
Willow, 37, 386
Wine, 253
Wintergreen, 326
Wisdom of the Body, The
    (Cannon), 106
Witch hazel, 326, **326,** 373
Wok, **262**
Wolpe, Joseph, 134
Wood element, 164, 165
Wordsworth, William, 102
Workaholics, 146
World Health Organization, 54
Worms, 298, 308
Worry, **29**
Wound healing, 249, 253, 301,
    303, 304, 317, 323, 325,
    327
Wremen, Germany, **241**
Wrist
    gout and, 367
    pain in, 75
Writing in journals, 141
Wushu, 224
Wyethia, 340

for chronic pain, 385
for constipation, 357
corpse pose in, 216, **220**
for depression, 360
for diabetes, 362
for diverticulitis, 364
extended-angle pose in, **217**
getting started in, 216-218
hatha, 104, 216
for hay fever, 369
for headache, 371
for heart disease, 373
for indigestion, 377
for insomnia, 378
for irritable bowel syndrome,
    379
knee-up pose in, **218**
meditation in, 216, 221
for menopausal problems, 380
for menstrual problems, 382
for migraine, 383
for osteoporosis, 384
polarity therapy and, 176, 178
poses in, 216-218
pregnancy and, 337
seated forward bend in, **219**
shoulder stand in, **214**
single forward bend in, **219**
for sore throat, 389, **389**
spinal-twist pose in, **220**
sun salutation and warm-up
    in, **215-216**
triangle pose in, **217**
for varicose veins, 391
warrior pose in, **218**
Yoga Sutras, 214
Yogis, **117**
Yogurt, **250,** 253
Youngest Science, The (Thomas),
    98
Your Maximum Mind (Benson),
    109
Yo-yo syndrome, 267

Walking, **194,** 195, 197-198
Walleye, 90
Warrior pose, **218**
Warts, 92, 93
    hypnotherapy for, 120
Water cures, 78
Water Dreaming at Mikanji, **131**
Water element, 164, 177
Water intake, 245, 254, **255**
Watermelon, **273**
Water therapy. *See*
    Hydrotherapy.
Water-walking, **209**
Wave hands like clouds, **233, 236**
Waxed produce, 257
Weight, losing of:
    evening primrose for, 305
    exercise for, **267**
    reflexology for, 170
    sand baths for, **213**
    yoga for, 220
    See also Diet, dieting; Obesity.

X-rays, 73
Yang. *See* Yin and yang.
Yarrow, 327, **327**
Yee, Franklin K., 25-26
*Yellow Emperor's Classic of Internal
    Medicine, The,* 42, 156
Yin and yang, 42-44, **44,** 49-50,
    52, 270
    of foods, 270, 271
    shiatsu and, 164
    t'ai chi and, 231, **236**
Yoga, **53,** 101, **117,** 124, 214-
    221, **214-220,** 336-337, **372**
    as ancient practice, 214
    for arteriosclerosis, 343
    for arthritis, 344-345
    for asthma, 346
    Ayurvedic medicine and,
        55-56
    back-lift in, **219**
    for back pain, 9-10, 348
    benefits of, 218-221
    big toe pose in, **217**
    bound-angle pose in, **220**
    for bronchitis, 351
    for cancer, 353

Zen, 100, 101-102, 104, 105,
    222
Zinc, 276, 282-283, 339, 344,
    348, 349, 350, 355, 356,
    362, 376, 387, 389, 390
    food sources of, 280
    main role of, 280
    therapeutic uses of, 287
Zones. *See* Meridians.
Zone therapy, 170

Sources

Readers looking for more information on the various healing methods in this book can turn to the following organizations. Some are prepared to give referrals to practitioners in your area. Most ask that you include a self-addressed, stamped envelope.

Activity Therapies
National Coalition of Arts Therapies
  Associations (NCATA)
c/o Cynthia Briggs, Chairperson
2000 Century Plaza, Suite 108
Columbia, MD 21044

Alexander Technique
North American Society of Teachers
  of the Alexander Technique
P.O. Box 3992
Champagne, IL 61826-3992

Aromatherapy
Aromatherapy Institute and
  Research (AIR)
P.O. Box 2354
Fair Oaks, CA 95628

National Association of Holistic
  Aromatherapy (NAHA)
P.O. Box 17622
Boulder, CO 80308-7622

Ayurvedic Medicine
Himalayan International Institute of
  Yoga Science and Philosophy of
  the U.S.A.
RR1, Box 400
Honesdale, PA 18431

Bach Flower Remedies
Ellon Bach U.S.A., Inc.
644 Merrick Road
Lynbrook, NY 11563

Flower Essence Society
P.O. Box 459
Nevada City, CA 95959

Bioenergetics
International Institute
  for Bioenergetic Analysis
144 East 36th Street
New York, NY 10016

Biofeedback
Association for Applied
  Psychophysiology and
  Biofeedback
10200 West 44th Avenue, Suite 304
Wheat Ridge, CO 80033

Chiropractic
American Chiropractic Association
  (ACA)
1701 Clarendon Boulevard
Arlington, VA 22209

International Chiropractic
  Association (ICA)
1110 North Glebe Road, Suite 1000
Arlington, VA 22201

Dream Analysis
Association for the Study of Dreams
P.O. Box 1600
Vienna, VA 22183

Exercise
IDEA: The Association for
  Fitness Professionals
6190 Cornerstone Court East
Suite 204
San Diego, CA 92121-3773

Eye Therapies
American Optometric Association
243 North Lindbergh Boulevard
St. Louis, MO 63141

Optometric Extension Program
2912 Daimler Street
Santa Ana, CA 92705

Hellerwork
Hellerwork Inc.
406 Berry St.
Mount Shasta, CA 96067

Herbal Medicine
American Botanical Council
P.O. Box 201660
Austin, TX 78720-1660

Holistic Medicine
American Holistic Medical
  Association
4101 Lake Boone Trail, Suite 201
Raleigh, NC 27607

Center for Holistic Medicine
78 Fifth Avenue
New York, NY 10011

New Center for Wholistic Health
  Education and Research
50 Maple Place
Manhasset, NY 11030-1927

Homeopathy
National Center for Homeopathy
801 N. Fairfax Street
Alexandria, VA 22314

Hypnosis
American Society of Clinical
  Hypnosis (ASCH)
2200 East Devon Avenue, Suite 291
Des Plaines, IL 60018

Macrobiotics
Kushi Institute
P.O. Box 7
Becket, MA 01223

Martial Arts
Wushu Resources U.S.A.
P.O. Box 210159
San Francisco, CA 94121

Massage
American Massage Therapy
  Association
National Information Office
1130 West North Shore Avenue
Chicago, IL 60626

Meditation
Insight Meditation Society
1230 Pleasant Street
Barre, MA 01005

Naturopathy
American Association of
  Naturopathic Physicians
P.O. Box 20386
Seattle, WA 98102

John Bastyr College
144 N.E. 54th Street
Seattle, WA 98105

National College of Naturopathic
  Medicine
11231 S.E. Market Street
Portland, OR 97216

Osteopathy
American Academy of Osteopathy
P.O. Box 750
Newark, OH 43058

American Osteopathic Association
142 East Ontario Street
Chicago, IL 60611

Physical Therapy
American Physical Therapy
  Association
P.O. Box 37257
Washington, DC 20013

Polarity
American Polarity Association
4101 Lake Boone Trail, Suite 201
Raleigh, NC 27607

Psychotherapies
American Psychiatric Association
1400 K Street Northwest
Washington, DC 20005

National Association of Social
  Workers
750 First Street Northeast, Suite 700
Washington, DC 20002

Reflexology
International Institute of
  Reflexology
P.O. Box 12642
St. Petersburg, FL 33733

Reike
Reike Alliance
P.O. Box 41
Cataldo, ID 83810

Rolfing
International Rolf Institute
P.O. Box 1868
Boulder, CO 80306

Rosen Method
Rosen Institute
825 Bancroft Way
Berkeley, CA 94710

Rubenfeld Synergy
The Rubenfeld Center
115 Waverly Place
New York, NY 10011

Self-help
National Self-Help Clearinghouse
25 West 43rd Street, Room 620
New York, NY 10036

Shamanism
The Foundation for Shamanic
 Studies
P.O. Box 670, Belden Station
Norwalk, CT 06852

Shiatsu/Acupressure
American Oriental Bodywork
 Association
50 Maple Place
Manhasset, NY 11030-1927

T'ai Chi
A Taste of China
111 Shirley Street
Winchester, VA 22601

Therapeutic Touch
Nurse Healers — Professional
 Associates, Inc.
175 Fifth Avenue, Suite 2755
New York, NY 10010

*Traditional Chinese Medicine
 and Acupuncture*
American Association of
 Acupuncture and Oriental
 Medicine
4101 Lake Boone Trail, Suite 201
Raleigh, NC 27607

Trager Work
The Trager Institute
10 Old Mill Street
Mill Valley, CA 94941

Vegetarian Diets
Department of Nutrition
 School of Public Health
 Loma Linda University
Loma Linda, CA 92350

Yoga
American Yoga Association
3130 Mayfield Road
Cleveland Heights, OH 44118

Credits and Acknowledgments Grateful acknowledgment is made for permission to excerpt or adapt featured material taken from the following works:

Alcoholics Anonymous World Services, Inc. *The Twelve Steps.* Copyright © 1939, 1955, 1976. **The American Journal of Clinical Hypnosis.** "Cholecystectomy with Self-Hypnosis" by Victor Rausch, D.D.S. Volume 22, Number 3, January 1980. Copyright © 1980 American Society of Clinical Hypnosis. **Brunner/Mazel, Inc.** *Self-Hypnosis: The Complete Manual for Health and Self-Change,* Second Edition, by Dr. Brian M. Alman and Dr. Peter T. Lambrou. Copyright © 1992 by Brunner/Mazel, Inc. **Centerline Press.** *F. Matthias Alexander: The Man and His Work* by Lulie Westfeldt. Text Copyright © 1964 by Lulie Westfeldt. **Doubleday Dell Publishing Group Inc.** *The Allergy Discovery Diet* by John E. Postley, M.D. with Janet M. Barton. Copyright © 1990 by John E. Postley, M.D. and Janet M. Barton. Used by permission of Doubleday, a division of Bantam Doubleday Dell Publishing Group, Inc. **Eating Well (TM) Inc.** May/June 1991 "Primal Prescription" by John Willoughby. Copyright © 1991 by John Willoughby. **Element Books Ltd.** *The Elements of Shamanism* by Nevill Drury. Copyright © 1989 by Nevill and Susan Drury Publishing Pty Ltd. **HarperCollins Publishers.** *The Art of Survival* Edited by Dr. M.L. Gharote and Maureen Lockhart. Copyright © 1987 by Dr. M.L. Gharote and Maureen Lockhart. *The Case of Nora: Body Awareness as Healing Therapy* by Moshe Feldenkrais. Copyright © 1977 by Moshe Feldenkrais. **Harvard University Press.** *The Navaho* by Clyde Kluckhohn and Dorothy Leighton. Copyright © 1946, by the President and Fellows of Harvard College, 1974 by Florence Kluckhohn and Dorothea Leighton. **Health Media Inc.** March/April 1987 "Medical Self Care. Self-Care in the Information Age," by Tom Ferguson, M.D. **Houghton Mifflin Company.** *Health and Healing* by Andrew Weil. Copyright © 1983, 1988 by Andrew Weil. *Natural Health, Natural Medicine* by Andrew Weil, M.D. Copyright © 1990 by Andrew Weil, M.D. **Overeaters Anonymous, ® Inc.** *The Great American Wife.* Copyright © 1980 by Overeaters Anonymous, ® Inc. **Penguin USA,** **Inc.** *Head First: The Biology of Hope* by Norman Cousins. Copyright © 1989 by Norman Cousins. Used by permission of the publisher, Dutton, an imprint of New American Library, a division of Penguin Books USA Inc. *The Youngest Science: Notes of a Medicine Watcher* by Lewis Thomas. Copyright © 1983 by Lewis Thomas. Used by permission of Viking Penguin, a division of Penguin Books USA Inc. **Random House, Inc.** *Dr. Dean Ornish's Program for Reversing Heart Disease* by Dr. Dean Ornish, M.D. Copyright © 1990 by Dr. Dean Ornish, M.D. **Shelter Publications, Inc.** *Galloway's Book on Running.* Copyright © 1983 by Jeff Galloway. **Simon & Schuster, Inc.** *A Leg to Stand On* by Oliver Sacks. Copyright © 1984 by Oliver Sacks. Reprinted by permission of Summit Books, a division of Simon & Schuster, Inc., and Gerald Duckworth & Co. Ltd. **St. Martin's Press, Inc.** *Healers on Healing* Edited by Richard Carlson, Ph.D. and Benjamin Shield. Copyright © 1989 by Richard Carlson, and Benjamin Shield. Reprinted by special permission from Jeremy P. Tarcher, Inc. **Station Hill Press.** *Job's Body: A Handbook for Bodywork*, by Deane Juhan. Copyright © 1987 by Deane Juhan. **The New York Times.** "How Tools of Medicine Can Get in the Way" by Lawrence K. Altman, M.D. May 12, 1992. Copyright © 1992 by The New York Times Company. **The Overlook Press.** *The Overlook Martial Arts Reader* edited by Randy F. Nelson. Copyright © 1989 by Randy F. Nelson. "A State of Grace: Understanding the Martial Arts" by Don Ethan Miller. Reprinted by permission of Don Ethan Miller. **Vegetarian Times, Inc.** "The Natural Doc" by Victoria Moran. *Vegetarian Times*, August, 1990. **World Publications.** *Dr. Sheehan on Running* by George A. Sheehan, M.D. Copyright © 1975 by *Runner's World Magazine*. **W.W. Norton & Company, Inc.** *Encounters with Qi, Exploring Chinese Medicine*, by David Eisenberg, M.D., with Thomas Lee Wright. Copyright © 1985 by David Eisenberg and Thomas Lee Wright.

ILLUSTRATIONS

3 *calligraphy* John Stevens. 8 *calligraphy* John Stevens. 9 Mojgan Azimi. 10 Robert Grant. 13 Penny Gentieu. 14 Rooney Johansson. 16 *calligraphy* John Stevens. 16-17 *border* Cynthia Watts Clark. 19 Sam Abell, © 1992 National Geographic Society. 20 Rick Smolan. 22 David Parker/Science Photo Library/Photo Researchers, Inc. 23 Jean François Allaux. 25 Sam Abell, © 1992 National Geographic Society. 26 *top & middle* James A. McInnis; *bottom* Noel Allum. 28 *both* Ilhami/Sipa Press. 29 Jean François Allaux. 30 The Bettmann Archive. 31 Douglas Kirkland/Sygma. 32 *top* Mark Peters/Sipa Press; *bottom* Tourneret/Sipa Press. 33 R. Schefold. 34 Peter Menzel. 36 Courtesy of the Denver Art Museum, Denver, Colorado/ Photo by Ben Benschneider courtesy of Time-Life Books, Inc. 37 *top* Susanne Page; *lower inset* Michal Heron/Woodfin Camp & Associates. 38 Stephen Trimble. 39 Jean François Allaux. 40-41 *all* Ted Wood. 42 New York Public Library Picture Collection. 43 Phil Schermeister/ AllStock. 44 The Plastic Source. 45 Robert Harding Picture Library. 46 *top* Peter Chadwick/Octopus Publishing Group Ltd; *illustration* Michael Reingold. 47 *top* Wellcome Institute Library, London; *bottom* Marais Grussen/ Sipa Press. 49 Jeffrey Aaronson. 50 David Henderson/ Eric Roth Studio. 51 Alain Nogues/Sygma. 52 Nik Douglas. 53 Giorgio Tavaglione. 54 from MANDALA by José and Miriam Argüelles © by José and Miriam Argüelles and Shambhala Publications; reprinted by permission of Shambhala Publications, Inc., Boston. 55 *top* Henry Hilliard; *bottom* Dilip Mehta/Contact Stock/Woodfin Camp & Associates. 56 Stephanie Maze. 57 Dilip Mehta/Contact Stock/Woodfin Camp & Associates. 58-59 *all* Marcia Keegan. 60 Hahnemann University. 61 Henry Groskinsky. 62 Culver Pictures. 63 Jean François Allaux. 64-65 *all* Brian Seed. 67 Peter Chadwick/Octopus Publishing Group Ltd. 68 Paul Biddle & Tim Malyon/Science Photo Library/ Photo Researchers, Inc. 69 Michael Reingold. 71 The British School of Osteopathy. 72 Palmer College of Chiropractic. 73 Peter Chadwick/Octopus Publishing Group Ltd; *illustration* Michael Reingold. 74-75 *all* Peter Chadwick/Octopus Publishing Group Ltd. 76 *top* UPI/Bettmann; *bottom* Culver Pictures. 77 Dan Heringa. 78 The J. Allan Cash Photolibrary. 80 Mary Evans Picture Library. 81 François Gauthier/Sipa Press. 82 Steve McCurry/Magnum. 83 Jack Reznicki. 85 Pierre Boulat/Woodfin Camp & Associates. 86 *calligraphy* John Stevens. 86-87 *border* Cynthia Watts Clark. 88 Dona Burns-Pizer. 89 Michael Freeman. 91 Roy Morsch/The Stock Market. 92 Jean François Allaux. 93 Timm Rautert/Visum. 94 The Bettmann Archive. 95 *top* Frank Fournier/Contact Stock/ Woodfin Camp & Associates; *middle* Steve McCurry/ Magnum; *bottom* Terence Spencer/Colorific! 97 *all* Noel Allum. 98 Jean François Allaux. 99 *top* © SPL/Science Source/Photo Researchers, Inc.; *bottom* G. Hadjo, CNRI/Science Photo Library/Photo Researchers, Inc. 100 *top* The Bettmann Archive; *bottom* From the Manly P. Hall Collection of the Philosophical Research Society. 100-101 Dilip Mehta/Contact Stock/Woodfin Camp & Associates. 102 Michael A. Keller/The Stock Market. 103 *left* Nik Douglas; *top & bottom right* Reprinted by permission of Princeton University Press © 1979 by Princeton University Press. 105 Robert Frerck/The Stock Market; *bottom* Michael S. Yamashita. 106 John G. Horey. 107 Louie Psihoyos/Matrix. 108 *both* David Madison. 110 Torin Boyd. 111 Benjamin Ailes/Floatation Tank Association/ Photo courtesy of *Newsweek.* 112-113 *all* David Madison. 114 Will & Deni McIntyre/Photo Researchers, Inc. 115 *both* Vandystadt/Allsport. 117 Hartley Film Foundation. 118 *both* From GETTING WELL AGAIN by O. Carl Simonton, S. Matthews-Simonton, James Creighton © 1978 by O. Carl Simonton and Stephanie Matthews-Simonton. Used by permission of Bantam Books, a divi-

sion of Bantam Doubleday Dell Publishing Group, Inc. 119 David Cannon/Allsport. 120 The Granger Collection, New York. 121 Howard S. Friedman. 122 *all* Bart Bartholomew/Black Star. 125 National Guild of Hypnotists, Photography by Steven Bachand. 126 Photograph © 1991, The Art Institute of Chicago. All Rights Reserved. 127 Louie Psihoyos/Matrix. 128 *top* James A. McInnis; *bottom* National Museum of the American Indian. 130 *top* Impact Photos; *bottom* Penny Tweedie/Colorific! 131 *top* Michael Kluvanek/South Australian Museum; *bottom* Impact Photos. 132 Freud Museum, London. 133 *both* The Wilhelm Reich Museum. 134 *top* Rick Friedman/Black Star; *bottom* Andrew Sacks/Black Star. 136 Ann Chwatsky/Phototake. 138 from SPONTANEOUS PAINTING AND MODELLING, © 1971 by E.M. Lyddiatt, published by Constable & Company Limited, London. 139 Ellerbrock & Schafft/Bilderberg. 140 *top* Ed Quinn; *bottom* Gale Zucker/Stock, Boston. 141 *top* Frank Fournier/Contact Stock/Woodfin Camp & Associates; *bottom* David Burnett/Contact Stock/Woodfin Camp & Associates. 142 Polly Brown/Actuality Inc. 143 *both* From THE BODY VICTORIOUS by Lennart Nilsson, published by Dell Publishing Company, New York. 144 Gianfranco Gorgoni/Contact Stock. 145 Jean François Allaux. 147 *all* Mary Ellen Mark/Library. 148 *both* Paul Fusco/Magnum. 150-151 *all* Joel Gordon. 152 *calligraphy* John Stevens. 152-153 *border* Cynthia Watts Clark. 154 International Institute of Reflexology. 155 Max Aguilera-Helweg. 156 *both* Elizabeth Hathon. 157 Noel Allum. 158 Michael Reingold. 158-159 *all* Jan Cobb. 160-161 *all* Jan Cobb. 162-163 *all* Jan Cobb. 164 Dona Burns-Pizer. 165 Noel Allum. 166 *all* Noel Allum. 168-169 *all* Jan Cobb. 170 The Plastic Source. 171 The Plastic Source. 172-173 *all* Jan Cobb. 174-175 *all* Jan Cobb. 176 *photographs* Jan Cobb; *illustration* Dona Burns-Pizer. 177 Noel Allum. 178 *all* Noel Allum. 179 Jean François Allaux. 180 NASTAT. 181 *photographs* Noel Allum; *illustration* The Plastic Source. 182 *all* Noel Allum. 183 Jean François Allaux. 184 © Bonnie Freer 1992. 185 Joel Gordon. 187 Joel Gordon. 188 © Karsh, Ottawa/ Woodfin Camp & Associates. 189 *photo* Dan McCoy/ Rainbow; *illustration* Michael Reingold. 190 *calligraphy* John Stevens. 190-191 *border* Cynthia Watts Clark. 193 © 1978 Charles B. (Chuck) Rogers, Jr. 194 Shelby Thorner/ David Madison Photography. 195 *all* Noel Allum. 197 Shelly Katz/*Time* Magazine. 198 *top* David Brownell; *bottom* Karen Keeney. 199 Keith Gunnar/Bruce Coleman Inc. 200-201 *all* Bruce Curtis. 202-203 *all* Bruce Curtis. 204-205 *all* Bruce Curtis. 206 Joyce Tenneson. 207 by Winfield Parks © 1973 National Geographic Society. 208 Carol Guzy/Black Star. 209 Carol Lee/St. Croix. 210 Lester Sloan/Woodfin Camp & Associates. 212 *top* Carlos Angel/Gamma Liaison; *bottom* Jonathan Blair/Woodfin Camp & Associates. 212-213 *bottom* Mike Yamashita. 213 *right* Nathan Benn/Woodfin Camp, Inc. 214 Dilip Mehta/ Contact Stock/Woodfin Camp & Associates. 215 *all* Bruce Curtis. 216-217 *all* Bruce Curtis. 218-219 *all* Bruce Curtis. 220 *all* Bruce Curtis. 222 R. Norman Matheny/*The Christian Science Monitor.* 223 Doug Menuez/Reportage. 224 *left* Pat LaCroix/The Image Bank; *right* Courtesy of Roxby Press, London. 225 *all* Courtesy of Roxby Press, London. 226 *top* Alon Reininger/Woodfin Camp & Associates; *bottom* Alon Reininger/Contact Stock/Woodfin Camp & Associates. 227 Ed Kashi. 228. Chris Johns/AllStock. 229 Jean François Allaux. 230 Andrew Grant. 231 *all* Joseph Quever. 232-233 *all* Joseph Quever. 234-235 *all* Joseph Quever. 236-237 *all* Joseph Quever. 238 *calligraphy* John Stevens. 238-239 *border* Cynthia Watts Clark. 241 Wolfgang Kunz/Bilderberg. 242 *top* Nathan Benn/Woodfin Camp & Associates; *bottom* Tobey Sanford. 243 Harriet Pertchik. 245 John Running. 246 Jean François Allaux. 248 The Granger Collection, New York. 249 *top* Jerry

Howard/Positive Images; *bottom* William Whitehurst/The Stock Market. **250** Jasper Partington/Octopus Publishing Group Ltd. **251** *top* Louie Psihoyos/Woodfin Camp & Associates; *bottom* Tom Tracy. **252** *left* G.K. & Vikki Hart/The Image Bank; *right* Obremski/The Image bank. **253** Jean François Allaux. **255** Zao Longfield/The Image Bank. **256** *top* Martin Culik/Rodale Press; *bottom* Mitch Mandel/Rodale Press. **258** Jacques Chenet/Woodfin Camp & Associates. **260-261** *all* Robert Grant. **262** Jerry Howard/Positive Images. **264** Nancy Coplon. **265** Bruce Curtis. **267** Rick Friedman/Black Star. **269** *both* Jerry Simpson. **270-271** *both* Studio Marcialis. **271** Michael Holford. **272** Stephanie Maze. **273** *top left* Terry Madison/The Image Bank; *middle right* Elyse Lewin/The Image Bank; *middle left* Amanda Adey/Stockphotos Inc.; *bottom right* Brett Froomer/The Image Bank. **274** New York Public Library Picture Collection. **275** Gordon Gahan, Photographer/© National Geographic Society. **276** Kellogg Company. **277** Mark S. Wexler. **278** Murray Alcosser/The Image Bank. **279** *left* Charles Gold; *right* M. Pedone/Puglia/The Image Bank. **281** *top left* Murray Alcosser/The Image Bank; *bottom left & right* H. Armstrong Roberts. **282** *top* David Parker/Science Photo Library/Photo Researchers, Inc.; *bottom* Jeremy Burgess/Science Photo Library/Photo Researchers, Inc. **283** Christopher Springmann. **285** Nick Kelsh. **286** M.J. Klein, M.D. **287** Dennis Kunkel/CNRI/Phototake. **288** *calligraphy* John Stevens. **288-289** *border* Cynthia Watts Clark. **290** Robert Golden. **291** Heather Angel. **292-293** G.I. Bernard/NHPA. **293** *right* Mark J. Plotkin. **295** Jean François Allaux. **296** Grant Heilman/Grant Heilman Photography, Inc. **297** Eleanor B. Wunderlich. **298** *top* Studio Marcialis; *bottom* David M. Stone: Photo/Nats. **299** Eleanor B. Wunderlich. **300** Bob Gossington/Bruce Coleman Inc. **301** Eleanor B. Wunderlich. **302** *top* Studio Marcialis; *bottom* W.H. Hodge/Peter Arnold, Inc. **303** Eleanor B. Wunderlich. **304** Eleanor B. Wunderlich. **305** *top* L. West/Bruce Coleman Inc.; *bottom* Walter Chandoha. **306** *illustration* Marilena Pistoia from F. Bianchini-F. Corbetta LE PIANTE DELLA SALUTE, Arnoldo Mondadori Editore © 1975. **307** Laura Riley/Bruce Coleman Inc. **308** *illustration* Marilena Pistoia from F. Bianchini-F. Corbetta LE PIANTE DELLA SALUTE, Arnoldo Mondadori Editore © 1975. **309** *top* Norman O. Tomalin/Bruce Coleman Inc.; *bottom* Dr. Willmar Schwabe. **310** Murray Alcosser/The Image Bank. **311** David M. Stone: Photo/Nats. **312** Hans Reinhard/Bruce Coleman Inc. **313** *top* Michel Viard/Peter Arnold, Inc.; *bottom illustration* by Marilena Pistoia from F. Bianchini-F. Corbetta LE PIANTE DELLA SALUTE, Arnoldo Mondadori Editore © 1975. **314** *top* Heather Angel; *illustration* Marilena Pistoia from F. Bianchini-F. Corbetta LE PIANTE DELLA SALUTE, Arnoldo Mondadori Editore © 1975. **315** Studio Marcialis. **316-317** *illustrations* Marilena Pistoia from F. Bianchini-F. Corbetta LE PIANTE DELLA SALUTE, Arnoldo Mondadori Editore © 1975. **318** *illustration* Marilena Pistoia from F. Bianchini-F. Corbetta LE PIANTE DELLA SALUTE, Arnoldo Mondadori Editore © 1975. **319** Pat & Roe Hagan/Bruce Coleman Inc. **320** Studio Marcialis. **321** *top* Studio Marcialis; *bottom* Betsy Fuchs: Photo/Nats. **322** *illustration* Marilena Pistoia from F. Bianchini-F. Corbetta LE PIANTE DELLA SALUTE, Arnoldo Mondadori Editore © 1975. **323** *top* John A. Lynch: Photo/Nats; *bottom* Walter Chandoha. **324** *illustration* Marilena Pistoia from F. Bianchini-F. Corbetta LE PIANTE DELLA SALUTE, Arnoldo Mondadori Editore © 1975. **325** John Markham/Bruce Coleman Inc. **326** *illustration* Marilena Pistoia from F. Bianchini-F. Corbetta LE PIANTE DELLA SALUTE, Arnoldo Mondadori Editore © 1975. **327** John Markham/Bruce Coleman Inc. **328** Robert Conrad. **329** Noel Allum. **330-331** *both* The Dr. Edward Bach Centre. **332** *calligraphy* John Stevens. **332-333** *border* Cynthia Watts Clark. **335** Joel Gordon. **337** Foto Marburg/Art Resource, N.Y. **339** David Scharf/Peter Arnold, Inc. **340** Nathan Benn/Woodfin Camp & Associates. **342** *top* From THE INCREDIBLE MACHINE by Lennart Nilsson, published by Boehringer Ingelheim International GmbH, courtesy of the National Geographic Society; *bottom* Alfred Pasieka/Peter Arnold, Inc. **344** Ethan Hoffman/Picture Project. **347** *all* Jan Cobb. **348** Sal DiMarco, Jr./*Time* Magazine. **349** John Huet/Leo de Wys, Inc. **351** *both* Bruce Curtis. **352** Hank Morgan/Rainbow. **354** Douglas Kirkland/Sygma. **355** Biozentrum/Science Photo Library/Photo Researchers, Inc. **357** Henryk Kaiser/Leo de Wys, Inc. **359** Bill Binzen. **360** Françoise Sauze/Science Photo Library/Photo Researchers, Inc. **362** Craig Stafford/*Time* Magazine. **365** Peggy & Yoram Kahana/Peter Arnold, Inc. **366** Linda Bohm/Leo de Wys, Inc. **367** Harry Przekop, Jr./Medichrome Division/The Stock Shop Inc. **369** *both* From THE BODY VICTORIOUS by Lennart Nilsson, published by Dell Publishing Company, New York. **370** Steven Mays/Rebus, Inc. **371** Brian Hill. **372** *both* Andrew Eccles/Rebus, Inc. **374** Steve McCurry/Magnum. **375** Dan McCoy/Rainbow. **377** Schmid/Langsfeld/The Image Bank. **378-379** *all* Bruce Curtis. **381** Noel Allum. **382** Noel Allum. **384** Douglas Kirkland/Sygma. **385** Barbara J. Rosen/Images Press. **387** Noel Allum. **389** Bruce Curtis. **391** Bill Binzen/The Stock Market.

Efforts have been made to contact the holder of the copyright for each picture. In several cases these have been untraceable, for which we offer our apologies.